THE CORONARY CIRCULATION IN HEALTH AND DISEASE

THE CORONARY CIRCULATION IN HEALTH AND DISEASE

Melvin L. Marcus, M.D.

Professor of Medicine
Director of Coronary Physiology Laboratory
University of Iowa

McGRAW-HILL BOOK COMPANY

New York St. Louis San Francisco Auckland Bogotá Guatemala
Hamburg Johannesburg Lisbon London Madrid Mexico Montreal New Delhi
Panama Paris San Juan São Paulo Singapore Sydney Tokyo Toronto

This book was set in Times Roman by Dharma Press; the editors were Joseph J. Brehm and Maggie Schwarz, the production supervisor was Ave McCracken.
R.R. Donnelley & Sons Company was printer and binder.

Notice

Medicine is an everchanging science. As new research and clinical experience broaden our knowledge, changes in treatment and drug therapy are required. The editors and the publisher of this work have made every effort to ensure that the drug dosage schedules herein are accurate and in accord with the standards accepted at the time of publication. Readers are advised, however, to check the product information sheet included in the package of each drug they plan to administer to be certain that changes have not been made in the recommended dose or in the contraindications for administration. This recommendation is of particular importance in regard to new or infrequently used drugs.

THE CORONARY CIRCULATION IN HEALTH AND DISEASE

1 2 3 4 5 6 7 8 9 0 DOC DOC 8 9 8 7 6 5 4 3

ISBN 0-07-040293-0

Library of Congress Cataloging in Publication Data

Marcus, Melvin L.
The coronary circulation in health and disease.

Includes index.
1. Coronary heart disease. 2. Coronary arteries.
I. Title. [DNLM: 1. Coronary circulation. 2. Coronary disease—Physiopathology. 3. Coronary vessels—Physiopathology. WG 300 M322c]
RC685.C6M35 1983 616.1'23 83-754
ISBN 0-07-040293-0

TO MY MOTHER, BESSIE,
WHO ENCOURAGED ME
TO PURSUE EXCELLENCE,
AND TO MY WIFE, CARLA

CONTENTS

PREFACE

Coronary heart disease is the predominant cardiovascular affliction in the industrialized world. Because of the prevalence and severity of coronary disease, many physicians and scientists have focused their attention to this area.

The evaluation and treatment of patients with heart disease must be founded upon a thorough understanding of the function of the coronary circulation in normal and pathological states. In 1950, Donald Gregg published *The Coronary Circulation in Health and Disease*, a classic treatise on coronary physiology that has continued to serve as a major reference text in this field.* Although other volumes on the coronary circulation have been published subsequent to Dr. Gregg's book, a comprehensive text written by a single author has not been published since 1950. Contributed texts are almost always plagued by fragmentation, gaps, and inconsistencies. The present monograph provides the reader with an integrated, comprehensive summary of the present state of knowledge concerning the regulation of the coronary circulation in health and disease. It is directed toward physicians involved in the care of patients with heart disease (internists, cardiologists, radiologists, cardiac surgeons, anesthesiologists) and basic scientists (physiologists, pharmacologists, bioengineers, anatomists, etc.) interested in problems that involve the coronary circulation.

The volume is divided into six parts. Parts 1 and 2 contain one chapter each on coronary anatomy and methods of measuring coronary blood flow. The anatomic description of the coronary vasculature is closely linked to the functional capacity of the circulation. Part 2, on methods of measuring coronary blood flow, focuses on approaches in current use. Part 3 deals with basic mechanisms that regulate coronary flow under normal conditions. Throughout the six chapters in Part 3 I have emphasized the critical role these basic regulatory mechanisms play in determining the clinical manifestations of disease processes that affect the coronary circulation. Part 4, which is comprised of seven chapters, centers on the manner in which specific disease processes (coronary occlusion, coronary spasm, coronary stenosis, etc.) disturb the functional capacity of the coronary circulation. Part 5 calls attention to significant differences in the regulation of blood flow to the right

*Dr. Gregg kindly allowed me to use this title for the present book.

and left ventricles. The six chapters in Part 6 describe the manner in which various medical and surgical therapies alter the functional characteristics of the coronary circulation.

The roots of this book stem from my years in medical school at the University of Wisconsin where three individuals—Richard Wasserberger, Professor of Medicine; George G. Rowe, Professor of Medicine; and Thomas C. Meyer, Professor of Pediatrics—provoked my initial interest in cardiology. My training in cardiovascular research began under the tutelage of Stephen E. Epstein, Chief of the Cardiology Branch at the National Institutes of Health. My interest in the coronary circulation was fostered by François M. Abboud, Chairman of the Department of Medicine and Director of the Cardiovascular Center at the University of Iowa. Dr. Abboud provided my colleagues and me with superb laboratory facilities, generous financial support, constant guidance, and a stimulating, challenging atmosphere in which we have been able to pursue a wide range of studies concerning the regulation of the coronary circulation. The information contained in this volume is a reflection of the work I have done and the knowledge I have gained at the Cardiovascular Center at the University of Iowa.

Although a monograph supposedly represents the efforts of an individual, many people often contribute to such works. *The Coronary Circulation in Health and Disease* was immensely improved as a result of the efforts of four reviewers: Julien I.E. Hoffman, Professor of Pediatrics, University of California, San Francisco; Joseph C. Greenfield, James Duke Professor of Medicine and Chief of the Cardiology Division at Duke University; Donald E. Heistad, Professor of Medicine, University of Iowa; and Richard E. Kerber, Professor of Medicine, University of Iowa and Associate Director of the Cardiology Division. Each of these colleagues reviewed the entire volume and made numerous suggestions for additions, deletions, and revisions which were incorporated into the final manuscript.

For over a decade I have learned a great deal about the coronary circulation by studying the published works of Drs. Julien I.E. Hoffman and Joseph C. Greenfield and their coworkers. In addition, numerous formal and informal meetings with these two outstanding coronary physiologists have played a major role in shaping my views concerning a host of basic concepts that relate to the regulation of the coronary circulation. In the course of reviewing this monograph, Dr. Hoffman and Dr. Greenfield encouraged me to reexamine my views in many areas relevant to this field. In so doing, they have contributed even further to this work.

Drs. Donald E. Heistad and Richard E. Kerber have been close colleagues and collaborators since I came to the University of Iowa in 1973, and I have come to place great value on their criticism. Hence, I deeply appreciate the time and effort they devoted to reviewing the manuscript. Their many suggestions significantly improved the book.

I have received valuable criticism concerning selected chapters from James Willerson, Professor of Medicine and Chief of the Cardiology Division, Southwestern Medical School; Lewis Becker, Associate Professor of Medicine at Johns Hopkins Medical School; Paul Cannon, Associate Professor of Medicine at Columbia Medical School; Carl White, Associate Professor of Medicine, University of Iowa; Robert Bache, Professor of Medicine, University of Minnesota; and William C. Chilian, Assistant Research Scientist, University of Iowa.

During the past decade I have been privileged to participate in the education of many young investigators and senior research associates who came to the Cardiovascular Center to study the regulation of the coronary circulation. These young people have been a constant source of stimulation to me. In many instances they have significantly influenced my views on many controversial areas that relate to the coronary circulation. In this regard, I am particularly thankful to Thomas Mueller, James Martins, Sidney Klopfenstein, Joseph Gascho, Charles Eastham, David Harrsion, Roger Wangler, Kevin Peters, Samon Koyanagi, Tesuji Inou, John Rumberger, Natsea Pandian, David Gutterman, Andrew Feiring, Tarek Husayni, and William Chilian.

I want to thank Dr. Allyn Mark, Professor of Medicine and Chief of the Cardiology Division at the University of Iowa for arranging to decrease my clinical assignments so I would have sufficient time to complete this book.

I am also grateful to Linda Godfrey, Director of Medical Graphics, University of Iowa, who designed the illustrations for the book, and to my secretaries, Beverly Layton and Maureen Kent who assisted me in preparing the manuscript.

Finally, it has been a pleasure to work with McGraw-Hill Book Company. Special thanks should be given to Robert P. McGraw, Richard Laufer, and Maggie Schwarz. They provided me with excellent counsel regarding many aspects of this project, and assigned a superb copyeditor, Irene Curran, to assist me. Irene worked diligently to enhance the accuracy and clarity of the presentation.

Many talented individuals have made significant contributions to this volume. I am indebted to all of them and deeply appreciate their unselfish efforts on my behalf.

Melvin L. Marcus

PART **ONE**

CORONARY ANATOMY

CHAPTER **1**

ANATOMY OF THE CORONARY VASCULATURE

Each segment in the coronary vasculature has specific anatomic characteristics which enable the vascular segment to perform its functional role. The various individual vascular components act in concert to permit the coronary circulation to respond effectively to a wide variety of physiologic stimuli.

GENERAL FUNCTIONS OF THE VASCULATURE

All segments of the coronary vasculature (epicardial vessels, capillaries, venules, etc.) act as conduits, metabolic units, and semipermeable membranes, but only selected vascular segments contribute significantly to the resistance and capacitance of the vasculature. For example, the epicardial coronary arteries contribute importantly to coronary capacitance, but under most conditions they have only a small effect on total coronary vascular resistance. In contrast, the small transmural coronary arterial vessels (100 μm in diameter) play a dominant role in regulating total coronary vascular resistance. Before describing the anatomic characteristics of various vascular segments in the coronary tree, I will briefly review the specific functions of various segments of the vasculature.

Conduit Function

All vessels in the body act as conduits; that is, they facilitate the transport of blood. Synthetic conduits have fixed configurations and are relatively unresponsive to external stimuli. Vessels are much more versatile. Besides maintaining the blood within a confined space, blood vessels can dilate and constrict, change permeability, and grow or degenerate in response to a myriad of stimuli.

Resistance Function

Under normal conditions in the human left ventricle, a 90 mmHg pressure head will drive 90 to 180 ml of blood per minute through the coronary vasculature. This ratio (driving pressure/coronary blood flow = coronary vascular resistance) can be altered markedly in either direction. Powerful coronary vasoconstrictors such as angiotensin [1], vasopressin [2], and thromboxane A_2 [3] can increase coronary vascular resistance substantially. Potent coronary dilators such as adenosine [4] can decrease coronary vascular resistance to as little as one-sixth of the usual resting value. These alterations in coronary vascular resistance can occur within seconds. Although changes in the caliber of large epicardial coronary vessels contribute to these alterations in total coronary vascular resistance [5], major changes in resistance are mediated primarily by intramural coronary vessels 10 to 140 μm in diameter [6,6a].

Capacitance Function

When the left ventricle contracts, blood in the venules is moved toward the coronary sinus [7] and blood in the intramural coronary arteries is forced retrograde into the large epicardial coronary vessels [8,9]. Because blood flow in the proximal epicardial coronary arteries is usually anterograde throughout systole [7], the retrograde flow must be masked by dilation of large epicardial coronary vessels. These vessels store energy and blood, and thus act as a functional capacitance during systole.

Function as Semipermeable Membranes

Vessels may be thought of as having semipermeable membranes at two levels. First, the endothelium is a semipermeable membrane between the blood column and the vessel wall. Substances such as lipids, glucose and oxygen gain access to the wall of the blood vessel by passing from the vascular space through the endothelium into the vessel wall. A major theory of atherogenesis [10], the insudation theory, depends on the assumption that lipids carried in the blood enter the vascular wall. Second, there is a semipermeable membrane at the capillary level that links the vascular and interstitial spaces. Although some exchange between the vascular and interstitial space occurs in larger vessels [11], the bulk of the exchange processes occur in capillaries and perhaps venules. Oxygen, electrolytes, and nutrients leave the vessels and enter the interstitial space of the myocardium, while CO_2 and metabolites leave the interstitium and enter the vascular space from the interstitium. The exchange of substances through the plasma membrane and endothelial clefts of capillaries is accomplished by both passive diffusion and vesicular transport [12,13].

Function as Metabolic Units

All vascular segments act as metabolic units. Coronary vessels can grow and repair damaged components [14], synthesize and degrade numerous molecules, some of which are vasoactive [15], maintain the functional integrity of their cellular components and respond to pathologic challenges. Thus, the vascular wall is a microcosm of metabolic activity.

The following sections of this chapter will describe the anatomic characteristics of specific vascular segments in the coronary hierarchy.

EPICARDIAL CORONARY VESSELS

Distribution

The epicardial coronary arteries originate from ostia in the left and right sinuses of Valsalva (Figure 1-1). In adult humans, the main left coronary artery is 2 to 5.5 mm in diameter (mean $\sim$ 4 to 4.7 mm) and varies in length from 2 to 40 mm (mean $=$ 13 mm) [16–20]. The major branch vessels of the left main are the left anterior descending artery and the circumflex coronary artery. A large intermediate or obtuse marginal vessel occasionally arises from the main left coronary artery; more often, this branch originates from the proximal circumflex. The left anterior descending coronary artery in humans has many septal perforating branches

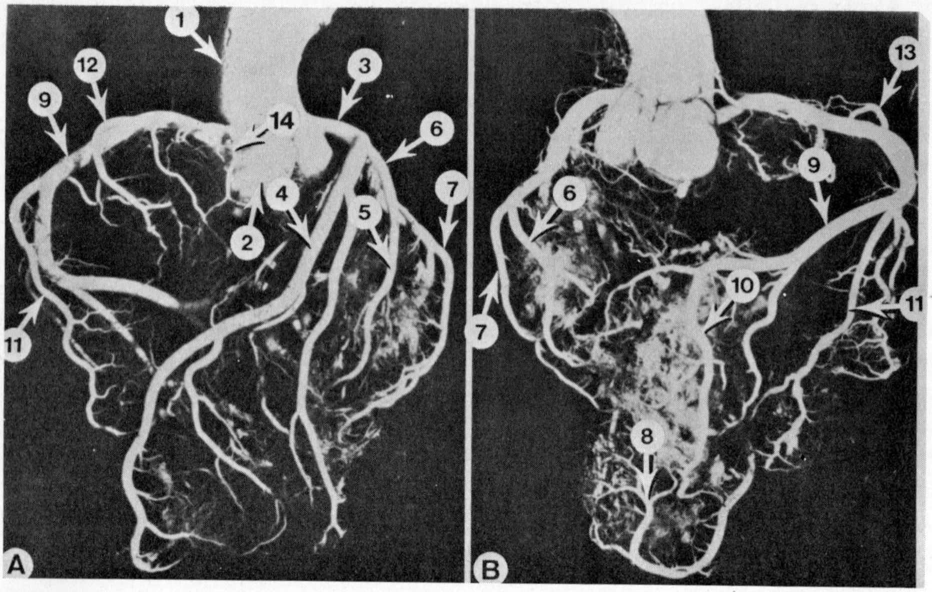

FIGURE 1-1
Extramural coronary arteries. Plastic cast of the coronary arteries (male, 15 years) injected with Geon under low pressure in order to fill only the extramural arterial vessels. *(a)* Anterior surface of the heart. *(b)* Posterior surface of the heart. 1. Aorta. 2. Aortic valve. 3. Left main coronary artery. 4. Left anterior descending branch (LADB). 5. Left diagonal branch. 6. Left circumflex branch. 7. Left marginal branch, ascending portion of the LADB. 9. Right coronary artery. 10. Posterior descending branch. 11. Right marginal branch. 12. Anterior branch of the right coronary artery. 13. Main atrial branch. 14. Third coronary atery. *(From G Baroldi and G Scomazzoni* [*16*].)

(mean = 13: range 16 to 23) [16–20] which perfuse the interventricular septum. In addition, the left anterior descending artery and its diagonal branches usually supply a larger mass of the left ventricular myocardium than the circumflex or the right coronary arteries [16–20].

The right coronary artery in adult humans is 1.5 to 5.5 mm in diameter (mean = 3.2 to 4.1 mm) at its origin [16–20]. In 86 percent of people, the inferior wall of the left ventricle is perfused by a posterior descending branch which arises from the right coronary artery. Numerous variations in the distribution of the large epicardial coronary arteries have been carefully described [16–25a]. Congenital abnormalities in the coronary arteries will be discussed in Chapter 15.

Histology

The wall of the epicardial and large intramural coronary vessels is composed of three coats: tunica intima, tunica media, and tunica adventitia. The *tunica intima* is several cell layers thick. The innermost layer of this coat is the vascular endothelium. The tunica intima and tunica media are separated by a continuous internal elastic membrane. The *tunica media* makes up the bulk of the arterial wall and is composed of alternating lamellae of smooth muscle cells and elastic tissue which are disposed circularly around the vessel. The outermost portion of the media is perfused by a separate vascular network, the vasa vasorum [7,26]. Recent studies of vasa vasorum in the thoracic aorta [26] indicate that this vascular bed responds to neural and humoral stimulation and is altered by disease processes. It is possible that the vasa vasorum in the large coronary vessels play some role in the pathenogenesis of coronary atherosclerosis. The *tunica adventitia*, an outer layer, is composed of areolar tissue mixed with collagenous tissue, fat, and elastic fibers. The tunica adventitia contains lymphatic channels and nerve fibers in route to the smooth muscle cells in the tunica media.

The architecture of large epicardial coronary arteries differs significantly from that of similar-sized vessels that serve skeletal muscle. In large epicardial coronary arteries, the wall-to-lumen ratio is 1:15; in vessels of similar external diameter that perfuse skeletal muscle, i.e., posterior tibial artery, the wall-to-lumen ratio is 1:6 [26a]. This difference in architecture may help to explain why vasoconstrictor responses of large coronary vessels to several stimuli, such as adrenergic stimulation, are less prominent than those observed in vessels that serve skeletal muscle (see Figure 6-3). In addition, age, sex, and ethnic background affect the architectural characteristics of large epicardial coronary arteries in humans [26b,26c].

Species Differences

Dog In the dog, the circumflex coronary artery supplies the largest mass of cardiac muscle. Average values of the mass of the ventricle perfused by major coronary vessels are circumflex 39 percent, left anterior descending 32 percent, and the right coronary artery 17 percent [27]. In addition, in the dog, the first septal perforator arises very proximally and supplies 12 percent of left ventricular mass [27]. The posterior descending coronary artery in the dog invariably arises from the circumflex [18].

Pig The distribution of the major epicardial coronary arteries is similar to the most common pattern (right dominant system) observed in humans [28]. However, in the pig, the septum is mainly supplied by a single large septal perforating branch.

Rat In the rat, the left anterior descending artery and its main branches supply the largest portion of the left ventricle. Also, within a short distance from the left coronary artery the major conduit vessels become subepicardial.

Monkey The pattern of the coronary vasculature in nonhuman primates is similar to that observed in humans.

Interdigitation of Perfusion Fields

The perfusion fields of large epicardial coronary vessels interdigitate with each other to a great extent. This is dramatically illustrated in Figure 1-2. This macroscopic interdigitation is of great concern in studies of experimental myocardial infarction. Unless special techniques are employed to outline the perfusion field or "risk area" of the coronary artery to be occluded, it is nearly impossible to determine if a given intervention alters infarct size (see Chapter 9). In addition to macroscopic interdigitation, recent studies suggest that capillary loops from adjacent vascular beds interdigitate and may provide dual circulatory support to single myocardial cells [29].

Specific Functions of the Epicardial Coronary Vessels

Like all vessels, epicardial arteries act as conduits, semipermeable membranes, and metabolic units. The large surface coronary vessels also contribute to total resistance and capacitance of the coronary vasculature. These arteries slightly decrease total coronary artery resistance by dilating in response to nitroglycerin [5,30,31,31a] and other stimuli (see Figure 1-3). Epicardial coronary vessels can modestly increase total coronary vascular resistance by constricting in response to alpha-adrenergic stimulation [5,31,32] (see Figure 1-4) and ergonovine [33]. Although small changes in the diameter of large coronary arteries are of limited importance in normal coronary vessels, active constriction or dilation of these vessels in the presence of superimposed atherosclerosis can importantly modify the physiological significance of obstructive lesions (see Chapter 11). The large quantity of elastic fibers in the epicardial coronary vessels permits them to contribute to coronary capacitance. During early systole, the epicardial coronary vessels expand and store blood and energy (Figures 1-3 and 1-4).

INTRAMURAL CORONARY VESSELS

Distribution

Intramural coronary vessels penetrate perpendicularly into the myocardium from the epicardial vessels. In humans the longest intramyocardial vessels (4 to 6 cm) originate from the left anterior descending coronary artery and perfuse the anterior two-thirds of the interventricular septum [16–20]. Usually one of the proximal two or three septal perforators of the left anterior descending artery is particularly large (0.5 to 1.2 mm proximal diameter). The perforating branches of the posterior descending coronary artery which perfuse the posterior one-third of the interventricular septum are also relatively long. All other perforating branches are relatively short (0.8 to 1.4 cm), as they course directly down to the subendocardium.

The intramural coronary arteries form a dense vascular network in the wall of the left ventricle (see Figure 1-5). In humans, these penetrating branches form

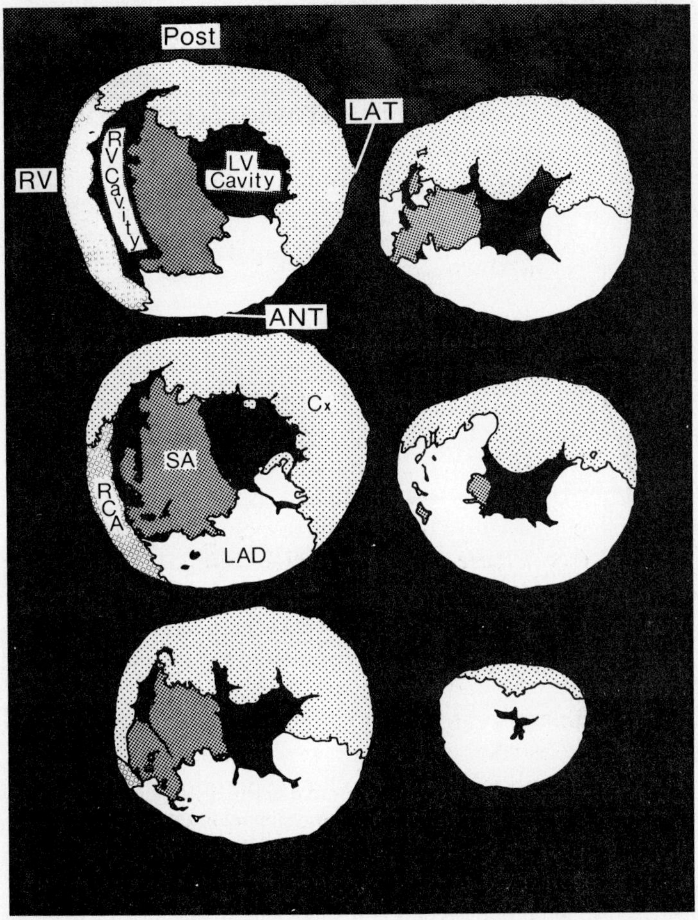

FIGURE 1-2
Perfusion fields of the four major coronary vessels. RCA = right coronary artery; SA = sepal artery; Cx = circumflex coronary artery; LAD = left anterior descending coronary artery. The six contiguous heart slices are from the ventricles of a dog. The top left slice is from the base of the heart. The bottom right slice is from the apex. The vascular fields were outlined by perfusing all four vessels simultaneously at 100 mmHg with four different colored batches of Microphil [27]. The irregularity and interdigitation of the vascular perfusion fields is obvious. The exact pattern varies considerably in different dogs. RV = right ventricle: ANT = anterior; POST = posterior; LAT = lateral; RV cavity = right ventricular cavity; LV = left ventricular cavity. (*Courtesy of C Scheel, Professor of Physiology, Osteopathic School of Medicine, Kirksville, Missouri.*)

2.8 → 3.15

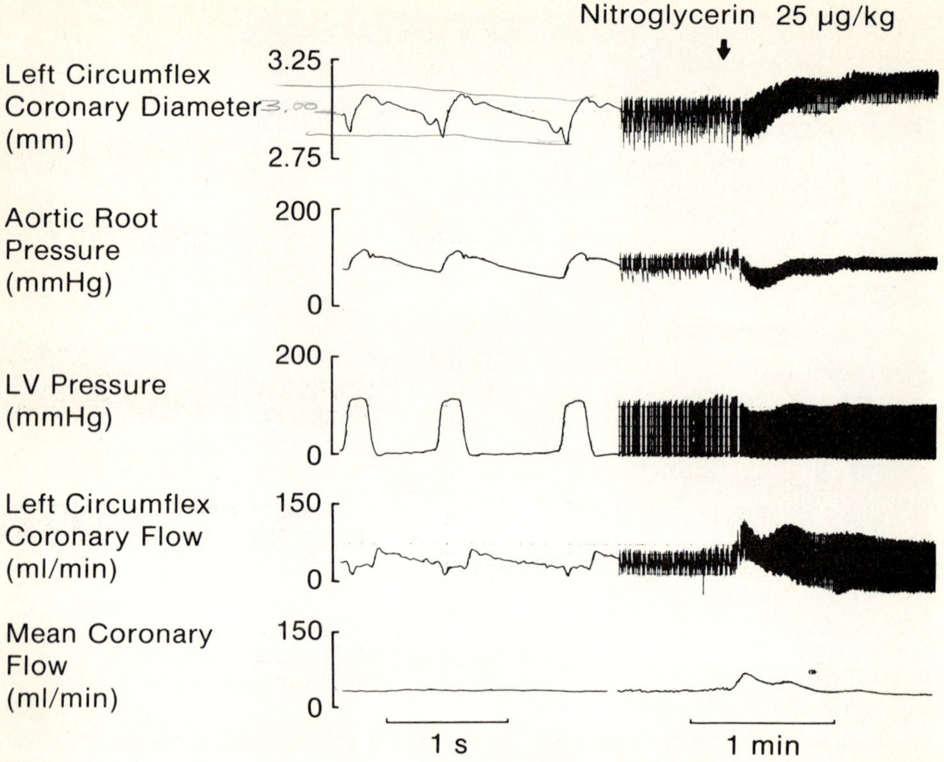

FIGURE 1-3
Effects of intravenous administration of nitroglycerin on systemic hemodynamics, left circumflex coronary diameter and coronary blood flow. Coronary diameter was continuously monitored with sonomicrometer crystals which were chronically implanted. Note that during early systole, coronary diameter increases by about 10 percent. During administration of nitroglycerin, although aortic pressure falls, coronary artery diameter increases by about 10 percent. This indicates that nitroglycerin produces active dilation of large epicardial coronary arteries. LV = left ventricle. (*Modified from SF Vatner et al* [5].)

a subendocardial plexus with intercommunicating anastomoses that are 100 to 200 μm in diameter [23]. In the dog, Wüston et al. [34] have shown that the vascular volume of the intramyocardial arteries in the subendocardium is significantly greater than that of the subepicardial (Figure 1-6).

Species Differences

The first septal perforating artery in the dog is of special significance to investigators. It is large (1 to 3 mm in diameter, 3 to 7 cm in length) and supplies 12 percent of the left ventricular mass. Because it originates very proximally, when the left main coronary artery is canulated, the orifice of the first septal perforator can be easily occluded. Unless special care is taken to avoid occlusion of this

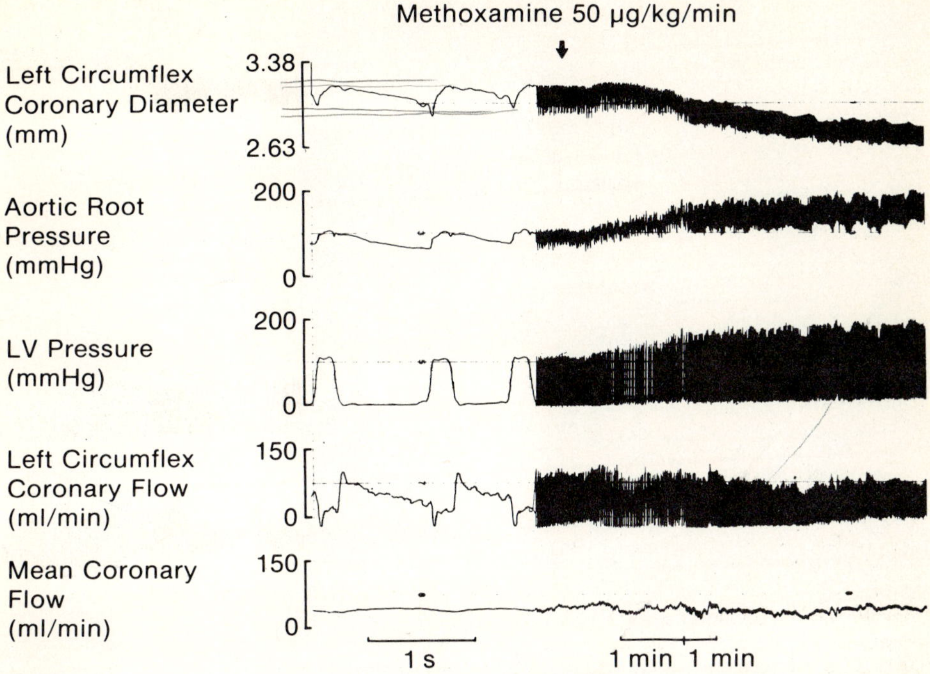

FIGURE 1-4
Effects of intravenous administration of methoxamine on systemic hemodynamics, left circumflex coronary diameter and coronary blood flow. Note that during early systole coronary artery diameter increases by about 10 percent. During administration of methoxamine, although aortic pressure increases substantially, left circumflex coronary diameter decreases by 15 to 20 percent. This indicates that methoxamine, an alpha agonist, produces active coronary constriction in the large epicardial coronary arteries. LV = left ventricle. (*Modified from SF Vatner et al* [5].)

vessel, severe septal ischemia occurs. Ligation of the left anterior descending coronary artery and its first septal perforator is associated with a high incidence (88 percent) of ventricular fibrillation [35]. Finally, the first septal perforator provides a unique model for studying phasic coronary blood flow in intramyocardial coronary vessels [8] and for evaluating intramural collateral vessels (see Chapter 10).

Special Functions

The intramural coronary arteries and arterioles play a dominant role in regulating coronary vascular resistance. Because direct measurements of pressure within intramural coronary vessels in the left ventricle have not been made, the precise distribution of the resistance is unknown. Measurements of pressure in subepicardial coronary vessels in the right ventricle of the rabbit have recently been reported by Nellis et al. [6]. These studies indicate that a substantial pressure

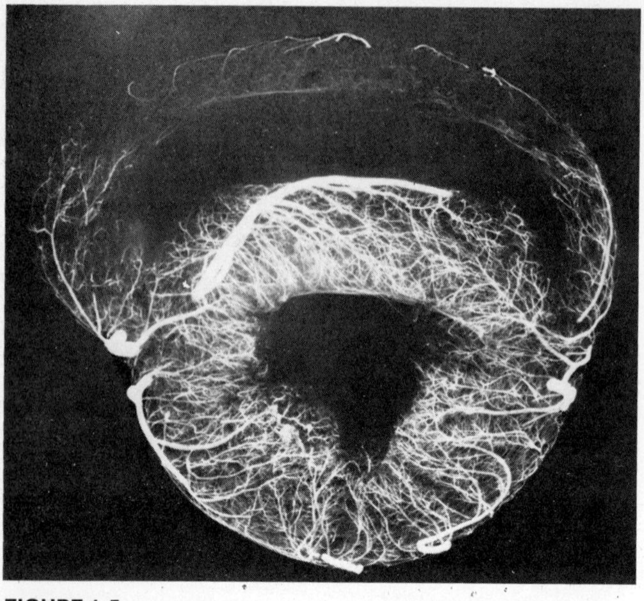

FIGURE 1-5
A coronary arteriogram of a dog's heart (basal slice). The arterial vessels were filled with a barium mixture at systemic pressure. The figure demonstrates the great density of arterial vessels in the wall of the left ventricle. (*Courtesy of S Koyanagi, University of Iowa.*)

gradient exists between the conduit coronary vessels and the arterial branches that are 10 to 140 μm in diameter (Figure 1-7). The extent to which intramural vessels contribute to coronary capacitance remains to be defined. Although some exchange of substances between the vascular and interstitial space occurs in these vessels [11], it is probably small.

Because compressive forces are greater in the subendocardium than in the subepicardium, the perfusion pressure must be lower in the subendocardial intramural coronary vessels. This is compensated for in two ways: (1) total vascular volume is greater and minimal vascular resistance is lower in endocardial vessels [34]; (2) the subendocardial vessels under normal conditions may be slightly dilated. Even so, the autoregulatory capacity of subendocardial vessels in the left ventricle is substantially less than that of subepicardial vessels (see Chapter 4).

THE PRECAPILLARY SPHINCTERS

Histology

Precapillary sphincters have been identified in human and dog hearts [36,37]. These vessels have three coats: intima, media, and adventitia. They are distinguished from arterioles solely by the characteristics of the media. In an arteriole,

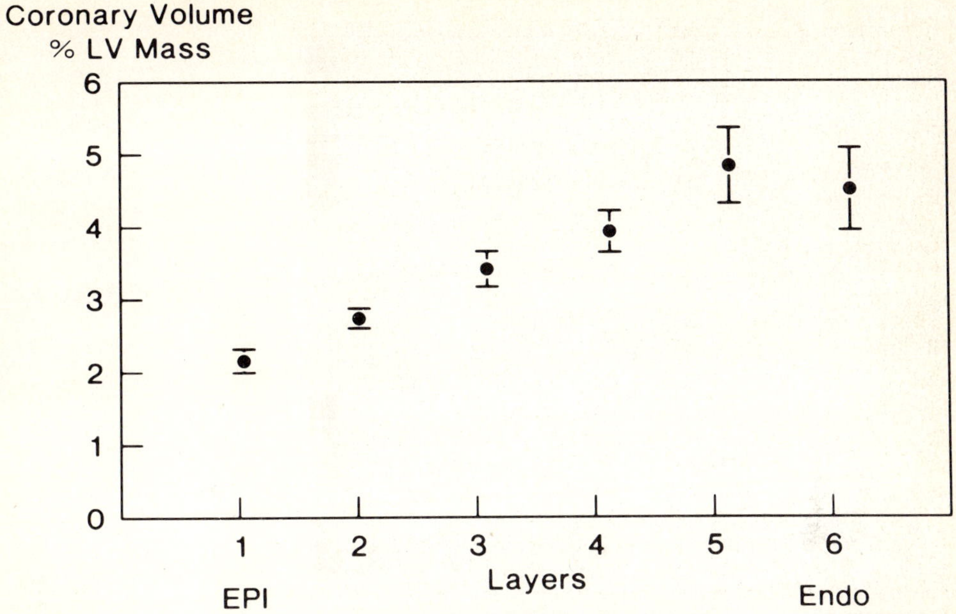

FIGURE 1-6
Volume of arterial vessels in various transmural layers of the dog's left ventricle. The arterial volume of the endocardial (Endo) layers is twofold greater than that observed in epicardial (Epi) layers. LV = left ventricle. (*Redrawn from data presented by B. Wüsten et al* [*34*].)

the media contains a continuous ring of smooth muscle which is usually composed of several overlapping smooth muscle cells. In contrast, in the precapillary sphincter, the smooth muscle layer in the media is not continuous and only 1 to 3 smooth muscle cells usually are present in the media. Often the precapillary sphincter is innervated. The precapillary sphincter and its nerve constitute a functional unit [36,37].

Specific Functions

Precapillary sphincters may regulate the density of open capillaries. The available studies indicate that under normal conditions at any one instant in time, not all the capillaries in the myocardium are open [38–41]. Under normal conditions, in other vascular beds, the precapillary sphincters and the arterioles exhibit vasomotor tone which is manifest by periodic closure of the capillaries [38]. Indirect studies in the myocardium suggest that such periodic vasomotion, or "twinkling," may be present in the coronary bed [39–41]. Several stimuli, such as hypoxia, cause relaxation of the precapillary sphincters; hence, the density of open capillaries increases and minimal diffusion distance decreases during severe hypoxia [42].

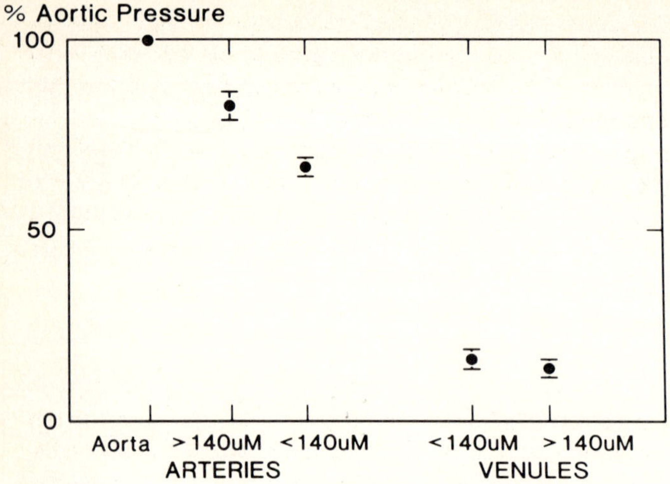

FIGURE 1-7
Relative pressure in various segments in the coronary vasculature. A substantial pressure drop is evident in vessels larger than arterioles. This indicates that relatively large arteries in the coronary vasculature control a significant portion of total coronary vascular resistance. (*Redrawn from data originally presented by SH Nellis et al* [6].)

CAPILLARIES

Distribution

Capillary density in the left and right ventricles is 2 to 5 $\times$ 10^5 capillary per square millimeter; capillary diameter averages 4.4 to 5.2 μm; the capillary/fiber ratio in adult humans and in animals is 1:1, and the intercapillary distance is 14 to 19 μm [43–49]. Capillary density in the heart is greater than that in most other organs [43].

Several disease states alter capillary density. For example, pressure-induced left ventricular hypertrophy decreases capillary density by 20 to 30 percent [50–53]; exercise conditioning increases capillary density by 10 to 20 percent [54].

Histology

Capillaries throughout the body are broadly categorized in three groups: continuous, fenestrated, and discontinuous [43]. In the heart, brain, skeletal muscle, and gut, the capillaries are of the continuous type. The endocardial cells of the basal membrane form a continuous barrier to the interstitial space. In addition, the interendothelial clefts are relatively tight. Occluding junctions are spotty; 30-Å separations in many regions allow passage of small molecules via the interendothelial clefts. The endothelial cell is thickened in the region of the nucleus (3 μm). This segment comprises 8 percent of the surface area of the capillary wall [45]. The remaining portion of the endothelial cell is very thin (0.1 to 0.3 μm) [45]. The ends of the capillary cells overlap and form a cleft. In addition, around each capillary is a pericyte. Although the pericyte nucleus surrounds only a small portion of the capillary, the dendritic processes of the pericytes surround a large segment of the capillary wall. The pericytes contain fibrils which may act to alter capillary size [55].

Specific Functions

Capillaries act primarily as semipermeable membranes. Oxygen, electrolytes, and nutrients leave and simultaneously CO_2 and metabolites enter the vascular space via the capillaries. The exchange of these substances is mediated by several transport processes, including passive diffusion and pinocytosis [12,13]. In addition, recent studies indicate that molecules with molecular weights equal to horseradish peroxidase (molecular weight = 40,000) pass into the interstitial space via interendothelial pores [56]. This mechanism of capillary transport is controversial [45].

CORONARY COLLATERAL VESSELS

Collateral channels connect large coronary arterial vessels to one another and are broadly classified into two major groups: (1) preexisting, or native, collaterals and (2) mature, or stimulated collaterals. A detailed description of the coronary collateral vessels is presented in Chapter 10.

CORONARY VEINS

Distribution

The heart has three separate venous systems [57-62]. The largest system primarily drains the left ventricle. These epicardial veins converge and drain into the coronary sinus, which lies in the left posterior atrioventricular groove and empties into the right atrium. The second system of anterior superficial veins drains mainly the right ventricle. These veins usually empty into the right atrium at a site separate from the coronary sinus. A third system, the thebesian veins, is composed of small venules which enter directly into all four cardiac chambers. These veins are quantitatively significant with respect to the venous drainage of the atria and the interatrial septum and, to a much lesser extent, the left and right ventricles and interventricular septum.

Three features of the coronary venous system in the dog are of special importance to investigators. First, there are prominent interconnections between large coronary veins [57]. Hence, the blood draining from any specific vein does not contain effluent that arises exclusively from the apparent drainage field of the vessel. The magnitude of these interconnections in the dog is best demonstrated by selectively occluding either the coronary sinus or the anterior cardiac veins. Occlusion of the coronary sinus decreases left main coronary inflow by only 8 percent [57]; occlusion of the anterior veins decreases right coronary inflow by 20 percent [57]. Even if the coronary sinus and anterior veins are both occluded, survival is common and ventricular function is reasonably well preserved for several hours [57]. Furthermore, the ratio of flow draining via the coronary sinus and anterior cardiac veins and the oxygen saturation in these venous channels varies with different hemodynamic perturbations [60]. These large interconnections between the venous channels in the heart must be considered when venous blood samples from small veins are obtained in studies of myocardial ischemia [63]. Second, the most proximal portion of the coronary sinus is a continuation of the interventricular, or great cardiac, vein. In the dog, 95 percent of blood in the great cardiac vein arises from the left anterior descending coronary artery [61]. However, only 65 percent of the left anterior descending inflow drains into the great cardiac vein [57,61]. Nonetheless, the great cardiac vein provides an opportunity to separate venous flow which drains from the perfusion field of the left anterior descending coronary artery from that of other portions of the left ventricle. Third, several cardiac veins arising from the left ventricle enter the coronary sinus very close to its right atrial orifice or enter into the right atrium at a separate site. Finally, a significant amount of blood from the right side of the septum drains either directly into the right ventricle or via anterior cardiac veins. Therefore, coronary sinus blood regularly underestimates total coronary flow to the left ventricle by 10 to 15 percent [57,58]. Total left ventricular coronary venous outflow can be assessed by employing right heart bypass and collecting all coronary venous blood that enters the right side of the heart from any route.

Although the coronary venous system in humans has not been studied in as much detail as that of the dog, a few general statements can be made: (1) there are large connections between the major venous channels in the heart; (2) about 85 percent of coronary sinus flow arises from the left ventricle [66,67]; (3) venous drainage to the great cardiac vein comes almost exclusively from the left anterior descending coronary artery [64-67]. This fortuitous arrangement has permitted investigators to estimate regional left ventricular flow in humans [64,65].

Specific Functions

It is likely that veins contribute to the capacitance of the coronary vasculature. During systole, some venous blood is forced into the coronary sinus and some is stored in the venous system. In addition, venous volume probably increases during vasodilation [68]. Under normal conditions, venous tone probably does not contribute significantly to total coronary vascular resistance [68a].

BLOOD VOLUME OF THE CORONARY VASCULATURE

Under control conditions, the total volume of left ventricular coronary vessels (i.e., coronary arteries, capillaries, and venules less than 100 μm in diameter) has been estimated at 6 to 15 ml/100 g of left ventricular mass [68–70a]. Severe hypoxia can increase this volume about twofold. Also, blood volume within the wall of the left ventricle can significantly alter diastolic wall thickness [70a]. In one recent study [71], during maximal coronary dilation the volume of small vessels (capillaries, arterioles, and venules) within the left ventricle of a dog was reported to be approximately 27 percent of total tissue volume. The epicardial coronary arteries and veins contain a very small fraction (less than 5 percent) of total blood volume in the coronary vasculature. The volume of the intramural coronary arteries in the left ventricle is about 3ml/100 g of left ventricle [34,71]. The density of the vasculature in the right ventricle is similar to that in the left ventricle [71]. The volume of the vasculature in the right and the left atria is not known. Although one can be certain that a substantial percentage of the left and right ventricular walls is occupied by the coronary vasculature, the exact value under various conditions remains controversial.

The volume of blood in the coronary vessels has two important effects which are often forgotten. First, the fluid and the distending pressure in the vessels contribute to "stiffness" of the left ventricular wall [72,73]. This "garden hose" effect can alter global left ventricular function and diastolic wall thickness. Second, the volume may serve as a reservoir. The amount of blood pumped into the coronary vessels per cardiac cycle is about 10 to 15 percent of the total volume in the system. Thus, for a few cardiac cycles, the stored blood in the vasculature could theoretically buffer the effects of sudden reductions in coronary inflow.

SUMMARY

The anatomic characteristics of the coronary vasculature provide the foundation that permits the vascular bed to respond promptly and dramatically to a wide range of perfusion pressures and metabolic requirements.

REFERENCES

1 Britton S, Di Salvo J: Effects of angiotensin I and angiotensin II on hindlimb and coronary vascular resistance. *Am J Physiol* 225: 1226, 1973.

2 West JW,Guzman SV: Coronary dilation and constriction visualized by selective angiography. *Circ Res* 7: 527, 1959.

3 Ellis EF, Oelz O, Roberts LJ II, Payne NA, Sweetman BJ, Nies AS, Oates JA: Coronary arterial smooth muscle contraction by a substance released from platelets: Evidence that it is thromboxane A_2. *Science* 193: 1135, 1976.

4 Schrader J, Haddy FJ, Gerlach E: Release of adenosine, inosine and hypoxanthine from the isolated guinea pig heart during hypoxia, flow-autoregulation and reactive hyperemia *Pfluegers Arch European J Physiol* 369: 1, 1977.

5 Vatner SF, Pagani M, Manders WT, Pasipoularides AD: Alpha adrenergic vasoconstriction and nitroglycerin vasodilation of large coronary arteries in the conscious dog. *J Clin Invest* 65: 5, 1980.

6 Nellis SH, Liedtke AJ, Whitesell L: Small coronary vessel pressure and diameter in an intact beating rabbit heart using fixed-position and free-motion techniques. *Circ Res* 49: 342, 1981.

6a Tillmans H, Steinhausen M, Leinberger H, Thederan H, Kubler W: Pressure measurements in the terminal vascular bed of the epimyocardium of rats and cats. *Circ Res* 49: 1202, 1981.

7 Gregg DE: *The Coronary Circulation in Health and Disease.* Philadelphia, Lea & Febiger, 1950.

8 Chilian WM, Bohling BA, Marcus ML: Capacitance function of epicardial coronary arteries. *Fed Proc* 40: 603, 1981, no. 2133.

9 Spaan JAE, Breuls NPW, Laird JD: Diastolic-systolic coronary flow differences are caused by intramyocardial pump action in the anesthetized dog. *Circ Res* 49: 584, 1981.

10 Wissler RW, Vesselinovitch D, Getz GJ: Abnormalities of the arterial wall and its metabolism in atherogenesis. *Progr Cardiovasc Dis* 18: 341, 1976.

11 Duling BR, Berne RM: Longitudinal gradients in periarteriolar oxygen tension: A possible mechanism for the participation of oxygen in local regulation of blood flow. *Circ Res* 27: 669, 1970.

12 Landis EM, Pappenheimer JR: Exchange of substances through the capillary walls, in *Handbook of Physiology Circulation,* WF Hamilton (ed). Washington, DC, American Physiological Society, 1963, sect 2, vol II, chap 29, p 961.

13 Renkin EM: Multiple pathways of capillary permeability. *Circ Res* 41: 735, 1977.

14 Schaper W: *The Collateral Circulation of the Heart.* Amsterdam, North Holland, 1971.

15 Dusting GJ, Moncada S, Vane JR: Prostaglandins, their intermediates and precursors: Cardiovascular actions and regulatory roles in normal and abnormal circulatory systems. *Prog Cardiovas Dis* 21: 405, 1979.

16 Baroldi G, Scomazzoni G: Coronary circulation in the normal and the pathologic heart. Washington, DC, Office of the Surgeon General, Dept of the Army, 1967.

17 Vieweg WVR, Alpert JS, Hagan AD: Caliber and distribution of normal coronary arterial anatomy. *Catheterization Cardiovas Diag* 2: 269, 1976.

18 James TH: *Anatomy of the Coronary Arteries.* New York, Harper & Row, 1961

19 Gensini GG: *Coronary Arteriography.* Mount Kisco, NY, Futura, 1975, p 261.

20 MacAlpin RN, Abassi AS, Grollman JH, Eber L: Human coronary artery size during life. *Circulation* 46 (suppl. II): 6, 1972.

21 McAlpine W: *Heart and Coronary Arteries.* New York, Springer-Verlag, 1975.

22 Baltaxe HA, Amplatz K, Levin DC: *Coronary Angiography.* Springfield, Ill, Charles C Thomas, 1973, p 43.

23 Fulton WFM: *The Coronary Arteries: Arteriography, Microanatomy, and Pathogenesis of Obliterative Coronary Artery Disease.* Springfield, Ill, Charles C Thomas, 1965.

24 Gross L: *The Blood Supply to the Heart in its Anatomical and Clinical Aspects.* Introduction by Horst Oertel. New York, Paul B. Hoeber, 1921.

25 Paulin S: Coronary angiography. *Acta Radiol* (suppl 233) 1964.

25a Farrer-Brown G: Normal and diseased vascular pattern of the myocardium in the human heart. *Brit Heart J* 30: 527, 1968.

26 Heistad DD, Marcus ML, Law EG, Armstrong ML, Ehrhardt JC, Abboud FM: Regulation of blood flow to the aortic media in dogs. *J Clin Invest* 62: 133, 1978.

26a Gerova M, Gero J, Barta E, Dolezel S, Smiesko V, Levicky V: Neurogenic and myogenic control of conduit coronary a.: A possible interference. *Basic Res Cardiol* 76: 503, 1981.

26b Vlodaver Z, Kahn H, Neufeld HN: The coronary arteries in early life in three different ethnic groups. *Circulation* 39: 541, 1969.

26c Neufeld HN, Wagenvoort CA, Edwards JE: Coronary arteries in fetuses, infants, juveniles and young adults. *Lab Invest* 11: 837, 1962.

27 Scheel KW, Ingram LA, Gordey R: The relationship between myocardial perfusion territory and coronary flow. *Fed Proc* 40: 546, 1981.

28 Christensen GC, Campeti FD: Anatomic and functional studies of the coronary circulation in the dog and pig. *Am J Vet. Res* 20: 18, 1959.

29 Okun EM, Factor SM, and Kirk ES: End-capillary loops in the heart: An explanation for discrete infarctions without border zones. *Science* 206: 565, 1979.

30 Macho P, Hintze TH, Vatner SF: Regulation of large coronary arteries by increases in myocardial metabolic demands in conscious dogs. *Circ Res* 49: 594, 1981.

31 Tomoike H, Ootsubo H, Sakai K, Kikuchi Y, Nakamura M: Continuous measurement of coronary artery diameter in situ. *Am J Physiol* 240: H73, 1981.

31a Brown BG, Petersen RB, Pierce CD, Bolson EL, Dodge HT: Dynamics of human coronary stenosis: Interactions among stenosis flow, distending pressure and vasomotor tone, In *Coronary Artery Disease*, WP Santamone, F Bove (ed). Baltimore, Urban and Schwarzenberg, 1982.

32 Gerova M, Barta E, Gero J: Sympathetic control of major coronary artery diameter in the dog. *Circ Res* 44: 459, 1979.

33 Heupler FA, Proudfit WL, Razavi M, Shirey EK, Greenstreet R, Sheldon WC: Ergonovine maleate provocative test for coronary arterial spasm. *Am J Cardiol* 41: 631, 1978.

34 Wüsten B, Buss DD, Deist H, Schaper W: Dilatory capacity of the coronary circulation and its correlation to the arterial vasculature in the canine left ventricle. *Basic Res Cardiol* 72: 636, 1977.

35 Borer JS, Harrison LA, Kent KM, Levy R, Goldstein RE, Epstein SE: Beneficial effect of lidocaine on ventricular electrical stability and spontaneous ventricular fibrillation during experimental myocardial infarction. *Amer J Card* 37: 860, 1976.

36 Provenza DV, Scherlis S: Coronary circulation in dog's heart. Demonstration of muscle sphincters in capillaries. *Circ Res* 7: 318, 1959.

37 Provenza DV, Scherlis S: Demonstration of muscle sphincters as a capillary component in the human heart. *Circulation* 20: 35,1959.

38 Johnson PC: The myogenic response, in *Handbook of Physiology*, DF Bohr, AP Somlyo, HV Sparks, Jr (eds). Bethesda, Maryland, American Physiological Society, 1980, vol 2, sect 2, The cardiovascular system, chap 15, p 409.

39 Marcus ML, Kerber RE, Ehrhardt JC, Falsetti HL, Davies DM, Abboud FM: Spatial and temporal heterogeneity of left ventricular perfusion in awake dogs. *Am Heart J* 94: 749, 1977.

40 Weiss HR, Sinha AK: Regional oxygen saturation of small arteries and veins in the canine myocardium. *Circ Res* 42: 119, 1978.

41 Sestier FJ, Mildenberger RR, Klassen GA: Role of autoregulation in spatial and temporal perfusion heterogeneity of canine myocardium. *Am J Physiol* 235: 464, 1978.

42 Henquell L, Honig CR: Intercapillary distances and capillary reserve in right and left ventricles: Significance for control of tissue pO_2. *Microvascular Res* 12: 35, 1976.

43 Krogh A: *The Anatomy and Physiology of Capillaries*. New York, Hafner, 1959.

44 Bruns RR, Palade GE: Studies on blood capillaries. I. General organization of blood capillaries in muscle. *J Cell Biol* 37: 244, 1968.

45 Berne RM, Rubio R: Coronary circulation, in *Handbook of Physiology*, RM Berne (ed). Bethesda, Maryland, American Physiological Society, 1979, vol 1, sect 2, The cardiovascular system, chap 25, p 873.

46 Bassingthwaighte JB, Yipintsoi T, Harvey RB: Microvasculature of the dog left ventricular myocardium. *Microvasc Res* 7: 229, 1974.

47 Martini J, Honig CR: Direct measurement of intercapillary distance in beating rat heart in situ under various conditions of O_2 supply. *Microvascular Res* 1: 244, 1969.

48 Roberts JT, Wearn JT: Quantitative changes in the capillary-muscle relationship in human hearts during normal growth and hypertrophy. *Am Heart J* 21: 617, 1941.

49 Schafer DE, Johnson JA: Permeability of mammalian heart capillaries to sucrose and inulin. *Am J Physiol* 206: 985, 1964.

50 Lund DD, Tomanek RJ: Myocardial morphology in spontaneously hypertensive and aortic constricted rats. *Am J Anat* 152: 141, 1978.

51 Rakusan K: Quantitative morphology of capillaries of the heart. Number of capillaries in animal and human hearts under normal and pathological conditions. *Methods Achiev Exp Pathol* 5: 272, 1971.

52 Murray PA, Baig H, Fishbein MC, Vatner SF: Effects of experimental right ventricular hypertrophy on myocardial blood flow in conscious dogs. *J Clin Invest* 64: 421, 1979.

53 Rembert JC, Kleinman LH, Fedor JM, Wechsler AS, Greenfield JC: Myocardial blood flow distribution in concentric left ventricular hypertrophy. *J Clin Invest* 62: 379, 1978.

54 Tomanek RJ: Effects of age and exercise on the extent of the myocardial capillary bed. *Anat Record* 167: 55, 1970.

55 Forbes MS, Rennels ML, Nelson E: Ultrastructure of pericytes in mouse heart. *Am J Anat* 149: 47, 1977.

56 Karnovsky MJ: The ultrastructural basis of capillary permeability studied with peroxidase as a tracer. *J Cell Biol* 35: 213, 1967.

57 Gregg DE, Shipley RE: Studies of the venous drainage of the heart. *Am J Physiol* 151: 13, 1947.

58 Rayford CR, Khouri EM, Lewis FB, Gregg DE: Evaluation of use of left coronary artery inflow and O_2 content of coronary sinus blood as a measure of left ventricular metabolism. *J Appl Physiol* 14: 817, 1959.

59 Friesinger GC, Schaefer J, Gaertner RA, Ross RS: Coronary sinus drainage and measurement of left coronary artery flow in the dog. *Am J Physiol* 206: 57, 1964.

60 Lafontant RR, Feinberg H, Katz LN: Partition of coronary flow and cardiac oxygen extraction between coronary sinus and other coronary drainage channels. *Circ Res* 11: 686, 1962.

61 Roberts DL, Nakazawa HK, Klocke FJ: Origin of great cardiac vein and coronary sinus drainage within the left ventricle. *Am J Physiol* 230: 486, 1976.

62 Nakazawa HK, Roberts DL, Klocke FJ: Quantitation of anterior descending vs circumflex venous drainage in the canine great cardiac vein and coronary sinus. *Am J Physiol* 234: H163, 1978.

63 Owen P, Thomas M, Young V, Opie L: Comparison between metabolic changes in local venous and coronary sinus blood after acute experimental coronary arterial occlusion. *Am J Cardiol* 25: 562, 1970.

64 Ganz W, Tamura K, Marcus HS, Donoso R, Yoshida S, Swan HJC: Measurement of coronary sinus blood flow by continuous thermodilution in man. *Circulation* 44:181, 1971.

65 Pepine CJ, Mehta J, Webster WW Jr, Nichols WW: In vivo validation of a thermodilution method to determine regional left ventricular blood flow in patients with coronary disease. *Circulation* 58: 795, 1978.

66 Hood WB Jr: Regional venous drainage of the human heart. *Brit Heart J* 30: 105, 1968.

67 Parsonnet V: The anatomy of the veins of the human heart with special reference to normal anastomotic channels. *J Med Soc NJ* 50: 446, 1953.

68 Crystal GJ, Downey HF, Bashour FA: Small vessel and total coronary blood volume during intracoronary adenosine. *Am J Physiol* 241: H194, 1981.

68a Armour JA, Klassen GA: Epicardial coronary venous pressure. *Can J Physiol Pharmacol* 59: 1250, 1981.

69 Weiss HR, Winbury MM: Nitroglycerin and chromonar on small-vessel blood content of the ventricular walls. *Am J Physiol* 226: 838, 1974.

70 Rakušan K, Braasch W, Du Mesnil de Rochemont W: The total capacity of the vascular bed and the capacity of the terminal vascular bed of a normal heart muscle of a dog. *Physiol Bohemoslov* 18: 7, 1969.

70a Gaasch WH, Bernard SA: The effect of acute changes in coronary blood flow on left ventricular end-diastolic wall thickness. An echocardiographic study. *Circulation* 56: 593.

71 O'Keefe DD, Hoffman JIE, Cheitlin R, O'Neill MJ, Allard JR, Shapkin E: Coronary blood flow in experimental canine left ventricular hypertrophy. *Circ Res* 43: 43, 1978.

72 Salisbury PF, Cross CE, Ieben PA: Influence of coronary artery pressure upon myocardial elasticity. *Circ Res* 8:794, 1960.

73 Olsen CO, Attarian DE, Jones RN, Hill RC, Sink JD, Lee KL, Wechsler AS: The coronary pressure-flow determinants of left ventricular compliance in dogs. *Circ Res* 49: 856, 1981.

PART TWO

METHODS OF MEASURING CORONARY BLOOD FLOW

CHAPTER 2

METHODS OF MEASURING CORONARY BLOOD FLOW

New, important insights concerning control mechanisms in the coronary circulation have been tightly coupled to the development of approaches to measuring coronary flow. This chapter will review methods of measuring coronary blood flow in current use.

TIMED VENOUS COLLECTION

Collecting coronary venous blood with a graduated cylinder and a stopwatch is the oldest method of measuring coronary blood flow. This approach, introduced by Langendorf in 1895 [1] is still widely used to estimate coronary flow in several types of preparations.

Flow to an isolated perfused heart is often measured by timed venous collection. The heart is excised, and the proximal aorta is perfused from a pressurized reservoir with an oxygenated crystalloid solution, a crystalloid solution containing washed red cells or oxygenated blood. All of the perfusate entering the right heart is collected, measured, and returned to the reservoir. Perfusion with oxygenated crystalloid solutions is employed in biochemical studies to prevent blood constituents from altering substances released by the myocardium. Unfortunately, perfusion with crystalloid solutions is associated with exceedingly high flows [2], may cause edema, and possibly produces subendocardial ischemia. Also, when hearts are perfused with constant pressure, the phasic flow pattern in epicardial coronary arteries is altered [3].

Changes in left ventricular flow of an intact heart can be assessed by securing a cannula in the coronary sinus and collecting the venous effluent [4]. This procedure is almost always limited to studies in open-chest preparations. If any obstruction in the cannula develops, venous blood from the left ventricle will preferentially drain into coronary venous channels that do not enter the coronary sinus [4]. Under such conditions, the coronary sinus drainage will drastically underestimate left ventricular blood flow. In addition, in the dog 5 to 10 percent of flow entering the coronary sinus originates in the right ventricle and 10 to 15 percent of flow from the left ventricle does not enter the coronary sinus [4,5].

Total coronary blood flow to an in situ heart can be determined by employing right heart bypass and collecting the coronary venous blood that enters the right atrium and right ventricle [6]. Such measurements accurately collect 98 to 99 percent of coronary blood flow. The only flow not measured enters the left ventricle via the thebesian veins.

Regional coronary flow can be estimated by cannulating one of the superficial veins on the surface of the heart and collecting the effluent. By measuring both the flow and the concentration of various substances in the effluent draining an ischemic area of the myocardium, investigators have tried to gain insight into the metabolic state of ischemic cardiac muscle [7]. This approach is very crude because (1) the perfusion field of the artery and the drainage field of the vein may not overlap perfectly, and (2) there are extensive, large anastomoses in the coronary venous system [4]. Consequently, the blood returning to a superficial vein is a mixture of venous drainage from various regions, and the contribution from each region probably varies under different conditions.

Collateral flow can be measured with timed venous collection of blood if a small cannula is placed distal to the point of complete occlusion of the large coronary artery [8]. This approach has problems: (1) the retrograde flow drains against atmospheric pressure, which is certainly less than the coronary resistance beyond the occlusion, and (2) the distal circulation of the occluded vessel can divert blood away from the cannula [9]. Despite these problems, measurements of retrograde flow have provided considerable insight into the function of the coronary collateral circulation [10].

Advantages of Timed Venous Collection

Timed venous collection is a simple, inexpensive, relatively accurate method of measuring coronary blood flow that can be employed in both small and large animals. Mean coronary blood flow can be measured continuously. *The validity of new approaches for measuring mean coronary flow often rests on the demonstration that timed venous collection and the new method yield similar values over a wide range of blood flows.*

Disadvantages of Timed Venous Collection

With few exceptions, timed venous collection can be employed only when the heart is either excised or exposed; hence, this approach has rarely been used in humans [11]. Because coronary venous flow is predominantly systolic, continuous measurements of the coronary venous effluent provide no information about the phasic character of coronary arterial inflow. Timed venous outflow cannot be used to examine the transmural distribution of flow or to assess perfusion to the atria or the right ventricle separately. Finally, because there are numerous large anastomoses within the coronary venous system, the precise origin of the coronary venous drainage is often uncertain.

ELECTROMAGNETIC FLOW METERS

Principle

Faraday's induction law, that is, a conductor moving in a magnetic field produces electric current, is the principle on which electromagnetic flow meters are based. Faraday tried to apply the principle on a grand scale. Standing on Waterloo Bridge, he attempted to measure the electromagnetic force generated by the River Thames as it passed through the earth's magnetic field [12]. In 1936, Kolin recognized an important practical application of Faraday's law, that is, measuring blood flow in unopened blood vessels [13]. Martson obtained the first recordings of phasic coronary blood flow with a noncannulating electromagnetic flow probe in 1959 [14].

Many major improvements have been made in the design of the electromagnetic flow meters and probes. The early bulky direct-current devices were replaced by smaller, more efficient units which used alternating current (sinusoidal wave form) to energize the magnet. Current designs employ a square-wave current (240 to 480 cps) [15]. The flow signal is intermittently sampled at the peak plateau phase of the square wave. This operation is called gating. As a result of these improvements, the confounding effects of two extraneous electric currents, the transformer emf (electromotive force) and cardiac action potential, have been minimized [16]. Perivascular and extracorporeal electromagnetic flow probes are the two types most often used (Figure 2-1).

Perivascular Flow Meters

When initially introduced, perivascular probes were the only means of measuring coronary blood flow in an unopened vessel. Although some have argued that vessel dissection may interrupt sympathetic innervation to coronary vessels, studies made by Johannsen et al. [17] indicate that this problem is of no functional significance. When these probes are used in acute experiments, three problems related to probe-vessel contact arise. First, if the probe does not fit snugly around the vessel throughout the study period, the quality of the flow signal will be variable. This problem is exaggerated if the experiment involves major alterations in coronary diameter secondary to variable distending pressures or interventions such as nitroglycerin and methoxamine, which directly alter the diameter of conduit coronary vessels [18]. Second, if the probe fits too tightly around the vessel, a hemodynamically significant stenosis will be produced. This problem should be suspected if a marked increase in flow (reactive hyperemia) does not occur following release of a 20-s occlusion of the coronary vessel. Third, several studies suggest that the calibration of an acutely placed electromagnetic flow probe may change during the course of a single experiment [19,19a]. *For these reasons, flow measurements obtained with acutely placed perivascular electromag-*

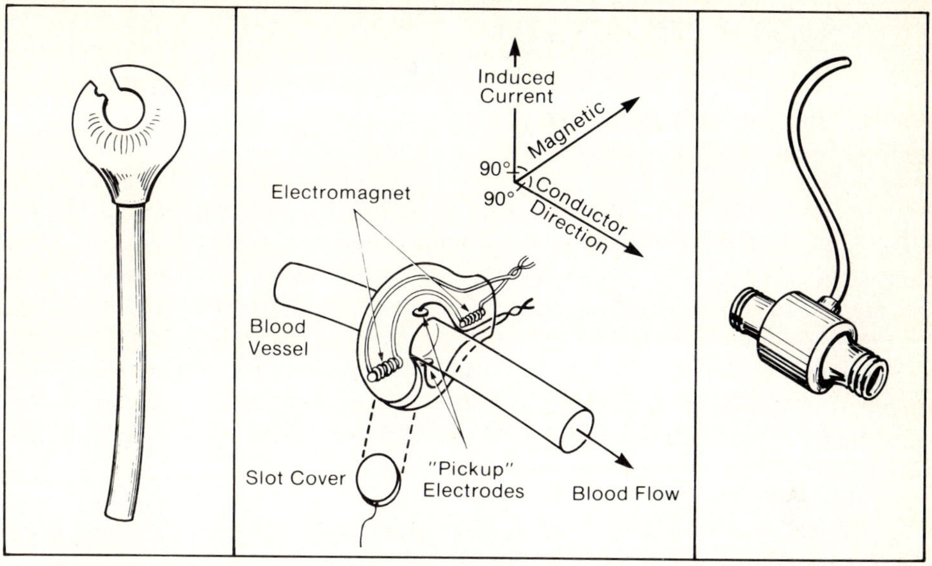

Perivascular EMF Probe | Diagram of Perivascular EMF Probe | Extracorporeal EMF Probe

FIGURE 2-1
Electromagnetic flow (emf) probes. The center illustration is of the basic design of a perivascular emf probe. The magnetic field, induced by tiny electromagnetics, is perpendicular to the induced current measured by the "pickup" electrodes.

netic flow meters should be carefully scrutinized and, if possible, compared with simultaneous flow measurements obtained by another technique.

When perivascular electromagnetic flow probes are implanted chronically, the ingrowth of fibrous tissue fosters excellent probe-vessel contact. The flow signals and their stability are excellent. Significant coronary stenosis can be detected by obtaining coronary reactive hyperemic responses by postmortem coronary angiography or postmortem casts of the vessel. Signals from implanted probes can be monitored by telemetry [20].

Extracorporeal Flow Meters

These probes are commonly used to measure flow in cannulas perfusing coronary arteries or draining coronary veins. Because of probe construction, contact with the blood stream is excellent. In addition, calibration can be readily performed by pumping blood at known flow rates through the cannula.

Advantages of Electromagnetic Flow Meters

The key advantage of the electromagnetic flow meter is its high frequency response. Without interfering with the blood column, the electromagnetic flow meter can measure rapid changes in flow with equal sensitivity in the backward and forward directions [12, 16]. Furthermore, the electromagnetic flow meter integrates flow across the entire vessel and is insensitive to alterations in the velocity profile if the flow is axisymmetric. Electromagnetic flow probes can be used in both acute and chronic animal experiments. The calibration of an electromagnetic flow probe is independent of density, viscosity, and temperature of the fluid and of whether flow is laminar or turbulent. Calibration curves pass through zero and are remarkably linear over a broad range. In addition, flow in non-particle-containing conductive fluids can be measured. By using various probe configurations, measurements can be obtained in vessels that vary in size from about 0.15 to several centimeters in diameter.

Because of these numerous attributes, the electromagnetic flow probe is the most widely used method of measuring phasic coronary blood flow. This instrument has permitted rapid advancement of knowledge concerning regulation of the coronary circulation.

Disadvantages of Electromagnetic Flow Meters

The major disadvantage of electromagnetic flow probes is that the zero-flow determination varies considerably. Therefore, it is crucial to obtain mechanical zero intermittently throughout the course of each experiment. Also, the calibration of electromagnetic flow probes is slightly dependent on blood hematocrit and critically dependent on probe-vessel contact. Consequently the device should be calibrated by pumping the animal's blood at known flow rates through the vessel with the probe in the same location that it was during the study. The probes are relatively expensive and difficult to repair. Because perivascular probes must encircle the vessel being studied, the coronary artery must be dissected prior to probe placement. This procedure is unacceptable in humans because of the risk of damaging perforating branches of the epicardial coronary arteries. Electromagnetic flow meters can be placed on coronary bypass grafts in patients at the time of cardiac surgery [21].

ULTRASONIC FLOW METERS

Principle

When sound waves are passed through a column of blood containing moving particles, two characteristics of the transmitted sound are altered: transmit time and Doppler shift. The ultrasonic flow probe initially introduced by Kalmus [22] measured changes in transit time. Modern ultrasonic flow meters detect changes in the Doppler effect [23] (Figure 2-2). Franklin has played a major role in developing ultrasonic flow meters for use in cardiovascular physiology [24–28].

The classic example of the Doppler effect is the sound you note if you stand at a stationary point as a train comes toward and goes away from you. A dramatic change in the sound frequency (Doppler effect) will occur as the train passes. The

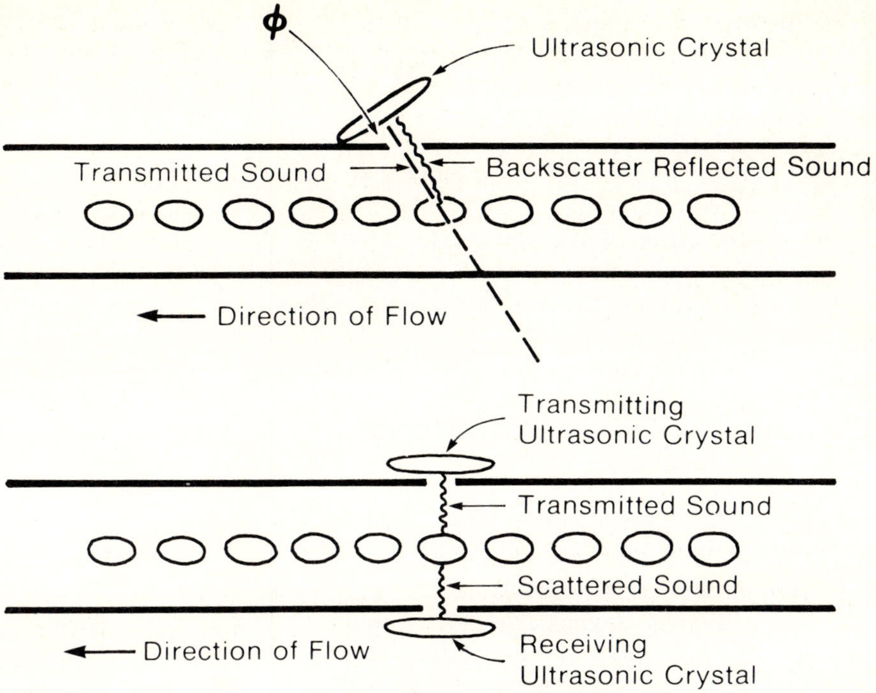

FIGURE 2-2
(*Top*) Diagram of a single-crystal Doppler blood velocity probe. For any given blood flow velocity, the magnitude of the Doppler shift depends upon the frequency of the transmitted sound and the angle ϕ between the crystal and the blood stream. (*Bottom*) A diagram of a two-crystal Doppler velocity probe. This arrangement requires placement of a cuffed probe around the vessel with the two crystals 108° apart.

magnitude of the Doppler effect is proportional to the train's velocity. In practice, high-frequency sound passed through a blood vessel is transmitted and received by piezoelectric crystals; changes in the velocity of blood flow alter the Doppler shift. Sophisticated electronic circuits precisely determine the Doppler shift and provide a continuous record of blood flow velocity.

When ultrasonic flow meters based on the Doppler shift are employed, two important parameters must be considered. First, with single-crystal probes, the magnitude of the Doppler shift is dependent on the angle between the piezoelectric crystal and the blood column. Maximal shift occurs when this angle is 45 degrees [29,30]. When two-crystal Doppler flow probes are employed, the angle between the crystals and the blood column is not a problem (Figure 2-2). Second, to convert measurements of blood flow velocity to absolute flow, the cross-sectional area of the vessel must be known and the velocity profile must be relatively flat [29,30].

Another problem with the ultrasonic approach concerns the relationship between sound frequency, sound penetration, and the magnitude of the Doppler shift. As the frequency of transmitted sound decreases, sound penetration increases but the magnitude of the Doppler shift with respect to a given velocity decreases [29]. Therefore, to determine the velocity in the center of the large vessel such as the dog aorta, transmitted frequencies of 3 to 6 MHz must be employed to achieve adequate penetration. To measure velocity in the left anterior descending coronary artery of the rat [31], transmitted frequencies of 20 MHz are needed so that the minute flow in this tiny vessel (0.15 mm outer diameter) will produce a Doppler shift that is readily detectable.

The waveform of the emitted sound is also important. If continuous sinusoidal waves are employed (continuous wave Doppler), the system cannot discriminate between forward and reverse flow, but velocity across the entire vessel is integrated [23]. Pulsed ultrasound permits discrimination between forward and reverse flow [29,30] and also provides the potential for measuring vessel diameter and the velocity profile of the blood column because velocity is measured in discrete sample volumes of the blood stream [29]. In addition, a single crystal that emits and receives can be used if the emitted sound is pulsed [30].

Types of Ultrasonic Flow Meters

Several ultrasonic flow probe configurations (intravascular, perivascular, extracorporeal) are available. Signals from perivascular probes can be monitored with telemetry [27,28]. In addition, two unique Doppler probe designs have been described.

A piezoelectric crystal can be mounted at the tip of a coronary arteriographic catheter. Under fluoroscopic control, such a device can be positioned in the orifice of the right or main left coronary arteries or a vein bypass graft in humans [32–34]. Phasic coronary blood flow velocity can be measured, and responses to vasoactive stimuli can be assessed [32–34].

A piezoelectric crystal can be mounted in a suction cup (Figure 2-3). Such probes can be placed on epicardial coronary vessels without dissection of the coronary artery. This approach, developed at the University of Iowa [35], can be used to measure phasic and mean coronary blood velocity in patients during open heart surgery. In addition, a similar device has been utilized to measure blood flow velocity in the left anterior descending coronary artery of the rat and in the spetal artery of the dog [31,36]. Such measurements cannot be obtained by any other approach.

Advantages of Ultrasonic Flow Meters

Ultrasonic and electromagnetic flow probes share many attributes. With both systems, the frequency response is good, calibration curves are linear and pass through zero, and phasic blood flow can be measured in unopened vessels.

Ultrasonic systems offer several advantages over electromagnetic flow meters. Most important, "zero" with the ultrasonic flow probe is stable and can be accurately determined without mechanical occlusion of the vessel. Also, ultrasonic probes can be miniaturized so that blood flow velocity in vessels 100 to 200 μm can

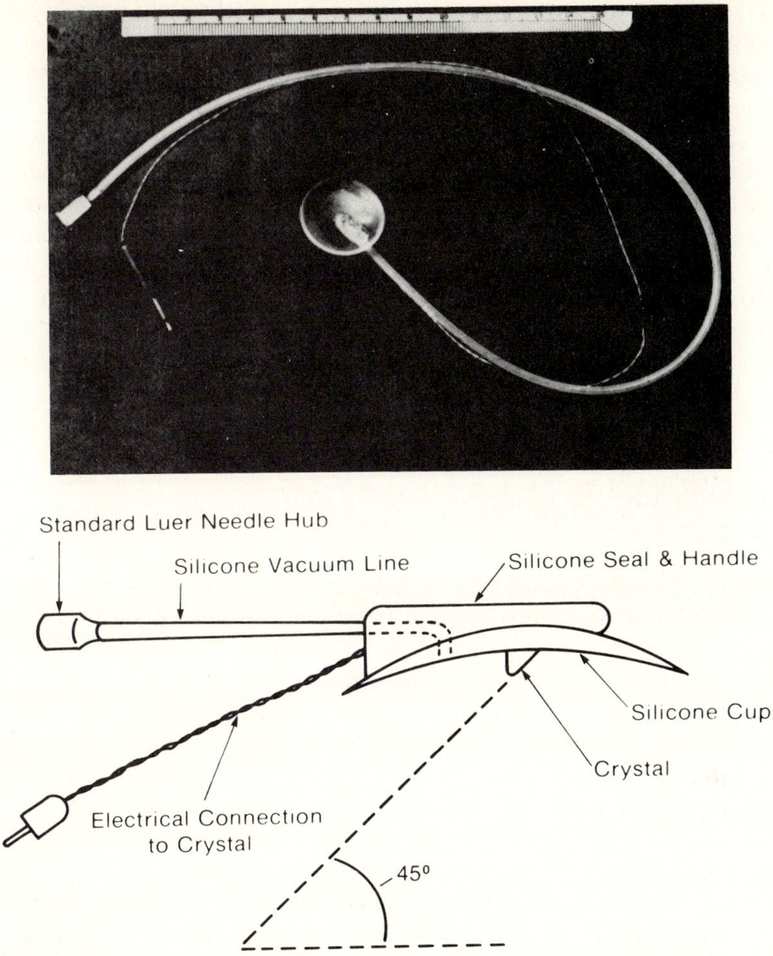

FIGURE 2-3
Photograph and diagram of a single-crystal Doppler probe. The device shown was developed at the University of Iowa to measure coronary blood flow velocity in patients at the time of cardiac surgery. The crystal is coupled to the coronary vessel with a small suction cup. (*From M Marcus et al* [35].)

be assessed. The calibration of the ultrasonic probe is hematocrit-independent, and the probes are simple and inexpensive to construct. Finally, ultrasonic probes provide the only available means of measuring phasic coronary blood flow velocity in the coronary arteries in humans.

Disadvantages of Ultrasonic Flow Meters

The principle disadvantage of ultrasonic flow meters is that blood flow velocity rather than blood flow is measured. Although changes in blood flow can be accurately estimated, absolute flow cannot be determined without knowledge of the angle between the blood column and the crystal and the cross-sectional area of the vessel. Angiographic studies by Gould et al. [36a] have shown that, even when two-crystal Doppler probes are chronically implanted, the cross-sectional area of the vessel within the probe is not fixed. A second disadvantage is that velocity is not integrated across the vessel with pulsed Doppler probes; instead, it is measured in a specific segment of the bloodstream that varies with the sample volume that is characteristic of the instrument. Therefore, changes in the velocity profile can affect the calibration of the probe. In addition, there are a few minor disadvantages: (1) ultrasonic probes work only if the fluid being studied contains particles such as red blood cells, (2) extraneous radio signals can interfere with probe function, (3) relatively few ultrasonic systems are commercially available.

LABELED MICROSPHERES

Principle

When particles that cannot recirculate because of capillary entrapment are injected into the systemic circulation, their distribution in body organs will be proportional to organ blood flow provided that certain criteria are met. These criteria relate to the number of particles injected, the adequacy of mixing in arterial blood, hemodynamic effects and rheological characteristics of the particles, and the magnitude of arteriovenous shunting. Buckberg et al. [37] have shown that for accurate ($\pm$ 10 percent at the 95 percent confidence level) determination of tissue perfusion, the tissue segment analyzed should contain at least 400 microspheres. In the dog left ventricle, this criterion is satisfied by injecting 0.5 to 1×10^6 microspheres into the left atrium and analyzing tissue samples that weigh more than 0.5 g. Adquate mixing of spheres with systemic blood is always accomplished by injecting the particles into the left atrium [37–39]. With this injection site, the spheres must traverse two mixing chambers (left atrium and left ventricle) before distribution. Some studies indicate that acceptable mixing for measurement of myocardial perfusion can usually be achieved if spheres are injected into the left ventricle [37,40]. This question, however, is not completely resolved [40a]. Many studies have shown that small microspheres (9 to 15 μm) do not alter systemic or regional hemodynamics, provided that concentration of the agent commonly employed to minimize aggregation of microspheres (Tween-80) is not greater than 0.1 percent [41]. Spheres produced by the New England Nuclear Corporation can be adequately dispersed without the addition of Tween-80. The rheological characteristics of microspheres are not sufficiently different from those of red cells to cause important artifactual distortion of regional perfusion measurements in the myocardium, provided that sphere size is 15 μm or less [42–44]. Finally, arteriovenous shunting of microspheres in the myocardium is not a major problem, particularly if spheres 15 μm in diameter are employed [44a]. Even over a period of weeks, losses of 15-μm microspheres from the myocardium average only about 3 percent. Cosigny et al. [44a] have recently reexamined the extent of microsphere loss in the myocardium under a variety of conditions. They found that when microspheres which averaged 9 μm in diameter were utilized, early arteriovenous shunting (first 2 min) averaged 3.6 percent and late arterial shunting (1 to 2 h) averaged 11 percent. Type of anesthesia, maximal coronary dilation, myocardial infarction, or decreases in coronary perfusion pressure did not alter arteriovenous shunting in a major way. Crystal et al. [45] demonstrated that when coronary perfusion pressure is 100 mmHg greater than left ventricular pressure, shunting of 9-μm microspheres increases significantly. Long-term arteriovenous shunting is also a major problem when 9-μm microspheres are employed. Cosigny et al. [44a] reported that long-term (1 to 21 days) losses of 9-μm microspheres from the myocardium averaged about 14 percent (ranged 2 to 40 percent). Direct measurements indicate that the actual diameter of microspheres that are lost from the myocardium by arteriovenous shunts rarely exceeds 10 μm. Because shunting of small microspheres (average diameter 9 μm) in the myocardium can be a problem, most investigators who study myocardial perfusion prefer the 15-μm size, even though the ratio of subendocardial to subepicardial left ventricular perfusion may be slightly increased versus that measured with spheres 9 μm in diameter [42].

Microsphere perfusion measurements are calibrated in one of two ways. The oldest approach is to inject a known number of spheres and independently measure systemic cardiac output at the time of microsphere injection [46]. Tissue perfusion is expressed as a percentage of total cardiac output. Alternatively, a reference arterial sample may be drawn at a known flow rate at the time of microsphere injection [42,46a]. The reference blood supplies a "surrogate organ," and tissue flows can be expressed as a ratio of flow to the surrogate organ. The reference sample technique is simple to apply and the most widely used approach for calibrating microsphere flows.

Differential Gamma Spectroscopy

To permit multiple measurements of tissue perfusion in a single animal, microspheres are labeled with various gamma-emitting isotopes: ^{125}I, ^{153}Gd, ^{57}Co, ^{114}In, ^{51}Cr, ^{113}Sn, ^{85}Sr, ^{95}Nb, ^{46}Sc, ^{54}Mn, and ^{65}Zn (Figure 2-4). The isotopes are incorporated into the substance that forms the spheres, and hence the label cannot be eluted from their surface.

Gamma emissions from the various isotopes can be separated by differential spectroscopy [42,46]. This process requires that reference blood and tissue samples obtained following the death of the animal be placed in a gamma counter. If no more than six different isotopes are employed, adequate separation can be achieved by a curve-stripping technique [42]. If more than six labels are employed, a least-squares approximation technique [47] must be employed to achieve acceptable separation. With either approach, the accuracy of separation is enhanced if the radioactivity in the tissue sample associated with each isotope is similar. A detailed description of this methodology has recently been published [42]. New systems currently being developed (germanium crystal [48,48a] and fluorescence separation techniques [48b]) will permit separation of 20 or more types of labeled microspheres.

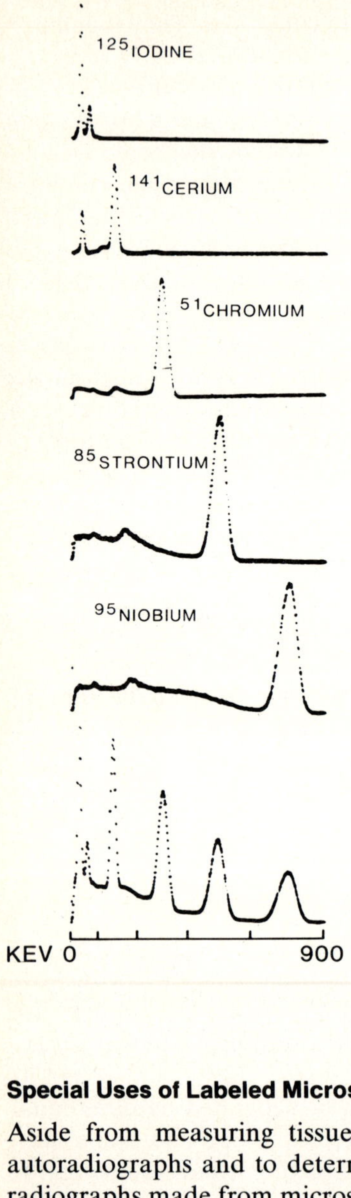

FIGURE 2-4
Energy spectra of several gamma-emitting isotopes. Microspheres labeled with different gamma-emitting isotopes can be used to obtain multiple measurements of blood flow in a single animal preparation. The energy spectrum shown at the bottom of the figure was obtained from a mixture of the five isotope spectra shown above. (*Redrawn from data originally presented by MA Heyman et al* [*42*].)

Special Uses of Labeled Microspheres

Aside from measuring tissue perfusion, microspheres can be used to obtain autoradiographs and to determine the perfusion field of a specific vessel. Autoradiographs made from microspheres usually employ low-energy gamma emitters such as ^{99m}Tc and ^{141}Ce [49]. Although the resolution of the autoradiographs is crude compared with what can be obtained with diffusible indicators labeled with beta emitters [50], the autoradiographs enhance the spatial resolution of this method. Microspheres can also be used to identify the perfusion field of a vessel if spheres are either selectively injected or excluded from a specific vascular bed [51]. Albumin microspheres labeled with ^{99m}Tc can be injected directly into coronary vessels or bypass grafts to determine the perfusion field of the vessel [52]. The distribution of radioactivity is recorded with a gamma camera.

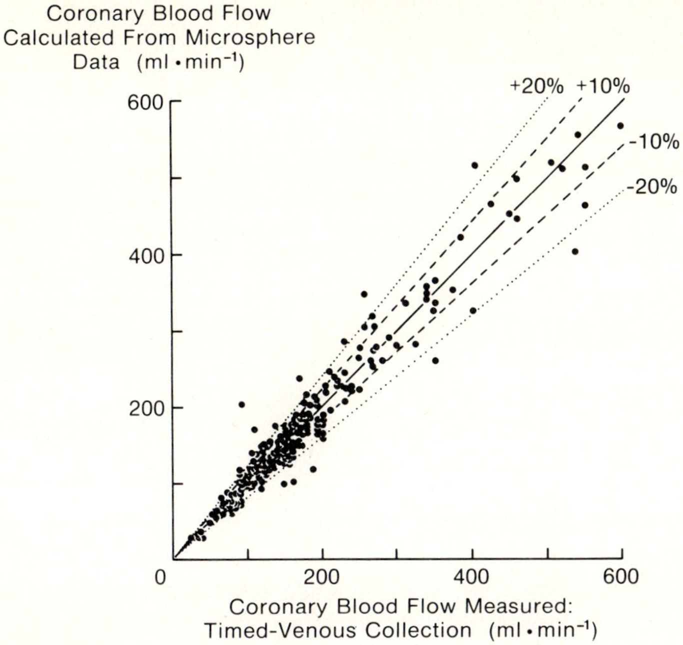

FIGURE 2-5
Correlation between two methods of measuring left ventricular blood flow: microspheres and timed venous collection. The excellent correlation between these two methods over a broad range flow supports the validity of microsphere measurements of left ventricular coronary blood flow. Percent values and dotted lines represent over- and underestimates of flow. (*Redrawn from data originally presented by J Utley et al* [6].)

Advantages of Labeled Microspheres

The microsphere technique, introduced by Rudolph and Heyman in 1967 [46], has permitted an enormous advancement in knowledge concerning the regulation of the coronary circulation. This technique is the only method that allows repeated accurate measurements (Figure 2-5) of the transmural distribution of left ventricular perfusion and blood flow to the atria and the right ventricle. In addition, one can simultaneously measure total and regional flow to all the organs of the body [42]. The microsphere approach has been modified for use in small animals, such as the rat [40] and in unborn animal fetuses [46], and it can be employed in anesthetized and awake animal preparations. Although the method measures "steady state" rather than phasic blood flow, it can be used to measure changes in mean flow which occur at 20-s intervals [53]. In addition, with microspheres, flow can be measured without disturbing systemic or regional hemodynamics.

Disadvantages of Labeled Microspheres

The major disadvantage of the microsphere method is that it cannot be used in humans to obtain quantitative measurements of perfusion. In animal studies, the microsphere method has several limitations. First, the results of an experiment cannot be obtained until the animal is killed. The frequency response of the measurement is slow (i.e., 10–30 s). The maximum number of flow measurements that can be obtained at present in a single animal is nine [47]. In contrast, with electromagnetic or Doppler flow probes, the frequency response is almost infinite and an unlimited number of measurements can be obtained in a single animal. There are two additional disadvantages of the labeled microsphere method: it is expensive to introduce and employ in a laboratory, and many precautions must be observed to prevent undue exposure from the radioactivity.

Several recent studies have suggested that substantial numbers of spheres are "lost" from areas of infarction within 24 h following coronary occlusion [54–56]. Although these studies were initially of great concern, the importance of this issue has been overemphasized. Murdock and Cobb [56] have shown that the quantitative importance of "apparent microsphere loss" in an area of infarction is inconsequential. Typically, flows in such areas of infarcted myocardium are 5 to 10 ml/mm/100 g. Even if the flow measurement is associated with a ± 50 percent error, the absolute difference in flow is of minimal physiological significance. The reported studies concerning microsphere loss have demonstrated only a decrease in microsphere density rather than an actual loss of spheres from the area of infarction [44a]. Much of the data could be explained by the usual evolution of tissue weight (an initial increase secondary to edema followed by a decrease as a result of fibrosis) that occurs in the course of infarction [57]. Studies by Koyanagi et al. [58] and White et al. [59] indicate that the apparent loss of spheres from infarcted myocardium is minimized if large numbers of microspheres (1×10^7) are injected. Although all these observations cannot be completely reconciled, it is my opinion that microsphere loss from infarcted myocardium is not a significant limitation of this method.

DIFFUSIBLE INDICATORS

Principle

If a diffusible indicator is infused into the arterial circulation, the concentration of the substance in an organ will depend upon the integrated arterial concentration of the indicator, the organ extraction ratio of the indicator and organ blood flow [60]. This principle can be used to measure tissue blood flow provided the tracer in the amount used is physiologically inert, tissue uptake does not depend on a metabolic process, and recirculation is prevented. Several indicators (^{42}K, ^{86}Rb, ^{201}Tl $^{3}H_2O$, ^{125}I, or ^{131}I-antipyrine and ^{14}C-antipyrine) which are physically inert in minute quantities have been used to measure myocardial perfusion [44,50,61–70]. Three of these tracers (^{42}K, ^{86}Rb, and ^{201}T) are less than ideal because tissue uptake depends on the viability of myocardial cells. The effects of indicator recirculation are minimized by removing the organ from the body within 15 to 90 s following injection of the tracer. If recirculation is not prevented, organs that have an extraction ratio greater than the total body extraction ratio will accumulate indicator with time; organs with relatively low extraction ratios will give up indicator as recirculation proceeds [60].

Advantages of Diffusible Indicators

The geometric resolution of diffusible indicators is impressive. If the concentration of a tracer is determined by quantitative autoradiography [50], the perfusion in tissue segments less than 50 μm^2 can be determined even if regional perfusion is extremely low (Figure 2-6). This is several orders of magnitude better than the geometric resolution that can be achieved with microspheres. In addition, the accuracy of regional perfusion measurements with diffusible indicators is not affected by rheological factors.

Disadvantages of Diffusible Indicators

The disadvantages of the diffusible indicators are so great that this technique is seldom used in studies related to coronary circulation. Because recirculation of the indicator must be prevented or accounted for in some manner, with rare exception [69], only one flow measurement can be made in each animal. Furthermore, because the heart must be excised within seconds following tracer administration, the animal preparation must be studied in the anesthetized state. Additional problems include the precision of the partition coefficient, the relative concentra-

FIGURE 2-6
Photograph and quantitative analysis of an autoradiograph. The autoradiograph was obtained from a left ventricular segment which contained normally perfused and ischemic cardiac muscle. By using quantitative densitometry, flow across the tissue segment can be assessed. The data shown in the right panel were obtained from a thin (less than 1 mm) horizontal segment in the center of the autoradiograph shown on the left. (*Modified from data originally presented by PM Malsky et al* [50].)

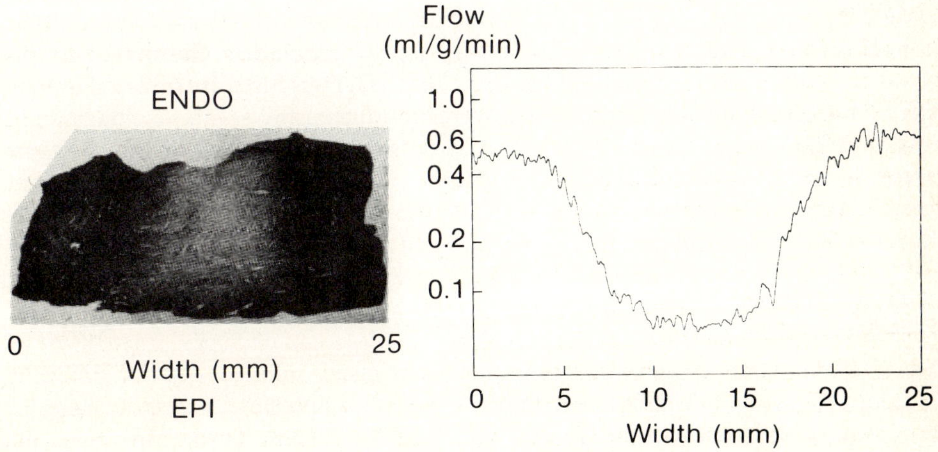

tion of the indicator in plasma and in red cells, diffusional shunting, and possible effects of capillary surface area on diffusion [6,70a].

Prior to the development of the labeled microsphere technique, most studies concerning regional myocardial perfusion employed a diffusible indicator. The labeled microsphere technique has almost completely replaced diffusible indicators in studies of regional myocardial perfusion.

CLEARANCE METHODS

Principle

Inert gas clearance techniques for measuring coronary flow are based on an approach Kety and Schmidt introduced [71–73] for measuring cerebral blood flow. Because the inert gases are diffusible indicators, in a strict sense, the clearance methods represent a modification of the diffusible indicator principle. Eckenhoff et al. [74] modified the technique of Kety and Schimidt for use in the coronary circulation. If an inert gas is introduced into the systemic circulation (saturation), the arterial concentration of the gas will rise faster than the coronary sinus concentration. If the heart is fully saturated with an inert gas and tracer input ceases, the arterial concentration of the indicator will fall more rapidly than the venous concentration (desaturation). In either case, the integrated difference in gas concentration between the arterial and the coronary sinus blood is proportional to coronary flow per unit weight [75,76], provided certain criteria are met (Figure 2-7). The requirements that must be fulfilled are (1) the partition coefficient for the inert gas must be known and adjusted for hematocrit if tracer solubility in red cells and plasma is not identical; (2) representative venous blood must be sampled from the entire area under study; (3) coronary flow must be stable during the measurement period (usually 5 to 20 min); (4) all tissue regions under study must be fully saturated (or desaturated) during the measurement period; (5) the total difference in the venous and arterial gas concentrations must be precisely quantitated until tissue saturation (or desaturation) is 98 to 99 percent complete; and (6) the indicator should be physiologically inert. The use of an inert gas with minimal solubility in blood, such as heluim or argon, which is nearly completely eliminated in one passage through the lung is particularly advantageous because recirculation is effectively eliminated. Although measurements during the saturation phase take less time, Klocke has argued that measurements during desaturation may be more accurate because small differences in arterial and venous gas concentrations are more easily quantified when gas concentrations are near zero than when they are high [75,76]. This is only so if the gas employed is not present in air.

Practical Considerations of Clearance Techniques

Since 1948, when Eckenhoff et al. [74] first used inhaled nitrous oxide to measure coronary flow in humans, the clearance principle has formed the basis for numerous approaches to assessing myocardial perfusion. Three aspects of the

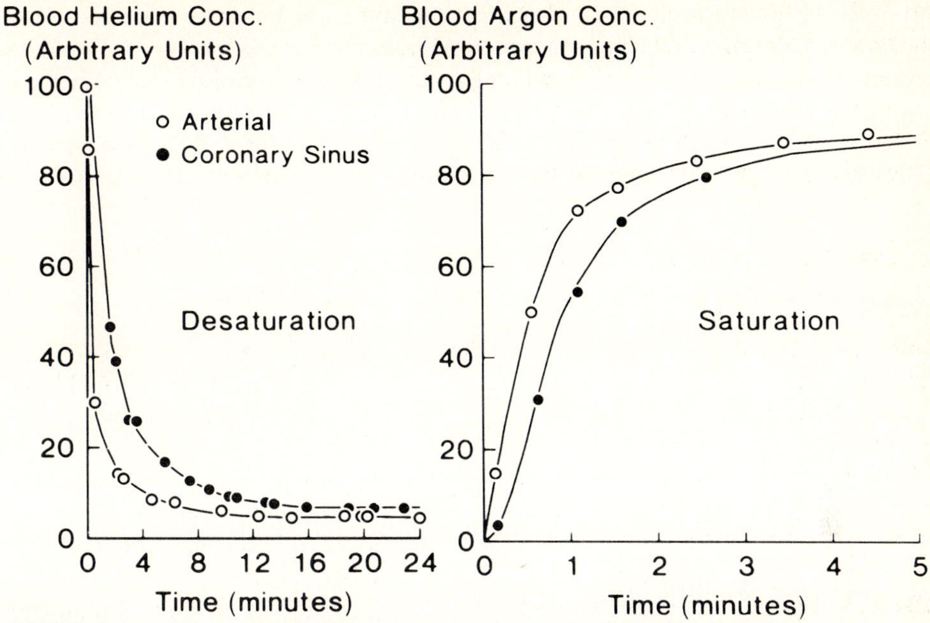

FIGURE 2-7
Arterial and coronary sinus measurements of inert gas concentrations (Conc) during desaturation and saturation. By determining the arterial coronary sinus differences in gas saturation, coronary blood flow can be calculated from equations originally developed by Kety [73]. (*Redrawn from data originally presented by FJ Klocke et al* [75] *and von M Tauchert* [83].)

procedure have been varied: delivery of the indicator, the tracer employed, and the method of analyzing the tracer.

The indicator can gain access to the myocardium by a depo injection [77–79], intracoronary injection [80,80a], injection into the left atrium or left ventricle, and inhalation [74–76]. Depo injection can be performed only in anesthetized open-chest animals or humans at cardiac surgery [77–79]. With the depo deposition technique, the rate of indicator removal is influenced by the size of the depo, repeated injections may cause tissue damage, and the clearance rate cannot be directly translated to absolute flow rates [81]. Intracoronary injections of ^{131}Xe is an invasive procedure that must be done in conjunction with coronary angiography [80]. Most clearance techniques in current use employ an inert gas indicator that is inhaled and thereby transported to the pulmonary venous blood [74–76].

The substances that have been employed as tracers include inert gases (nitrous oxide) [74], hydrogen [76], helium [75,76], argon [82,83], radioactive cations (^{24}Na [77], Na^{131}I [78], ^{85}Kr [79]), and ^{131}I-iodo-antipyrine [84].

Many approaches have been used to quantify the clearance of the indicator. These include implanted platinum electrodes for hydrogen clearance [85,85a], various detectors for measuring the activity of radioactive indicators (scintillation probes and multicrystal scintillation cameras [80]), and several methods of measuring the concentration of inert gases (Van Slyke analysis and gas chromatography [75,82]). Only two approaches for measuring coronary blood flow with clearance techniques are used at present: inhalation of a nonradioactive inert gas, such as helium, hydrogen, or argon and the detection of changes in arterial and coronary sinus gas concentrations with gas chromatography, and intracoronary injection of ^{133}Xe and detection of the radioactivity with a multicrystal gamma camera.

Advantages and Disadvantages of Nonradioactive Gas Clearance

The major advantage of this approach is that it can be used in humans to measure flow per gram in the left ventricle. The method is theoretically sound and has been convincingly validated at flow rates less than 200 ml/min × 100 g [75,86] (Figure 2-8). Also, if coronary venous samples are obtained from the great cardiac vein and the distal coronary sinus, the flow through the anterior portion of the left ventricle can be separated from total left ventricular flow. *A significant share of our knowledge concerning pharmacologic and physiological factors which regulate coronary flow in humans rests upon flow measurements made with clearance techniques* [87,88].

There are numerous disadvantages to measurements of coronary blood flow with inert gas clearance. The frequency of the response is very slow. A single measurement takes 5 to 30 min. During this time period flow must remain constant. The assumption that coronary sinus effluent contains flow only from the left ventricle is not completely valid [4,5]. Hood has shown that 17 percent of the veins that enter into the coronary sinus in humans do not arise from the left ventricle [89]. Furthermore, in 0.2 percent of patients without congenital heart disease and 10 to 20 percent of patients with atrial septal defect, an anomalous left superior vena cava drains into the coronary sinus [90]. Also, veins from the inferior-posterior wall of the left ventricle enter the distal 2 cm of the coronary sinus, and this blood cannot be sampled without contamination with right atrial blood [87]. Furthermore, there are numerous anastomoses in the coronary venous system [4,5]. Tricuspid valve disease, cardiac arrhythmias, any cause of right atrial hypertension, rapid coronary sinus withdrawal, or placement of the coronary sinus catheter within 2 cm of the ostium of the coronary sinus can lead to contamination of coronary sinus blood by right atrial blood [87,91]. Great care must be taken in the analysis of the minute quantities of gas that are present in the blood sample. Flow rates are reported in flow per gram rather than absolute flow. Thus, absolute resistance cannot be calculated unless an accurate estimate of left ventricular mass is available. Finally, the technique cannot measure flow to the right ventricle, atria, or the transmural distribution of myocardial perfusion.

Advantages and Disadvantages of Radioactive Inert Gas Clearance

When the ^{133}Xe clearance method was introduced by Cannon et al. in 1972 [80], it was the only way to estimate regional myocardial blood flow in unanesthetized

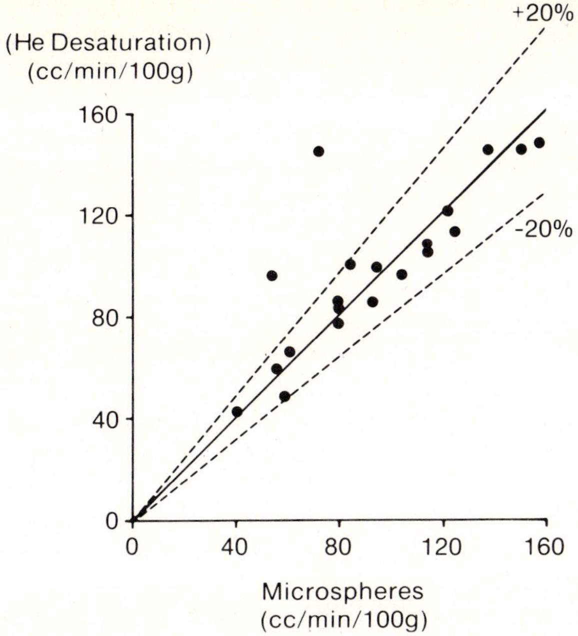

FIGURE 2-8
Relationship between measurements of left ventricular perfusion in dogs measured with He (helium) desaturation or washout and microspheres. Flow measurements with these techniques yield comparable flows at flow rates less than 160 ml/min/100 g. Percent values and dotted lines represent over- and underestimates of flow. (*Modified from a figure originally presented by P Schanzenbacher et al* [*86*].)

humans (Figure 2-9). Flow per gram could be estimated with this approach, in major regions of the left ventricle, the right ventricle, and the right atrium [80]. Unfortunately, this technique has numerous limitations [92-101]. It requires coronary angiography and intracoronary injection of ^{133}Xe [80,92–101]; thus it is not without potential morbidity and mortality. The ^{133}Xe clearance rates are determined with a curve stripping approach which is not theoretically sound [97,102]. A typical washout curve has at least two specific slopes (fast and slow). Consequently, investigators have related flow rates to the fast component, the slow component (compartmental analysis), or the area under the curve (stochastic analysis) [97,102]. Although the stochastic analysis is the only approach that is theoretically sound, investigators have often utilized some type of compartmental analysis because it is simpler and under some conditions it works reasonably well. With either type of analytical approach, flow is reported per gram rather than in absolute terms. Validation studies have yielded conflicting results with respect to the accuracy of measurements of myocardial blood flow with ^{133}Xe clearance [94,96,97]. The solubility of ^{133}Xe in fat is eight times greater than its solubility in cardiac muscle [92]. Thus, with repeated flow measurements with ^{133}Xe, accumulation of the isotope in fat can be a significant problem. For this reason, most studies are limited to only two flow measurements. Coronary flow rates greater than 200 ml/min/100 g cannot be accurately measured [103]. The equipment required to perform sophisticated ^{133}Xe clearance studies is very expensive [101]. Finally, this technique cannot measure the transmural distribution of left ventricle perfusion. Because of these limitations, the ^{133}Xe clearance technique is not widely used.

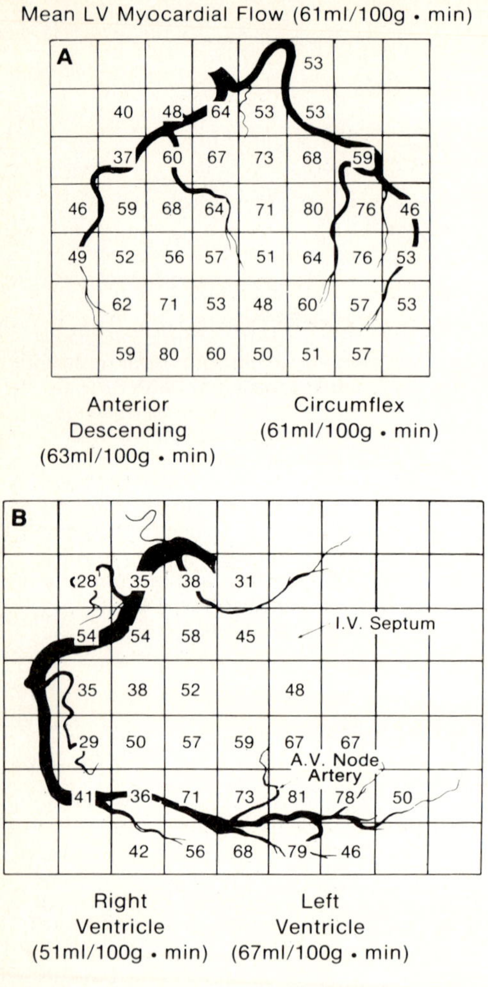

FIGURE 2-9
(*a*) Regional coronary blood flow measurements obtained with ^{133}Xe clearance. By superimposing the patient's coronary arteriographic and scintigraphic data, a regional coronary blood flow map can be constructed. (*b*) Right coronary artery. Note that right ventricular flow is less than left ventricular flow. LV = left ventricle; IV septum = interventricular septum. (*Data originally presented by PJ Cannon et al* [*80*].)

Heat Clearance

A special application of the clearance approach involves heat dissipation. When this method is applied to measure myocardial blood flow, a temperature-sensitive probe is placed in the heart muscle and heated with a steady current. Increases in blood flow in the tissue surrounding the probe decrease the temperature of the probe and vice versa [103a,103b]. Under ideal conditions, this method can provide continuous recording of blood flow in relatively discrete regions of the myocardium. Technical problems related to probe size and design, calibration difficulties, and confounding effects of tissue blood volume and blood flow on heat clearance have hindered acceptance of this method.

VIDEODENSITOMETRY

Principle

When radiographic contrast material is infused into an artery, mean blood flow velocity can be determined by measuring the transit time of the contrast agent. The cross-sectional area of the vessel can be assessed with biplane angiograms. Blood flow can be assessed with videodensitometry by obtaining the product of mean blood flow velocity times the cross-sectional area of the vessel being examined [104–113].

In practice, following injection of contrast into a vessel, density at two points along the vascular segment is simultaneously measured (Figure 2-10). From this data, mean transit time is determined and mean blood flow velocity can be calculated. This information, in combination with the cross-sectional area of the

FIGURE 2-10
Measurements of coronary blood flow by videodensitometry. By measuring density in two regions of interest along a vessel during passage of a bolus of contrast medium, transit time can be obtained. Blood flow velocity can be calculated from transit time. Blood flow velocity × cross-sectional area of the vessel = coronary blood flow. (*Redrawn from data originally presented by W Rutishauser* [*108*].)

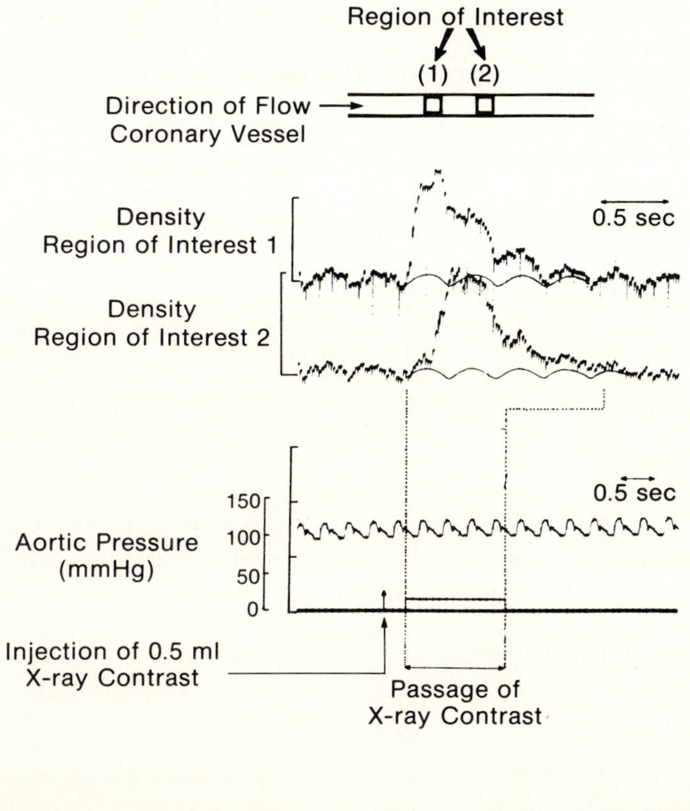

vessel, is used to ascertain mean blood flow [104-113]. Measurements can be made off line from cine- or videoangiograms.

Advantages of Videodensitometry

This system permits accurate measurements of mean coronary blood flow in individual coronary arteries or coronary artery bypass grafts in unanesthetized patients (Figure 2-11) [104–113]. At present, the contrast medium must be injected into the arterial system. However, with computerized x-ray tomography, such measurements can be obtained following intravenous injection of the contrast agent [114,115].

Disadvantages of Videodensitometry

Background alterations and density, which vary during the cardiac and respiratory cycles and when the capillary circulation is filled with contrast, must be recorded and subtracted from the angiogram. This requires relatively expensive equipment [104–113]. In addition, selective intraarterial injection of contrast agents can alter transit time of the contrast agent [116]. This problem can be minimized by injecting small quantities of contrast intravenously [114–115]. Finally, the method does not measure the transmural distribution of flow, and the frequency response is too slow to measure the phasic pattern of coronary flow. When ultrafast computerized x-ray tomographs become available, it may be possible to measure the transmural distribution of myocardial perfusion in humans with this method.

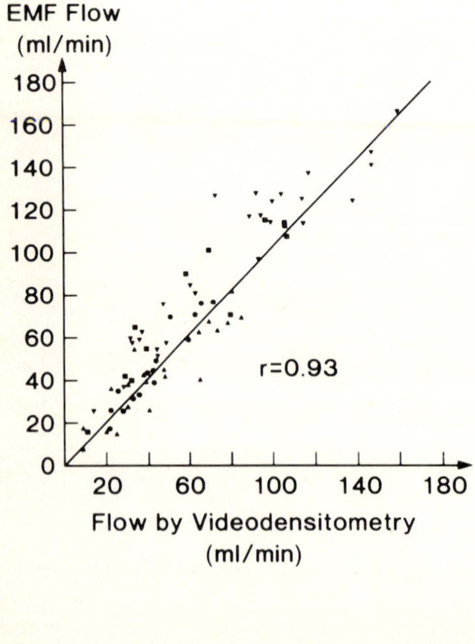

FIGURE 2-11
Correlation between two methods of measuring coronary blood flow: electromagnetic flow (emf) probes and videodensitometry. The excellent correlation between these two methods suggests that coronary blood flow can be measured accurately with videodensitometry. (*Redrawn from data originally presented by W Rutishauser* [*108*].)

Although videodensitometry has been infrequently applied to study the coronary circulation in humans, advances in computerized x-ray tomography should stimulate interest in this approach [114-115].

THERMODILUTION TECHNIQUES

Principle

When a fluid miscible in blood and of a lower temperature than blood is infused into a vessel, the downstream temperature of the fluid-blood mixture can be used to predict blood flow [117].

In 1971, Ganz et al. [117] introduced a thermal dilution method for measuring coronary sinus flow in humans which is now widely used (Figure 2-12). In the original description of the method, Ganz et al. set forth several conditions which must be met if valid measurements are to be obtained. The injectate must be infused at an adequate rate (35 to 55 ml/min) by a specially designed catheter to ensure good mixing with coronary sinus blood. The catheter system employed should be insulated to minimize heat exchange during catheter transit of the injectate. The thermomisters in the system must be sensitive and carefully calibrated. Recirculation of the thermal indicator should be minimized by limiting the duration of infusion of the injectate to 20 to 30 s. Finally, the catheter position in the coronary sinus must be extremely stable for multiple measurements of flow to be comparable. This technique can measure flow from the anterior portion of the left ventricle separately if the catheter is placed in the most proximal segment of the coronary sinus [117–118], i.e., at the juncture where the great cardiac vein joins the coronary sinus.

FIGURE 2-12
Measurements of coronary sinus flow with the thermodilution technique. Injection of contrast media produces coronary dilation. The increase in coronary flow is reflected by an increase in coronary sinus temperature. A.P. = aortic pressure; cor. sin. flow = coronary sinus flow. (*Redrawn from data presented by W Ganz et al [117].*)

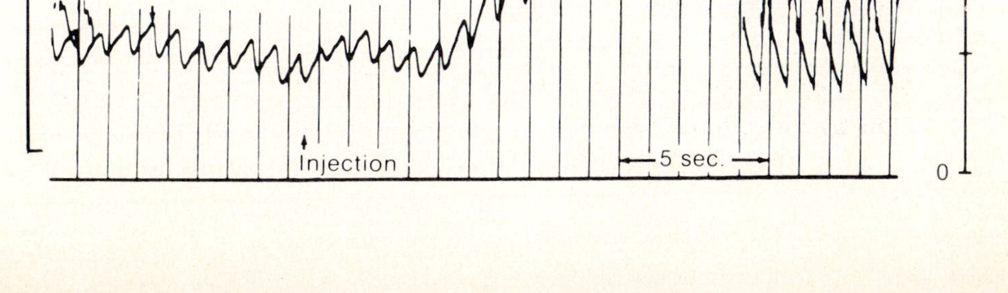

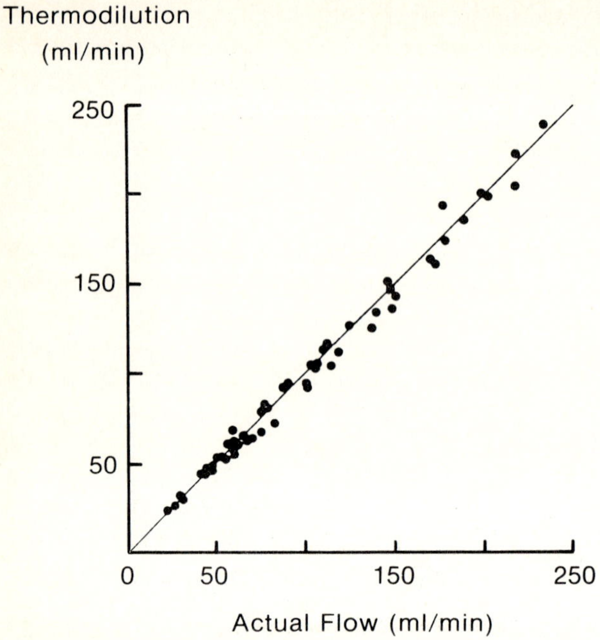

FIGURE 2-13
Correlation between two methods of measuring coronary blood flow: thermodilution and timed venous collection. In this study the thermodilution catheter was secured in the coronary sinus. Under these conditions there is an excellent correlation between measurements of coronary blood flow with the thermodilution technique and timed venous collection. $n = 54$; $Y = 0.99x + 0.3$; $r = 0.99$. (*Redrawn from data presented by W Ganz et al* [*120*].)

Although the thermodilution technique for measuring coronary sinus flow has been in use for over a decade, serious questions about the validity of the method exist. The validation studies with models are convincing [117]. Thus, the mathematical formulations employed are sound. The validation studies in animals are controversial. Studies which have secured the thermodilution catheter in the coronary sinus [117,119–121] have reported an excellent correlation between coronary blood flow measured with the coronary sinus thermodilution method and other approaches, such as electromagnetic flow meters and timed venous collection (Figure 2-13). These experiments may not be relevant to clinical practice, however, because under normal conditions the thermodilution catheter is not "secured" in the coronary sinus. Validation studies which have positioned the coronary sinus catheter in a more realistic fashion have reported exceedingly poor correlations between coronary blood flow measured with the thermodilution approach and other methods such as krypton clearance [122] and the electromagnetic flow meters [91]. The worst correlations occur with interventions that vary a

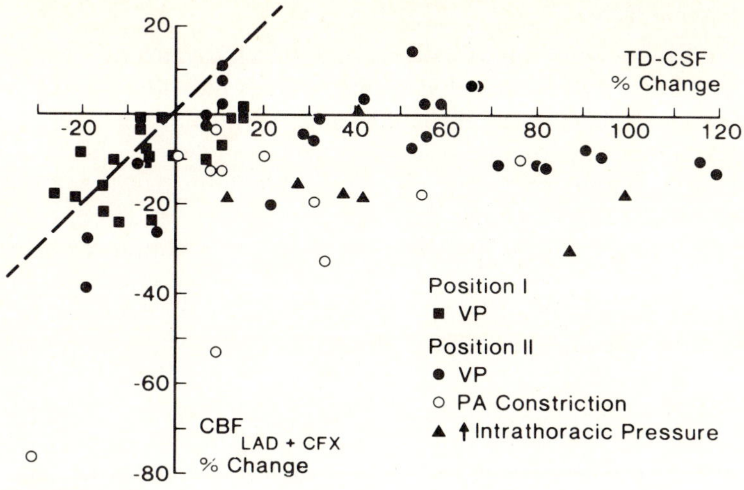

FIGURE 2-14
Correlation between two methods of measuring coronary blood flow (CBF); thermodilution (TD-CSF) and electromagnetic flow probes placed on the left anterior descending (LAD) and circumflex (CFX) coronary arteries. The thermodilution catheter was not secured in the coronary sinus. Measurements were made with the thermodilution catheter in two different positions in the coronary sinus. Position 1 was more proximal than position II. VP = increased venous pressure; PA = pulmonary artery. Under the conditions of this study, coronary blood flow was not measured accurately with the thermodilution method. (*Redrawn from data originally presented by DG Mathey et al* [91].)

right atrial pressure over a wide range [91] (Figure 2-14). Under such conditions, coronary sinus reflux is frequent. Finally, no animal studies have been done to validate the coronary sinus thermodilution technique in the presence of chronic occlusive coronary disease and myocardial infarction. Such validation studies are needed because coronary disease almost certainly alters the pattern of the venous inflow into the coronary sinus.

In my view, the thermodilution technique probably yields valid measurements of flow in the great cardiac vein if the method is carefully applied in patients with normal coronary vessels. Total coronary sinus flow cannot be assessed and measurements of coronary blood flow in patients with severe coronary disease are probably not quantitative when the thermodilution technique is employed.

Advantages of Thermodilution

The thermodilution technique is a simple and relatively inexpensive method of measuring coronary sinus or great cardiac vein blood flow in awake humans. Because the body acts as a large heat sink, multiple measurements of flow can be made at short intervals. The frequency response of the measurements is sufficient to measure changes in flow which occur in 2 to 3 s [117].

Disadvantages of Thermodilution

Thermodilution requires coronary sinus catheterization, which at times can be difficult. Because this approach assumes that coronary sinus blood flow is representative of left ventricular flow, it has all the limitations which accompany this assumption (see above). Recirculation must be minimized, and factors which may independently change the temperature of coronary sinus blood, such as alterations in cardiac work or pharmacologic coronary dilation, should be considered. Total coronary sinus flow cannot be measured because the thermodilution catheter must be placed at least 2 cm distal to the ostium of the coronary sinus to avoid contamination with right atrial blood. The tramsmural distribution of left ventricular perfusion cannot be assessed, and flow to the atria or right ventricle cannot be measured.

Serious problems with the validity of the method under various conditions persist. In the presence of certain conditions, such as severe coronary artery disease, chronic myocardial infarction, cardiac dysrhythmias, increased right atrial pressure, and major changes in intrapleural pressures, flow measurements with thermodilution may be seriously in error [191,122]. Finally, repeated measurements of coronary sinus flow at sequential catheterizations may not be comparable because the position of the catheter in the coronary sinus is difficult to reproduce.

POSITRON EMISSION TOMOGRAPHY

Principle

In essence, when positron emission tomography is utilized to measure coronary blood flow it is an elaborate diffusible indicator technique. Consequently, the general principle is identical to that of diffusible indicators. If the arterial input function is known, the concentration of an indicator in the tissue will depend upon tissue blood flow and the organ extraction ratio [60]. As with other diffusible indicators, the recirculation must be eliminated.

In practice, a positron-emitting radionuclide, such as ^{13}N-ammonia, is injected into the venous circulation, and the arterial input function is measured by withdrawing an arterial blood sample or an "arterialized venous sample" [123,124]. A radionuclide such as ^{13}N-ammonia is selected for this application because it is nearly completely extracted in one pass through the systemic circulation; recirculation is consequently minimal [123–127]. The absolute amount of the radionuclide in multiple regions of the myocardium is then measured with a positron camera gated to the cardiac cycle [127] (Figures 2-15 and 2-16). To quantitatively determine the amount of the positron-emitting indicator in the heart, the positron emissions must be corrected for attenuation, radioactive decay, and loss of complete recovery related to object size [127].

Studies with positron-emitting radionuclides (^{13}N-ammonia and ^{68}Ga-labeled albumin microspheres) in animals have reported an excellent correlation between flows estimated from positron emissions and those obtained with gamma-emitting

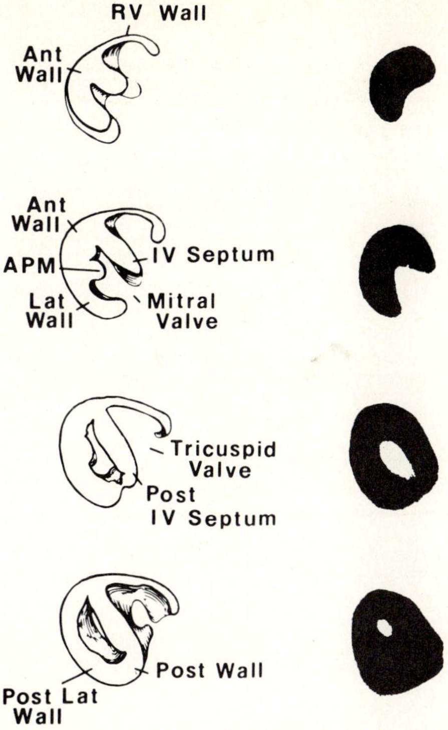

FIGURE 2-15
Tomographic scintigrams of a dog left ventricle and a diagram of the corresponding cross-sectional slices. The tomogram was obtained with a positron camera. The radionuclide was ^{13}N-ammonia. RV = right ventricle; Ant Wall = anterior wall; APM = anterior papillary muscle; Lat Wall = lateral wall of the left ventricle; IV Septum = interventricular septum; Post Wall = posterior wall of the left ventricle; Post Lat Wall = posterior lateral wall of the left ventricle. (*From HR Schelbert, E Henze, and ME Phelps* [*128*].)

carbonized microspheres [124-127] (Figure 2-17). A few studies in patients have demonstrated encouraging results [125].

Advantages of Positron Emission Tomography

Positron emission tomography is an extremely powerful approach which may permit accurate, repeated measurements of the regional distribution of coronary blood flow in awake humans. At present, no other method of obtaining such quantitative data in patients exists.

Disadvantages of Positron Emission Tomography

The equipment (a positron camera and a cyclotron for generating positron-emitting isotopes) and personnel needed to perform these studies are extraordinary (Figure 2-17). The minimal cost of establishing such a laboratory is several million dollars [123]. In addition, many practical and theoretical problems are unresolved. The resolution of current positron cameras is about 1 to 2 cm^2. The frequency response of these flow measurements is relatively slow, i.e., seconds to minutes. An ideal positron-emitting indicator for measuring coronary flow has not

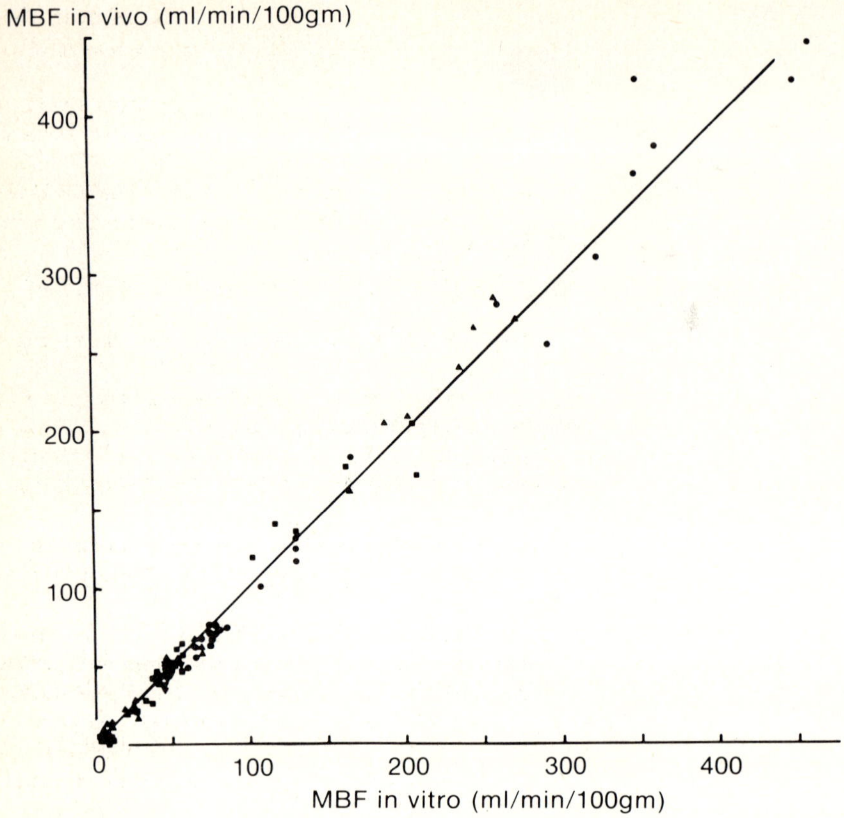

FIGURE 2-16
Correlation between two methods of measuring myocardial blood flow (MBF): positron emission tomography (in vivo) and microspheres (in vitro). The excellent correlation suggests that coronary blood flow can be accurately measured with positron emission tomography. $n = 84$; $Y = 0.7 + 0.99x$; $r = 0.99$; SEE = 12 ml/min/100 g. (*Redrawn from data presented by G Wisenberg et al* [*127*].)

been identified. Such a substance would have to be distributed in tissues on the basis of flow alone and not be affected by alterations in metabolism. Furthermore, recirculation must be prevented. In addition, validation studies performed under clinically relevant conditions are needed.

The potential uses of positron emission tomographic measurements of coronary blood flow in research and in clinical practice are enormous.

SUMMARY

Technological advances have permitted the development of many useful methods of measuring coronary blood flow.

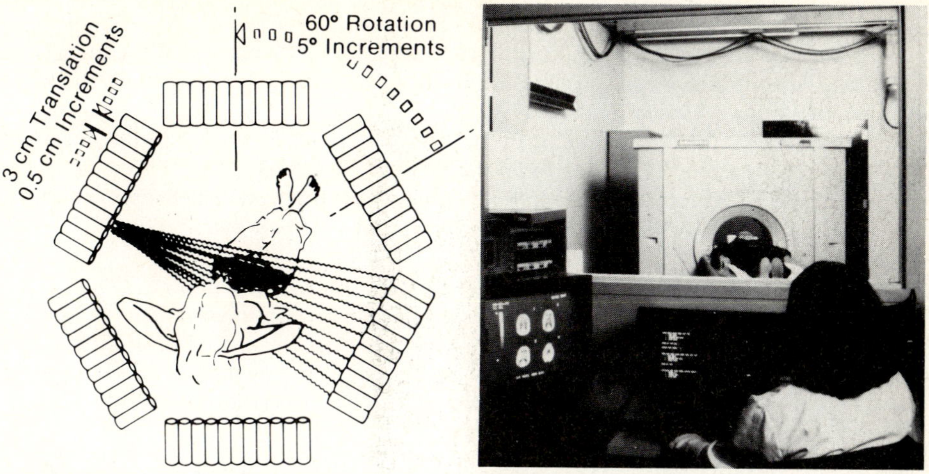

FIGURE 2-17
Diagram and photograph of a positron camera. (*Courtesy of H Schelbert, Nuclear Medicine Department, University of California.*)

There is a great need to develop approaches for studying the coronary microcirculation in the beating heart. Methods of measuring coronary blood flow in humans are still relatively crude in comparison with the precise techniques available in the animal laboratory. In the past few years, however, three new approaches (pulsed Doppler [35], videodensitometry coupled with computerized x-ray tomography [114,115], and positron emission tomography [123]) have been introduced, and these should permit significant advances in knowledge in this decade about the regulation of the coronary circulation in humans.

REFERENCES

1 Langendorff O: Untersuchungen am überlebenden Säugethierherzen. *Pflügers Arch ges Physiol* 61: 291, 1895.

2 Bhan AK, Scheuer J: The effects of physical training on cardiac myosin ATPase activity. *Am J Physiol* 228: 1178, 1975.

3 Panerai RB, Chamberlain JH, Sayers BMcA: Characterization of the extravascular component of coronary resistance by instantaneous pressure-flow relationships in the dog. *Circ Res* 45: 378, 1979.

4 Gregg DE, Shipley RE: Studies of the venous drainage of the heart. *Am J Physiol* 151: 13, 1947.

5 Rayford CR, Khouri EM, Lewis FB, Gregg DE: Evaluation of use of left coronary artery inflow and O_2 content of coronary sinus blood as a measure of left ventricular metabolism. *J Appl Physiol* 14: 817, 1959.

6 Utley J, Carlson EL, Hoffman JIE, Martinez HM, Buckberg GD: Total and regional myocardial blood flow measurements with 25 micron, 15 micron, and 9 micron, and filtered 1–10 micron diameter microspheres and antipyrine in dogs and sheep. *Circ Res* 34: 391, 1974.

7 Owen P, Thomas M, Young V, Opie L: Comparison between metabolic changes in local venous and coronary sinus blood after acute experimental coronary arterial occlusion *Am J Cardiol* 25: 562, 1970.

8 Mautz FR, Gregg DE: Dynamics of collateral circulation following chronic occlusion of coronary arteries. *Proc Soc Exptl Biol Med* 36: 797, 1937.

9 Loser WR, Diemer HP, Lochner W: Pharmacological alterations of coronary collateral circulation: Implication to the steal-phenomenon. *European J Physiol* 373: 219, 1978.

10 Gregg DE: The natural history of collateral development. *Circ Res* 35: 335, 1974.

11 Goldstein RE, Michaelis LL, Morrow AG, Epstein SE: Coronary collateral function in patients without occlusive coronary artery disease. *Circulation* 51: 118, 1975.

12 Wetterer E: Flowmeters: Their theory, construction, and operation, in *Handbook of Physiology*, WF Hamilton (ed). Washington, DC, American Physiology Society, 1963, vol 2, sect 2, Circulation, p 1294.

13 Kolin A: An electromagnetic flowmeter: Principle of the method and its application to bloodflow measurements. *Proc Soc Exptl Biol Med* 35: 53, 1936.

14 Marston EL, Barefoot CA, Spencer MP: Non-cannulating measurements of coronary blood flow. *Surg Forum* 10: 636, 1959.

15 Spencer MP, Denison AB Jr: Square-wave electromagnetic flowmeter for surgical and experimental application, in *Methods in Medical Research*, HD Bruner (ed). Chicago, Year Book Medical, 1960, vol 8, p 321.

16 Mills CJ: Measurement of pulsatile flow and flow velocity, in *Cardiovascular Fluid Dynamics*, DH Bergel (ed). London, Academic Press, 1972, vol 1, chap 3, pp 71–77.

17 Johannsen UJ, Mark AL, Marcus ML: Responses to cardiac sympathetic nerve stimulation during maximal coronary dilation produced by adenosine. *Circ Res* 50: 510, 1982.

18 Vatner SF, Pagani M, Manders WT, Pasipoularides AD: Alpha adrenergic vasoconstriction and nitroglycerin vasodilation of large coronary arteries in the conscious dog. *J Clin Invest* 65: 5, 1980.

19 Carlson EL, Selinger SL, Utley J, Hoffman JIE: Intramyocardial distribution of blood flow in hemorrhagic shock in anesthetized dogs. *Am J Physiol* 230: 41, 1976.

19a Dobson A, Sellers AF, McLeod FD: Performance of a cuff-type blood flowmeter in vivo. *J Appl Physiol* 21: 1642, 1966.

20 Vatner SF, Franklin D, Higgins CB, Patrick T, Braunwald E: Left ventricular response to severe exertion in untethered dogs. *J Clin Invest* 51: 3052, 1972.

21 Greenfield JC Jr, Rembert JC, Young WG Jr, Oldham HN Jr, Alexander JA, Sabiston DC Jr: Studies of blood flow in aorta-to-coronary venous bypass grafts in man. *J Clin Invest* 51: 2724, 1972.

22 Kalmus HP, Hedrich AL, Pardue DR: The acoustic flowmeter using electronic switching. *IRE (Inst Radio Engrs) Trans Ultrasonics Eng* UE-1: 49, 1954.

23 Woodcock JP: *Theory and Practice of Blood Flow Measurement*. Woburn, Mass, Butterworth, 1975.

24 Franklin DL, Baker DW, Rushmer RF: Pulsed ultrasonic transit time flowmeter. *IRE (Inst Radio Engrs) Trans Bio-Med Electron* 9: 44, 1962.

25 Franklin DL, Schlegel E, Rushmer RF: Blood flow measured by Doppler frequency shift of back-scattered ultrasound. *Science* 134: 564, 1961.

26 Franklin D, Watson NW, Pierson KE, Van Citters RL: Technique for radiotelemetry of blood flow from unrestrained animals. *Am J Med Electron* 5: 24, 1966.

27 Franklin D, Patrick T, Kemper S, Vatner SF: A system for radiotelemetry of blood pressure, blood flow and ventricular dimensions from animals: A summary report. Proceedings of the International Telemetry Conference, Washington, DC, September 1971, p 244.

28 Franklin D, Vatner SF, Higgins CB, Patrick T, Kemper WS, Van Citters RL: Measurement and radiotelemetry of cardiovascular variables in conscious animals: Techniques and applications, in *Research Animals in Medicine.* Washington, DC, Government Printing Office, 1973, p 1119.

29 Peronneau PA, Bournat J-P, Bugnon A, Barber A, Xhaard M: Theoretical and practical aspects of pulsed Doppler flowmetry: Real-time application to the measure of instantaneous velocity profiles in vitro and in vivo, in *Cardiovascular Applications of Ultrasound,* RS Reneman (ed). *Proc Internatl Sym* (Janssen Pharmaceutica, Beerse, Belgium, May 29–30, 1973), New York, American Elsevier, 1974, chap 6, p 66.

30 Hartley CJ, Cole JS: An ultrasonic pulsed doppler system for measuring blood flow in small vessels. *J Appl Physiol* 37: 626, 1974.

31 Wangler RD, Peters KG, Laughlin DE, Tomanek RJ, Marcus ML: A method for continuously assessing coronary blood flow velocity in the rat. *Am J Physiol* 241: H816, 1981.

32 Cole JS, Hartley CJ: The pulsed Doppler coronary artery catheter: Preliminary report of a new technique for measuring rapid changes in coronary artery flow velocity in man. *Circulation* 56: 18, 1977.

33 Benchimol A, Desser KB: Measurement of phasic aortocoronary bypass graft blood flow velocity in conscious man. *Am J Cardiol* 32: 895, 1973.

34 Benchimol A, Desser KB: Phasic aortocoronary bypass graft blood velocity during ventricular arrhythmias in man. *Am J Cardiol* 40: 315, 1977.

35 Marcus M, Wright C, Doty D, Eastham C, Laughlin D, Krumm P, Fastenow C, Brody M: Measurements of coronary velocity and reactive hyperemia in the coronary circulation of humans. *Circ Res* 49: 877, 1981.

36 Chilian WM, Marcus ML: Phasic coronary blood flow velocity in intramural and epicardial coronary arteries. *Circ Res* 50: 775–781, 1982.

36a Gould KL, Kelley KO: Physiologic significance of coronary flow velocity and changing stenosis geometry during coronary vasodilation in awake dogs. *Circ Res* 50: 695, 1982.

37 Buckberg GD, Luck JC, Payne DB, Hoffman JIE, Archie JP, Fixler DE: Some sources of error in measuring regional blood flow with radioactive microspheres. *J Appl Physiol* 31: 598, 1971.

38 Archie JP Jr, Fixler DE, Ullyot DJ, Hoffman JIE, Utley JR, Carlson EL: Measurement of cardiac output with and organ trapping of radioactive microspheres. *J Appl Physiol* 35: 148, 1973.

39 Marcus ML, Heistad DD, Ehrhardt JC, Abboud FM: Total and regional cerebral blood flow measurement with 7-10-, 15-, 25-, and 50-μm microspheres. *J Appl Physiol* 40(4): 501, 1976.

40 Wangler RD, Peters KG, Marcus ML, Tomanek RJ: Effects of duration and severity of arterial hypertension on cardiac hypertrophy and coronary vasodilator reserve. *Circ Res* 51: 10, 1982.

40a Wicker P, Tarazi RC: Importance of injection site for coronary blood flow determinations by microspheres in rats. *Am J Physiol* 242: H94, 1982.

41 Millard RW, Baig H, Vatner SF: Cardiovascular effects of radioactive microsphere suspensions and Tween 80 solutions. *Am J Physiol* 232: H331, 1977.

42 Heymann MA, Payne BD, Hoffman JIE, Rudolph AM: Blood Flow Measurements With Radionuclide-Labeled Particles. *Prog Cardiovas Dis* 20: 55, 1977.

43 Yipintsol T, Dobbs WA Jr, Scanlon PD, Knopp TJ, Bassingthwaighte JB: Regional distribution of diffusible tracers and carbonized microspheres in the left ventricle of isolated dog hearts. *Circ Res* 33: 573, 1973.

44 Tripp MR, Meyer MW, Einzig S, Leonard JJ, Swayze CR, Fox IJ: Simultaneous regional myocardial blood flows by tritiated water and microspheres. *Am J Physiol* 232: H173, 1977.

44a Consigny PM, Verrier ED, Payne BD, Edelist C, Jester J, Baer RW, Vlahakes GJ, Hoffman JIE: Acute and chronic microsphere loss from canine left ventricular mycardium. *Am J Physiol* 242: H392, 1982.

45 Crystal GJ, Boatwright RB, Downey HF, Bashour FA: Shunting of microspheres across the canine coronary circulation. *Am J Physiol* 236: H7, 1979.

46 Rudolph AM, Heymann MA: The circulation of the fetus in utero: Methods for studying distribution of blood flow, cardiac output and organ blood flow. *Circ Res* 21: 163, 1967.

46a Makowski EL, Meschia G, Droegemueller W, Battaglia FC: Measurement of umbilical arterial blood flow to the sheep placenta and fetus in utero: Distribution to cotyledons and the intercotyledonary chorion. *Circ Res* 23: 623, 1968.

47 Baer RW, Verrier ED, Vlahakes GJ, Payne BD, Hoffman JIE: Validation of eight sequential myocardial blood flow determinations with radioactive microspheres using least-squares analysis. *Circulation* 62 (suppl 3): 65, 1980.

48 Winkler B, Nienaber C, Stammler G, Schaper W: High precision measurement of acute collateral blood flow with tracer microspheres and a well type GE-detector. *Circulation* 64(suppl. 4): 118, 1981.

48a Kaufman L, Rowan W, Payne B, Hoffman J, Hirk R, Schoenmaekers W, Kamp D: Large high purity germanium well detector in biomedical applications. *IEEE Trans Nucl Sci* NS28: 117, 1981.

48b Hoffman J: Personal Communication. San Francisco, University of California, Department of Pediatrics, August 1981.

49 Heistad DD, Marcus ML, Gourley JK, Busija DW: Effect of adenosine and dipyridamole on cerebral blood flow. *Am J Physiol* 9: H775, 1981.

50 Malsky PM, Vokonas PS, Paul SJ, Robbins SL, Hood WB Jr: Autoradiographic measurement of regional blood flow in normal and ischemic myocardium. *Am J Physiol* 232: H576, 1977.

51 Hirzel HO, Sonnenblick EH, Kirk ES: Absence of a lateral border zone of intermediate creatine phosphokinase depletion surrounding a central infarct 24 hours after acute coronary occlusion in the dog. *Circ Res* 41: 673, 1977.

52 Ritchie JL, Hamilton GW, Gould KL: Myocardial imaging with indium-113m and technetium-99m labeled macroaggregated albumin. *Am J Cardiol* 35: 380, 1975.

53 Busija DW, Heistad DD, Marcus ML: Effect of sympathetic nerves on cerebral vessels during acute, moderate increases in arterial pressure in dogs and cats. *Circ Res* 46: 696, 1980.

54 Capurro NL, Goldstein RE, Aamodt R, Smith HJ, Epstein SE: Loss of microspheres from ischemic canine cardiac tissue: An important technical limitation. *Circ Res* 44: 223, 1979.

55 Jugdutt BI, Hutchins GM, Bulkley BH. Becker LC: The loss of radioactive microspheres from canine necrotic myocardium. *Circ Res* 45: 746, 1979.

56 Murdock RH Jr, Cobb FR: Effects of infarcted myocardium on regional blood flow measurements to ischemic regions in canine heart. *Circ Res* 47: 701, 1980.

57 Reimer KA, Jennings RB: The changing anatomic reference base of evolving myocardial infarction. *Circulation* 60: 866, 1979.

58 Koyanagi S, Eastham CL, Harrison DG, Marcus ML: Transmural variation in the relationship between myocardial infarct size and risk area. *Am J Physiol* 242: H867, 1982.

59 White FC, Sanders M, Andres J, Bloor CM: Reduction of tracer microsphere loss from ischemic myocardium. *Circulation* 57 & 58 (suppl II): 36, 1978, no. 132.

60 Sapirstein LA: Regional blood flow by fractional distribution of indicators. *Am J Physiol* 193: 161, 1958.

61 Love WD, Burch GE: Differences in the rate of Rb^{86} uptake by several regions of the myocardium of control dogs and dogs receiving L-norepinephrine or pitressin. *J Clin Invest* 36: 479, 1957.

62 Levy MN, De Oliveira JM: Regional distribution of myocardial blood flow in the dog as determined by Rb^{86}. *Circ Res* 9: 96, 1961.

63 Cutarelli R, Levy MN: Intraventricular pressure and the distribution of coronary blood flow. *Circ Res* 12: 322, 1963.

64 Palmer WH, Fam WM, McGregor M: The effect of coronary vasodilatation (dipyridamole-induced) on the myocardial distribution of tritiated water. *Canadian J Physiol Pharmacol* 44: 777, 1966.

65 Moir TW, DeBra DW: Effect of left ventricular hypertension, ischemia and vasoactive drugs on the myocardial distribution of coronary flow. *Circ Res* 21: 65, 1967.

66 Griggs DM Jr, Nakamura Y: Effect of coronary constriction on myocardial distribution of iodoantipyrine-^{131}I. *Am J Physiol* 215: 1082, 1968.

67 Howe BB, Winbury MM: Effect of acute coronary occlusion on myocardial nutritional circulation in swine. *Am J Physiol* 216: 1069, 1969.

68 Downey JM, Downey HF, Kirk ES: Effects of myocardial strains on coronary blood flow. *Circ Res*, 34: 286, 1974.

69 Downey JM, Kirk ES: Distribution of coronary blood flow across the canine heart wall during systole. *Circ Res* 34: 251, 1974.

70 Mueller TM, Marcus ML, Ehrhardt JC, Chaudhuri T, Abboud FM: Limitations of thallium-201 myocardial perfusion scintigrams. *Circulation* 54: 640, 1976.

70a Carlin R, Chien S: Partition of xenon and iodoantipyrine among erythrocytes, plasma, and myocardium. *Circ Res* 40: 497, 1977.

71 Kety, SS, Schmidt CF: The determination of cerebral blood flow in man by the use of nitrous oxide in low concentrations. *Am J Physiol* 143: 53, 1945.

72 Kety SS, Schmidt CF: The nitrous oxide method for the quantitative determination of cerebral blood flow in man: Theory, procedure and normal values. *J Clin Invest* 27: 476, 1948.

73 Kety SS: The theory and applications of the exchange of inert gas at the lungs and tissues. *Pharmacol Rev* 3: 1, 1951.

74 Eckenhoff JE, Hafkenschiel JH, Harmel MH, Goodale WT, Lubin M, Bing RJ, Kety SS: Measurement of coronary blood flow by the nitrous oxide method. *Am J Physiol* 152: 356, 1948.

75 Klocke FJ, Bunnell IL, Greene DG, Wittenberg SM, Visco JP: Average coronary blood flow per unit weight of left ventricle in patients with and without coronary artery disease. *Circulation* 50: 547, 1974.

76 Klocke FJ, Koberstein RC, Pittman DE, Bunnell IL, Greene DG, Rosing DR: Effects of heterogeneous myocardial perfusion on coronary venous H_2 desaturation curves and calculations of coronary flow. *J Clin Invest* 47: 2711, 1968.

77 Salisbury PF, Cross CE, Oblath RW, Rieben PA: Local circulation in heart muscle studied with Na^{24} clearance method. *J Appl Physiol* 17: 475, 1962.

78 Kirk ES, Honig CR: Nonuniform distribution of blood flow and gradients of oxygen tension within the heart. *Am J Physiol* 207: 661, 1964.

79 Sullivan JM, Taylor WJ, Elliott WC, Gorlin R: Regional myocardial blood flow. *J Clin Invest* 46: 1402, 1967.

80 Cannon PJ, Dell RB, Dwyer EM Jr: Measurement of regional myocardial perfusion in man with ^{133} Xenon and a scintillation camera. *J Clin Invest* 51: 964, 1972.

80a Ross RS, Ueda K, Lichtlen PR, Rees JR: Measurement of myocardial blood flow in animals and man by selective injection of radioactive inert gas into the coronary arteries. *Circ Res* 15: 28, 1964.

81 Hoffman JIE, Buckberg GD: Transmural variations in myocardial perfusion, in *Progress in Cardiology*, PN Yu, JF Goodwin (eds). Philadelphia, Lea & Febiger, chap 3, p 37.

82 Strauer BE: *Hypertensive Heart Disease*, Berlin, Springer-Verlag, 1980.

83 Tauchert von M: Koronarreserve und Maximaler Sauerstoffverbrauch des Menschlichen Herzens. *Basic Res Cardiol* 68: 183, 1973.

84 Krasnow N, Levine HJ, Wagmen RJ, Gorlin R: Coronary blood flow measured by I^{131}-iodo-antipyrine. *Circ Res* 12: 58, 1963.

85 Weiss HR, Cohen JA, McPherson LA: Blood flow and relative tissue PO_2 of brain and muscle: Effect of various gas mixtures. *Am J Physiol* 203: 839, 1976.

85a Aukland K, Kiil F, Kjekshus J: Relationship between ventricular pressures and right and left myocardial blood flow. *Acta Physiol Scand* 70: 116, 1967.

86 Schanzenbacher P, Klocke FJ: Inert gas measurements of myocardial perfusion in the presence of heterogeneous flow documented by microspheres. *Circulation* 61: 590, 1980.

87 Klocke FJ: Coronary blood flow in man. *Prog Cardiovas Dis* 19: 117, 1976.

88 Rowe GG: Pharmacology of the coronary circulation. *Ann Rev Pharmacol* 1968: 8, 95–112.

89 Hood WB Jr: Regional venous drainage of the human heart. *Brit Heart J* 30: 105, 1968.

90 Gensini GG, Caldini P, Casaccio F, Blount SG Jr: Persistent left superior vena cava. *Am J Cardiol* 4: 677, 1959.

91 Mathey DG, Chatterjee K, Tyberg JV, Lekven J, Brundage B, Parmley WW: Coronary sinus reflux: A source of error in the measurement of thermodilution coronary sinus flow. *Circulation* 57: 778, 1978.

92 Maseri A, Pesola A, L'Abbate A, Contini C, Michelassi C, D'Angelo T: Contribution of recirculation and fat diffusion to myocardial washout curves obtained by external counting in man: Stochastic versus monoexponential analysis. *Circ Res* 35: 826, 1974.

93 Carlin R, Chien S: Effect of hematocrit on the washout of xenon and iodoantipyrine from dog myocardium. *Circ Res* 40: 505, 1977.

94 Morgan SM, Fisher JD, Horwitz LD: Validation of regional myocardial flow measurements with scintillation camera detection of xenon-133. *Invest Radiol* 13: 132, 1978.

95 Maseri A, L'Abbate A, Michelassi C, Pesola A, Pisani P, Marzilli M, De Nes M, Mancini P: Possibilities, limitations, and technique for the study of regional myocardial perfusion in man by xenon-133. *Cardiovas Res* 11: 277, 1977.

96 Sciacca RR, Weiss MB, Blood DK, Brennan DL, Cannon PJ: Comparison of regional myocardial blood flow measurements with ^{133}Xe and radioactive microspheres in dogs with coronary artery constrictions. *Cardiovas Res* 13: 330, 1979.

97 L'Abbate A, Maseri A, Ballestra AM, Michelassi C, Marzilli M, Camici P, Trivella MG: Stochastic and exponential analysis of precordial washout curves for myocardial blood flow measurement: Experimental evaluation. *Circ Res* 49: 41, 1981.

98 Lichtlen PR, Englel HJ, Handeshagen H: Clinical application and results of the assessment of coronary blood flow by the regional xenon residue detection technique. *Nucl Med* 17: 161, 1978.

99 Ross RS, Veda K, Lichtlen PR, Rees JR: Measurement of myocardial blood flow in animals and man by selective injection of radioactive inert gas into the coronary arteries. *Circ Res* 15: 28, 1964.

100 Holman BL, Adams DF, Jewit F, Eldh E, Iodoine J, Cohn PF, Gorlin R, Adelstein SJ: Measuring regional myocardial blood flow with ^{133}xenon and the Anger camera. *Radiology* 112: 99, 1974.

101 Cannon PJ: Measurement of coronary blood flow and evaluation of regional myocardial perfusion by intracoronary injection techniques, in "Cardiovascular Nuclear Medicine," *Prog Nucl Med* vol 6, pp 85–111, Basel, Karger, 1980.

102 Glass HI, de Garreta AC: The quantitative limitations of exponential curve fitting. *Phys Med Biol* 16: 119, 1971.

103 Engel HJ: Assessment of regional myocardial blood flow by the precordial ^{133}xenon clearance technique, in *The Pathophysiology of Myocardial Perfusion,* W Schaper (ed). Amsterdam, Elsevier/North-Holland Biomedical Press, 1979, 58.

103a Grayson J, Coulson RL, Winchester B: Internal calorimetry—assessment of myocardial blood flow and heat production. *J Appl Physiol* 30:251, 1971.

103b Grayson J, Irvine M: Myocardial infarction in the monkey: Studies on the collateral circulation after acute coronary occlusion. *Cardiovasc Res* 2: 170, 1968.

104 Rutishauser W, Simon H, Stacky JP, et al: Evaluation of roentgen cinedensitometry for flow measurements in models and in the intact circulation. *Circulation* 36: 951, 1967.

105 Rutishauser W, Bussman W, Noseda G, et al: Blood flow measurement through single coronary arteries by roentgen densitometry: Part I. A comparison of flow measured by radiologic technique applicable in the intact organism and by electromagnetic flowmeter. *Am Heart J* 109: 12, 1970.

106 Rutishauser W, Bussmann W, Noseda G, Meier W, Wellauer J: *Blood flow measurement through single coronary arteries by roentgendensitometry.* Part I: A comparison of flow measured by a radiologic technique applicable in the intact organism and by electromagnetic flowmeter. *Am J Roentgenol* 109: 12, 1970.

107 Rutishauser W, Noseda G, Bussmann W, Preter B: *Blood flow measurement through single coronary arteries by roentgendensitometry.* Part II: Right coronary artery flow in conscious man. *Am J Roentgenol* 109: 21, 1970.

108 Rutishauser W: Usefulness and limitations in roentgendensitometric coronary artery blood flow measurements, in *Myocardial Blood Flow in Man: Methods and Significance in Coronary Disease,* A Maseri (ed). *Proc Internatl Sym* Laboratorio di Fisiologia Clinica C.N.R., Pisa, and Council on Clinical Science of the Internatl Soc Cardiol, auspices of World Health Organization, Pisa, June 10–12, 1971, Turin, Minerva Medica, 1972, chap 2, p 175.

109 Smith HC, Frye RL, Davis GD, Pluth JR, Sturm RE, Wood EH: Simultaneous Indicator Dilution Curves at Selected Sites in the Coronary Circulation and Determination of Blood Flow in Coronary Artery-Saphenous Vein Grafts by Roentgen-videodensitometry, in *Proc. Internatl Sym on Cine- and Videodensitometry*, Kiel, Georg Thieme, 1971.

110 Assad-Morell JL, Frye RL, Connolly DC, Gau GT, Pluth JR, Barnhorst DA, Wallace RB, Davis GD, Elveback LR, Danielson GK: Relation of intraoperative or early postoperative transmural myocardial infarction to patency of aortocoronary bypass grafts and to diseased ungrafted coronary arteries. *Am J Cardiol* 35: 767, 1975.

111 Chesebro JH, Ritman EL, Frye RL, Smith HC, Connolly DC, Rutherford BD, Davis GD, Danielson GK, Pluth JR, Barnhorst DA, Wallace RB: Videometric analysis of regional left ventricular function before and after aortocoronary artery bypass surgery. *J Clin Invest* 58: 1339, 1976.

112 Hamby RI, Aintablian A, Wisoff BG, Hartstein ML: Comparative study of the postoperative flow in the saphenous vein and internal mammary artery bypass grafts. *Am Heart J* 93: 306, 1977.

113 Weisz D, Hamby RI, Aintablian A, Voleti C, Fogel R, Wisoff BG: Late coronary bypass graft flow: Quantitative assessment by roentgendensitometry, *Ann Thoracic Surg* 28: 429, 1979.

114 Brundage BH, Lipton MJ, Herfkens RJ, Berninger WH, Redington RW, Chatterjee K, Carlsson E: Detection of patent coronary bypass grafts by computed tomography: A preliminary report. *Circulation* 61: 826, 1980.

115 Boyd DP, Gould RG, Quinn JR, Sparks R, Stanley RH, Herrmannsfeldt WG: A proposed dynamic cardiac 3-D densitometer for easy detection and evaluation of heart disease. *IEEE Trans Sci* NS-26: 2724, 1979.

116 Gould KL, Lipscomb K, Hamilton GW: A physiologic basis for assessing critical coronary stenosis. *Am J Cardiol* 33: 87, 1974.

117 Ganz W, Tamura K, Marcus HS, Donoso R, Yoshida S, Swan HJC: Measurement of coronary sinus blood flow by continuous thermodilution in man. *Circulation* 44: 181, 1971.

118 Pepine CJ, Mehta J, Webster WW Jr, Nichols WW: In vivo validation of a thermodilution method to determine regional left ventricular blood flow in patients with coronary disease. *Circulation* 58: 795, 1978.

119 Van Devanter SH, Mills RM, Lesch M: Thermodilution measurement of coronary sinus blood flow during cardiopulmonary bypass. *Surg Forum* 26: 225, 1975.

120 Ganz W, Tamura K, Marcus HS, Donoso R, Yoshida S, Swan HJC: "Measurement of coronary sinus blood flow in man by constant infusion thermodilution," in *Myocardial Blood Flow in Man: Methods and Significance in Coronary Disease, Proc Internatl Sym*, A Maseri (ed). Laboratorio di Fisiologia Clinica C.N.R., Pisa, and Council on Clinical Science of the Internatl. Soc. Cardiol., auspices of World Health Organization, Pisa, June 10–12, 1971, Turin, Minerva Medica, 1972, p 159.

121 Ganz W, Swan HJC: Measurement of blood flow by thermodilution. *Am J Cardiol* 29: 241, 1972.

122 Weisse AB, Regan TJ: A comparison of thermodilution coronary sinus blood flows and krypton myocardial blood flows in the intact dog. *Cardiovas Res* 8: 526, 1974.

123 Ter-Pogossian MM, Raichle ME, Sobel BE: Positron-emission tomography. *Scientific American* 243: 139, 1980.

124 Schelbert HR, Phelps ME, Hoffman EJ, Huang S-C, Selin CE, Kuhl DE: Regional myocardial perfusion assessed with N-13 labeled ammonia and positron emission computerized axial tomography. *Am J Cardiol* 43: 209, 1979.

125 Walsh WF, Harper PV, Resnekov L, Fill H: Noninvasive evaluation of regional myocardial perfusion in 112 patients using a mobile scintillation camera and intravenous nitrogen-13 labeled ammonia. *Circulation* 54: 266, 1976.

126 Gould KL, Schelbert HR, Phelps ME, Hoffman EJ: Noninvasive assessment of coronary stenoses with myocardial perfusion imaging during pharmacologic coronary vasodilation. *Am J Cardiol* 43: 200, 1979.

127 Wisenberg G, Schelbert HR, Hoffman EJ, Phelps ME, Robinson GD, Selin CE, Child J, Skorton D, Kuhl DE: In vivo quantitation of regional myocardial blood flow by positron emission computed tomography. *Circulation* 63: 1281, 1981.

128 Schelbert HR, Henze E, Phelps ME: Emission tomography of the heart. *Seminars in Nuclear Medicine* 10: 355, 1980.

PART **THREE**

BASIC REGULATORY MECHANISMS IN THE CORONARY CIRCULATION

CHAPTER **3**

METABOLIC REGULATION OF CORONARY BLOOD FLOW

There is a close linkage between oxygen demand and coronary blood flow in the myocardium. This coupling is necessary because the myocardium is almost completely dependent on aerobic metabolism. Oxygen stores are meager [1,1a], and normally the oxygen content of coronary venous blood is very low. If coronary blood flow is not sufficient to supply the oxygen demands of the myocardium, only a few compensatory mechanisms can be marshaled to preserve cell viability: the number and size of open capillaries can increase [2], glycogen stores can be consumed [3], oxygen in blood stored in the vasculature dissolved in the interstitial fluid and combined with myoglobin can be utilized [1], and active contraction can cease [4]. Under normal conditions, these compensatory mechanisms can preserve cell viability for 20 min in the presence of severe ischemia [5] and for longer periods of less intense ischemia.

Usually coronary blood flow closely parallels myocardial oxygen demand. This relationship overrides most perturbations which produce coronary constriction. Although there are many potent neural, humoral, and pharmacologic coronary constrictors, they rarely produce myocardial ischemia because they are not sufficiently powerful to compete effectively with metabolically mediated coronary vasodilation.

RELATIONSHIP BETWEEN MYOCARDIAL OXYGEN CONSUMPTION AND CORONARY BLOOD FLOW

A large volume of data supports the concept that left ventricular coronary blood flow and left ventricular myocardial oxygen consumption are closely coupled (Figure 3-1) [6–12]. This relationship is linear over a broad range of coronary flow rates (10 to 600 ml/min/100 g in the dog) [6–11]. Furthermore, all species that have been studied, including humans [12] exhibit this phenomenon.

Studies of regional myocardial blood flow and myocardial oxygen consumption demonstrate that the close parallelism between coronary blood flow and oxygen consumption extends transmurally in the left ventricle. Under normal conditions, the subendocardial layers of the left ventricle utilize more oxygen than the subepicardial layers (Figure 3-2) [13,13a]; as expected, coronary flow per gram in the subendocardium is 10 to 30 percent greater than flow in the subepicardium (Figure 3-2) [13a,14]. Studies of the relationship between oxygen consumption and perfusion in the left atrium also demonstrate a close relationship between these two variables (Figure 3-3) [15].

Changes in oxygen demand produce alterations in coronary vascular resistance in less than 1 s. Schwartz et al. [16] have shown that if the oxygen requirements of one cardiac cycle in the left ventricle are increased, in the following cycle coronary vascular resistance will decrease and coronary flow will rise (see Figure 3-4). Occlusion of a coronary vessel for 1 s in both animals and humans produces a large decrease in coronary vascular resistance which is evident immediately following release of the occlusion [1,17]. *Thus, the close coupling between myocardial oxygen consumption and coronary blood flow is adjusted on a second-to-second basis. This relationship is the dominant mechanism that regulates coronary blood flow.*

Mechanisms of Increasing Oxygen Delivery to the Myocardium

If the hemoglobin concentration, oxyhemoglobin dissociation curve and cardiac myoglobin are normal, oxygen delivered to the myocardium can be augmented by increasing coronary blood flow, augmenting oxygen extraction, or decreasing the average diffusion distance between capillaries and myocytes. Because coronary blood flow can increase by five- to sixfold in several animal species and humans [17–19], coronary dilation is the primary mechanism for increasing oxygen delivered to the myocardium. Although increases in oxygen extraction are limited because coronary venous saturation is normally about 30 percent of the arterial

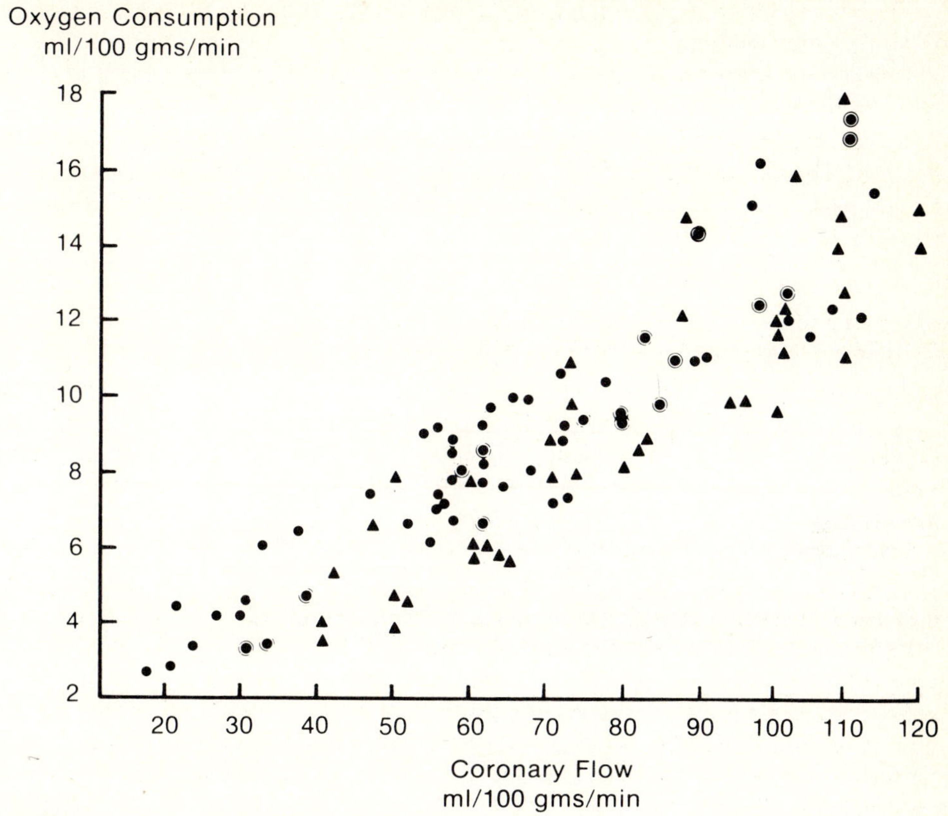

FIGURE 3-1
Relationship between left ventricular myocardial oxygen consumption and left ventricular coronary blood flow. Over a broad range there is a close correlation between left ventricular myocardial oxygen consumption and left ventricular coronary blood flow. ⊙ = experimental procedure (hemorrhage or intravenous epinephrine); ▲ = intracoronary infusion of 2,3-dinitrophenol; • = intracoronary infusion of 2,4-dinitrophenol; 0 = control. (*Redrawn from data presented by RM Berne and R Rubio* [*11*].)

FIGURE 3-2
Coronary blood flow and myocardial oxygen consumption (MVO_2) in the subepicardial (Epi) and subendocardial (Endo) layers of the left ventricle. The increase in subendocardial blood flow reflects increased subendocardial oxygen consumption. (*Redrawn from data presented by J Vinten-Johansen and HR Weiss* [*13a*].)

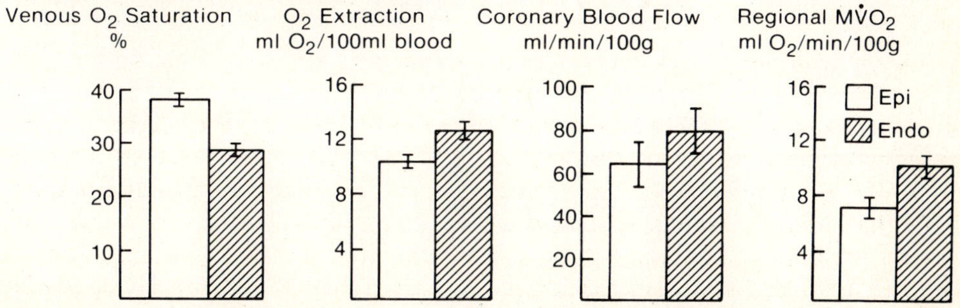

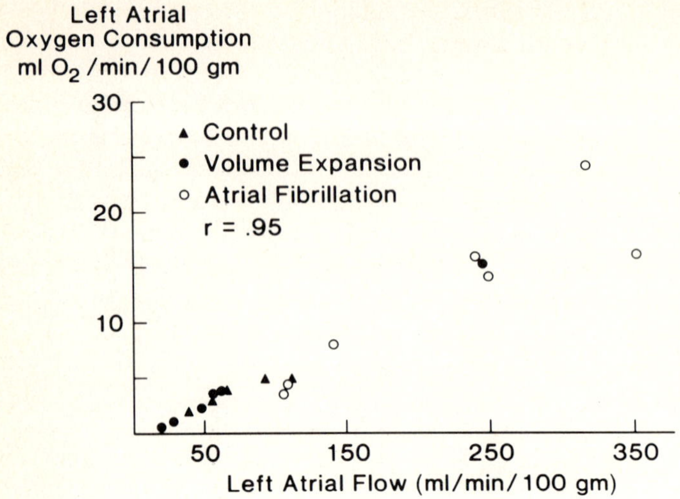

FIGURE 3-3
Oxygen consumption and blood flow in the left atrium. In atrial tissue there is a close correlation between oxygen consumption and blood flow. Note that electrically induced atrial fibrillation markedly increased left atrial blood flow and oxygen consumption. (*Based on data originally presented by CW White et al* [*15*].)

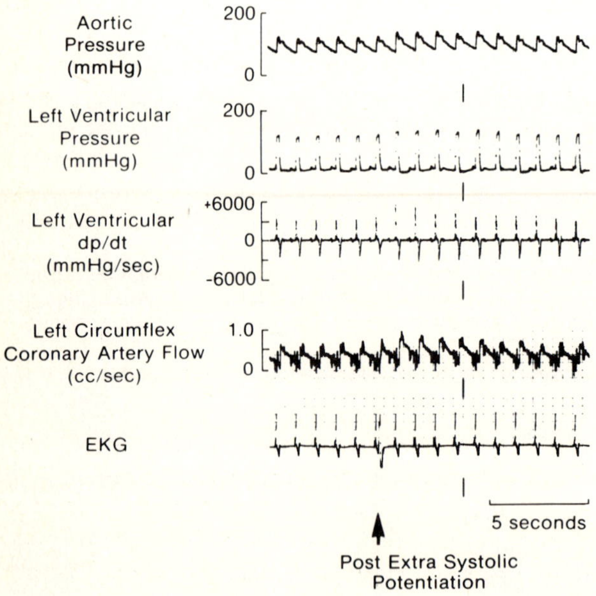

FIGURE 3-4
Effects of a transient increase in myocardial contractility on coronary blood flow. Postextrasystolic potentiation was utilized to increase myocardial contractility. Note that within one cardiac cycle coronary blood flow increases in response to an increase in myocardial oxygen consumption. (*Data originally presented by GG Schwartz et al* [*16*].)

saturation [20], excitement, exercise, ischemia, and alpha-adrenergic stimulation increase oxygen delivery to the myocardium, in part by increasing oxygen extraction [20–22]. At maximal coronary flow rates, in an adult dog with a 100-g left ventricle and a normal hematocrit, increasing oxygen extraction in coronary sinus blood from 70 to 90 percent will increase the amount of oxygen delivered to the left ventricle by 24 ml/min/100 g. This is about two to three times normal left ventricular oxygen consumption. Under most conditions, coronary sinus oxygen saturation remains relatively stable because increases in oxygen demand by the left ventricle are met by augmenting coronary blood flow. However, the myocardium can increase oxygen supply by increasing either coronary blood flow or oxygen extraction. *The signal which determines whether increases in oxygen demand by the myocardium will be met by an increase in coronary flow or an increase in oxygen extraction is unknown.*

Oxygen delivery at the cellular level can be enhanced by decreasing diffusion distance. This is accomplished by increasing the number of "open capillaries" in the myocardium. Such an effect in the myocardium has been observed during hypoxia [2]. The importance of this mechanism remains to be elucidated.

Determinants of Myocardial Oxygen Consumption

The determinants of myocardial oxygen consumption have been elucidated [23]. The three major determinants are heart rate, myocardial contractility, and wall stress (volume × chamber pressure ÷ wall thickness). Shortening, activation, and basal metabolic requirements are minor determinants of myocardial oxygen consumption. The relative contribution of various determinants of myocardial oxygen consumption is dependent on the level of cardiac stress (see Figure 3-5). In the intact circulation, most perturbations of the system will affect multiple variables simultaneously. For example, paroxysmal atrial tachycardia increases heart rate, decreases left ventricular volume and wall stress, decreases shortening, and has variable effects on myocardial contractility and arterial pressure. Because coronary blood flow is coupled to myocardial oxygen consumption, the effects of paroxysmal atrial tachycardia on coronary flow will reflect the aggregate result of all variables on myocardial metabolism. Because of this complex relationship it is often difficult to predict accurately the effect of a given hemodynamic stress on coronary blood flow.

EFFECTS OF SPECIFIC FACTORS ON CORONARY BLOOD FLOW

The relative effects of specific interventions on coronary blood flow have obvious clinical significance. Unfortunately, a single perturbation almost always produces concomitant changes in other determinants of myocardial oxygen consumption. Furthermore, the effects of any given intervention on coronary flow depends on prevailing conditions such as baseline coronary flow, blood viscosity,

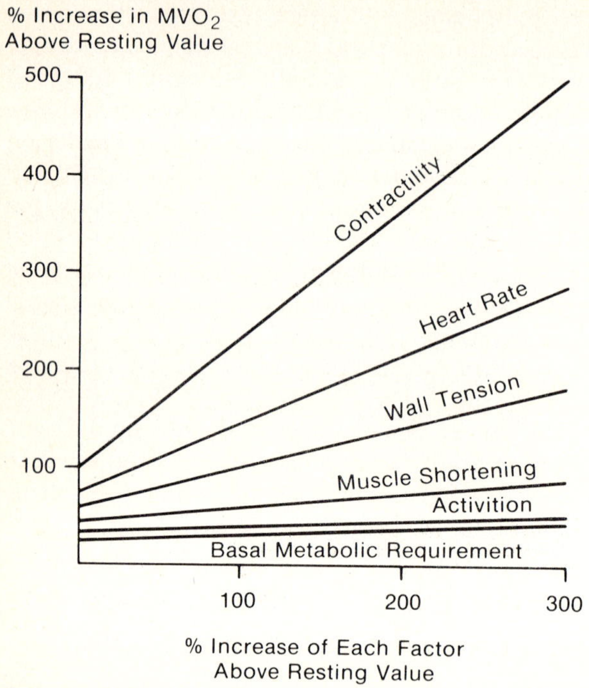

FIGURE 3-5
Relationship between changes in various parameters and myocardial oxygen consumption (MVO_2). This stylized diagram roughly approximates the relative importance of each factor on myocardial oxygen consumption.

and the presence of disease processes which may modulate the response of the coronary circulation. Hence, the available data permit one only to approximate the effects of specific perturbations on coronary flow.

Heart Rate

Increases in heart rate are associated with coronary dilation. The magnitude of this effect is moderate. For example, if heart rate in the awake dog is increased from 90 to 200 beats per minute by ventricular pacing, coronary blood flow increases twofold [24,25]. In patients with normal coronary vessels, increasing heart rate by 60 beats per minute with pacing causes coronary flow to increase from 123 to 230 ml/min [26]. Vatner has estimated that tachycardia is responsible for about one-third of the coronary dilation associated with maximal exercise in dogs [27]. Thus, it is not surprising that in patients with coronary obstructive disease exercise is more effective than tachycardia alone in producing manifestations of myocardial ischemia.

Tachycardia has other effects on the coronary circulation. In epicardial coronary arteries, tachycardia increases the percent of coronary flow that occurs in systole [28]. Also, the ratio of endocardial to epicardial flow in the left ventricle decreases from 1.3:1 to about 1.2:1 if heart rate is markedly increased by pacing [24,25].

Myocardial Contractility

When the inotropic state of the heart increases, myocardial oxygen consumption rises and the coronary vessels dilate [29,30]. Coronary blood flow increased by about one-third when contractility as assessed by measurement of left ventricular *dp/dt* increased twofold as a result of postextrasystolic potentiation [29]. This potent inotropic intervention has no effect on heart rate and only small effects on wall stress and shortening. When wall stress and heart rate were held constant and ventricular contractility was increased by an infusion of norepinephrine, a 30 percent increase in contractility was associated with an 18 percent increase in coronary blood flow [30]. Most potent inotropic agents such as catecholamines, dopamine, and calcium increase coronary blood flow [30]. Patients with coronary obstructive disease frequently develop manifestations of myocardial ischemia in response to an increase in the inotropic state of the left ventricle.

Wall Stress

Increasing wall stress in the left ventricle, right ventricle, or the left atrium [15,30,31] decreases coronary vascular resistance and increases coronary blood flow. In the left ventricle, a 60 percent increase in wall stress increased coronary blood flow by 10 percent if heart rate, left ventricular contractility, and mean aortic pressure were held constant [30].

Shortening

Since 1910, it has been known that shortening causes only small changes in myocardial oxygen consumption in comparison with changes in wall tension [32]. Thus, it follows that muscle shortening should have little effect on coronary blood flow. Carefully controlled experiments have shown that if aortic pressure, heart rate, and contractility are kept relatively constant, a threefold increase in left ventricular stroke volume (muscle shortening) is associated with a 20 percent increase in coronary flow [32a,33] and a 20 percent increase in left ventricular oxygen consumption [33a]. The marked difference in the effects of shortening and tension generation of myocardial metabolism and coronary flow contribute to the clinical profile of patients with coronary obstructive disease. In patients with coronary disease, vigorous isometric exercise, which primarily increases the aortic pressure, wall stress, and heart rate, often precipitates angina. In the same patients, walking, which primarily increases stroke volume and heart rate, may not precipitate angina. This clinical relationship is complex because isometric exercise increases coronary driving pressure to a greater extent than isotonic exercises.

Activation

Electrical activation of cardiac membranes increases myocardial oxygen consumption by less than 1 percent [34]. Hence, activation plays an insignificant role in regulation of the coronary circulation.

Basal Metabolic Requirements

When the heart is quiescent, energy is needed to maintain the metabolic integrity of cardiac cells. Many years ago, McKeever et al. demonstrated that one-quarter of resting coronary flow is required to meet the basal metabolic requirements of the myocardium [35].

Excitement and Exercise

Excitement produces an array of hemodynamic changes which tend to increase coronary flow. When awake, well-conditioned dogs are exposed to a sudden loud noise, their heart rate and blood pressure increase substantially. In response to excitement, coronary flow increases threefold and coronary sinus oxygen saturation decreases (Figure 3-6) [20]. The increase in myocardial oxygen consumption that occurs in association with a sudden excitatory stimulus is similar to that which accompanies moderately intense exercise. Excitement often precipitates manifestations of myocardial ischemia (angina pectoris, transient heart failure, arrhythmias) in patients which severe coronary obstructive disease.

Exercise increases all the principal determinants of myocardial oxygen consumption, that is, contractility, wall stress, and heart rate. In free-ranging chronically instrumented dogs, coronary blood flow increases three- to fivefold during peak exercise (Figure 3-7) [36]. Occasionally, treadmill exercise in dogs will induce a four- to fivefold rise in coronary flow [37–41]. Studies of regional myocardial

FIGURE 3-6
Effects of spontaneous excitement on coronary blood flow (C.B.F.) in a chronically instrumented dog. Excitement was produced by a sudden loud noise in a previously quiet room. Excitement was associated with prompt and striking increase in coronary blood flow. A.P. = aortic pressure. (*Redrawn from data originally presented by CR Rayford et al* [20].)

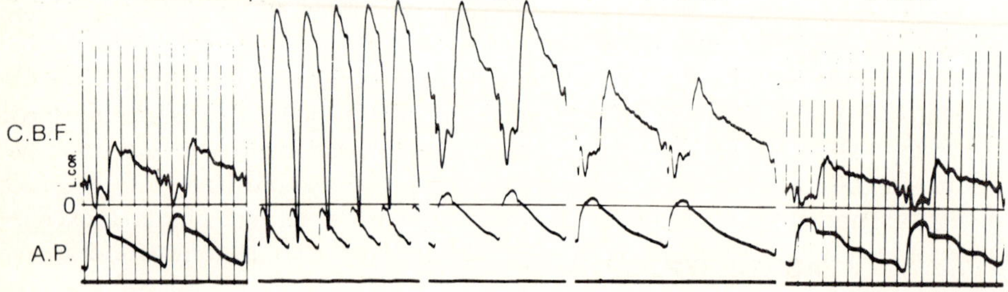

	Control	25 Sec.	55 Sec.	71 Sec.	5 Min.
Heart Rate	98	250	117	77	72
Mean A.P.	115	122	137	126	113
Mean CBF ML/Min.	94	314	340	200	74

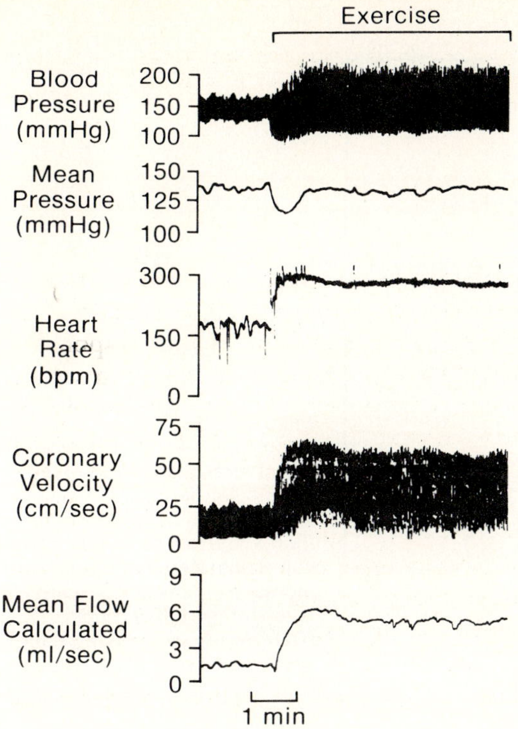

FIGURE 3-7
Effects of exercise on coronary blood flow. The data presented were obtained by telemetry from a dog pulling a sled in the snow. Intense exercise was associated with marked tachycardia and a fourfold increase in calculated coronary blood flow. (*Redrawn from data presented by RL Van Citters and DL Franklin* [*36*].)

perfusion during exercise suggest that flow to all layers and regions of the left ventricle increase nearly uniformly during exercise (see Figure 3-8) [37–41].

Measurements of coronary flow in patients indicate that the most intense exercise that can be achieved under study conditions augments coronary flow by 460 percent [42]. The level of coronary dilation achieved during exercise in humans is usually less than the maximal dilatory capacity that can be obtained with pharmacologic dilation of the coronary bed [43]. Because exercise induces the greatest increase in myocardial oxygen demand encountered under clinical conditions, angina pectoris is usually first noted during exercise in patients with ischemic heart disease. This occurs because an obstructed coronary vessel cannot dilate sufficiently to deliver adequate flow to provide for the oxygen needs of the myocardium during exercise.

CORONARY REACTIVE HYPEREMIA

Intense myocardial ischemia produces maximal coronary dilation. Therefore, when a coronary artery is occluded for 10 to 30 s, release of the occlusion and restoration of normal perfusion pressure is followed by a marked increase in coronary flow which gradually dissipates in less than 1 min (see Figures 3-9 and 3-10) [17–19,44–49]. This vascular response to transient myocardial ischemia

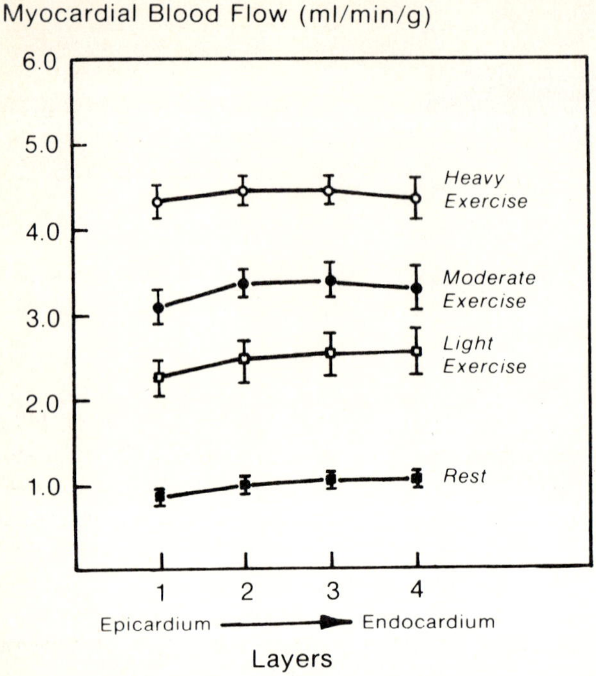

FIGURE 3-8
Effects of treadmill exercise on the transmural distribution of left ventricular perfusion. Treadmill exercise was associated with more than a fourfold increase in left ventricular perfusion. A similar increase in flow occurred to all layers of the left ventricle. (*Redrawn from data originally presented by RJ Bache et al* [*41*].)

FIGURE 3-9
Coronary reactive hyperemia following release of a transient coronary occlusion in a dog. There was a marked increase in coronary blood flow following release of the occlusion which gradually dissipates. F.D. = calculated flow debt; flow repayment = reactive hyperemic component (R.H.) and baseline flow (indicated by values below the dotted lines. (*Redrawn from data originally presented by JD Coffman and DE Gregg* [*18*].)

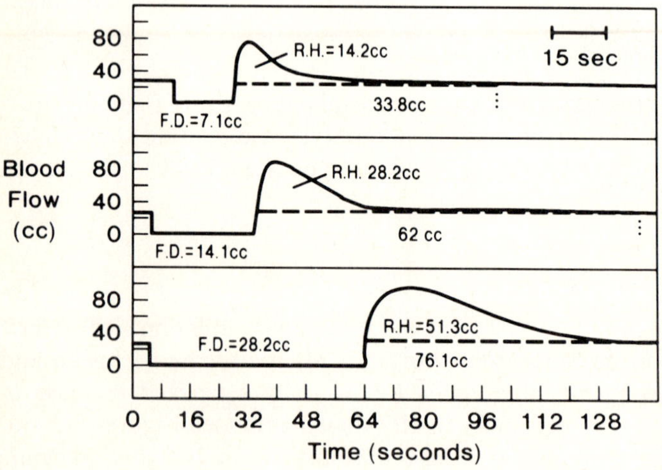

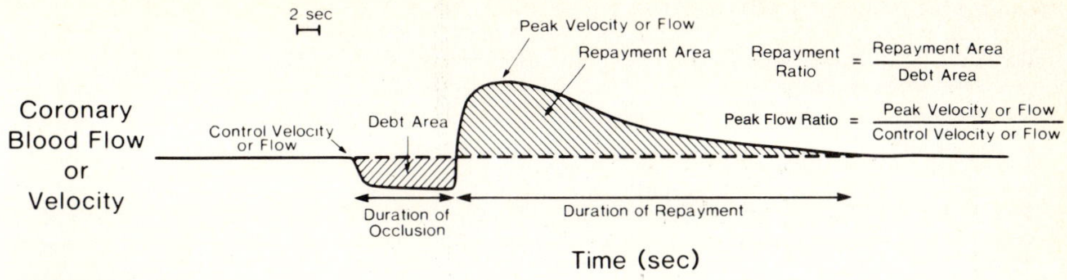

FIGURE 3-10
Standard measurements used to analyze reactive hyperemic responses.

is called coronary reactive hyperemia. Recent studies by Schwartz et al. [49a] indicate that even coronary occlusions as brief as 200 milliseconds in duration can produce coronary reactive hyperemic responses (see Figure 3-11). In all organs that have been tested including brain, skeletal muscle, and kidney, transient ischemia is followed by reactive hyperemia.

Although coronary reactive hyperemia was first described by Katz and Linder [49b], the quantitative characteristics of coronary reactive hyperemia in dogs were first determined by Coffman and Gregg [18]. They noted that the peak-flow response in anesthetized dogs followed a coronary occlusion of 15 to 20 s. Longer coronary occlusions increase the duration of the hyperemic response and the total repayment volume. These data have been confirmed in many laboratories [17–19,44–48]. The peak flow following a coronary occlusion of 15 s in a normal dog is primarily dependent on minimal coronary vascular resistance and the prevailing coronary driving pressure [50].

FIGURE 3-11
Effects of a transient coronary occlusion on coronary blood flow in an awake dog. The occlusion of the coronary vessel was limited to a portion of diastole in a single cardiac cycle. This brief occlusion nonetheless elicited a modest hyperemic response. *(Based on data originally presented by GG Schwartz et al* [49a].)

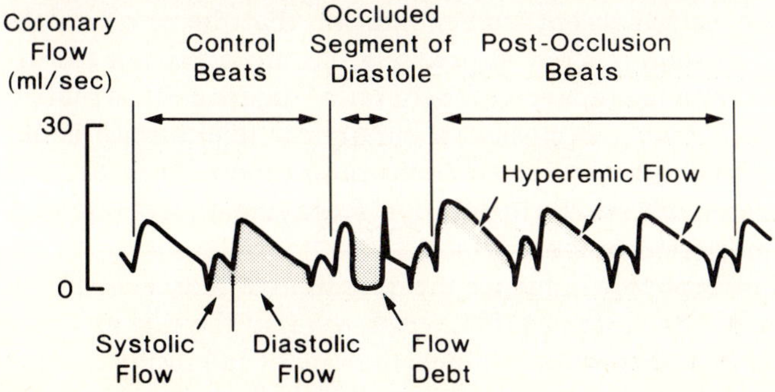

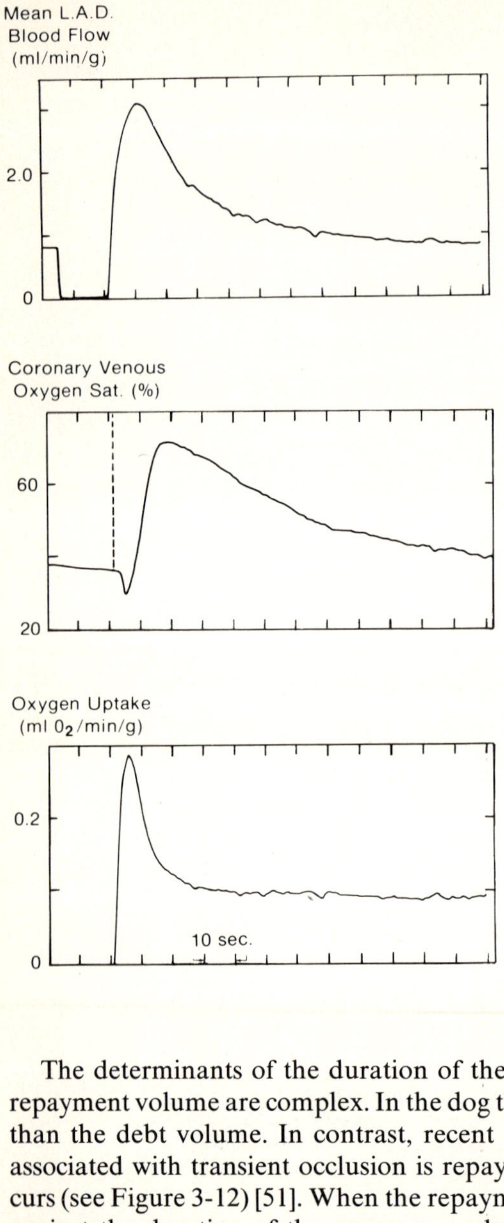

FIGURE 3-12
Alterations in coronary venous oxygen saturation (Sat.) and oxygen uptake during a coronary reactive hyperemic response. Because coronary venous saturation rises markedly during the reactive hyperemic response, oxygen debt is not overpaid. L.A.D. = left anterior descending coronary artery. (*Redrawn from data originally presented by JH Ruiter et al* [*51*].)

The determinants of the duration of the reactive hyperemic response and the repayment volume are complex. In the dog the repayment volume is always greater than the debt volume. In contrast, recent studies indicate that the oxygen debt associated with transient occlusion is repayed precisely, i.e., no overpayment occurs (see Figure 3-12) [51]. When the repayment/debt ratio (Figure 3-10) is plotted against the duration of the coronary occlusion, a curvilinear relationship is observed (17–19,44–48). The maximal repayment/debt ratio (about 4) in the dog occurs with coronary occlusions of 15 to 20 s in duration. Repayment/debt ratios are less with either longer or shorter occlusions [47].

Various metabolic factors probably influence the quantitative characteristics of coronary reactive hyperemia. Olsson et al. [52] have shown that the rate at which the reactive hyperemic response dissipates parallels the rate of fall in myocardial

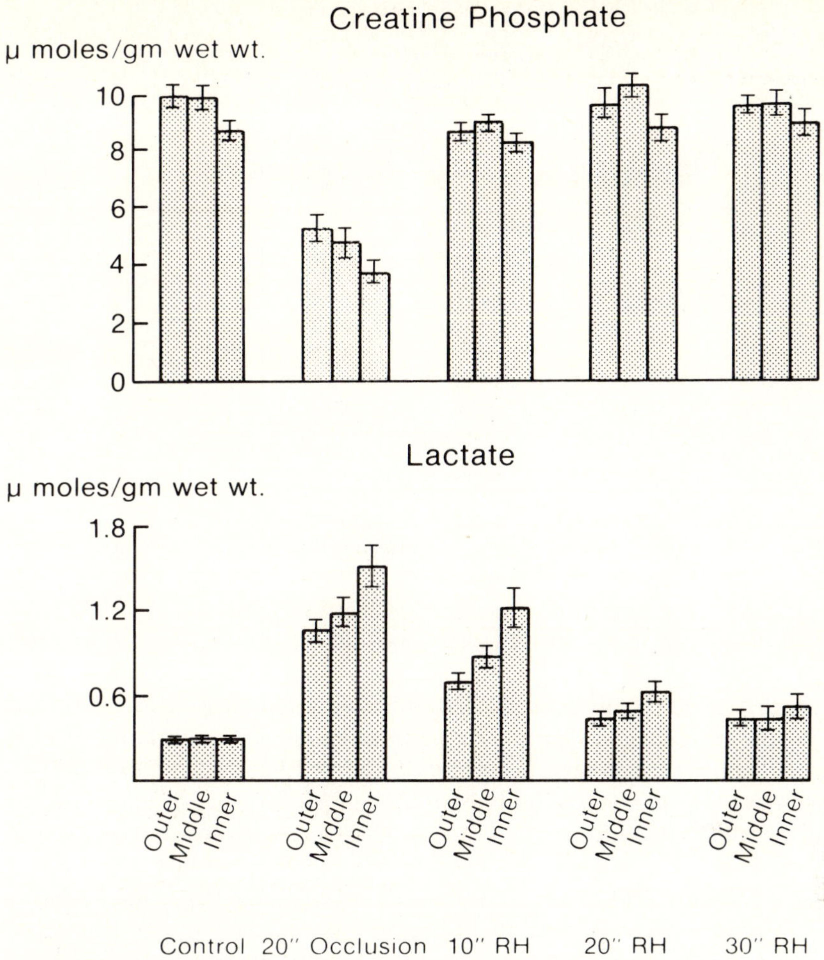

FIGURE 3-13
Alterations in tissue levels of creatine phosphate and lactate during the course of a coronary reactive hyperemia (RH) response. During occlusion, creatine phosphate declines and lactate increases. Both substances return to normal by 30 s following release of the occlusion. Metabolic abnormalities were greatest in the inner third of the left ventricle. Outer = outer third of the left ventricle. Inner = inner third of the left ventricular wall; middle = middle third of the left ventricular wall. (*Redrawn from data originally presented by RB Dunn et al* [53].)

levels of adenosine. Abnormalities in myocardial levels of lactate and high-energy phosphates produced by transient coronary occlusion return to normal by the end of the hyperemic response (Figure 3-13) [53].

Neural mechanisms probably have little effect on the coronary reactive hyperemic response. Schwartz and Stone [54] have shown that sympathetic tone can alter the repayment/debt ratio of the coronary reactive hyperemic response; however, the effect of sympathetic tone on this response was small. Bache et al.

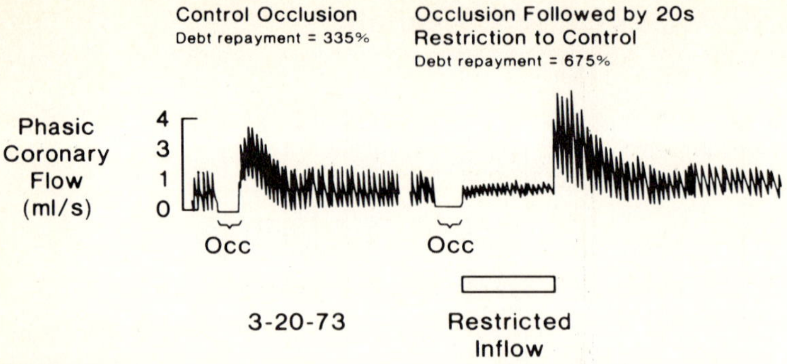

FIGURE 3-14
Effects of restricted inflow on the coronary reactive hyperemic response in an awake dog. If inflow is restricted to the level of control flow for 20 s following release of a 5-s coronary occlusion, the coronary reactive hyperemic response is augmented; that is, repayment is increased from 335 to 675 percent and peak flow following release of restricted inflow is increased significantly. Studies with microspheres indicate that during the period of restricted inflow, subendocardial perfusion in the left ventricle is inadequate. Occ = coronary occlusion. (*From RJ Bache et al* [55].)

reported [54a] that neurohumoral influences had no effect on coronary reactive hyperemia.

If flow is restricted to resting levels for 20 s following release of a 15-s coronary occlusion [55], the reactive hyperemic response is augmented, presumably because subendocardial ischemia persists during the period of restricted inflow (see Figure 3-14). On the other hand, if a limited volume of reflow is permitted following release of a 10-s coronary occlusion and then restricted flow is imposed for 10 s, on complete release of the occlusion the reactive hyperemic response is markedly attenuated (see Figure 3-15) [1,19,46]. Apparently, local metabolism or washout of a vasodilator substance may be the critical element that governs the magnitude of debt repayment and duration of the reactive hyperemic responses.

Factors That Modulate the Coronary Reactive Hyperemic Response

Since 1960, five factors have been shown to modify the coronary reactive hyperemic response: coronary driving pressure, myocardial metabolism, coronary vasomotor tone, Ca^{2+} blockers, and disease states.

Coronary Driving Pressure Following release of a 15- to 20- s coronary occlusion, the coronary bed is maximally dilated. Under such conditions, small changes in the driving pressure markedly increased coronary blood flow (Figure 3-16) [50]. Consequently, peak-flow rates following a release of a 20-s occlusion are pressure dependent. When perfusion pressure is less than 40 mmHg, the reactive hyperemia response to a 20-s coronary occlusion is negligible [50].

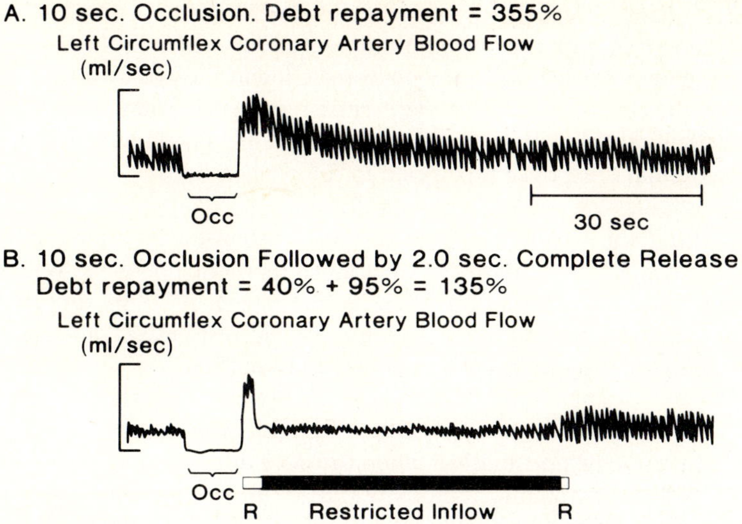

FIGURE 3-15
Effects of transient complete release followed by restricted inflow on the characteristic of coronary reactive hyperemia in an awake dog. If a brief period of complete release follows a transient coronary occlusion, restricted inflow does not augment the coronary reactive hyperemic response. In fact, the reactive hyperemic response is remarkably attenuated. Debt repayment decreases from 355 to 135 percent. Occ = coronary occlusion; R = complete release. (*From RJ Bache et al* [*46*].)

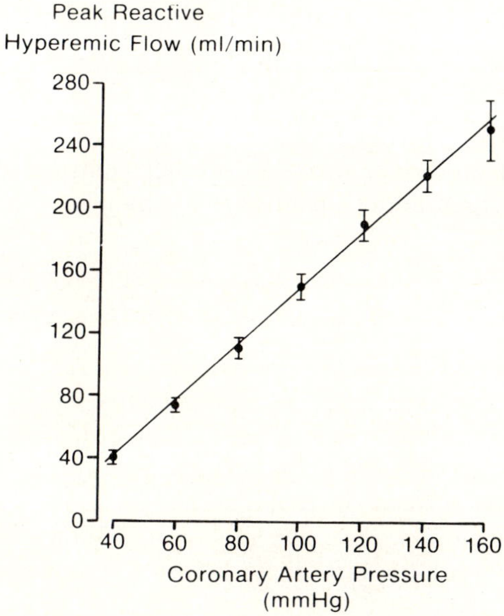

FIGURE 3-16
Effects of coronary artery pressure and peak reactive hyperemic flow. At each pressure, the duration of the coronary occlusion was similar. The data indicate that coronary artery pressure is a major determinant of peak reactive hyperemic flow. (*Redrawn from data originally presented by WP Dole et al* [*50*].)

Myocardial Metabolism Increases in myocardial metabolism produced by catecholamines or postextrasystolic potentiation increased repayment volume and the duration of the hyperemic response following transient coronary occlusion [49]. During hypothermia, the coronary reactive hyperemia response is attenuated [56]. These data support the hypothesis that the repayment volume associated with the coronary reactive hyperemia response is coupled to the oxygen debt.

Coronary Vasomotor Tone Alterations in coronary vasomotor tone unrelated to myocardial metabolism affect the coronary reactive hyperemic response. When drugs which produce intense vasodilation, such as adenosine, ATP, or dipyridamole, are administered, the coronary reactive hyperemic response is inversely related to the extent of pharmacologic coronary vasodilation [57].

Ca^{2+} Blockers It has recently been shown that Ca^{2+} blocking drugs diminish coronary reactive hyperemic responses even when the dose administered does not alter baseline coronary flow or systemic hemodynamics [57a]. The specificity of this effect has not been defined (see Chap. 22).

Disease States Two common disease states, cardiac hypertrophy and coronary stenosis, produce major decreases in the coronary reactive hyperemic response (see Chapters 11 and 13). These disease processes alter the transmural distribution of myocardial perfusion.

Regional Differences in the Coronary Reactive Hyperemic Response

Coronary reactive hyperemic responses in the left and right ventricles are similar [17]. In the right atrium, the coronary reactive hyperemic response is much smaller than that observed in the right or left ventricles [15]. The explanation for this difference is unknown.

Preliminary studies with microspheres [58,59] suggest that the time course of the reactive hyperemic response is different in various layers of the left ventricular myocardium (subepicardial flow peaks sooner than subendocardial flow).

Species Variability in the Coronary Reactive Hyperemic Response

In large mammals, the characteristics of coronary reactive hyperemia are remarkably similar [17–19,44]. Quantitative studies of coronary reactive hyperemia in human beings have recently been reported from our laboratory (see Figures 3-17 and 3-18) [17]. These studies indicate that in humans the coronary reactive hyperemic response is similar to that observed in other large animals with one exception: in patients, the duration of the coronary reactive hyperemic response is much shorter (Figure 3-19). Other studies with humans in our laboratory indicate

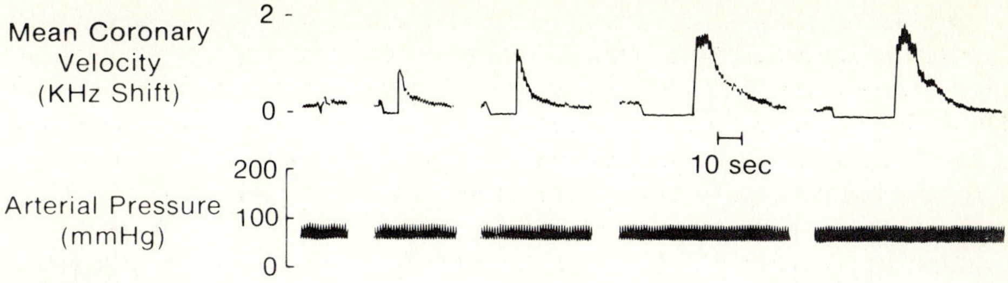

FIGURE 3-17
Coronary reactive hyperemic responses in a patient. The responses were obtained from a right ventricular branch of the right coronary artery. The coronary artery was angiographically normal and the right ventricle was also normal. Transient coronary occlusion did not alter arterial pressure or heart rate. In this patient, the maximal reactive hyperemic response occurred following a 20-s coronary occlusion. (*Data originally presented by M Marcus et al* [17].)

FIGURE 3-18
Quantitative characteristics of coronary reactive hyperemic responses in humans. Duration of response, repayment ratio, and peak to resting velocity ratio all increased as a function of the duration of the coronary occlusion. Maximal responses occurred with an occlusion of 15 to 20 s. The integers above the zero line in the bottom panel refer to the number of patients studied at each occlusion time. In all patients the coronary vessel studied was angiographically normal and perfused a normal ventricle. Responses of the right and left coronary vessels were similar. (*Redrawn from data originally presented by M Marcus et al* [17].)

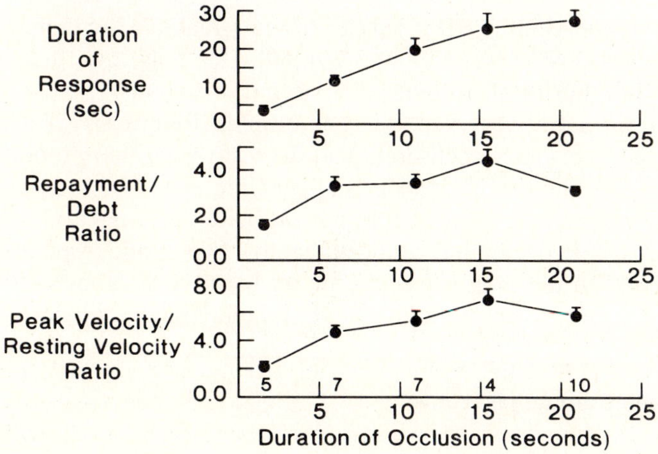

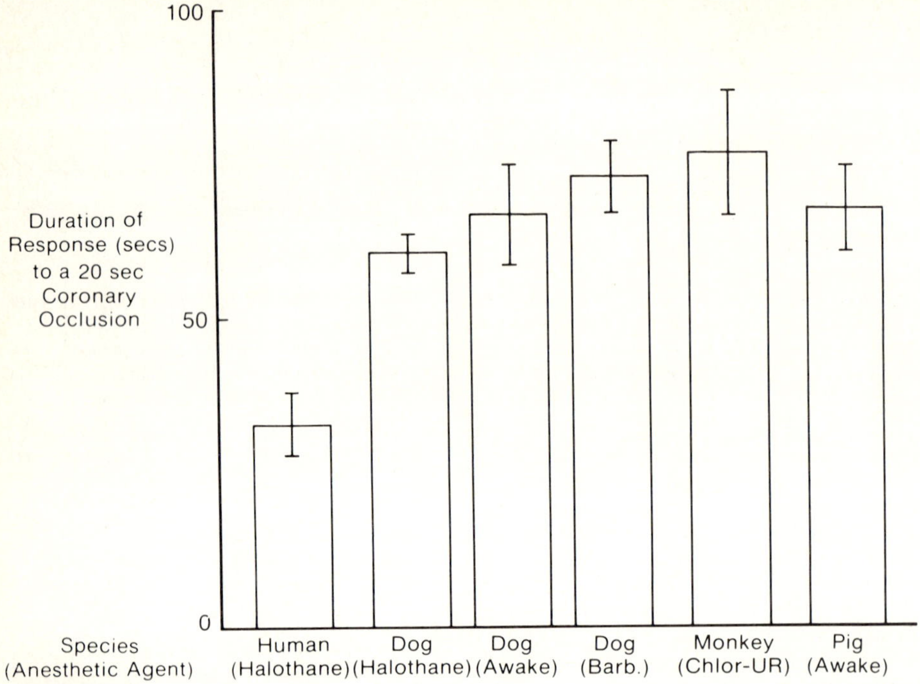

FIGURE 3-19
Effects of species, type of anesthesia, and state of consciousness on the duration of the coronary reactive hyperemic response to a 20-s coronary occlusion. In humans the duration of the coronary reactive hyperemic response is much shorter than that observed in several other mammalian species. The anesthetic agent employed or the state of consciousness has little effect on the duration of the coronary reactive hyperemic response. Barb = pentobarbital anesthesia; Chlor-Ur = chloralose-urethane anesthesia. (*Data in the pig are based on original studies presented by TM Fedor et al* [19]. *All other data were collected at the University of Iowa.*)

that age and gender have no appreciable effect on the coronary reactive hyperemic response to a 20-s coronary occlusion (see Figure 3-20) [60].

In the rat, and perhaps in other small animals, the coronary reactive hyperemic response is vastly different from that observed in larger animals (Figure 3-21) [61]. In particular, following a 20-s coronary occlusion, peak-to-resting coronary blood flow velocity ratio is about 2 in the rat, whereas it is approximately 4 to 6 in large animals. The debt/repayment ratio is about 1.5 in the rat, whereas it is 4 to 6 in large animals. This striking difference in the coronary reactive hyperemic response of the rat is probably related to the high resting coronary blood flow (about 450 ml/min/100 g) [61] and oxygen consumption observed in the rat [62].

Practical Applications of the Coronary Reactive Hyperemic Response

Because 15- to 20-s coronary occlusion reliably produces maximal coronary dilation, this response has been used as a tool in laboratory investigations. If the

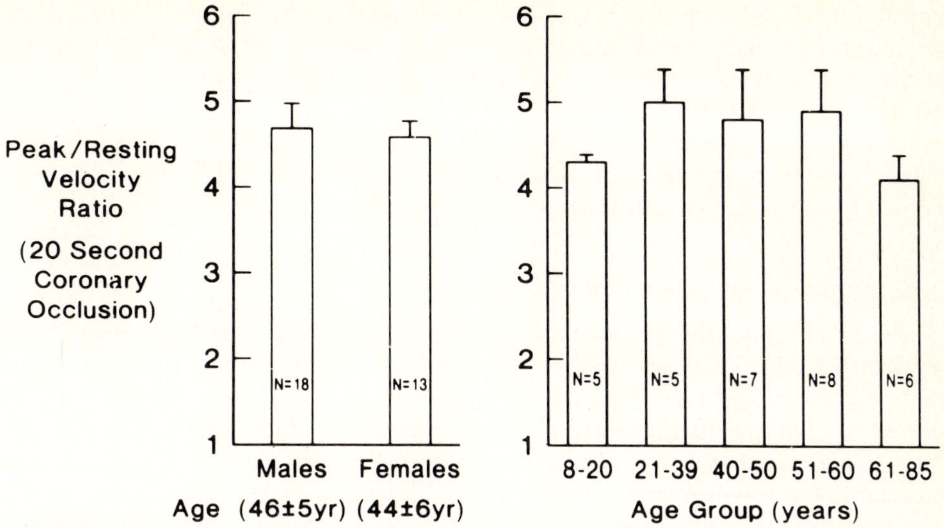

FIGURE 3-20
Effects of gender (*left*) and age (*right*) on the peak/resting velocity ratio following release of a 20-s coronary occlusion. All vessels included in the analysis were angiographically normal and perfused a normal ventricle. In humans, gender and age have no significant effect on the quantitative characteristics of the coronary reactive hyperemic response. The data in the graph to the right suggest that coronary reserve is not adversely affected by age. The integers in the bars indicate the number of patients studied in each subgroup. Age in males and females is presented as the mean ± 1 standard error. (*Based on data originally presented by C Eastham et al* [*60*].)

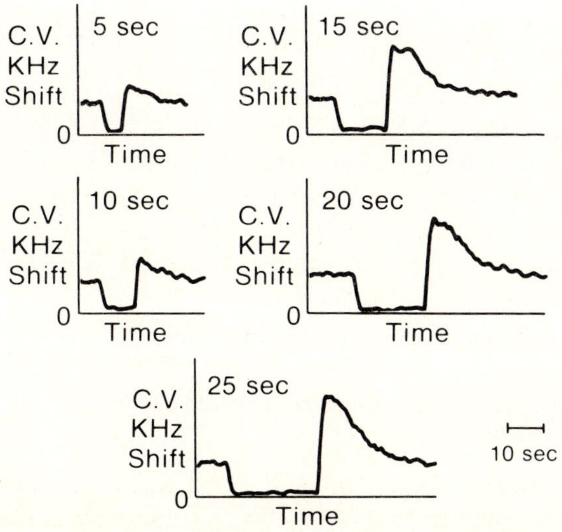

FIGURE 3-21
Coronary reactive hyperemic responses obtained in the left anterior descending coronary artery of a 7-month-old anesthetized Wistar-Kyoto rat. The reactive hyperemic responses in the rat are much smaller than those obtained in a larger mammal. (*Redrawn from data originally presented by KG Peters et al* [*61*].)

coronary reactive hyperemic response is attenuated in a normal animal, one should suspect that the measuring device (electromagnetic or Doppler flow probe) is constricting the coronary vessel. The coronary reactive hyperemic response can be used to assess coronary reserve in disease states such as cardiac hypertrophy and coronary obstruction (see Chapters 11 and 13). Finally, the extent of coronary dilation produced by vasoactive compounds can be compared to the dilator response to transient myocardial ischemia.

MEDIATORS OF METABOLIC VASODILATION

For over 50 years, investigators have sought to identify the mediator which links myocardial metabolic activity and coronary vascular resistance. Although many potential mediators have been suggested (see Figure 3-22), none has been established beyond question. Indeed, most investigators, including Robert Berne [63], have concluded that several mediators acting in concert probably link changes in myocardial metabolism and vasomotor tone in the coronary circulation.

Over the years, criteria have evolved (see Table 3-1) for establishing a substance as a mediator of metabolically induced coronary dilation. The criteria are formidable; hence, it is not surprising that the data supporting any proposed mediator are not sufficient to satisfy all of the criteria listed in Table 3-1.

Several of the proposed mediators are no longer under serious consideration. Following release of the 20-s coronary occlusion, when coronary dilation is maximal, oxygen saturation in the coronary arterial blood is normal and the oxygen saturation in coronary venous blood approaches that in the arterial circulation (see Figure 3-12) [51]. Yet, intense coronary dilation persists. This dramatic dissociation between the oxygen content of coronary arterial and venous blood and coronary vascular resistance is incompatible with the hypothesis that alterations in oxygen tension mediate the relationship between myocardial metabolism and coronary blood flow. Increases in myocardial metabolism are not correlated with significant increases in K^+, Ca^{2+}, or osmolality of coronary sinus blood [64–67].

TABLE 3-1
CRITERIA FOR ESTABLISHING THE SUBSTANCE WHICH MEDIATES THE COUPLING OF VASCULAR RESISTANCE AND MYOCARDIAL METABOLISM

Potent dilator.
Adequate endogenous source.
Access to vascular smooth muscle.
Concentration at the active site is reached under physiologic conditions and is sufficient to produce maximal dilation.
Coronary vascular responses are appropriately altered by substances which alter the concentration of the mediator at the active site.
Does not exhibit tachyphylaxis.

When coronary sinus blood obtained from hypoxic hearts is reoxygenated (a process that should not alter K^+, Ca^{2+}, or osmolality) and infused into a test coronary artery, vasodilation does not occur [64]. In addition, measurements of tissue levels of K^+ with electrodes indicate that when myocardial metabolism is increased by an increase in heart rate, tissue levels of K^+ rise and then fall even though coronary dilation persists [68,69]. Thus, in the myocardium, changes in interstitial K^+, Ca^{2+}, or osmolality are unlikely to mediate the coronary dilation that occurs in response to an increase in myocardial metabolism.

All the potential mediators under serious consideration (see Figure 3-22) are potent coronary dilators, and an endogenous source of the mediator is present [63,70–73]. Thus, criteria 1 and 2 listed in Table 3-1 are satisfied. In addition, aden-

FIGURE 3-22
Diagram illustrating potential mediators which may couple myocardial cellular metabolism and coronary vascular resistance. These potential mediators are divided into unlikely and likely categories on the basis of presently available evidence. The metabolic pathway of the most likely mediator (adenosine) is also illustrated. ATP = adenosine triphosphates; ADP = adenosine diphosphate; IMP = inosine monophosphate; AMP = adenosine monophosphate; K^+ = potassium ions; Ca^{++} = calcium; CO_2 = carbon dioxide; H^+ = hydrogen ion.

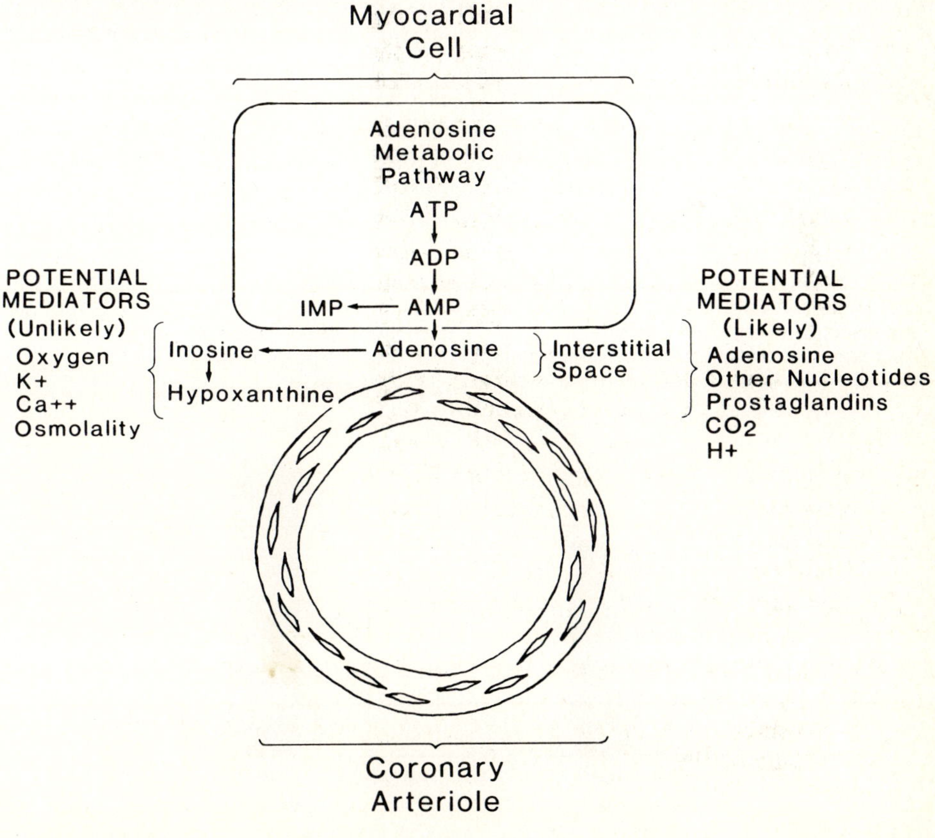

osine, CO_2, H^+, and prostaglandins have access to coronary vascular smooth muscle (criterion 3). None of the proposed mediators completely satisfies criteria 4 and 5. A critical problem relates to measuring the concentration of the proposed mediator in either the interstitial or perivascular space (the site of action) and correlating this concentration with alterations in coronary vascular resistance. In isolated cell preparations, the intracellular and extracellular concentrations of a potential mediator are measurable [74]; in the intact heart, such measurements are exceedingly difficult. Present methods permit only indirect measurements of the perivascular concentration of the proposed mediators. Two approaches that have been utilized are measurements of the mediator in coronary sinus blood or a pericardial perfusate [75–77]. The issue is further complicated because the proposed mediators are very labile in vivo [63,70–73].

The data supporting prostaglandins as a mediator which couples myocardial oxygen consumption and coronary vascular resistance are very controversial. This area will be reviewed in Chapter 7.

The volume of information presently available concerning adenosine as the proposed mediator vastly exceeds that available for other proposed substances. Berne and Rubio have recently reviewed these studies [11,63] and have concluded that "adenosine fulfills most of the criteria for the physiological regulation of coronary blood flow." Many elegant, carefully controlled studies support the view that adenosine plays a major role in the regulation of coronary vascular resistance.

There are at least six major challenges to the adenosine hypothesis which are presently unanswered. First, xanthines block coronary dilator responses to adenosine infusions but only slightly alter the characteristics of coronary reactive hyperemic responses (Figure 3-23) [78–82,85]. This suggests that adenosine may not be

FIGURE 3-23
Effects of theophylline (Theoph) and adenosine deaminase (Aden Deam) on the quantitative characteristics of coronary reactive hyperemic responses following a 20-s coronary occlusion. Both agents decrease the repayment/debt ratio by about one-third and do not alter the peak/resting flow ratio. (*Based on data originally presented by D Saito et al* [85].)

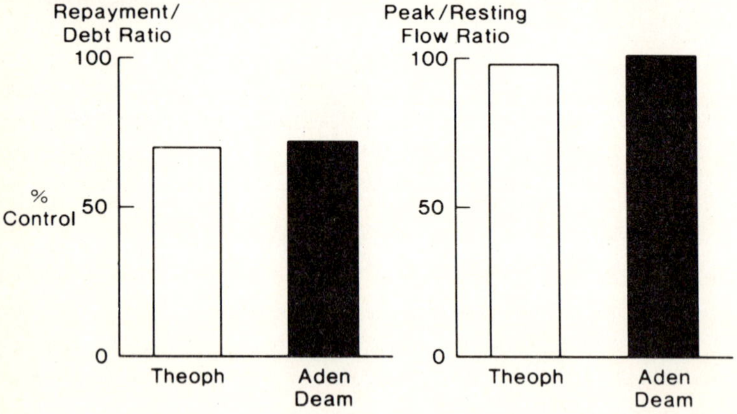

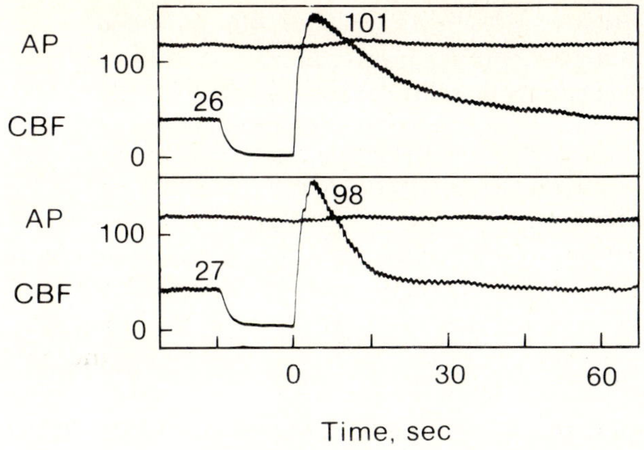

FIGURE 3-24
(*Top*) Coronary reactive hyperemic response before and (*bottom*) following adenosine deaminase. The coronary reactive hyperemic response is only slightly modified following adenosine deaminase. The peak response is unchanged, but the duration of the response is shortened. AP = aortic pressure; CBF = coronary blood flow.

involved in the coronary dilation following transient coronary occlusion. One explanation for these observations is that the vasodilator responses to adenosine are augmented by tissue acidosis, which probably accompanies transient coronary occlusion. [83,84] . However, it has not been conclusively shown that this effect can fully account for the failure of xanthines to markedly influence coronary reactive hyperemic responses [84a]. Second, intracoronary infusions of adenosine deaminase have only a small effect on the repayment/debt ratio and virtually no effect on the peak/resting velocity ratio of a coronary reactive hyperemic response (Figures 3-23 and 3-24) [85]. Again, this suggests that adenosine is not the crucial mediator that links changes in myocardial metabolism to changes in coronary vascular resistance. Third, intracoronary infusion of adenosine deaminase does not alter resting coronary flow [85]. Thus, under normal conditions adenosine may not play a key role in the regulation of coronary blood flow. Fourth, recent studies indicate that a large fraction of adenosine in the myocardium is not present in the interstitial space but rather resides in a "protected pool" within myocytes [74,86–89]. Thus, correlations between tissue levels of adenosine and changes in coronary vascular resistance do not provide convincing evidence that adenosine is the mediator that couples changes in myocardial metabolism to changes in coronary vascular resistance. Direct measurements of adenosine in the interstitial space are needed. Fifth, Hester et al. [90] have shown that infusions of massive amounts of adenosine in skeletal muscle do not alter reactive hyperemia responses. Sixth, DeWitt et al. [91] have shown a striking dissociation between alterations in coronary sinus levels of adenosine and changes in coronary vascular resistance in response to prolonged infusions of norepinephrine. In summary, these six unresolved challenges to the adenosine hypothesis indicate that many questions concerning the mediator which couples changes in myocardial metabolism to alterations in coronary vascular resistance remain unanswered.

Despite these important challenges to the adenosine hypothesis, adenosine remains the most promising mediator that links changes in myocardial metabolism to alterations in coronary blood flow.

The quest for the mediator that couples myocardial oxygen consumption to coronary vascular resistance continues. Future investigators should give special consideration to assessing the concentration of the proposed mediator at the active site and relating temporal changes in the concentration of the mediator to temporal changes in coronary vascular resistance.

REFERENCES

1 Eikens E, Wilcken DEL: Reactive hyperemia in the dog heart: Effects of temporarily restricting arterial inflow and of coronary occlusions lasting one and two cardiac cycles. *Circ Res* 35: 702, 1974.

1a Kanaide H, Yoshimura R, Makino N, Nakamura M: Regional myocardial function and metabolism during acute coronary occlusion. *Am J Physiol* 242 (Heart Circ Physiol 11): H980-H989, 1982.

2 Martini J, Honig CR: Direct measurement of intercapillary distance in beating rat heart in situ under various conditions of O_2 supply. *Microvascular Res* 1: 244, 1969.

3 Jennings RB: Early phase of myocardial ischemic injury and infarction. *Am J Cardiol* 24: 753, 1969.

4 Tennant K, Wiggers CJ: Effect of coronary occlusion on myocardial contraction. *Am J Physiol* 112: 351, 1935.

5 Jennings RB, Sommers HM, Smyth GA, Flack HA, Linn H: Myocardial necrosis induced by temporary occlusion of a coronary artery in the dog. *Arch Path* 70: 68, 1960.

6 Shipley RE, Gregg DE: The cardiac response to stimulation of the stellate ganglia and cardiac nerves. *Am J Physiol* 143: 396, 1945.

7 Eckenhoff JE, Hafkenschiel JH, Landmesser CM, Harmel M: Cardiac oxygen metabolism and control of the coronary circulation. *Am J Physiol* 149: 634, 1947.

8 Khouri EM, Gregg DE, Rayford CR: Effect of exercise on cardiac output, left coronary flow and myocardial metabolism in the unanesthetized dog. *Circ Res* 17: 427, 1965.

9 Rubio R, Berne RM: Regulation of coronary blood flow. *Prog Cardiovas Dis* 18: 105, 1975.

10 Restorff W von, Bassenge E: Transient effects of norepinephrine on myocardial oxygen balance. *Pfluengers Arch* 370: 131, 1977.

11 Berne RM, Rubio R: Coronary circulation, in *Handbook of Physiology*, RM Berne (ed). Bethesda, Maryland, American Physiological Society, 1979, vol 1, sect 2, The cardiovascular system, chap 25, p 873.

12 Lombardo TA, Rose L, Taeschler M, Tuluy S, Bing RJ: The effect of exercise on coronary blood flow, myocardial oxygen consumption and cardiac efficiency in man. *Circulation* 7: 71, 1953.

13 Weiss HR, Sinha AK: Regional oxygen saturation of small arteries and veins in the canine myocardium. *Circ Res* 42: 119, 1978.

13a Vinten-Johansen J, Weiss HR: Oxygen consumption in subepicardial and subendocardial regions of the canine left ventricle: The effect of experimental acute valvular aortic stenosis. *Circ Res* 46: 139, 1980.

14 Hoffman JIE: Determinants and prediction of transmural myocardial perfusion. *Circulation* 58: 381, 1978.

15 White CW, Kerber R, Weiss HR, Marcus ML: Effect of atrial fibrillation on wall stress, oxygen consumption and perfusion of the left atrium. *Circulation* (suppl 2) 64: IV-65, 1981, no. 225.

16 Schwartz GG, McHale PA, Greenfield JC: Coronary vasodilation after a single ventricular extra-activation in the conscious dog. *Circ Res* 50: 38, 1982.

17 Marcus M, Wright C, Doty D, Eastham C, Laughlin D, Krumm P, Fastenow C, Brody M: Measurements of coronary velocity and reactive hyperemia in the coronary circulation of humans. *Circ Res* 49: 877, 1981.

18 Coffman JD, Gregg DE: Reactive hyperemia characteristics of the myocardium. *Am J Physiol* 199: 1143, 1960.

19 Fedor JM, McIntosh DM, Rembert JC, Greenfield JC: Coronary and regional myocardial blood flow response to transient ischemia in awake domestic pigs. *Am J Physiol* 4: H435, 1978.

20 Rayford CR, Huvos A, Khouri EM, Gregg DE: Some determinants of coronary flow in intact dogs. *Physiologist* 4: 92, 1961.

21 Weiss HR: Effect of coronary artery occlusion on regional arterial and venous O_2 extraction, blood flow and O_2 consumption in the dog heart. *Circ Res* 47: 100, 1980.

22 Mohrman DE, Feigl EO: Competition between sympathetic vasodilation in the canine coronary circulation. *Circ Res* 42: 79, 1978.

23 Braunwald E: Control of myocardial oxygen consumption: Physiologic and clinical considerations. *Am J Cardiol* 27: 416, 1971.

24 Mueller TM, Marcus ML, Kerber RE, Young JA, Barnes RW, Abboud FM: Effect of renal hypertension and left ventricular hypertrophy on the coronary circulation in dogs. *Circ Res* 42:543, 1978.

25 Bache RJ, Vrobel TR, Arentzen CE, Ring WS: Effect of maximal coronary vasodilation on transmural myocardial perfusion during tachycardia in dogs with left ventricular hypertrophy. *Circ Res* 49: 742, 1981.

26 Ganz W, Yoshida S, Swan HJC: Coronary hemodynamics during progressive elevation of heart rate by pacing in subjects with normal coronary arteries and coronary artery disease, in *Myocardial Blood Flow in Man*, A Maseri (ed). Turin, Minerva Medica, p 310.

27 Vatner SF, Higgins CB, Franklin D, Braunwald E: Role of tachycardia in mediating the coronary hemodynamic response to severe exercise. *J Appl Physiol* 32: 380, 1972.

28 Pitt B, Gregg DE: Coronary hemodynamic effects of increasing ventricular rate in the unanesthetized dog. *Circ Res* 22: 753, 1968.

29 Ross J Jr, Sonnenblick EH, Kaiser GA, Frommer PL, Braunwald E: Electroaugmentation of ventricular performance and oxygen consumption by repetitive application of paired electrical stimuli. *Circ Res* 16: 332, 1965.

30 Graham TP Jr, Covell JW, Sonnenblick EH, Ross J Jr, Braunwald E: Control of myocardial oxygen consumption: Relative influence of contractile state and tension development. *J Clin Invest* 47: 375, 1968.

31 Fixler DE, Archie JP, Ullyot DJ, Buckberg GD, Hoffman JIE: Effect of acute right ventricular systolic hypertension on regional myocardial blood flow in anesthetized dogs. *Am Heart J* 85: 491, 1973.

32 Fenn WO: A quantitative comparison between the energy liberated and the work performed by the isolated sartorius muscle of the frog. *J Physiol* 58: 175, 1923.

32a Taylor RR, Cingolani HE, Graham TP, Clancy RL: Myocardial oxygen consumption, left ventricular fibre shortening and wall tension. *Cardiovasc Res* 1: 219, 1967.

33 Sarnoff SJ, Braunwald E, Welch GH Jr et al: Hemodynamic determinants of oxygen consumption of the heart with special reference to the tension-time index. *Am J Physiol* 192: 148, 1958.

33a Rooke GA, Feigl EO: Work as a correlate of canine left ventricular oxygen consumption, and the problem of catecholamine oxygen wasting. *Circ Res* 50: 273, 1982.

34 Klocke FJ, Braunwald E, Ross J Jr: Oxygen cost of electrical activation of the heart. *Circ Res* 18: 357, 1966.

35 McKeever WP, Gregg DE, Canney PC: Oxygen uptake of the nonworking left ventricle. *Circ Res* 6: 612, 1958.

36 Van Citters RL, Franklin DL: Cardiovascular performance of Alaska sled dogs during exercise. *Circ Res* 24: 33, 1969.

37 Ball RM, Bache RJ, Cobb FR, Greenfield JC Jr: Regional myocardial blood flow during graded treadmill exercise in the dog. *J Clin Invest* 55: 43, 1975.

38 Bassenge E, Kucharczyk M, Holtz J, Stoian D: Treadmill exercise in dogs under β-adrenergic blockage: Adaptation of coronary and systemic hemodynamics. *Pfluegers Arch* 332: 40, 1972.

39 Restorff WY, Holtz J, Bassenge E: Exercise induced augmentation of myocardial oxygen extraction in spite of normal coronary dilator capacity in dogs. *Pfluegers Arch* 372: 181, 1977.

40 Barnard RJ, Duncan HW, Livesay JJ, Buckberg GD: Coronary vasodilator reserve and flow distribution during near-maximal exercise in dogs. *J Appl Physiol Respirat Environ Exercise Physiol* 43: 988, 1977.

41 Bache RJ, Vrobel TR, Ring WS, Emery RW, Andersen RW: Regional myocardial blood flow during exercise in dogs with chronic left ventricular hypertrophy. *Circ Res* 48: 76, 1981.

42 Holmberg S, Serzysko W, Varnauskas E: Coronary circulation during heavy exercise in control subjects and patients with coronary heart disease. *Acta Med Scand* 190: 465, 1971.

43 Tauchert M, Hilger HH: Application of the coronary reserve concept to the study of myocardial perfusion, in *The Patho-Physiology of Myocardial Perfusion*, W Schaper (ed). Amsterdam, Amsterdam Elsevier/North-Holland Biomedical Press, p 141, 1979.

44 Olsson RA, Gregg DE: Myocardial reactive hyperemia in the unanesthetized dog. *Am J Physiol* 208: 244, 1965.

45 Olsson RA, Gregg DE: Metabolic responses during myocardial reactive hyperemia in the unanesthetized dog. *Am J Physiol* 208, 231, 1965.

46 Bache RJ, Cobb FR, Greenfield JC Jr: Limitations of the coronary vascular response to ischemia in the awake dog. *Circ Res* 35: 527, 1974.

47 Olsson RA: Myocardial reactive hyperemia. *Circ Res* 37: 263, 1975.

48 Giles RW, Wilcken DEL: Reactive hyperaemia in the dog heart: Evidence for a myogenic contribution. *Cardiovas Res* 11: 64, 1977.

49 Bache RJ, Cobb FR, Greenfield JC Jr: Effect of increased myocardial oxygen consumption on coronary reactive hyperemia in the awake dog. *Circ Res* 33: 588, 1973.

49a Schwartz GC, McHale PA, Greenfield JC Jr: Hyperemic response of the coronary circulation to brief diastolic occlusion in the conscious dog. *Circ Res* 50: 28, 1982.

49b Katz LN, Linder E: Quantitative relation between reactive hyperemia and the myocardial ischemia which it follows. *Am J Physiol* 126: 283, 1939.

50 Dole WP, Montville WJ, Bishop VS: Dependency of myocardial reactive hyperemia on coronary artery pressure in the dog. *Am J Physiol* 240: H709, 1981.

51 Ruiter JH, Spaan JAE, Laird JD: Transient oxygen uptake during myocardial reactive hyperemia in the dog. *Am J Physiol* 235: H87, 1978.

52 Olsson RA, Snow JA, Gentry MK: Adenosine metabolism in canine myocardial reactive hyperemia. *Circ Res* 42: 358, 1978.

53 Dunn RB, McDonough KM, Griggs DM Jr: High energy phosphate stores and lactate levels in different layers of the canine left ventricle during reactive hyperemia. *Circ Res* 44: 788, 1979.

54 Schwartz PJ, Stone HL: Tonic influence of the sympathetic nervous system on myocardial reactive hyperemia and on coronary blood flow distribution in dogs. *Circ Res* 41: 51, 1977.

54a Bache RJ, Cobb FR, Ebert PA, et al: Neurogenic influences on the coronary vascular response to ischemia in the awake dog. *J Thorac Cardiovasc Surg* 69: 421, 1975.

55 Bache RJ, Cobb FR, Greenfield JC Jr: Limitation of the coronary vascular response to ischemia in the awake dog. *Circ Res* 35: 527, 1974.

56 Badeer HS: Influence of cooling the heart on reactive hyperemia of the coronary bed in the heart-lung preparation. *Circ Res* 16: 19, 1965.

57 Eikens E, Wilcken DEL: Myocardial reactive hyperaemia in conscious dogs: Effect of dipyridamole and aminophylline on responses to four- and eight-second coronary artery occlusions. *Aust J Exp Biol Med Sci* 51: 617, 1973.

57a Bache RJ, Dymek DJ: Effect of diltiazem on myocardial blood flow. *Circulation* 65: I-19, 1982.

58 Bache RJ, Lambert PR: Transmural myocardial blood flow during coronary reactive hyperemia in the dog. *Circulation* 55/56 (suppl 3): III-37, 1977, no. 133.

59 Downey HF, Crystal GJ, Bashour FA: Transmural variations in myocardial blood flow during reactive hyperemia. *Physiologist* 24: 26, 1981.

60 Eastham C, Doty D, Wright C, Marcus M: Effects of age on coronary reserve in man. *Circulation* 62 (suppl 3): III-64, 1980.

61 Wangler RD, Peters KG, Marcus ML, Tomanek RJ: Effects of duration and severity of arterial hypertension on cardiac hypertrophy and coronary vasodilator reserve. *Circ Res* 51:10, 1982.

62 Gamble WJ, Conn PA, Edeljikumar A, Plenge R, Monroe RG: Myocardial oxygen consumption of blood perfused, isolated, supported rat heart. *Am J Physiol* 219: 604, 1979.

63 Berne RM: The role of adenosine in the regulation of coronary blood flow. *Circ Res* 47: 807, 1980.

64 Driscol TE, Berne RM: Role of potassium in regulation of coronary blood flow. *Proc Soc Exptl Biol Med* 96: 505, 1957.

65 Jelliffe RW, Wolf CR, Berne RM, Eckstein RW: Absence of vasoactive and cardiotropic substances in coronary sinus blood of dogs. *Circ Res* 5: 382, 1957.

66 Scott JB, Radawski D: Role of hyperosmolarity in the genesis of active and reactive hyperemia. *Circ Res* 28-29 (suppl 1): 26, 1971.

67 Sybers HD, Helmer PR, Murphy QR: Effects of hypoxia on myocardial potassium balance. *Am J Physiol* 220: 2047, 1971.

68 Kline RP, Morad M: Potassium efflux in heart muscle during activity: Extracellular accumulation and its implications. *J Physiol* (London) 280: 537, 1978.

69 Kunze DL: Rate-dependent changes in extracellular potassium in the rabbit atrium. *Circ Res* 41: 122, 1977.

70 Dusting GJ, Moncada S, Vane JR: Prostaglandins, their intermediates and precursors: Cardiovascular actions and regulatory roles in normal and abnormal circulatory systems. *Prog Cardiovas Dis* 21: 405, 1979.

71 Case RB, Felix A, Wachter M, Kyriakidis G, Castellana F: Relative effect of CO_2 on canine coronary vascular resistance. *Circ Res* 42: 410, 1978.

72 Case RB, Greenberg H: The response of canine coronary vascular resistance to local alterations in coronary arterial PCO_2. *Circ Res* 39: 558, 1976.

73 Case RB, Greenberg H, Moskowitz R: Alterations in coronary sinus pO_2 and O_2 saturation resulting from pCO_2 changes. *Cardiovas Res* 9: 167, 1975.

74 Belloni FL, Rubio R, Berne RM: Location of adenosine produced by hypoxic liver cells

Fed Proc 39: 270, 1980.

75 Rubio R, Berne RM: Release of adenosine by the normal myocardium in dogs and its relationship to the regulation of coronary resistance. *Circ Res* 25: 407, 1969.

76 Miller WL, Belardinelli L, Bacchus A, Foley DH, Rubio R, Berne RM: Canine myocardial adenosine and lactate production, oxygen consumption and coronary blood flow during stellate ganglia stimulation. *Circ Res* 45: 708, 1979.

77 Watkinson WP, Foley DH, Rubio R, Berne RM: Myocardial adenosine formation with increased cardiac performance in the dog. *Am J Physiol* 236: H13, 1979.

78 Afonso S: Coronary vasodilator responses to hypoxia and induced tachycardia before and after lidoflazine. *Am J Physiol* 216: 297, 1969.

79 Afonso S, Ansfield TJ, Berndt TB, Rowe GC: Coronary vasodilator responses to hypoxia before and after aminophylline. *J Physiol* 221: 589, 1972.

80 Bittar N, Pauly TJ: Myocardial reactive hyperemia responses in the dog after aminophylline and lidoflazine. *Am J Physiol* 220: 812, 1971.

81 Juhran W, Dietmann K: Zur Regelung der Coronardurchblutung im Akuten Sauerstoffmangel. *Pfluegers Arch* 315: 105, 1970.

82 Merrill GJ, Haddy FJ, Dabney JM: Adenosine, theophylline and perfusate pH in the isolated, perfused guinea pig heart. *Circ Res* 42: 225, 1978.

83 Raberger G, Schutz W, Draupp O: Coronary reactive hyperemia and coronary dilator action of adenosine during normal respiration and hypercapnic acidosis in the dog. *Clin Exp Pharmacol Physiol* 2: 373, 1975.

84 Merrill GF, Haddy FJ, Dabney JM: Adenosine, theophylline and perfusate pH in the isolated perfused guinea pig heart. *Circ Res* 42: 225, 1978.

84a Jones CE, Hurst TW, Randall JR: Effect of aminophylline on coronary functional hyperemia and myocardial adenosine. *Am J Physiol* 243: H480–H487, 1982.

85 Saito D, Steinhart CR, Nison DG, Ollsson RA: Intracoronary adenosine deaminase reduces canine myocardial reactive hyperemia. *Circ Res* 49: 1262, 1981.

86 Olsson RA, Saito D, Steinhart CR: Compartmentalization of the adenosine pool of dog and rat hearts. *Circ Res* 50: 617, 1982.

87 Schrader J, Gerlach E: Compartmentation of cardiac adenine nucleotides and formation of adenosine. *Pfluegers Arch* 367: 129, 1976.

88 Frick GP, Lowenstein JM: Vectorial production of adenosine by 5′-nucleotidase in the perfused rat heart. *J Biol Chem* 253: 1240, 1978.

89 Schrader J, Schutz W: Sites of adenosine production in the hypoxic heart (abstr). *Fed Proc* 38: 1037, 1979.

90 Hester RL, Guyton AC, Barber BJ: Reactive and exercise hyperemia during high levels of adenosine infusion. *Am J Physiol* 243: H181–H186, 1982.

91 DeWitt DF, Wangler RD, Sparks HV: Time-course of cardiac adenosine release during norepinephrine infusion. *Circ* (suppl II) 66: 154, 1982.

CHAPTER **4**

AUTOREGULATION IN THE CORONARY CIRCULATION

Blood flow to all segments of the circulation is dependent on arterial driving pressure. In the heart, three additional factors (extravascular compressive forces, diastolic chamber pressures, effects of increased pressure on myocardial metabolism) complicate the relationship between arterial pressure and coronary blood flow. In addition, in the left ventricle, transmural differences in vascular density [1], autoregulation [2], and critical closing pressure [3,4] further modify the pressure-flow relationship. All these modulating influences, acting in concert, contribute to pressure-flow relationships in the coronary circulation.

PRESSURE-FLOW RELATIONSHIPS IN THE INTACT CORONARY CIRCULATION

Acute increases in arterial pressure, and hence, left ventricular pressure and wall stress, augment myocardial metabolism and invariably increase coronary blood flow (see Chapter 3). Even though autoregulation tends to maintain coronary flow constant when pressure rises, the effects of increased wall stress on myocardial metabolism and myocardial oxygen consumption produce coronary dilation because the metabolic influences are dominant.

PRESSURE-FLOW RELATIONSHIPS IN PERFUSED HEARTS

In a perfused preparation, coronary driving pressure can be varied while left ventricular hemodynamics and oxygen consumption are stable [5-10]. Under such conditions, the pressure-flow relationship and the coronary circulation exhibit the typical features of autoregulation; that is, over a wide range of perfusion pressure, coronary flow remains relatively constant [2,3,5-11] (Figure 4-1). In normal dogs, the upper limit of autoregulation is 130 to 150 mmHg [12]. That is to say, when mean aortic driving pressure exceeds 130 to 150 mmHg, coronary flow begins to

FIGURE 4-1
Pressure-flow relationships in the coronary circulation during maximal coronary dilation (dotted line) and during normal coronary tone (solid circles). When normal tone is present, coronary flow remains relatively constant over a wide range of perfusion pressures. During maximal coronary dilation there is a steep relationship between coronary pressure and coronary flow. (*Redrawn from data originally presented by J Rouleau et al* [3].)

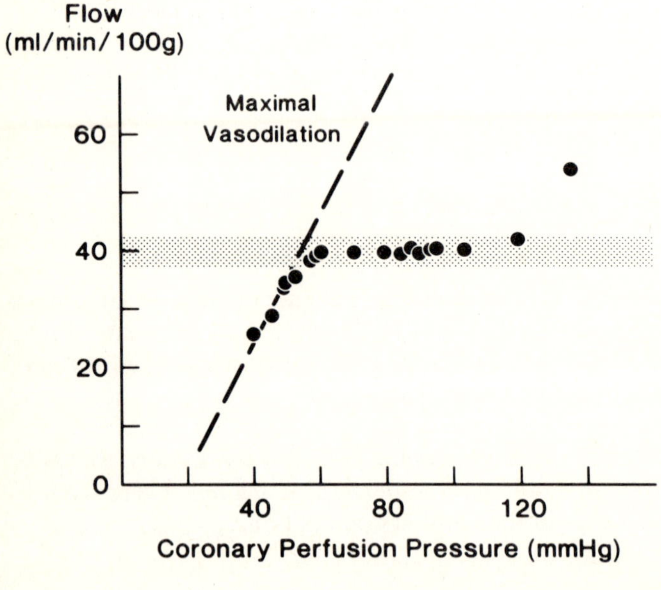

rise precipitously rather than remain relatively constant. The lower limit of autoregulation in the dog is 50 to 70 mmHg [2,5,11]. When mean coronary driving pressure decreases below 50 to 70 mmHg, coronary flow begins to fall sharply. If an abrupt change in coronary perfusion pressure occurs within the autoregulatory range, flow parallels the change in pressure transiently [5,10] but returns to near the control flow value within 5 to 15 s. Thus, autoregulation rapidly adjust coronary vascular resistance to maintain relatively constant myocardial perfusion.

Microsphere measurements have permitted investigators to determine the pressure-flow relationships in various layers of the left ventricle. Such studies demonstrate that autoregulation is more effective in the epicardial third than in the endocardial third of the left ventricular myocardium (see Figure 4-2) [2,12]. At both extremely high [12] and extremely low [2] perfusion pressures, the autoregulatory capacity of the subendocardium is exhausted before that of the subepicardium.

Factors That Modulate Autoregulation

Any intervention which impairs the function of smooth muscle in coronary vessels will attenuate autoregulation. Drugs which cause maximal relaxation of smooth muscle, such as adenosine, ATP, and dipyridamole, abolish autoregulation (see Figure 4-1). Partial coronary obstruction also impairs autoregulation (see Chapter 11), but this effect is apparent rather than real. If severe stenosis is present, the pressure downstream to the obstruction will be decreased. Thus, the

FIGURE 4-2
Pressure-flow relationships in the endocardial (*left*) and epicardial (*right*) thirds of the left ventricular myocardium. The ability of the epicardial vessels to autoregulate is substantially greater than that of the endocardial vessels. (*Redrawn from data originally presented by RA Guyton et al* [2].)

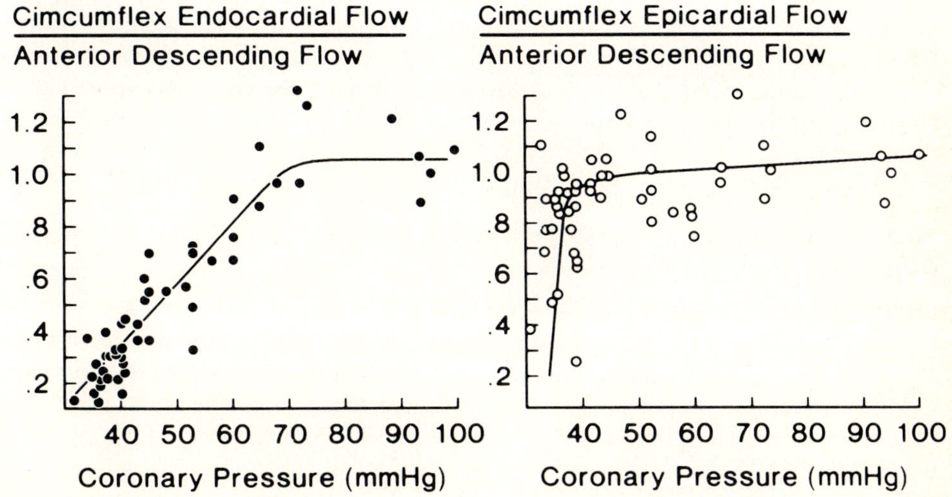

downstream vessels are on a lower portion of the autoregulatory curve than measurements of aortic pressure indicate. In addition, if pressure is lowered, the obstructed segment may collapse slightly because the distending pressure decreases [13,14]; this will augment the severity of the stenosis, and downstream pressure may fall farther [13,14]. In the presence of coronary occlusion, perfusion to the ischemic zone is strikingly pressure-dependent because native coronary collateral channels are maximally dilated and do not exhibit autoregulation (see Chapter 9). Chronic disease states may modify autoregulation. In the cerebral bed, chronic hypertension and concomitant vascular hypertrophy shift the autoregulatory curve to the right [15]. Thus, the threshold pressure below which cerebral flow will fall is higher in the presence of chronic hypertension. One might speculate that a similar effect may occur in the coronary bed. Finally, nonspecific depressants can markedly impair autoregulation. Loss of autoregulation has often been noted in prolonged experiments in anesthetized, open-chest or isolated heart preparations. In addition, a brief period of severe ischemia or severe hypertension can temporarily abolish autoregulation in the coronary circulation.

Mechanisms of Autoregulation

The mediator which couples changes in pressure to alterations in coronary vascular resistance remains elusive. It has often been assumed that a common mediator may couple myocardial metabolism and arterial driving pressure to vascular resistance. Most investigators in this area, however, have focused on the link between myocardial metabolism and coronary vascular resistance (see Chapter 3). The criteria for establishing the mediator that couples changes in perfusion pressure to alterations in coronary vascular resistance are similar to those described for a mediator linking myocardial oxygen consumption to coronary vascular resistance (see Table 3-1). To date, none of the proposed mediators satisfies all these criteria.

Autoregulation could, in part, be a myogenic response (see Chapter 6). The time course of the myogenic response observed in isolated vessels is similar to the time course of autoregulation observed in vivo. Although myogenic mechanisms have been demonstrated in several vascular beds [16], no study has shown conclusively that the coronary circulation is modulated by myogenic mechanisms (see Chapter 6).

EFFECTS OF DIASTOLIC CHAMBER PRESSURES ON CORONARY DRIVING PRESSURES

Intraventricular pressures are transmitted to the intramural coronary vessels. During diastole, it has been presumed that intraventricular pressure constitutes the primary source of extravascular coronary resistance. This source of resistance gains considerable importance when intraventricular diastolic pressure is increased or when arterial driving pressure is reduced. Both of these conditions exist when a failing ventricle is perfused by severely obstructed coronary arteries.

Because intraventricular pressures are transmitted to the subendocardium more so than to the subepicardium, alterations in diastolic chamber pressure exhibit their greatest effects on subendocardial perfusion.

EXTRAVASCULAR COMPRESSIVE FORCES

The heart and contracting skeletal muscle are the only organs that occlude their own blood supply. During systole, ventricular wall stress rises and intramural coronary vessels are compressed. As a consequence, arterial flow at peak systole is retrograde [17] and venous flow in the intramural venules is forced into the coronary sinus [18]. Extravascular compressive forces constitute a small component of total vascular resistance (Figure 4-3) [19–21]. If these compressive forces are completely eliminated, coronary vascular resistance decreases by 10 to 25 percent [19–21]. The extravascular compressive forces can be divided into two components: physical compression and shear caused by twisting of vascular channels as the heart contracts [21]. Under normal conditions, shear accounts for two-thirds of extravascular resistance (Figure 4-3) [21]. If ventricular pressure remains constant and coronary vasomotor tone is normal, changes in myocardial contractility have

FIGURE 4-3
Effects of extravascular compressive forces on coronary vascular resistance. Afterload-dependent extravascular forces, i.e., physical compression, are of lesser importance than afterload-independent extravascular compressive force, i.e., shear due to twisting of vascular channels as the heart contracts. (*Redrawn from data originally presented by JM Downey et al* [*21*].)

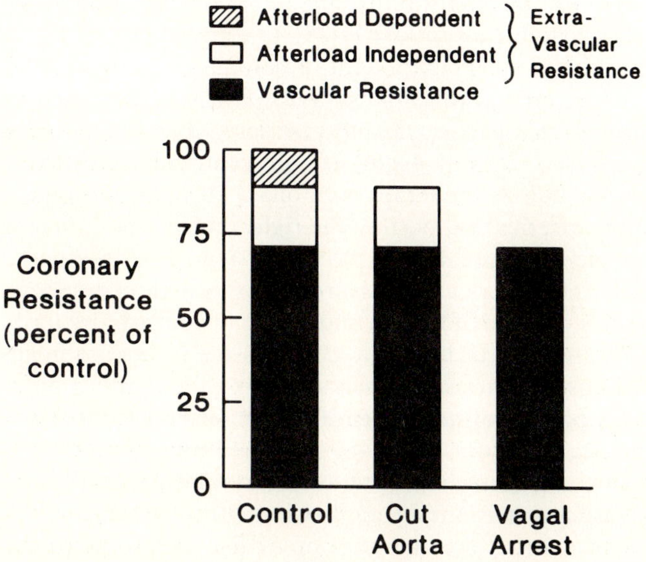

little effect on the component of coronary vascular resistance that is related to extravascular compressive forces [21a]. The importance of extravascular compressive forces is greatly magnified when coronary vessels are dilated. Marzilli et al. [21b] have shown that during maximal coronary dilation, alterations in myocardial contractility can have major effects on coronary vascular resistance and the transmural distribution of left ventricular perfusion. Under conditions of maximal coronary dilation, increases in myocardial contractility increase coronary vascular resistance and diminish subendocardial perfusion. Decreases in contractility have the opposite effect. Because the effects of extravascular components of coronary resistance are exaggerated during coronary dilation, these factors are very important in modulating myocardial perfusion during ischemia, when endogenous stimuli produce dilation of resistance vessels (see Chapter 10).

Effects of Extravascular Compressive Forces on Phasic Coronary Blood Flow in Epicardial Coronary Arteries

In the early 1950s, Gregg [22] and Wiggers [18] proposed alternative theories to explain the phasic character of coronary blood flow. Gregg suggested that extravascular compressive forces increased coronary vascular resistance in systole and limited systolic flow in vessels perfusing the left ventricle. Wiggers argued that the myocardium acted as a pump which forced blood retrograde into the conduit coronary arteries in systole and thereby limited systolic antrograde flow in arteries which supplied the left ventricle. These two theories are not mutually incompatible. Although this issue is not settled, I believe that both of these mechanisms modulate the phasic character of coronary blood flow.

The effects of extravascular compressive forces are most prominent in cardiac chambers that develop high systolic pressure. In chronically instrumented unanesthetized dogs, phasic flow in arteries that perfuse the left ventricle is markedly decreased in systole (diastolic/systolic flow ratio 6:1) [23]. In contrast, if pressure in the right ventricle is normal, the systolic component of coronary flow in arteries that perfuse the right ventricle is greater (diastolic/systolic flow ratio of 2:1) than that observed in coronary vessels that perfuse the left ventricle [23]. Similar results have been reported in humans (see Figure 4-4) [24]. If right ventricular pressure is increased by a disease process such as moderate pulmonary stenosis, the phasic pattern of flow in the coronary arteries that perfuse the right ventricle is similar to that observed in the left ventricle (Figure 4-4). If pulmonic stenosis is severe and the ventricular septum intact, right ventricular pressure can exceed aortic pressure. Under these conditions, there is reversal of flow in midsystole in epicardial arteries that supply the ventricle (Figure 4-4). In the atria, compressive forces are negligible. Phasic coronary blood flow in coronary vessels supplying the right atrium is dominant in systole [25]. This pattern of flow resembles that observed in peripheral arteries.

To minimize the effects of compressive forces on coronary vascular resistance, one can calculate coronary vascular resistance from flow and pressure measured in late diastole when compressive forces are minimal or as the reciprocal of the coronary pressure-flow relationship obtained during diastole.

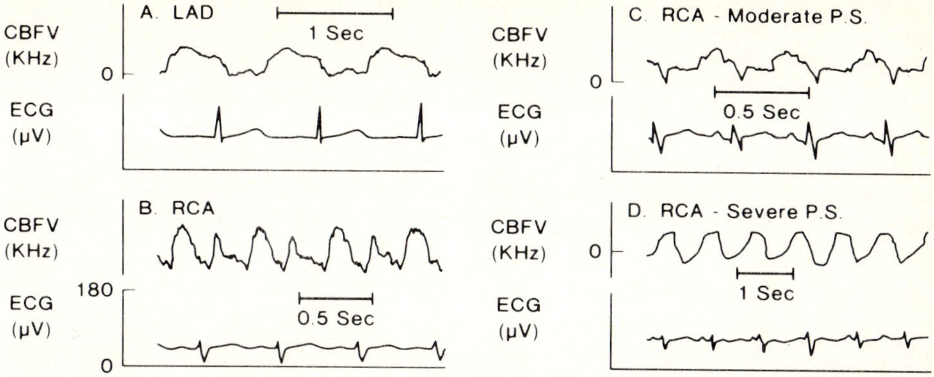

FIGURE 4-4
Phasic coronary blood flow velocity (CBFV) obtained in various coronary vessels under different conditions. In all patients the coronary vessels examined were angiographically normal. Under normal conditions, systolic coronary blood flow velocity is more prominent in vessels that perfuse a normal right ventricle. When right ventricular pressure increases secondary to moderate pulmonary stenosis (P.S.), coronary blood flow velocity recordings obtained in a vessel perfusing the right ventricle resemble those from the left anterior descending (LAD). When systolic right ventricular pressure exceeds left ventricular systolic pressure, (Severe P.S.) retrograde coronary blood velocity is noted during systole in vessels that perfuse the hypertensive right ventricle. RCA = right coronary artery. In the studies depicted, recordings were obtained from right ventricular branches of the right coronary artery. (*All data were collected at the University of Iowa.*)

Effects of Extravascular Compressive Forces on Phasic Coronary Blood Flow in Intramural Coronary Arteries

Recent studies by Chilian et al. [17] have assessed the phasic pattern of coronary blood flow velocity in intramyocardial coronary vessels. The results of these studies imply that phasic coronary blood flow in the epicardial arteries may not accurately reflect phasic myocardial perfusion. The phasic pattern of blood flow in intramyocardial vessels differs from epicardial vessels in three ways: (1) the amount of flow in systole is decreased by more than half, (2) midsystolic flow is persistently retrograde, and (3) the flow during diastole is increased by 20 percent (see Figure 4-5). Differences in the phasic pattern of coronary blood flow in epicardial and intramyocardial coronary vessels are exaggerated during coronary vasodilation (Figure 4-6), aortic insufficiency, right ventricular hypertension, tachycardia, and increases in the inotropic state of the left ventricle [26]. Spann et al. [27] have recently presented evidence which suggests that an intramyocardial pump displaces blood retrograde into the coronary arteries during systole. The observations of Spann et al. [27] and Chilian et al. [17,26] can only be reconciled by postulating the existence of a coronary capacitor of substantial importance. Although the compliance of epicardial vessels in comparison with other vessels of similar size is controversial [28-31a], coronary diameter does increase by about 5 percent in systole [32]. Furthermore, it is possible that some of the vessels in the superficial epicardium act in part as capacitors [33]. Although coronary capacitance has usually been dismissed as an unimportant aspect of coronary physiology

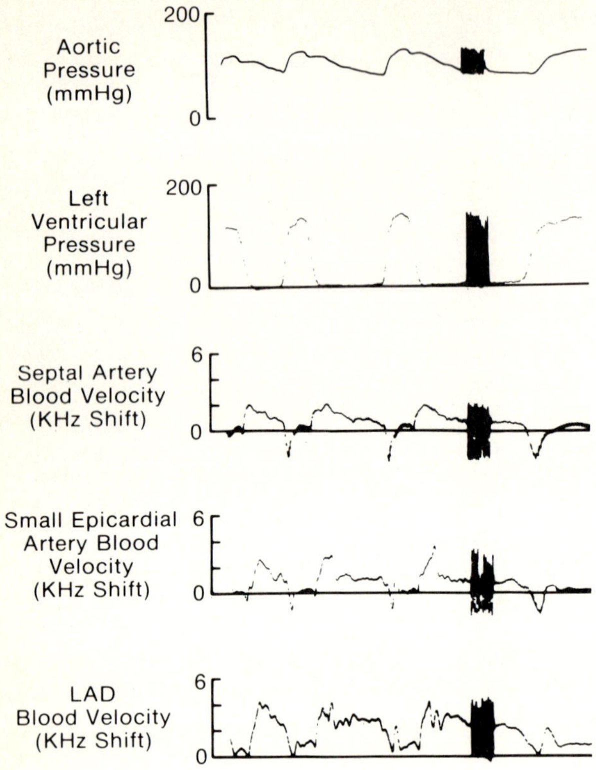

FIGURE 4-5
Phasic coronary blood flow velocity recordings in intramural (septal) and small epicardial artery and large epicardial coronary vessels (left anterior descending, LAD). During midsystole, when coronary blood flow was anterograde in the left anterior descending coronary artery it was retrograde in the septal artery and a small epicardial artery. Coronary blood flow velocity recordings from a small epicardial vessel were obtained within 0.5 cm of the point where the vessel penetrated into the wall of the left ventricle. The phasic configuration of these recordings are similar to those obtained in the septal artery. The presence of simultaneous anterograde and retrograde flow in different segments of the vessel is best reconciled by postulating the existence of a coronary capacitor. (*Data originally presented by WM Chilian et al* [26].)

[34], recent evidence suggests that this concept deserves additional attention [17,26,27,32,33,35,35a].

Effects of Extravascular Compressive Forces on Transmural Distribution of Coronary Blood Flow

Because extravascular compressive forces are not uniform across the left ventricular wall, these forces modulate the transmural distribution of myocardial perfusion in the left ventricle, particularly in systole. Several studies have shown that during systole very little blood is delivered to the endocardial third of the left ventricle (Figure 4-7) [36–37a]. Furthermore, because coronary blood flow is retrograde in midsystole [17], it is likely that the distribution of myocardial perfusion is variable in different portions of systole. This has not been systematically examined. When the transmural distribution of left ventricular perfusion throughout the cardiac cycle is measured in awake dogs, it is usually reported that the subendocardium receives more flow than the subepicardium.

In the right ventricle, where intraventricular pressure is lower, the transmural perfusion of flow in systole and diastole are similar [37b].

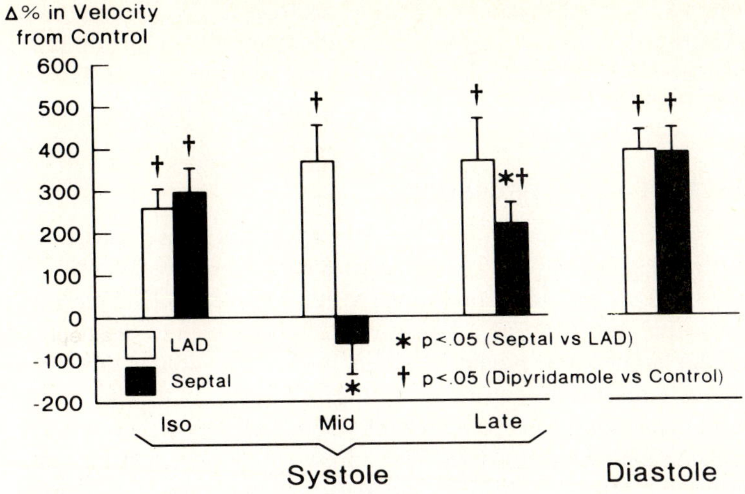

FIGURE 4-6
Quantitative characteristics of phasic coronary blood flow velocity during intense dilation produced by intravenous infusion of dipyridamole. Data are plotted as change in percent velocity versus control. Dipyridamole markedly increased left anterior descending (LAD) coronary blood flow velocity in all phases of systole (isovolumic, iso; mid- and late systole) as well as diastole. During midsystole, retrograde flow persisted in the septal artery (septal). (*Data originally presented by Chilian WM et al* [26].)

FIGURE 4-7
Transmural distribution of left ventricular perfusion throughout the cardiac cycle (control) and only during systole (systolic perfusion). During systole, perfusion to the inner layers of the left ventricle is markedly reduced. (*Redrawn from data originally presented by DS Hess and RJ Bache* [37].)

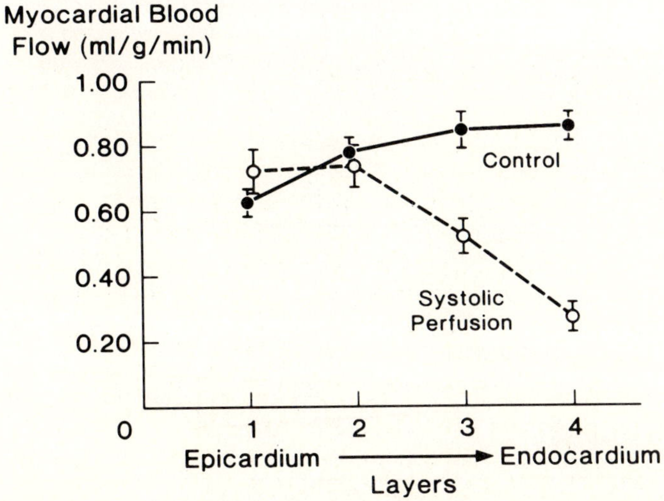

The two components of extravascular coronary resistance (shear and compression) have different effects on transmural flow. Shear forces are presumably distributed uniformly across the ventricular wall. Compressive forces are thought to be much greater in the subendocardium than in the subepicardium.

CRITICAL CLOSING (STOP-FLOW) PRESSURE

In 1954, Burton postulated that there should exist a transmural pressure below which active tension caused by smooth muscle contraction would cause physical closure of arterioles [38]. This zero-flow pressure is often referred to as the critical closing pressure of Burton [39]. Although Alexander [39a] has argued that critical closure in a Burtonian sense may never occur in maximally dilated coronary vessels, the concept of stop-flow, or critical closing, pressure in the heart and skeletal muscle [40,41] has been revived in recent years. Bellamy examined coronary pressure-flow data collected in Gregg's laboratory [41] and concluded that under normal conditions coronary blood flow ceases when coronary driving pressure is about 40 to 50 mmHg (Figure 4-8). Furthermore, Bellamy presented evidence that suggested that the pressure at which coronary flow stops is dependent on coronary vasomotor tone [41]. During intense coronary vasodilation, critical closing pressure decreases to about 12 to 18 mmHg (Figure 4-9). Studies by Ellis and Klocke [4] and Rouleau et al. [3] indicate that critical closing pressure may be higher in the subendocardial layers of the left ventricle than in the subepicardial layers (Figure 4-10). Experiments have also suggested mild coro-

FIGURE 4-8
Simultaneous recordings of circumflex coronary artery (Cir) blood flow, pressure and aortic pressure in a conscious chronically instrumented dog. During a spontaneous long diastole, circumflex coronary blood flow ceases when circumflex coronary pressure is about 50 mmHg. Note that under control conditions there is a small pressure gradient between the aorta and the proximal circumflex coronary artery. (*Data originally presented by RF Bellamy et al* [*40*].)

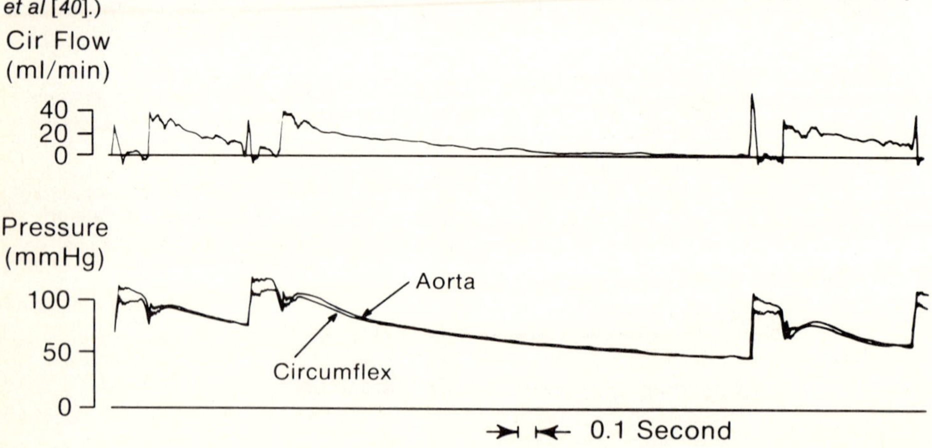

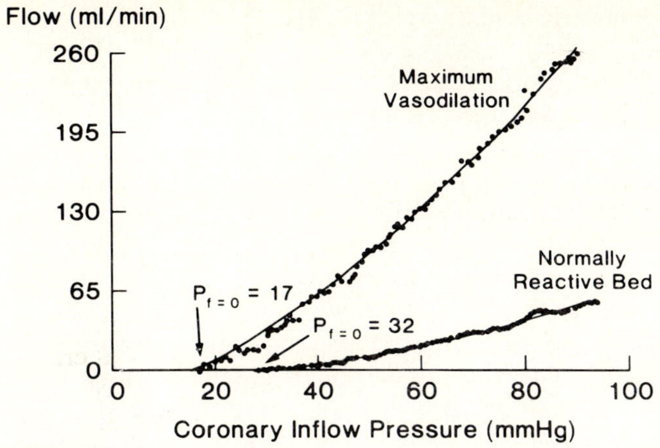

FIGURE 4-9
Pressure-flow relationship during a long diastole when coronary tone is normal (normally reactive bed) and during maximal coronary vasodilation. Note that the pressure-flow relationship is curvilinear and best fit by a second-order equation. During maximal coronary dilation, the pressure-flow relationship is steeper and the zero-flow pressure intercept is less than that noted with normal coronary tone. (*Courtesy of FJ Klocke, University of Buffalo Medical School* [49].)

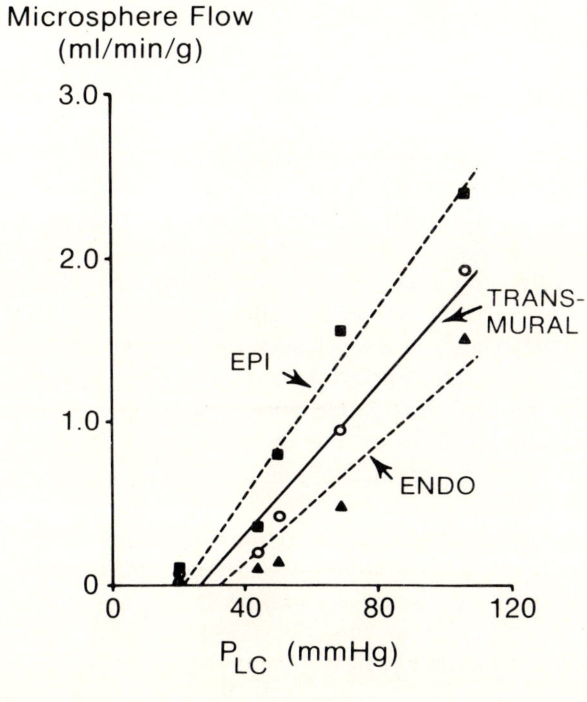

FIGURE 4-10
Pressure-flow relationships during a long diastole in the endocarcial third (ENDO) and the epicardial third (EPI) of the left ventricular wall. The endocardial pressure-flow relationship is less steep and shifted to the right compared with the epicardial pressure-flow relationship. The data suggest that critical closing pressure or pressure at zero flow is higher in the endocardium than in the epicardium of the left ventricle. Transmural = mean perfusion to all layers of the wall of the left ventricle. P_{LC} = pressure in the left circumflex coronary artery. (*Redrawn from data originally presented by AK Ellis and FJ Klocke* [4].)

nary stenosis [42,49], changes in alpha-adrenergic [43,44] and beta-adrenergic tone [44], increases in coronary sinus pressure [45], and anesthetic agents [45a] can alter critical closing pressure. Studies by Gascho et al. [46] indicate that moderate pressure-induced cardiac hypertrophy does not change critical closing pressure in the coronary circulation.

Why is the concept of critical closing pressure so important? The answer revolves around formulations for the calculation of coronary vascular resistance. Classically, coronary vascular resistance has been calculated by dividing coronary driving pressure by coronary flow. Coronary driving pressure was taken as mean aortic pressure minus the coronary sinus pressure, which was thought to be the effective coronary back flow pressure. Under most conditions, coronary sinus pressure is less than 10 mmHg, and hence it contributes little to calculated coronary vascular resistance. Recent studies which have measured critical closing pressure in the coronary circulation (see above) have implied that under some conditions critical closing pressure may be 30 to 50 mmHg [3,4,41–46,49]. If one assumes that the effective back pressure to coronary flow is not coronary sinus pressure (2 to 10 mmHg) but rather critical closing pressure (30 to 50 mmHg), the next logical step is to utilize critical closing pressure to determine effective coronary driving pressure. Thus, coronary driving pressure would equal mean aortic pressure minus critical closing pressure instead of mean aortic pressure minus coronary sinus pressure. This issue is further complicated by the finding that certain conditions may shift critical closing pressure to the right or left on the pressure axis without altering coronary conductance, i.e., the slope of the pressure-flow relationship in the coronary circulation (see Figure 4-11). Thus, if an intervention alters the ratio between pressure and flow in the coronary circulation, this may reflect a change in coronary vasomotor tone or a shift in the pressure-flow zero intercept, i.e., critical closing pressure.

Initially, critical closing pressure in the coronary circulation was interpreted in light of the "waterfall concept" of Permutt and Riley [47]. The flow over a waterfall will not change if the level of the river below the falls goes up or down, so long as the level of the river below the falls is lower than the level of the waterfall. By analogy, the waterfall concept as applied to the coronary circulation by Downey and Kirk [48] states that pressure-flow relationships in the coronary circulation will be unaltered by changes in coronary venous or outlet pressure until such pressures exceed the "level of the waterfall." In the coronary circulation, the level of the waterfall reflects the pressure at which a critical segment in the vascular tree closes and stops flow. According to this theory, diastolic left ventricular pressure or coronary sinus pressure would not influence the effective back pressure acting on the coronary circulation unless the waterfall pressure or height were exceeded (see Figure 4-11).

Three recent observations have raised doubt concerning the applicability of the waterfall concept to regulation of the coronary circulation. First, the lowest portion of the pressure-flow relationship in the coronary circulation is concave to the pressure axis (Figure 4-9), and the entire pressure-flow relationship during a long diastole is best fit by a second-order equation [49]. If a single waterfall pressure

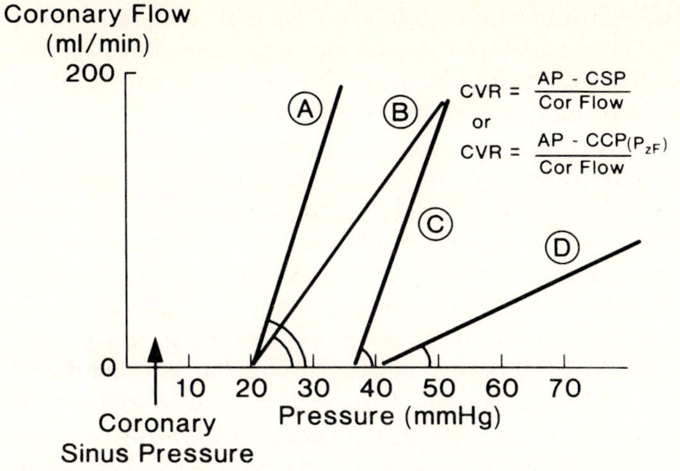

FIGURE 4-11
Diagram which illustrates the potential importance of critical closing pressure (CCP) or the pressure at zero flow (P_{zF}) on the calculation of coronary vascular resistance (CVR). The slopes of the lines reflect coronary conductance the inverse of coronary resistance: the pressure at zero flow represents critical closing pressure, or : P_{zf}. Line D depicts the normal situation. The coronary bed is not dilated because the pressure-flow relationship has a relatively shallow slope. Also, in line D, P_{zF} is almost 40 mmHg. Line A shows a theoretical pressure-flow relationship obtained in a maximally dilated coronary bed. The slope of line A is much steeper than that of line D, and P_{zF} is much lower in line A than in line D (approximately 20 mmHg). Lines B and C illustrate that either P_{zF} or conductance can be responsible for major changes in the pressure-flow relationships. This implies that without knowledge of P_{zF} calculations of resistance or conductance in the coronary bed may be seriously in error. In addition, it is obvious that coronary vasscular resistance will be much different if coronary driving pressure is aortic pressure (AP) — critical closing pressure P_{zF} instead of AP — coronary sinus pressure (CSP). Cor Flow = coronary flow.

existed in the wall of the left ventricle, the lowest portion of the coronary pressure-flow relationship would either be straight or convex to the pressure axis (see Figure 4-9). For the waterfall concept to be compatible with the concave nature of the pressure-flow relationship observed in the coronary circulation, a series of waterfalls across the left ventricle would have to be postulated. Data which have demonstrated that critical closing pressure is higher in the endocardial third than the epicardial third of the left ventricle [3,4] are compatible with the notion that a series of waterfalls may exist across the wall of the left ventricle. A second study which challenges the applicability of the waterfall concept to the coronary circulation has been reported by Bellamy [45]. In this study, it was demonstrated that mild increases in coronary venous pressure produced a rightward shift to the pressure-flow relationship in the coronary bed primarily by altering the zero flow intercept, or critical closing pressure. This result is incompatible with the waterfall concept. In Bellamy's studies, the lowest level of coronary sinus pressure examined was 11 mmHg. Recent studies suggest that when lower pressures are studied (5 to 12 mmHg) it can be shown that small increases in coronary venous pressure do not alter pressure-flow relationship in the coronary circulation [50,51]. Thus, if the waterfall concept is applicable to the coronary circulation, the level or height of the waterfall is probably less than 12 mmHg under normal conditions. Third, there is now unequivocal evidence that reverse flow occurs during systole in coronary arteries [17,26,27]. It is difficult to conceptualize a waterfall that would permit reverse flow, unless one assumes that the waterfall concept is only operative during diastole. In view of the observations cited above, I believe that the waterfall concept as *originally postulated* by Downey and Kirk to explain systolic coronary flow may not be applicable to the coronary circulation. Even if the original postulate was expanded to include a series of waterfalls across the ventricular wall and applied only to diastole, the concept may be of little importance, because the waterfall level, if it exists, is a value that may be only a few millimeters of mercury higher than coronary sinus pressure under normal conditions.

Despite the attention which studies of critical closing pressure currently receive, I believe that present notions about stop-flow pressure in the coronary circulation should be viewed with skepticism. If vasomotor tone in the coronary circulation is normal, current dogma suggests that critical closing pressure, or stop-flow pressure, is 40 to 50 mmHg. This conclusion is based on measurements of pressure and flow in epicardial arteries. It is premature to assume that pressure-flow relationships in proximal epicardial coronary arteries reflect pressure-flow relationships within the myocardium. If pressure-flow relationships at the root of the aorta are compared to pressure-flow relationships in the distal vessels in the limb, vast differences are immediately apparent. Just above the aortic valve, flow is zero throughout diastole, whereas in the periphery flow is continuous throughout the cardiac cycle. This occurs because capacitive forces can permit flow to continue in downstream vessels at a time that flow in the proximal artery has stopped. Eng et al. [35] have recently suggested that coronary capacitance masks the true critical closing pressure in the coronary circulation. Their results suggest that when vasomotor tone in the coronary circulation is normal and capacitance effects are minimized, critical closing pressure is only 2 to 5 mmHg greater than left ventricular end diastolic or coronary sinus pressure (Figure 4-12). This area is controversial because studies by Klocke et al. [49] and Downey et al. [52] do not support the notion that coronary capacitance has a major effect on critical closing pressure. Studies by Nellis et al. [53] indicate that large pressure gradients exist in the epicardial coronary arteries for various diameters. Hence, measurements of coronary pressure in a proximal epicardial artery probably greatly overestimate the pressure in coronary arteries less than 140 μm in diameter [53] (see Figure 1-6). Also, the importance of critical closing pressure in the presence of normal coronary driving pressure is unknown.

Hoffman [54] has called attention to three other difficulties that beset studies concerning measurements of critical closing pressure in the circulation. First, in practice, it is difficult to design experiments where very low flows and pressures in the coronary circulation will be present in the absence of myocardial ischemia.

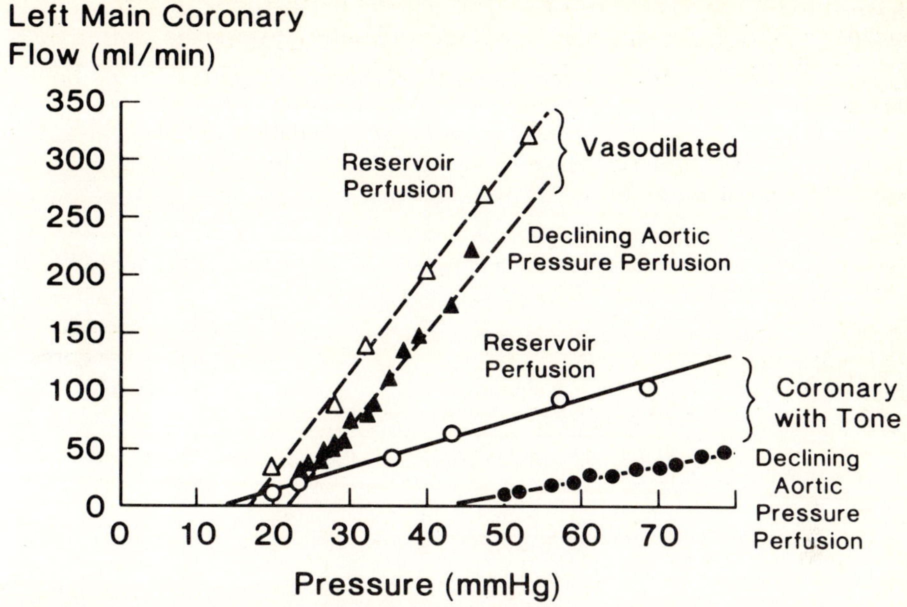

FIGURE 4-12
Pressure-flow relationships during a long diastole as obtained under two conditions: maximal coronary vasodilation (vasodilated) and normal coronary tone (coronary with tone). Aortic pressure was either allowed to decline normally (declining aortic perfusion pressure) or maintained constant at selected levels (reservoir perfusion). Reservoir perfusion minimizes coronary capacitance. When coronary capacitance is minimal, zero-flow pressure in the coronary circulation is decreased, particularly when coronary tone is normal. The data suggest that coronary capacitance contributes importantly to critical closing pressure or pressure at zero coronary flow. (*Redrawn from data originally presented by C Eng et al* [50].)

Second, under most conditions, when pressure and flow are both decreasing in the coronary circulation, tissue blood volume in the left ventricular wall is also declining significantly. These experimental difficulties are critical because ischemia and changes in tissue blood volume may be important independent determinants of the dependent variable being examined, critical closing pressure. Third, as coronary pressure is lowered it is likely that flow will be diverted to regions in the myocardium where "waterfall pressures" are lowest. Hence, pressure at which flow ceases may represent the lowest diastolic waterfall pressure.

In my view, current concepts concerning critical closing pressure should be regarded as tentative until additional experimental data which address the problems noted above become available.

METHODS OF CALCULATING CORONARY VASCULAR RESISTANCE

The formulations for computing coronary vascular resistance are controversial for several reasons: (1) intracoronary flow-dependent pressure gradients are pres-

TABLE 4-1
FORMULAS FOR CALCULATING CORONARY VASCULAR RESISTANCE

	Mean pressure/mean flow relationship
1	$\dfrac{\text{Mean aortic or coronary pressure (mmHg)}}{\text{Mean coronary flow (ml/min or ml/min/100 g)}}$
2	$\dfrac{\text{Mean aortic or coronary pressure} - \text{mean right atrial pressure}}{\text{Mean coronary flow}}$
3	$\dfrac{\text{Mean aortic or coronary pressure} - \text{Left ventricular end diastolic pressure}}{\text{Mean coronary flow}}$
4	$\dfrac{\text{Mean aortic or coronary pressure} - \text{Critical closing pressure}}{\text{Mean coronary flow}}$
	Late diastolic pressure/late diastolic flow relationship
1	$\dfrac{\text{Late diastolic aortic or coronary pressure (mmHg)}}{\text{Late diastolic coronary flow (mmHg)}}$
2	$\dfrac{\text{Late diastolic aortic or coronary pressure} - \text{Late diastolic right atrial pressure}}{\text{Late diastolic coronary flow}}$
3	$\dfrac{\text{Late diastolic aortic or coronary pressure} - \text{Late diastolic left ventricular pressure}}{\text{Late diastolic coronary flow}}$
4	$\dfrac{\text{Late diastolic aortic or coronary pressure} - \text{Critical closing pressure}}{\text{Late diastolic coronary flow}}$
	Pressure-flow relationships

Reciprocal of the slope of the relationship between coronary flow and aortic or coronary pressure

1 During diastole
  a Constant pressure perfusion
  b Declining pressure perfusion
2 During the entire cardiac cycle

ent; (2) extravascular compressive forces are prominent in systole; (3) diastolic coronary flow is impeded by diastolic ventricular pressure; (4) critical closing pressure may modify effective coronary driving pressure; (5) the relative importance of extravascular compressive forces, intraventricular diastolic pressure, and critical closing pressure varies in different transmural layers of ventricle; and (6) disease processes can modify all the factors 1 through 5 noted above for the entire ventricle or for localized regions of the ventricle. These considerations have led to many formulations for computing coronary vascular resistance (see Table 4-1). If a given intervention produces a major (± 50 percent) change in coronary vasomotor tone, the effect will be apparent regardless of the formula employed to calculate coronary vascular resistance. In contrast, when perturbations produce modest changes in coronary vascular resistance ($\pm$ 15 percent), the magnitude and direction of the change may depend on the formulation employed to compute coronary vascular resistance.

None of the present formulations for computing coronary vascular resistance is perfect. Whenever possible, confounding factors, such as end diastolic pressure and extravascular compressive forces, should be held relatively constant. Alternatively, the formula used to compute coronary vascular resistance should include variables that are likely to be changing during the experiment, such as left ventricular end diastolic pressure or right atrial pressure. Reasonably accurate measurements of coronary vascular resistance can be readily obtained in animal experiments because phasic and transmural coronary blood flow can be measured accurately. When coronary vascular resistance is measured in patients, the validity of the calculated values is less certain because computed resistance is usually based on measurements of mean coronary blood flow. Such calculations disregard the potential contributions of extravascular forces and coronary capacitance. In view of these limitations, little credence should be given to minor alterations ($\pm$ 15 percent) in coronary vascular resistance observed in clinical studies.

SUMMARY

This brief review emphasizes the critical importance of aortic pressure, autoregulation, extravascular compressive forces, and critical closing pressure on the regulation of the coronary circulation. Almost all interventions and disease processes that alter the coronary circulation also affect aortic pressure, autoregulation, extravascular compressive forces, and critical closing pressure. Hence, these factors modulate responses of the coronary circulation to almost all perturbations in the system.

REFERENCES

1 Wüsten B, Buss DD, Deist H, Schaper W: Dilatory capacity of the coronary circulation and its correlation to the arterial vasculature in the canine left ventricle. *Basic Res Cardiol* 72: 636, 1977.

2 Guyton RA, McClenathan JH, Newman GE, Michaelis, LL: Significance of subendocardial S-T segment elevation caused by coronary stenosis in the dog. *Am J Cardiol* 40: 373, 1977.

3 Rouleau J, Boerboom LE, Surjadhana A, Hoffman JIE: The role of autoregulation and tissue diastolic pressures in the transmural distribution of left ventricular blood flow in anesthetized dogs. *Circ Res* 45: 804, 1979.

4 Ellis AK, Klocke FJ: Effects of preload on the transmural distribution of perfusion and pressure-flow relationships in the canine coronary vascular bed. *Circ Res* 46: 68, 1979.

5 Berne RM: Cardiodynamics and the coronary circulation in hypothermia. *Ann NY Acad Sci* 80: 365, 1959.

6 Scott JB, Hardin RA, Haddy FJ: Pressure-flow relationships in the coronary vascular bed of the dog. *Am J Physiol* 199: 765, 1960.

7 Cross CE, Rieben PA, Salisbury PF: Coronary driving pressure and vasomotor tonus as determinants of coronary blood flow. *Circ Res* 9: 589, 1961.

8 Shaw RF, Mosher P, Ross J, Joseph JI, Lee ASJ: Physiological principles of coronary perfusion. *J Thoracic Cardiovasc Surg* 44: 608, 1962.

9 Mosher P, Ross J Jr, McFate PA, Shaw RF: Control of coronary blood flow by an autoregulatory mechanism. *Circ Res* 14: 250, 1964.

10 Driscol TE, Moir TW, Eckstein RW: Autoregulation of coronary blood flow: Effect of interarterial pressure gradients. *Circ Res* 15: 103, 1964.

11 Dole WP, Montville WJ, Bishop VS: Dependency of myocardial reactive hyperemia on coronary artery pressure in the dog. *Am J Physiol* 240: H709, 1981.

12 Boatwright RB, Downey HF, Bashour FA, Crystal GJ: Transmural variation in autoregulation of coronary blood flow in hyperperfused canine myocardium. *Circ Res* 47: 599, 1980.

13 Schwartz JS, Carlyle PF, Cohn JN: Effect of dilation of the distal coronary arteries in the dog. *Am J Cardiol* 43: 219, 1979.

14 Santamore WP, Walinsky P: Altered coronary flow responses to vasoactive drugs in the presence of coronary arterial stenosis in the dog. *Am J Cardiol* 45: 276, 1980.

15 Strandgaard S, Jones JV, MacKenzie ET, Harper AM: Upper limit of cerebral blood flow autoregulation in experimental renovascular hypertension in the baboon. *Circ Res* 37: 164, 1975.

16 Johnson PC: The myogenic response, in *Handbook of Physiology*, vol II, *The cardiovascular system. Vascular smooth muscle.* Bethesda, Maryland, American Physiological Society, 1980.

17 Chilian WM, Bohling BA, Marcus ML: Capacitance function of epicardial coronary arteries. *Fed Proc* 40: 603, 1981.

18 Wiggers CJ: The interplay of coronary vascular resistance and myocardial compression in regulating coronary flow. *Circ Res* 2: 271, 1954.

19 Sabiston DC Jr, Gregg DE: Effect of cardiac contraction on coronary blood flow. *Circulation* 15: 14, 1957.

20 Snyder R, Downey JM, Kirk ES: The active and passive components of extravascular coronary resistance. *Cardiovasc Res* 9: 161, 1975.

21 Downey JM, Downey HF, Kirk ES: Effects of myocardial strains on coronary blood flow. *Circ Res* 34: 286, 1974.

21a Bache RJ, Dymek DJ: Local and regional regulation of coronary vascular tone. *Prog Cardiovasc Dis* 24: 191, 1981.

21b Marzilli M, Goldstein S, Sabbah HN, Lee T, Stein PD: Modulating effect of regional myocardial performance on local myocardial perfusion in the dog. *Circ Res* 45: 634, 1979.

22 Gregg DE: *The Coronary Circulation in Health and Disease.* Philadelphia, Lea & Febiger, 1950.

23 Khouri EM, Gregg DE, Rayford CR: Effect of exercise on cardiac output, left coronary flow and myocardial metabolism in the unanesthetized dog. *Circ Res* 17: 427, 1965.

24 Marcus M, Wright C, Doty D, Eastham C, Laughlin D, Krumm P, Fastenow C, Brody M: Measurements of coronary velocity and reactive hyperemia in the coronary circulation of humans. *Circ Res* 49: 877, 1981.

25 White CW, Kerber RE, Weiss HR, Marcus ML: The effects of atrial fibrillation on atrial pressure-volume and flow relationships. *Circ Res* 51: 215, 1982.

26 Chilian WM, Marcus ML: Phasic blood flow velocity in intramural and epicardial coronary arteries. *Circ Res* 50: 775, 1982.

27 Span JAE, Breuls NPW, Laird JD: Diastolic-systolic coronary flow differences are caused by intramyocardial pump action in the anesthetized dog. *Circ Res* 49: 584, 1981.

28 Douglas JE, Greenfield JC Jr: Epicardial coronary artery compliance in the dog. *Circ Res* 27: 921, 1970.

29 Arts T, Kruger RTI, van Garven W, Lambregto GAC, Reneman RS: Propagation velocity and reflection of pressure wave in the coronary artery. *Am J Physiol* 237: H469, 1979.

30 Gow VS, Schonfeld D, Patel DJ: The dynamic elastic properties of the canine left circumflex coronary artery. *J Biomech* 7: 389, 1974.

31 Lewi PJ, Schaper WA: The estimation of coronary volume elasticity in the beating heart of the dog. *Pflugers Arch* 325: 191, 1971.

31a Gow BS, Hadfield CD: The elasticity of canine and human coronary arteries with reference to postmortem changes. *Circ Res* 45: 588, 1979.

32 Vatner SF, Pagani M, Manders WT, Pasipoularides AD: Alpha adrenergic vasoconstriction and nitroglycerin vasodilation of large coronary arteries in the conscious dog. *J Clin Invest* 65: 5, 1980.

33 Lee J, Downey JM, Chambers DE: Coronary artery capacitance. *Physiologist* 24: 26, 1981.

34 Mates RE, Gupta RL, Bell AC, Klocke FJ: Fluid dynamics of coronary artery stenosis. *Circ Res* 42: 152, 1978.

35 Eng C, Jentzer JH, Kirk ES: The effects of the coronary capacitance on the interpretation of diastolic pressure-flow relationships. *Circ Res* 50: 334, 1982.

35a Canty JM, Klocke F, Mates RE: Coronary capacitance calculated from in vivo measurement of diastolic coronary input impedance. *Fed Proc* 41: 1097, 1982.

36 Downey JM, Kirk ES: Distribution of the coronary blood flow across the canine heart wall during systole. *Circ Res* 34: 251, 1974.

37 Hess DS, Bache RJ: Transmural distribution of myocardial blood flow during systole in the awake dog. *Circ Res* 38: 5, 1976.

37a Rembert JC, Greenfield JC Jr, Alexander JA, Cobb FR: Transmural distribution of systolic myocardial blood flow in the awake dog, in *Cardiovascular System Dynamics*, J Baan, A Noodergraaf, J Raines (eds). London, MIT Press, 1978, p 40.

37b Hess DS, Bache RJ: Transmural right ventricular myocardial blood flow during systole in the awake dog. *Circ Res* 45: 88, 1979.

38 Burton AC: Relation of structure to function of walls of blood vessels. *Physiol Rev* 34: 619, 1954.

39 Burton AC: Physical principles of circulatory phenomena: The physical equilibria of the heart and blood vessels, in *Handbook of Physiology*, WF Hamilton (ed). Washington, DC, American Physiological Society, 1962, vol 1, sect 2, Circulation, chap 6, p. 85.

39a Alexander RS: Critical closure reexamined. *Circ Res* 40: 531, 1977.

40 Ehrlich W, Baer RW, Bellamy RF, Randazzo R: Instantaneous femoral artery pressure-flow relations in supine anesthetized dogs and the effect of unilateral elevation of femoral venous pressure. *Circ Res* 47: 88, 1980.

41 Bellamy RF: Diastolic coronary artery pressure-flow relations in the dog. *Circ Res* 43: 92, 1978.

42 Bellamy RF: Calculation of coronary vascular resistance. *Cardiovas Res* 5: 261, 1980.

43 Mueller TM, Sonel A, Fiore AC, Brown JW, Knoebel SB: Interaction of α and β_2 adrenergic tone on coronary diastolic flow-pressure relationship. *Circulation* 64 (suppl III): 63, 1980.

44 Vlahakes GJ, Baer RW, Uhlig PN, Verrier ED, Bristow JD, Hoffman JIE: β-adrenergic influence in the coronary circulation of conscious dogs. *Circulation* 64(suppl IV): 39, 1981.

45 Bellamy RF, Lowensohn HS, Ehrlich W, Baer RW: Effect of coronary sinus occlusion on coronary pressure-flow relations. *Am J Physiol* 239: H57, 1980.

45a Verrier ED, Edelist G, Consigny PM, Robinson S, Hoffman JIE: Greater coronary vascular reserve in dogs anesthetized with halothane. *Anesthesiology* 53: 445, 1980.

46 Gascho J, Alden B, Marcus M: Critical closing pressure in pressure induced left ventricular hypertrophy. *Circulation* 64 (suppl III): III-63, 1980.

47 Permutt S, Riley RL: Hemodynamics of collapsible vessels with tone: The vascular waterfall. *J Appl Physiol* 18: 924, 1963.

48 Downey JB, Kirk ES: Inhibition of coronary blood flow by a vascular waterfall mechanism. *Circ Res* 36: 753, 1975.

49 Klocke FJ, Weinstein IR, Klocke JF, Ellis AK, Kraus DR, Mates RE, Canty JM, Anbar RD, Romanowski RR, Wallmeyer KW, Echt MP: Zero-flow pressures and pressure-flow relationships during single long diastoles in the canine coronary bed before and during maximum vasodilation: Limited influence of capacitive effects. *J Clin Invest* 68: 970, 1981.

50 Eng C, Kirk ES: A vascular waterfall mechanism (VWM) affecting coronary collaterals and ischemic myocardium (IM). *Circulation* 64(suppl IV): IV-38, 1981.

51 Uhlig P, Baer R, Vlahakes G, Hoffman J: Effect of coronary sinus pressure elevation on coronary flow. *Circulation* 64(suppl IV): IV-38, 1981.

52 Downey J, Lee J, Chambers D: Coronary critical closing pressure corrected for coronary capacitance effects. *Physiologist* 24: 26, 1981.

53 Nellis SH, Liedtke AJ, Whitesell L: Small coronary vessel pressure and diameter in an intact beating rabbit heart using fixed-position and free-notion techniques. *Circ Res* 49: 342, 1981.

54 Hoffman JIE: Why is myocardial ischaemia so commonly subendocardial? *Clin Sci* (London) 61: 657, 1981.

CHAPTER **5**

TRANSMURAL DISTRIBUTION OF MYOCARDIAL PERFUSION

In 1967, Rudolph and Heyman [1] introduced the labeled microsphere technique. Although a few studies of transmural perfusion were performed prior to 1967 with diffusible indicators (see Chapter 2), the labeled microsphere technique afforded numerous investigators the opportunity to undertake extensive studies of regional myocardial perfusion. Since 1967, knowledge concerning the distribution of coronary flow to various cardiac chambers and to discrete layers of the ventricular walls has grown rapidly. A general understanding of the factors that regulate the transmural distribution of myocardial perfusion has emerged. It is now widely held that factors that regulate the distribution of coronary flow within the ventricular wall as well as total coronary flow are of critical importance in understanding mechanisms that regulate the coronary circulation.

TRANSMURAL DISTRIBUTION OF MYOCARDIAL PERFUSION: BASIC DETERMINANTS

The major determinants which effect the transmural distribution of coronary blood flow are vascular geometry, coronary vascular tone, coronary driving pressure, intramyocardial tissue pressure, and blood viscosity. Each is discussed below in some detail.

Vascular Geometry

The transmural distribution of the vasculature of the right ventricular free wall has not been extensively examined. Capillary density in the right ventricle is similar to that of the left ventricle [2,3].

Several types of studies have been directed toward assessing the transmural distribution of coronary vessels in the left ventricle (see Chapter 1). Although capillary density has been reported to be similar in the subendocardial and subepicardial thirds of the left ventricular wall [3–5], the concentration of alkaline phosphatase, an enzyme which occurs primarily in endothelial cells, is greatest in the inner layers of the left ventricular wall [6]. In addition, resistance vessels greater than 15 μm in diameter are more abundant in the left ventricular subendocardium than in the subepicardium (see Figure 1-6). Maximal diastolic conductance in the left ventricle is twofold greater in the inner sixth of the wall than the outer sixth [7,7a]. *Thus, in the normal left ventricle, the density of the vasculature is greatest in the subendocardium.* This anatomic arrangement compensates, in part, for the decrease in effective driving force to vessels in the inner layers of the wall of the left ventricle.

Vascular Tone

The vasomotor state of resistance vessels in various layers of the ventricle wall has an enormous effect on the transmural distribution of myocardial perfusion. This factor would be of lesser importance if the coronary vasculature responded in a homogenous way to pharmacologic, neural, humoral, and autoregulatory influences. Just the opposite is true. Coronary vessels in different layers of the left ventricular myocardium respond in a heterogenous fashion to drugs (see Chapter 22), neural stimuli (see Chapter 6), and humoral substances (see Chapter 8). Under normal conditions, in the left ventricle the metabolic requirements of the subendocardium are greater than those of the subepicardium (see Chapter 3). Finally, disease states often primarily involve the subendocardium. *The differential responsiveness of coronary vessels in various layers of the left ventricle to a host of stimuli promotes heterogenous vascular resistance across the wall of the left ventricle.*

Coronary Driving Pressure

Energy is required to drive blood through the conduit coronary vessels. Hence, the driving head of pressure is greater at the orifice of the left main coronary artery than in more distal surface branches of this vessel. At normal flow rates, the pressure gradient across large surface coronary vessels is 2 to 5 mmHg [8–9c]. At peak flow rates this gradient can exceed 20 mmHg [8]. In contrast, in the brain there is a 40 mmHg pressure gradient across relatively large vessels (3 mm to 300 μm in diameter [10-11]). Measurements of pressure in small subepicardial vessels (less than 140 μm) in the right and left ventricles indicate that the pressure gradient within coronary vessels proximal to the arterioles may be as great as 30 to 50 mmHg [9,12] (see Figure 1-6). Thus, a significant portion of total coronary vascular resistance is controlled by vessels much larger than arterioles. Consequently, aortic pressure substantially overestimates effective coronary driving pressure at a level in the coronary bed that is proximal to coronary arterioles. The magnitude of this overestimation at varying flow rates remains to be determined.

The effective driving pressure is intravascular pressure minus coronary venous or critical closing pressure (see Chapter 4). In the left ventricle, critical closing pressures vary in different layers of the ventricular wall and in different segments of the cardiac cycle (see Chapter 4).

Intramyocardial Tissue Pressure

Intramyocardial tissue pressure gradients modulate the transmural distribution of the coronary blood flow. It is unfortunate that no method of measuring intramyocardial pressure directly is completely satisfactory [13–20a]. Consequently, the transmural distribution of intramyocardial pressure remains controversial. Most investigators agree that during systole intramyocardial pressure is greater in the endocardial third of the left ventricle than in the epicardial third [21,22]. At peak systole, intramyocardial pressure in the deeper layers of the left ventricle is probably equal or greater than intracavitary pressure [21,22]. During diastole, intramyocardial pressures are much lower (4 to 20 mmHg) than those obtained in systole. Direct measurements indicate that during diastole, tissue pressures are not related to the depth in the left ventricular wall [15–17,21–23]. Regional flows, measured during a prolonged diastole, indicate that stop-flow pressure is greater in the deeper layers than in the more superficial layers of the left ventricle. This indirect assessment of tissue pressure implies that during diastole a significant gradient exists across the wall of the left ventricle [7,24,25]. Although there is general agreement that intramyocardial pressure in systole (and possibly diastole) is greatest in the deeper layers of the left ventricle, a precise definition of this transmural gradient under a variety of conditions is unavailable. Information pertaining to the transmural distribution of myocardial pressures in the right ventricle has not been reported.

If one assumes that aortic pressure adequately represents intravascular pressure in both superficial and deep coronary vessels, the autoregulatory capacity of the various layers of the left ventricle is heterogenous (Figure 4-2). Subendocardial vessels do not autoregulate as well as subepicardial vessels. It is likely, however, that this apparent shift in the autoregulatory capacity across the wall of the left ventricle does not reflect fundamental differences in the characteristics of the smooth muscle in superficial and deep vessels within the myocardium. The observed leftward shift of the autoregulatory curve (see Figure 4-2) of subendocardial vessels could occur because the effective driving pressure in these vessels is much less than that in the superficial vascular channels.

Blood Viscosity

Hydraulic principles indicate that blood viscosity must contribute to vascular resistance and, thereby, alter effective coronary driving pressure. In practice, changes in viscosity are inconsequential except during marked anemia or profound polycythemia (see Chapter 14). Stauer has shown that coronary reserve is normal in patients with hyperviscosity syndromes secondary to hyperproteinemia [26]. Only mild abnormalities in the transmural distribution of left ventricular perfusion can be induced by normovolemic polycythemia (see Chapter 15). Hence, under most circumstances, the effects of changes in blood viscosity on the transmural distribution of coronary blood flow can be neglected.

A broad outline of the factors which contribute to gradients of transmural coronary driving pressure and intramyocardial tissue pressures is available. A detailed quantitative description of these factors is needed.

TRANSMURAL DISTRIBUTION OF MYOCARDIAL PERFUSION UNDER NORMAL CONDITIONS

No major differences in the transmural distribution of myocardial perfusion of the left ventricle have been observed in mammals that range in size from less than 100 g to over 100 kg [27-30]. Studies of awake animals in the resting state have found that blood flow to the endocardial third of the left ventricle measured with microspheres exceeds perfusion to the epicardial third. In most studies in awake dogs, the subendocardial/subepicardial perfusion ratio is 1.1 to 1.4:1 (Figure 5-1) [2,22,27–31]. In the anesthetized dog with tachycardia, the ratio of flow to the subendocardial third and the subepicardial third of the left ventricle is usually 0.8 to 1.1:1 [32–36]. Although differences in heart rate may contribute to these discrepancies, at present, it is not certain why subendocardial/subepicardial flow ratios in the left ventricle are consistently lower in anesthetized than awake dogs. Flow is distributed evenly to various walls (septum, anterior, lateral, posterior) and apex-to-base segments of the left ventricle (Figure 5-1) [22,28,30–36].

There is no precise method for measuring the transmural distribution of myocardial perfusion in humans. In anesthetized primates, studies with labeled microspheres indicate that flow across the wall of the left ventricle is evenly distributed [36a]. In humans, crude estimates of the transmural distribution of left ventricular perfusion have been obtained with tomographic thallium 201 scintigrams [37] and studies of the distribution of $^{14}NH_4$[38] (see Figure 2-15). The data support the notion that blood flow is probably distributed homogeneously from the subepicardium to the subendocardium in the left ventricle of normal humans.

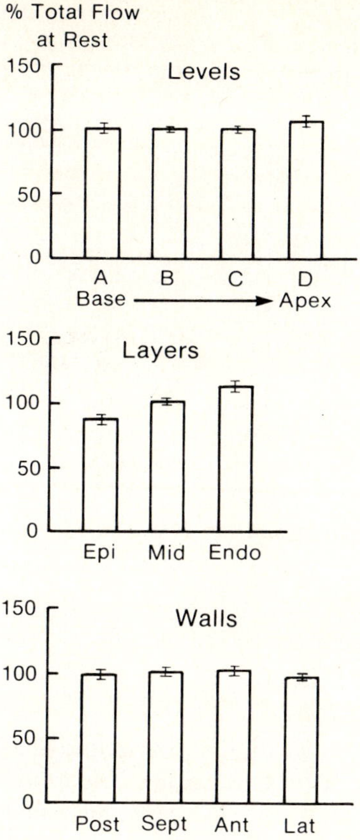

FIGURE 5-1
Relative perfusion to various regions of the left ventricle in awake dogs. (*Top*) Perfusion from base to apex and (*bottom*) to various walls of the left ventricle was remarkably uniform. The endocardial third of the left ventricular wall (Endo) receives more flow than the middle third (Mid) or epicardial (Epi) third (*middle*). Post = posterior wall; Sept = interventricular septum; Ant = anterior wall; Lat = lateral wall. (*Redrawn from data originally presented by TM Mueller et al* [*31*].)

Why is flow in the deeper layers of the left ventricular wall greater than that in the epicardium in most manuals? This reflects the gradient of metabolism that exists across the wall of the left ventricle (see Chapter 3). Calculated wall stress and oxygen consumption are greater in the deeper than in the superficial layers of the left ventricle (see Chapter 3).

The transmural distribution of flow to the right ventricle has been measured in awake dogs, lambs, and calves [2,29,39-42]. Perfusion of the right ventricular subendocardium is 10 to 20 percent greater than that of the right ventricular subepicardium in the awake dog.

Under normal conditions. the resting flow per gram in the right ventricle is about two-thirds of that in the left ventricle [2,39–42]. Flow per gram in the atria is about one-half of that in the right ventricle [43–45,50]. In absolute terms, because of differences in mass, the left ventricle, right ventricle, and atria receive 78 percent, 16 percent, and 6 percent, respectively, of total flow to the heart (Figure 5-2) [45,50].

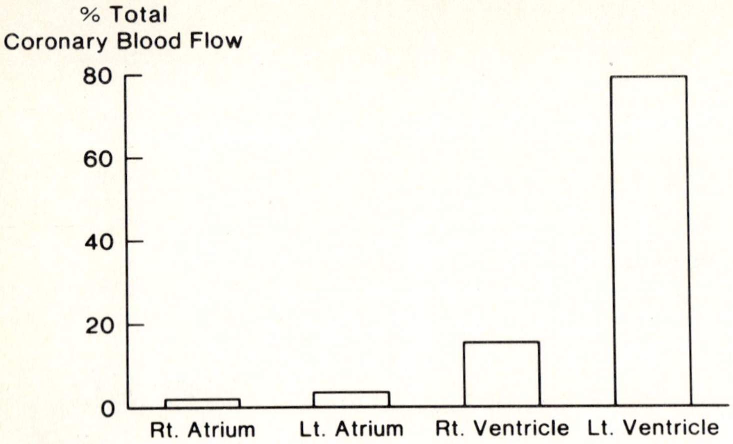

FIGURE 5-2
Distribution of coronary blood flow to the cardiac chambers in anesthetized dogs. The left ventricle receives about three-quarters of total coronary blood flow under normal conditions. (*Redrawn from data originally presented by CW White et al* [45].)

APPROACHES TO PREDICTING THE TRANSMURAL DISTRIBUTION OF MYOCARDIAL PERFUSION IN THE LEFT VENTRICLE

A simple equation for predicting the transmural distribution of myocardial perfusion in the left ventricle would have considerable practical value. Therefore, several investigators have attempted to develop a mathematical expression that would predict the transmural distribution of left ventricular perfusion under a variety of conditions.

In 1968, Griggs and Nakamura described a coronary ventricular pressure index [46]. The index was calculated by dividing the area under the coronary arterial pressure curve throughout the cardiac cycle by the area under the left ventricular pressure curve in systole (Figure 5-3). In essence, the index relates coronary supply (integrated coronary driving pressure) to an approximate index of myocardial oxygen demand. Under tightly controlled conditions, a marked fall in this index was associated with a relative decrease in subendocardial perfusion (Figure 5-4). *Subendocardial underperfusion occurred only when the autoregulatory capacity of subendocardial vessels had been exhausted* [46].

In 1972, Buckberg et al. [34] published an equation for predicting transmural left ventricular perfusion which was a slight modification of that suggested by Griggs and Nakamura. Buckberg et al. suggested that the DPTI/SPTI ratio (DPTI means Diastolic Pressure Time Index; SPTI means Systolic Pressure Time Index) might predict the transmural distribution of left ventricular perfusion under a variety of conditions (Figure 5-3). In anesthetized dogs, Buckberg et al. measured regional myocardial flow with labeled microspheres and varied the DPTI:SPTI ratio over a broad range with a variety of hemodynamic perturbations. At

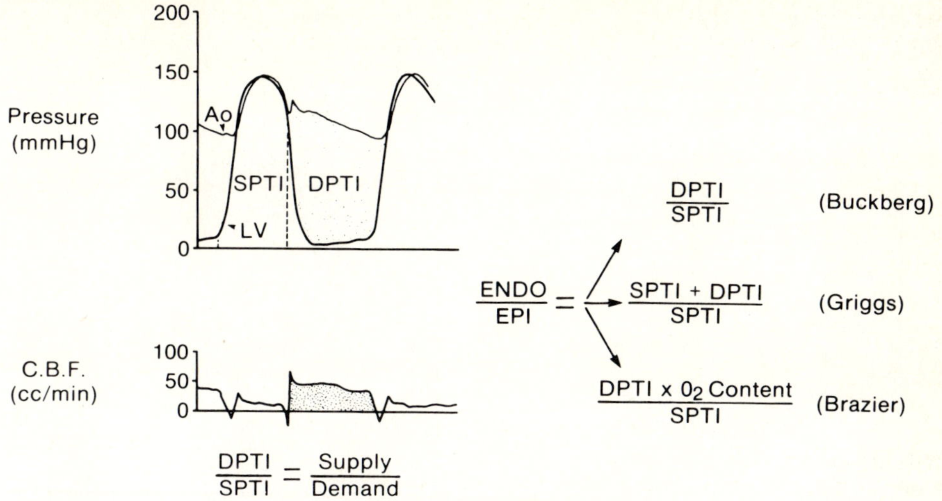

FIGURE 5-3
Three indices proposed to predict the transmural distribution of left ventricular perfusion in normal dogs. Conceptually, the systolic pressure time index (SPTI) relates to the demand for coronary blood flow (C.B.F.); the diastolic pressure time index (DPTI) relates to the supply of coronary blood flow which is delivered primarily during diastole. All three indices (34, 46, 47) are closely related. Ao = aortic pressure recording; LV = left ventricular pressure recording; ENDO = subendocardial layer of the left ventricle; EPI = subepicardial layer of the left ventricle; O_2 content = the arterial oxygen content. (*Based on an illustration originally presented by JIE Hoffman and GD Buckberg* [22].)

DPTI:SPTI ratios of less than 0.8, there was a linear relationship between the proposed index and the left ventricular subendocardial/subepicardial flow ratio (Figure 5-4). *In these experiments, a relative decrease in subendocardial flow occurred only after maximal dilation of the coronary bed had ensued.* In 1974, Brazier, Cooper, and Buckberg [47] modified this equation for predicting transmural perfusion in the left ventricle. The modified formulation included an estimate of arterial oxygen saturation in the denominator of the equation (Figure 5-3). This modification was required because it was found that anemia or hypoxia caused a leftward shift of the relationship between the DPTI/SPTI ratio and the subendocardial/subepicardial flow ratio in the left ventricle (Figure 5-5).

The proposed equations for predicting the transmural distribution of left ventricular perfusion have been very provocative. Many investigators have been stimulated to direct their research efforts to this important area. In addition, the formulations have crystallized the most critical determinants of the transmural distribution of left ventricular perfusion. Thus, these indices have served a useful purpose.

In 1976, Hoffman and Buckberg [22] listed several potential deficiencies of the DPTI/SPTI ratio. The index does not consider possible contributions of inertial factors, coronary capacitance (Chapter 4), or blood viscosity (Chapter 14). In 1976, the importance of coronary capacitance was less well appreciated than at

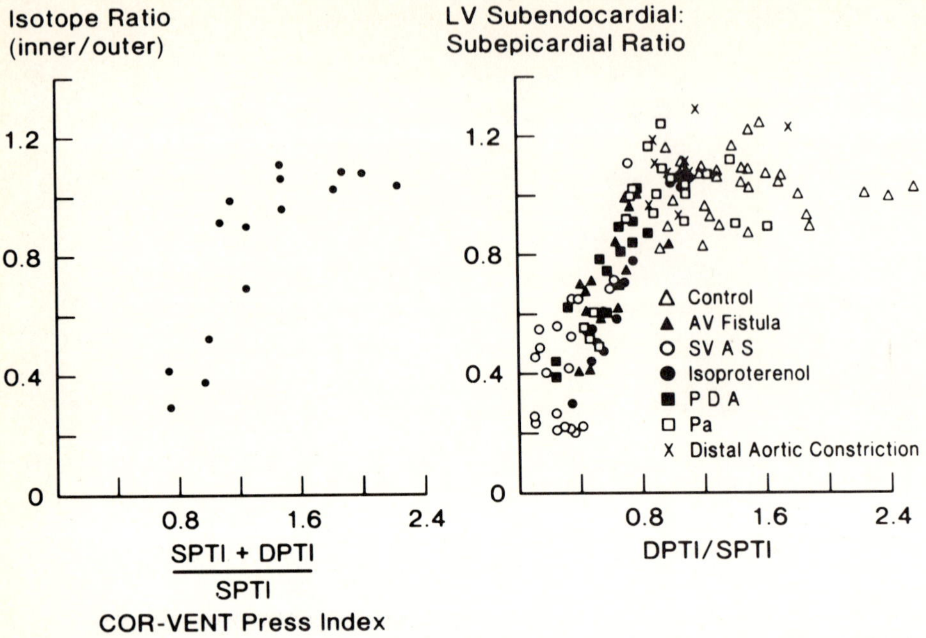

FIGURE 5-4
Relationship between two indices, Griggs (*left*) and Buckberg (*right*), and the transmural distribution of left ventricular perfusion in anesthetized dogs. When either index falls below a critical value, there is a linear relationship between the distribution of transmural perfusion to the wall of the left ventricle and the value of the index. This figure emphasizes the similarity of these two indices. Inner/outer ratio = the ratio of isotope concentration in the inner and outer halves of the left ventricular wall; left ventricular subendocardial: subepicardial ratio = the left ventricular ratio of perfusion to the subendocardial one-third of the left ventricle versus the subepicardial one-third of the left ventricle. SPTI = systolic pressure time index: DPTI = diastolic pressure time index; COR-VENT Press Index = coronary ventricular pressure index; AV Fistula = arterial venous fistula; SVAS = supravalvular aortic stenosis; isoproterenol = IV infusion of isoproterenol; PDA = patent ductus arteriosus; Pa = pacing. (*Redrawn from data presented by DM Griggs Jr and Y Nakamura (left)* [46] *and GD Buckberg et al (right)* [34].)

present. The equation proposed by Buckberg et al. assumes that stop-flow pressure in the coronary circulation is similar to left ventricular diastolic pressure and is relatively uniform across the left ventricular wall. Several studies [7,24,25] have shown that this assumption is invalid. The term used to estimate myocardial oxygen consumption, SPTI, is insensitive to the effects of changes in contractility on myocardial oxygen consumption and to the effects of chronic changes in left ventricular wall thickness on wall stress and oxygen consumption [48–49a]. In addition, recent studies have clearly shown that pathologic states such as cardiac hypertrophy can alter the transmural distribution of ventricular perfusion (Chapter 13). The index suggested by Buckberg et al. is useful only when coronary reserve has been exhausted. Recent studies indicate that drugs (Chapter 22), neural stimuli (Chapter 5), and pathological states such as cardiac hypertrophy

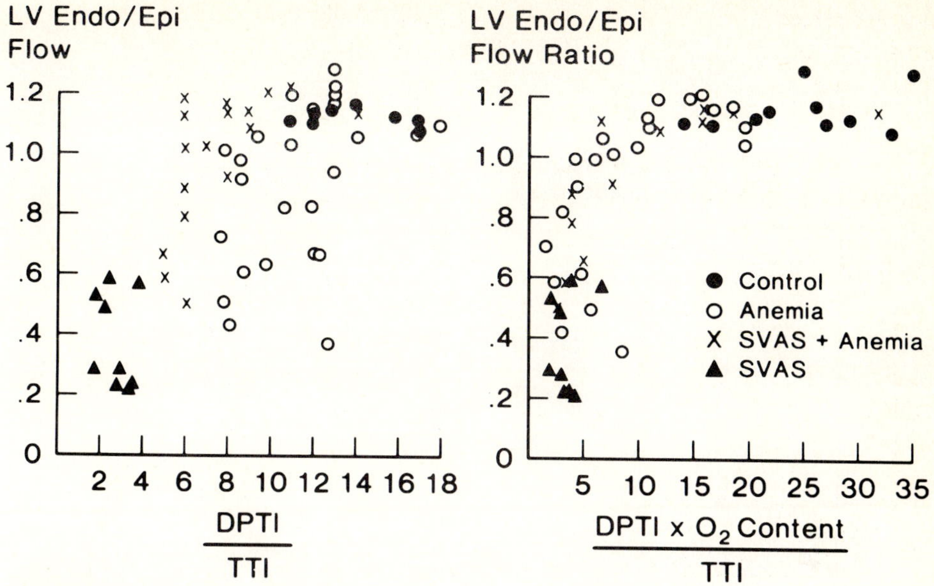

FIGURE 5-5
Relationship between two indices, Buckberg (*left*) and Brazier (*right*), and the transmural distribution of left ventricular perfusion in anesthetized dogs. Both parts of the figure present data from the same experiments analyzed in different ways. It is obvious that in the presence of large variations in the hemoglobin concentration, the Buckberg index cannot accurately predict the transmural distribution of left ventricular perfusion. Including arterial oxygen content (O_2 content) in the numerator of the formulation, as suggested by Brazier, corrects for this deficiency. LV Endo/Epi flow = the ratio of myocardial perfusion in the subendocardial third to the subepicardial third of the ventricle wall. SVAS = supravalvular aortic stenosis; TTI = tension time index; DPTI = diastolic pressure time index. (*Redrawn from data presented by J Brazier et al* [47].)

(Chapter 13) can alter the transmural distribution of left ventricular perfusion long before coronary reserve has been exhausted. *Thus, attempts to use an oversimplified formulation for predicting transmural left ventricular perfusion in patients with chronic heart disease are unwarranted at present. When sufficient knowledge is accumulated, it may be possible to develop a model that can accurately predict transmural distribution of left ventricular perfusion over a broad range of conditions.*

SPECIFIC STATES IN WHICH THE TRANSMURAL DISTRIBUTION OF LEFT VENTRICULAR PERFUSION IS ALTERED

The complexity of the mechanisms that control the transmural distribution of ventricular perfusion is vividly demonstrated by reviewing the effects of a single hemodynamic perturbation (change in heart rate) of the transmural distribution of left ventricular blood flow.

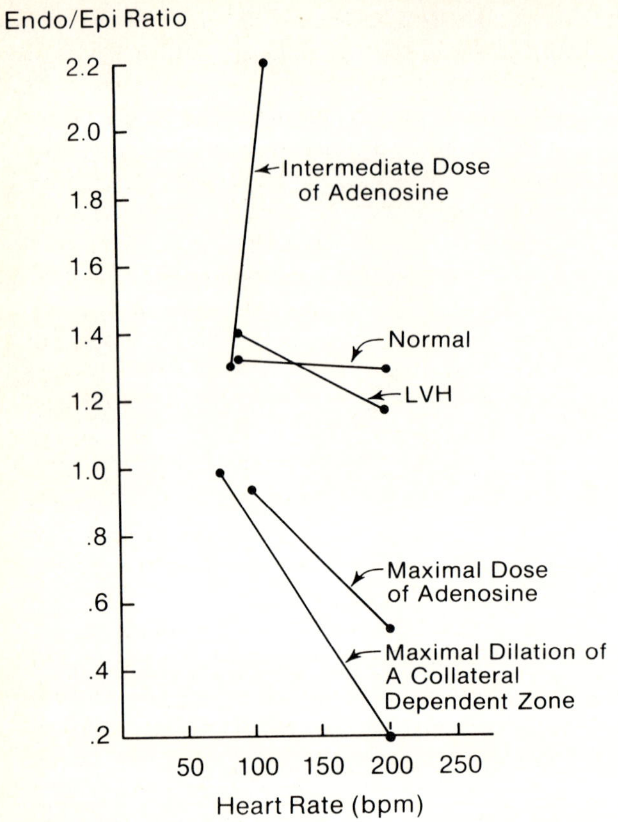

FIGURE 5-6
Effects of tachycardia produced during various conditions on the transmural distribution of left ventricular perfusion; Endo = subendocardial perfusion; Epi = subepicardial perfusion; Normal = normal awake dogs [31]; LVH = awake dogs with left ventricular hypertrophy secondary to renal hypertension (31). Maximal Dose of Adenosine = awake normal dogs paced during an intravenous infusion of a maximal dose of adenosine [54]. Collateral dependent zone = zone of myocardium supplied by mature collaterals in an isolated heart preparation in which maximal coronary dilation was achieved with an adenosine infusion [58]; Intermediate dose of adenosine = reflex tachycardia in awake dogs receiving an intermediate dose of adenosine [56]. bpm = beats per minute. The illustration emphasizes the wide range of alterations in the Endo/Epi ratio that occur when tachycardia is present under diverse conditions.

Effects of Tachycardia

When a normal left ventricle is subjected to tachycardia (80-200 beats per minute), coronary blood flow increases about twofold [3,34,50–55]. The effects on the transmural distribution of left ventricular perfusion are variable (Figure 5-6). If a normal awake dog is subjected to tachycardia, a mild alteration in the transmural distribution of left ventricular perfusion occurs. Typically, the ratio of subendocardial-to-subepicardial perfusion is 1.3:1 at a heart rate of 60 to 80 beats/min and 1.2:1 at a heart rate of 200 beats/min (Figure 5-6) [31,50,54–55]. If the coronary circulation is maximally dilated with adenosine, tachycardia is associated with relative underperfusion of the inner layers of the left ventricle (Figure 5-6) [31,54-56]. When an intermediate dose of adenosine is administered, coronary dilation is less intense and the reflex tachycardia that accompanies the adenosine infusion is associated with a marked increase in the subendocardial/subepicardial perfusion ratio in the left ventricle (Figure 5-5) [56]. (It should be noted that this increase in the subendocardial/subepicardial flow ratio during adenosine infusion primarily depends on the differential pharmacologic effects of intermediate doses of adenosine on transmural vessels rather than the associated changes in heart rate.) Coronary collateral flow under some conditions is impaired by tachycardia [57,58]. This limitation is greatest in the subendocardium and in native as opposed to mature or stimulated coronary collateral vessels [57,58]. (Tachycardia does not limit flow in mature coronary collaterals unless the coronary vessels are maximally dilated [see Chapter 10]). If left ventricular hypertrophy secondary to systemic hypertension is present, the effects of tachycardia on the ratio of perfusion to the subendocardium and subepicardium are slightly exaggerated (Figure 5-6) [31,55]. When tachycardia is present in dogs with marked anemia or acutely superimposed severe supravalvular stenosis, marked subendocardial perfusion abnormalities have been reported [51,59]. *The broad variations in transmural perfusion of the left ventricle that occur during the conditions described above (see Figure 5-6) underline the futility of applying simple formulations to predicting the transmural distribution of left ventricular perfusion.*

Intense, sudden strenuous exercise in patients with normal hearts is associated with transient S-T depression [60] and a transient decrease in left ventricular function [61]. In association with tachycardia, sudden severe exercise is associated with acute hypertension and a prolongation of the duration of systole. This clinical phenomenon is reminiscent of the "Anrep effect" described many years ago in animal studies [62–65]. In these earlier experiments a sudden increase in afterload was associated with a substantial decrease in left ventricular performance, which improved toward control within seconds to minutes [62–65]. Studies of regional left ventricular perfusion suggest that this initial decrease in left ventricular performance which accompanies a sudden increase in afterload is secondary to subendocardial underperfusion [66]. As the perfusion abnormalities abate, left ventricular performance improves [66]. Although these effects are interesting, the Anrep effect probably occurs rarely in humans because of the intensity of the stimulus required to elicit this response.

Other Hemodynamic States Associated with Abnormalities in the Transmural Distribution of Left Ventricular Perfusion

Many conditions have been associated with alterations in the transmural left ventricle perfusion [22,32,33]. In general, these situations alter one or more of the basic factors (vascular geometry, vasomotor tone, coronary driving pressure, tissue pressure or blood viscosity) that regulate transmural perfusion.

When coronary reserve is normal, transmural perfusion is usually not altered unless mutiple factors that determine the distribution of coronary blood flow are effected in an adverse fashion. For example, although tachycardia will modestly decrease relative perfusion to the subendocardium in normal hearts, intense tachycardia, anemia, and severe supravalvular aortic stenosis combined can profoundly decrease perfusion in the inner layers of a normal left ventricle. The opposite situation occurs in ventricles with limited coronary reserves. Under such conditions, often mild alterations in one parameter, i.e., mild tachycardia, will produce striking evidence of subendocardial ischemia (see Chapters 11 and 13).

SUMMARY

The principal factors that modulate the transmural distribution of left ventricular perfusion in animals have been identified and knowledge concerning their quantitative importance under a variety of conditions is rapidly accumulating. Because there is no method available to assess accurately the transmural distribution of perfusion in humans, statements concerning the distribution of coronary blood flow across the ventricular wall in patients are based on inference. Prudence dictates that these inferences should be regarded as rough estimates that must be confirmed by direct measurements of the transmural distribution of coronary blood flow in humans when appropriate methods become available. There is reason to believe that in the 1980s, relatively precise estimates of the transmural perfusion of left ventricular perfusion in humans will be obtainable with either positron emission tomography, enhanced computed x-ray tomography, or true tomographic scintigrams with gamma emitters (Chapter 2).

REFERENCES

1 Rudolph AM, Heymann MA: The circulation of the fetus in utero: Methods for studying distribution of blood flow, cardiac output and organ blood flow. *Circ Res* 21: 163, 1967.

2 Murray PA, Baig H, Fishbein MC, Vatner SF: Effects of experimental right ventricular hypertrophy on myocardial blood flow in conscious dogs. *J Clinic Invest* 64: 421, 1979.

3 O'Keefe DD, Hoffman JIE, Cheitlin R, O'Neill MJ, Allard JR, Shapkin E: Coronary blood flow in experimental canine left ventricular hypertrophy. *Circ Res* 43: 43, 1978.

4 Tomanek RJ: The role of prevention or relief of pressure overload on the myocardial cell of the spontaneously hypertensive rat. *Lab Invest* 40: 83, 1979.

5 Lund DD, Tomanek RJ: Myocardial morphology in spontaneously hypertensive and aortic constricted rats. *Am J Anat* 152: 141, 1978.

6 Dowell RT: Hemodynamic factors and vascular density as potential determinants of blood flow in hypertrophied rat heart. *Proc Soc Exp Biol Med* 154: 423, 1977.

7 Verrier ED, Baer RW, Hickey RF, Vlahakes GJ, Hoffman JIE: Transmural

pressure-flow relations during diastole in the canine left ventricle. *Circulation* 62: III-62, 1980.

7a Wusten B, Buss DD, Deist H, Schaper W: Dilatory capacity of the coronary circulation and its correlation to the arterial vasculature in the canine left ventricle. *Basic Res Cardiol* 72: 636, 1977.

8 Bellamy RF: Diastolic coronary artery pressure-flow relations in the dog. *Circ Res* 43: 92, 1978.

9 Nellis SH, Liedtke AJ, Whitesell L: Small coronary vessel pressure and diameter in an intact beating rabbit heart using fixed-position and free-motion techniques. *Circ Res* 49: 342, 1981.

9a Cohen MV, Kirk ES: Differential response of large and small coronary arteries to nitroglycerin and angiotensin. *Circ Res* 33: 445, 1972.

9b Fam WM, McGregor M: Effect of nitroglycerin and dipyridamole on regional coronary resistance. *Circ Res* 22: 649, 1968.

9c Winbury MM, Howe BW, Hefner MA: Effect of nitrates and other coronary dilators on large and small coronary vessels: An hypothesis for the mechanism of action of nitrates. *J Pharmacol Exp Ther* 168: 70, 1969.

10 Heistad DD, Marcus ML, Abboud FM: Role of large arteries in regulation of cerebral blood flow in dogs. *J Clin Invest* 62: 761, 1978.

11 Stromberg DD, Fox JR: Pressures in the pial arterial microcirculation of the cat during changes in systemic arterial blood pressure. *Circ Res* 31: 229, 1972.

12 Tillmanns H, Steinhausen M, Leinberger H, Thederan H, Kubler W: Pressure measurements in the terminal vascular bed of the epimyocardium of rats and cats. *Circ Res* 49: 1202, 1981.

13 Johnson JR, Di Palma JR: Intramyocardial pressure and its relationship to aortic blood pressure. *Am J Physiol* 125: 234, 1939.

14 Gregg DE, Eckstein RW: Measurements of intramyocardial pressure. *Am J Physiol* 132: 781, 1941.

15 D'Silva JL, Mendel D, Winterton MC: Determinants of intramyocardial pressure in the cat. *Am J Physiol* 207: 1117, 1964.

16 Salisbury PF, Cross CE, Rieben PA: Intramyocardial pressure and strength of left ventricular contraction. *Circ Res* 10: 608, 1962.

17 Kirk ES, Honig CR: Experimental and theoretical analysis of myocardial tissue pressure. *Am J Physiol* 207: 361, 1964.

18 Baird RJ, Manktelow RT, Shah PA, Ameli FM: Intramyocardial pressure: A study of its regional variations and its relationship to intraventricular pressure. *J Thorac Cardiovasc Surg* 59: 810, 1970.

19 Brandi G, McGregor M: Intramural pressure in the left ventricle of the dog. *Cardiovasc Res* 3: 472, 1969.

20 Archie JP: Determinants of intramyocardial pressure. *J Surg Res* 19: 338, 1973.

20a Stein PD, Marzilli M, Sabbah HN, Lee T: Systolic and diastolic pressure gradients within the left ventricular wall. *Am J Physiol* 238: H625, 1980.

21 Hoffman JIE: The effect of intramyocardial forces on the distribution of intramyocardial blood flow. *J Biomed Eng* 1: 33, 1979.

22 Hoffman JIE, Buckberg GD: Transmural variations in myocardial perfusion, in *Progress in Cardiology*, PN Yu, JF Goodwin (eds). Philadelphia, Lea & Febiger, 1976, chap 3, p 37.

23 Van Der Meer, JJ, Reneman RS: The relation of intramyocardial pressure (IMP) to coronary blood flow (CBF). Seventh European Conference Microcirculation, Aberdeen, 1972. Part I. *Bibl Anat* 11: 151, 1973.

24 Ellis AK, Klocke FJ: Effects of preload on the transmural distribution of perfusion and pressure-flow relationships in the canine coronary vascular bed. *Circ Res* 46: 68, 1979.

25 Rouleau J, Boerboom LE, Surjadhana A, Hoffman JIE: The role of autoregulation and tissue diastolic pressures in the transmural distribution of left ventricular blood flow in anesthetized dogs. *Circ Res* 45: 804, 1979.

26 Strauer B-E: Personal communication. Department of Medicine, University of Munich, June 1980.

27 Wangler RD, Peters KG, Marcus ML, Tomanek RJ: Effects of duration and severity of arterial hypertension on cardiac hypertrophy and coronary vasodilator reserve. *Circ Res* 51: 10, 1982.

28 Fedor M, McIntosh DM, Rembert JC, Greenfield JC Jr: Coronary and transmural myocardial blood flow responses in awake domestic pigs. *Am J Physiol* 235: H435, 1978.

29 Manohar M, Thurmon JC, Tranquilli WJ, Devous MD Sr, Theodorakis MC, Shawley RV, Feller DL, Benson JG: Regional myocardial blood flow and coronary vascular reserve in unanesthetized young calves with severe concentric right ventricular hypertrophy. *Circ Res* 48: 785, 1981.

30 Cobb FR, Bache RJ, Greenfield JC Jr: Regional myocardial blood flow in awake dogs. *J Clin Invest* 53: H1618, 1974.

31 Mueller TM, Marcus ML, Kerber RE, Young YA, Barnes RW, Abboud FM: Effect of renal hypertension and left ventricular hypertrophy on the coronary circulation in dogs. *Circ Res* 42: 543, 1978.

32 Hoffman JIE: Determinants and prediction of transmural myocardial perfusion. *Circulation* 58: 381, 1978.

33 Hoffman JIE, Buckberg GD: The myocardial supply: Demand ratio—a critical review. *Am J Cardiol* 41: 327, 1978.

34 Buckberg GD, Fixler DE, Archie JP, Hoffman JIE: Experimental subendocardial ischemia in dogs with normal coronary arteries. *Circ Res* 30: 67, 1972.

35 Tripp MR, Meyer MW, Einzig S, Leonard JJ, Swayze CR, Fox IJ: Simultaneous regional myocardial blood flows by tritiated water and microspheres. *Am J Physiol* 232: H173, 1977.

36 Falsetti HL, Carroll RJ, Marcus ML: Temporal heterogeneity of myocardial blood flow in anesthetized dogs. *Circulation* 52: 848, 1975.

36a Marcus ML, Armstrong ML, Heistad DD, Eastham CL, Mark AL: Comparison of three methods of evaluating coronary obstructive lesions: Postmortem arteriography, pathological examination and measurement of regional myocardial perfusion during maximal vasodilation. *Am J Cardiol* 49: 1699, 1982.

37 Vogel RA, Kirch DL, LeFree MT, Rainwater JO, Jensen DP, Steel PP: Thallium-201 myocardial perfusion scintigraphy: Results of standard and multi-pinhole tomographic techniques. *Am J Cardiol* 43: 787, 1979.

38 Schelbert HR, Phelps ME, Hoffman EJ, Huang S-C, Selin CE, Kuhl DE: Regional myocardial perfusion assessed with n-13 labeled ammonia and positron emission computerized axial tomography. *Am J Cardiol* 43: 209, 1979.

39 Domenech RJ, Ayuy AH: Total and regional coronary blood flow during acute right ventricular pressure overload. *Cardiovasc Res* 8: 611, 1974.

40 Fixler DE, Archie JP, Ullyot DJ, Buckberg GD, Hoffman JIE: Effect of acute right ventricular systolic hypertension on regional myocardial blood flow in anesthetized dogs. *Am Heart J* 85: 491, 1973.

41 Archie JP, Fixler DE, Ullyot DJ, Buckberg GD, Hoffman JIE: Regional myocardial blood flow in lambs with concentric right ventricular hypertrophy. *Circ Res* 34: 143, 1974.

42 Hess DS, Bache RJ: Transmural right ventricular myocardial blood flow during systole in the awake dog. *Circ Res* 45: 88, 1979.

43 Domenech RJ, Hoffman JIE, Noble MIM, Saunders KB, Henson JR, Subijanto S: Total and regional coronary blood flow measured by radioactive microspheres in conscious and anesthetized dogs. *Circ Res* 25: 581, 1969.

44 White CW, Marcus ML, Abboud FM: Distribution of coronary artery flow to the canine right atrium and sinoatrial node. *Circ Res* 40: 342, 1977.

45 White CW, Kerber RE, Weiss HR, Marcus ML: The effects of atrial fibrillation on atrial pressure-volume and flow relationships. *Circ Res* 51: 215, 1982.

46 Griggs DM Jr, Nakamura Y: Effects of coronary constriction on myocardial distribution of Iodoantipyrine-I^{131}. *Am J Physiol* 215: 1082, 1968.

47 Brazier J, Cooper N, Buckberg GD: The adequacy of subendocardial oxygen delivery: The interaction of determinants of flow, arterial oxygen content and myocardial oxygen need. *Circulation* 49: 968, 1974.

48 Braunwald E: Control of myocardial oxygen consumption: Physiologic and clinical considerations. *Am J Cardiol* 27: 416, 1971.

49 Rooke GA, Feigl EO: Work as a correlate of canine left ventricular oxygen consumption, and the problem of catecholamine oxygen wasting. *Circ Res* 50: 273, 1982.

49a Sasayama S, Ross J Jr, Franklin D, Bloor CM, Bishop S, Dilley RB: Adaptations of the left ventricle to chronic pressure overload. *Circ Res* 38: 172, 1976.

50 Neill WA, Phelps NC, Oxendine JM, Mahler DJ, Sim DN: Effect of heart rate on coronary blood flow distribution in dogs. *Am J Cardiol* 32: 306, 1973.

51 Vincent WR, Buckberg GD, Hoffman JIE: Left ventricular subendocardial ischemia in severe valvular and supravalvular aortic stenosis: A common mechanism. *Circulation* 49: 326, 1974.

52 Buckberg GD, Fixler DE, Archie JP, Henney RP, Hoffman JIE: Variable effects of heart rate on phasic and regional left ventricular muscle flow in anesthetized dogs. *Cardiovasc Res* 9: 1, 1975.

53 Domenech RJ, Goich J: Effect of heart rate on regional coronary blood flow. *Cardiovasc Res* 10: 224, 1976.

54 Bache RJ, Cobb FR: Effect of maximal coronary vasodilation on transmural myocardial perfusion during tachycardia in the awake dog. *Circ Res* 41: 648, 1977.

55 Bache RJ, Vrobel TR, Arentzen CE, Ring WS: Effect of maximal coronary vasodilation on transmural myocardial perfusion during tachycardia in dogs with left ventricular hypertrophy. *Circ Res* 49: 742, 1981.

56 Rembert JC, Boyd LM, Watkinson WP, Greenfield JC Jr: Effect of adenosine on transmural myocardial blood flow distribution in the awake dog. *Am J Physiol* 239: H7, 1980.

57 Flameng W, Schaper W, Lewi P: Multiple experimental coronary occlusion without infarction. *Am Heart J* 85: 767, 1973.

58 Flameng W, Wusten B, Winkler B, Pasyk S, Schaper W: Influence of perfusion pressure and heart rate on local myocardial flow in the collateralized heart with chronic coronary occlusion. *Am Heart J* 89: 51, 1975.

59 Holtz J, Bassenge E, Restorff WV, Mayer E: Transmural differences in myocardial blood flow and in coronary dilatory capacity in hemodiluted conscious dogs. *Basic Res Cardiol* 71: 36, 1976.

60 Barnard JR, et al: Ischemic response to sudden strenuous exercise in healthy men. *Circulation* 48: 936, 1973.

61 Foster C, Anholm JD, Hellman CK, Carpenter J, Pollock ML, Schmidt DH: Left ventricular function during sudden strenuous exercise. *Circulation* 63: 592, 1981.

62 von Anrep G: On the part played by the suprarenals in the normal vascular reactions of the body. *J Physiol* (London) 45: 307, 1912.

63 Knowlton FP, Starling EH: The influence of variations in temperature and blood pressure on the performance of the isolated mammalian heart. *J Physiol* (London) 44: 206, 1912.

64 Sarnoff SJ, Mitchell JH: The regulation of the performance of the heart. *Am J Med* 30: 747, 1961.

65 Monroe RG, Gamble WG, LaFarge CG, Juman AE, Stark J, Sanders GL, Phornphutkal C, Davis M: The Anrep effect reconsidered. *J Clin Invest* 51: 2573, 1972.

66 Walston A, Rembert JC, Fedor JM, Greenfield JC: Regional myocardial blood flow after sudden aortic constriction in awake dogs. *Circ Res* 42: 419, 1978.

CHAPTER **6**

NEURAL CONTROL OF THE CORONARY CIRCULATION

Early coronary physiologists had difficulty evaluating neural control mechanisms in the coronary circulation because stimulation of adrenergic or cholinergic nerves produced relatively weak direct effects coupled with potent indirect effects on coronary vascular resistance. In the past two decades, the development of selective receptor blockers and sophisticated experimental methods has permitted investigators to dissect the direct effects of cardiac nerve stimulation on the coronary circulation from indirect effects. Although many unanswered questions in this area remain, much of the controversy alluded to in earlier reviews of this subject [1,2] has been resolved.

INNERVATION OF CORONARY VESSELS

Sympathetic Nerves

The sympathetic nerves to the heart and coronary vessels arise from the three sympathetic ganglia (superior, middle, and inferior) and the first four thoracic sympathetic ganglia. The stellate ganglion, formed when the inferior cervical sympathetic ganglion merges with the first thoracic ganglion, is a major source of cardiac sympathetic nerves. The large epicardial coronary arteries and veins are densely innervated with sympathetic fibers [3–5]. In addition, intramural coronary arteries, capillaries, and venules receive substantial sympathetic innervation [6].

Parasympathetic Nerves

The vagi supply the heart and coronary vessels with efferent cholinergic nerves. Although vagal fibers to ventricular muscle are sparse, the conduction system and coronary vessels receive an abundant supply of cholinergic nerves [7–8].

Receptors

Coronary vessels contain $alpha_1$, $alpha_2$, $beta_1$, $beta_2$, and muscarinic-cholinergic receptors [9–21c]. $Beta_1$ receptors play a prominent role in the myocardium and conduction tissues. Present evidence suggests that the functional significance of $beta_1$ receptors in coronary vessels is very limited [14,15]. The density of the various receptor types in different segments of the coronary vascular bed has not been well defined.

DIRECT EFFECTS OF SYMPATHETIC NERVE STIMULATION ON THE CORONARY CIRCULATION

Alpha-Adrenergic Stimulation

Intracoronary or intravenous infusions of a specific alpha agonist, such as methoxamine or phenylephrine [11,19,22,23], can produce a twofold increase in coronary resistance. Likewise, electrical stimulation of sympathetic nerves during complete beta blockade constricts coronary vessels (Figure 6-1) [12,15,17,22,

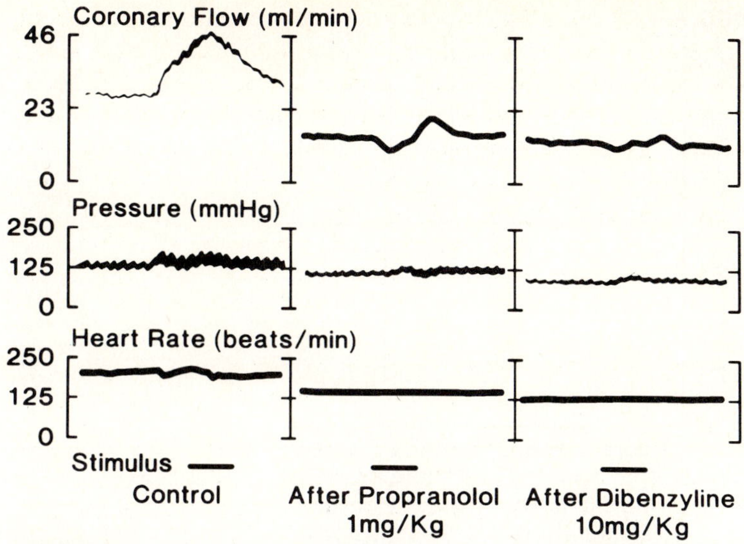

FIGURE 6-1
Effects of intense electrical sympathetic nerve stimulation (stimulus) on coronary flow. (*Left*) Without alpha or beta blockade sympathetic nerve stimulation is associated with coronary dilation. (*Center*) After beta blockade with propranolol sympathetic nerve stimulation produces coronary constriction. Following beta and alpha blockade (dibenzyline) sympathetic nerve stimulation has no effect on coronary blood flow. Pressure = mean arterial pressure. (*Redrawn from data originally presented by EO Feigl* [*24*].)

24–27]. It is of note, however, that when alpha receptors in coronary vessels are activated by intense sympathetic nerve stimulation in the presence of beta blockade, coronary vascular resistance increases only 10 to 25 percent. Thus, physiological activation of coronary alpha receptors produces only one-fourth of the coronary constrictor response that can be achieved with pharmacologic stimulation (Figure 6-2). In addition, the overall magnitude of alpha-adrenergic vasoconstriction in the coronary bed is small in comparison to that which occurs in skin and skeletal muscle (Figure 6-3) [28]. Both large epicardial vessels and intramural coronary arteries participate in the constrictor response to alpha-adrenergic stimulation [14,17,19,29]. Also, when sympathetic tone is increased by a physiological stimulus, such as activation of the baroreceptor reflex, alpha-adrenergic blockade or cardiac sympathectomy decreases coronary vascular resistance [24,26]. Thus alpha-adrenergic stimulation produces modest coronary constriction.

Under control conditions, alpha-adrenergic stimulation has little or no effect on the transmural distribution of coronary blood flow in the left ventricle [27,30,31].

In the past all investigators have focused their attention on $alpha_1$ receptors in the coronary circulation. It has recently been shown that $alpha_2$ receptors in the coronary circulation are present [31a,31b]. Activation of these receptors inhibits

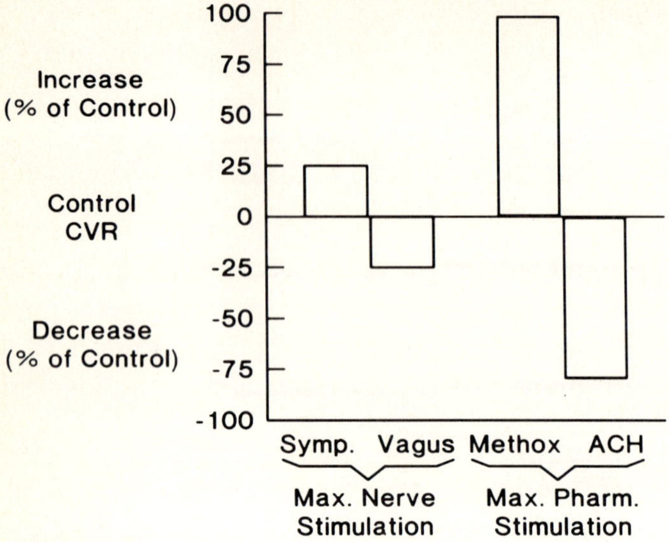

FIGURE 6-2
Effects of nerve stimulation versus pharmacologic stimulation on coronary vascular resistance (CVR). During beta blockade maximal (Max.) sympathetic (Symp.) nerve stimulation produced a 25 percent increase in coronary vascular resistance [24]. In contrast, infusion of the alpha agonist methoxamine (Methox) almost doubled coronary vascular resistance [19]. Maximal electrical stimulation of the vagus nerve when heart rate was held constant by pacing produced a 25 percent decrease in coronary vascular resistance [21]. Infusions of acetylcholine (ACH), with heart rate held constant, was associated with marked coronary dilation [42]. Thus, pharmacologic activation of coronary alpha and cholinergic receptors produced much more potent effects than neural activation of these receptors.

the release of norepinephrine from sympathetic nerves that innervate coronary vessels. The physiological importance of these alpha$_2$ receptors awaits further definition.

Beta$_2$ Stimulation

Pharmacologic stimulation of beta$_2$ receptors with isoproterenol during blockade of beta$_1$ receptors produces modest (about 10 to 25 percent) coronary dilation [9,12,14,15,34,35]. The dilation appears to occur predominantly in the subepicardial layers of the left ventricle (Figure 6-4) [34,35]. Although beta$_2$ receptors are not activated by norepinephrine released from nerve endings [15] these receptors can be stimulated by circulating epinephrine [12].

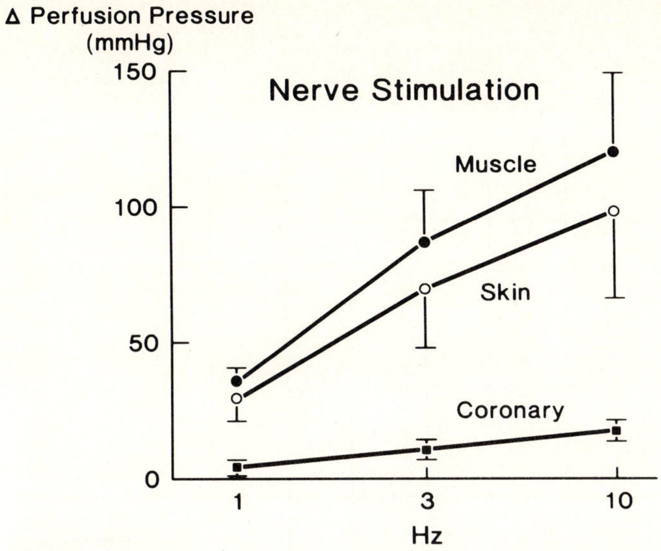

FIGURE 6-3
Effects of sympathetic nerve stimulation in three vascular beds during beta blockade. At all levels of stimulation (1,3,10 Hz) coronary constriction was much less than that observed in skin and muscle. The three vascular beds were perfused at constant flow. Therefore, increases in perfusion pressure are indicative of vasoconstriction. (*Redrawn from data originally presented by AL Mark et al* [22].)

INTEGRATED EFFECTS OF SYMPATHETIC NERVE STIMULATION ON THE CORONARY CIRCULATION

Sympathetic nerve stimulation increases heart rate and myocardial contractility and usually increases systemic pressure. Consequently, myocardial oxygen consumption rises substantially during sympathetic nerve stimulation (see Chapter 3). This increase in myocardial metabolism produces coronary dilation [15,24–26,37]. Simultaneously, sympathetic nerve stimulation activates alpha-adrenergic receptors which promote coronary constriction. The integrated response of the coronary circulation to sympathetic nerve stimulation depends on the temporal course over which these dilator and constrictor influences are activated and on their relative potencies. During the first few cardiac cycles following the onset of sympathetic nerve stimulation, there is little or no change in heart rate or myocardial contractility [36]. During this time period, sympathetic nerve stimulation produces net coronary constriction (see Figure 6-5) [36]. Within 2 to 6 s, heart rate, arterial pressure, and cardiac contractility increase and the coronaries dilate. *Thus, the response of the coronary vessels supplying the left ventricle to sympathetic nerve stimulation is biphasic: initial mild constriction followed within seconds*

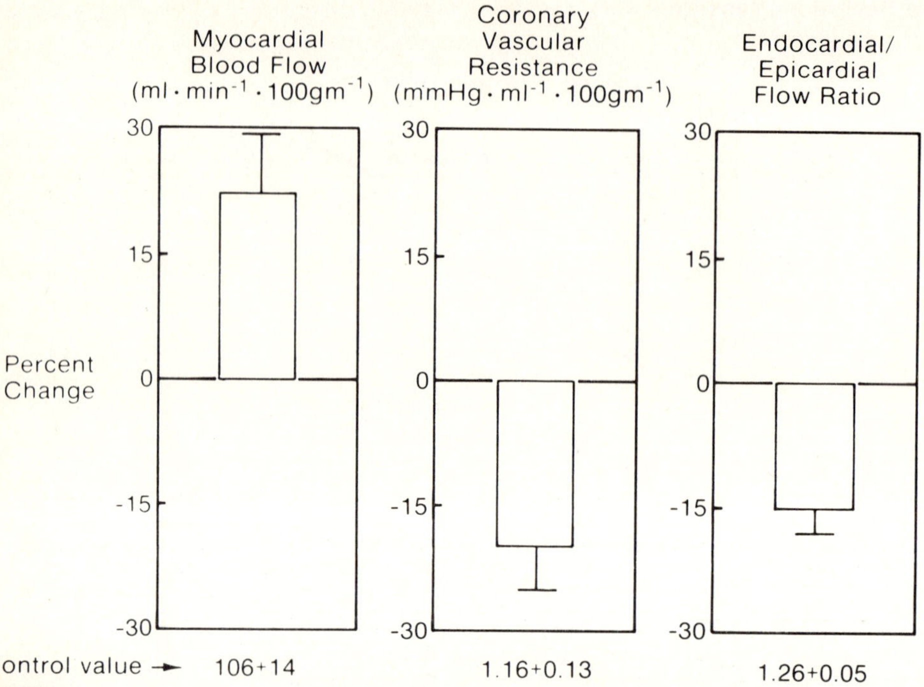

FIGURE 6-4

Effect of $beta_2$ stimulation on the coronary circulation. $Beta_2$ receptors were stimulated with isoproterenol; $beta_1$ receptors were blocked with practolol. $Beta_2$ stimulation increased coronary blood flow and decreased coronary vascular resistance modestly. The decrease in the ratio of left ventricular subendocardial to subepicardial flow during $beta_2$ dilation indicates that dilation was most prominent in the subepicardial vessels. (*Based on studies performed by B Johannsen and AL Mark at the University of Iowa.*)

by substantial coronary dilation. During continuous sympathetic nerve stimulation, the intracoronary infusion of an alpha blocker produces further coronary dilation [12,15,26]. This indicates that even though the net response to sympathetic nerve stimulation is coronary dilation. the constrictor effects of alpha-adrenergic stimulation are present. Sympathetic nerve stimulation in the absence of alpha blockade causes a small decrease in the ratio of subendocardial to subepicardial flow in the left ventricle. [27,30,31].

COMPETITION BETWEEN EFFECTS OF SYMPATHETIC NERVE STIMULATION AND OTHER FACTORS ON THE CORONARY CIRCULATION

Recent studies have demonstrated that under some conditions sympathetic nerve stimulation can compete with other potent factors that influence coronary vascular tone. Mohrman and Feigl [37] demonstrated that the increase of myocardial

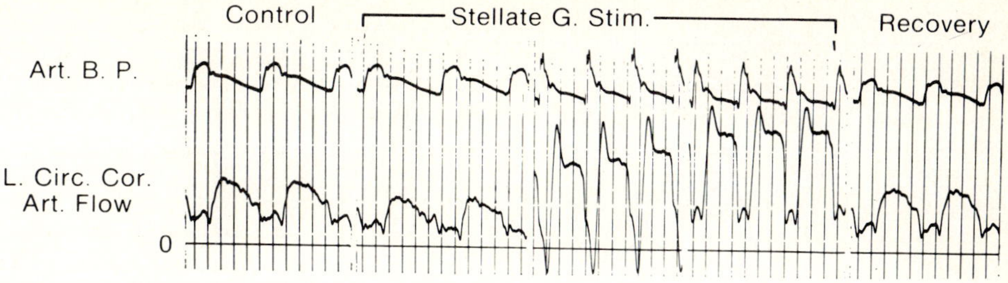

Heart Rate	110	110	176	166	122
Blood Pressure	120	120	118	108	113
Mean Cor. Flow/min	53	39	80	115	56

FIGURE 6-5
Effects of stellate ganglion stimulation (Stellate G. Stim.) on left circumflex coronary artery flow (L. Circ. Cor. Art. Flow) in a chronically instrumented awake dog. During the first few seconds following nerve stimulation there was no change in heart rate or arterial pressure (AP) but a decrease in coronary blood flow. Thereafter, heart rate, arterial pressure, and coronary blood flow increased substantially. Thus, sympathetic nerve stimulation produces a biphasic effect on coronary blood flow: initial coronary vasoconstriction followed by coronary dilation. Heart rate is reported in beats per minute; mean arterial pressure in millimeters of mercury (mmHg); mean coronary flow in milliliters per minute (ml/min). (*Redrawn from data originally presented by L Granata et al* [36].)

oxygen consumption associated with intracoronary infusion of norepinephrine was partially met by increasing oxygen extraction from coronary blood if alpha receptors are not blocked. One interpretation of this data is that alpha-adrenergic coronary constriction prevented the coronary circulation from meeting the additional oxygen requirements by dilation alone. Buffington and Feigl [38] have shown that sympathetic alpha receptor–mediated vasoconstriction operates even in the presence of coronary stenosis to limit oxygen delivery to the heart up to the point of cardiac failure. Murray and Vatner showed that during exercise, coronary vascular resistance is lower when alpha receptors to coronary vessels are blocked [39]. Johannsen et al. [35] noted that alpha-adrenergic stimulation can constrict coronary vessels that have been "maximally dilated" with adenosine. Vatner has recently presented data supporting the concept that alpha-adrenergic stimulation can prevent an augmentation in distending pressure from increasing the diameter of epicardial coronary vessels [19]. Together these studies indicate that sympathetic control of the coronary circulation is not always dwarfed by other potent regulators of coronary blood flow. Although the effects of sympathetic nerve stimulation on the coronary circulation are usually modest, future studies may identify conditions under which sympathetic nerves play a crucial role in the regulation of coronary blood flow.

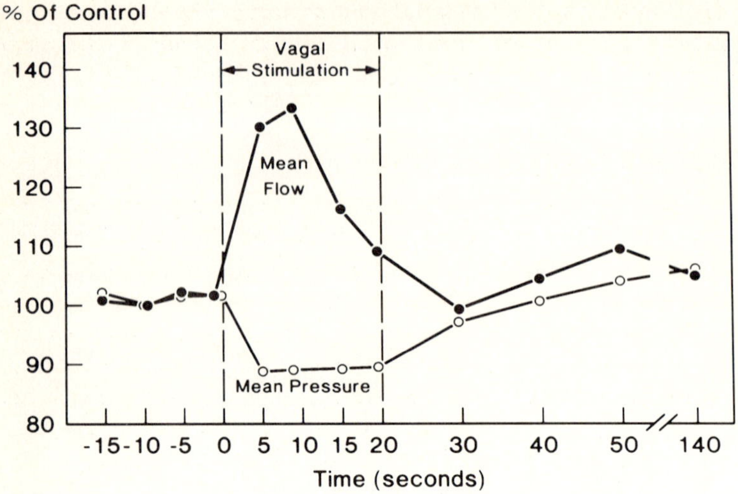

FIGURE 6-6
Effects of intense electrical stimulation of the vagus nerve (Vagal Stimulation) on coronary flow (Mean Flow) and mean arterial pressure (Mean Pressure). In these studies, heart rate was held constant by pacing. Vagal stimulation produced mild coronary dilation. (*Redrawn from data originally presented by EO Feigl* [*21*].)

DIRECT EFFECTS OF VAGAL STIMULATION ON THE CORONARY CIRCULATION

Intracoronary infusions of acetylcholine produce near maximal coronary dilation if heart rate is kept constant (Figure 6-2) [40–42]. In contrast, intense electrical stimulation of the vagus nerve produces only moderate coronary dilation (about 20 to 30 percent) if changes in heart rate are prevented (Figure 6-6) [21,40,43]. Infusions of acetylcholine produced dilation of large epicardial coronary arteries [43a]. Stimulation of muscarinic-cholinergic receptors in coronary vessels alters the transmural distribution of coronary blood flow [42]. Vessels in the subendocardial third of the left ventricle dilate more than vessels in the subepicardium. Thus, dilator responses to vagal stimulation or administration of acetylcholine involve both epicardial and intramural coronary vessels [42,43a]

INTEGRATED EFFECTS OF VAGAL STIMULATION ON THE CORONARY CIRCULATION

Vagal stimulation produces striking bradycardia, markedly decreases atrial contractility, and probably modestly decreases ventricular contractility [40,43–46]. Furthermore, if the bradycardia is marked, arterial pressure will fall. All these effects decrease myocardial metabolism (see Chapter 3). The effects of vagal stimulation on global hemodynamics occur within one cardiac cycle. Thus, although the direct effects of vagal stimulation are to produce mild coronary dilation, in the intact circulation vagal stimulation is associated with coronary constriction because of associated decreases in myocardial metabolism. Withdrawal of vagal tone in a normal, awake dog produces coronary dilation [47].

REFLEX CONTROL OF THE CORONARY CIRCULATION

Reflex effects on the coronary circulation are complex for many reasons. First, many reflexes produce alterations in coronary vascular resistance indirectly by changing cardiac metabolism or extravascular compressive forces. Second, the direct effects of the autonomic nervous system on the coronary circulation are usually modest. Third, some reflexes clearly elicit biphasic responses on coronary vascular resistance which have a distinct temporal course. Fourth, reflex effects are modified by the prevailing hemodynamic state. Fifth, anesthesia often markedly attenuates reflex effects [48]. Finally, under physiological conditions multiple reflexes can be activated simultaneously and they may interact [49]. Consequently, it is not surprising that reflex control of the coronary circulation is an area in coronary physiology that has been steeped in controversy.

Although many reflexes have been purported to have direct effects on the coronary circulation [50], the most important are the baroreceptor reflex, the pulmonary inflation reflex, the chemoreceptor reflex, and the Bezold-Jarisch reflex. The direct effects of other reflexes on coronary vascular resistance have not been well defined or are of dubious significance.

Baroreceptor Reflex

There are three distinct components to the baroreceptor reflex: the carotid, the aortic, and the low-pressure baroreceptors. Each component has separate afferents and exhibits specific effects on various segments of the circulation [51]. Only the effects of the carotid baroreceptors on the coronary circulation have been specifically examined.

Carotid hypotension decreases nerve traffic in the carotid sinus nerve (afferent limb of the reflex), and this results in vagal withdrawal and sympathetic stimulation. The resulting rise in heart rate and in arterial pressure increases myocardial metabolism and thereby decreases coronary vascular resistance to vessels which supply the left ventricle. In the presence of cholinergic and beta blockade, carotid hypotension is associated with systemic hypertension and coronary vasoconstriction [52,53]. Section of the cardiac sympathetic nerves prevents the coronary vasoconstriction that occurs in response to baroreflex activation [52]. Hence, in the left ventricle, coronary vasoconstrictor effects associated with activation of the carotid baroreceptor reflex are masked by a potent metabolic dilator stimulus [52,53]

Carotid sinus nerve stimulation produces bradycardia and systemic hypotension [33]. Although the resulting decrease in myocardial oxygen consumption would be expected to increase coronary vascular resistance, carotid sinus nerve stimulation causes a decrease in coronary vascular resistance which is

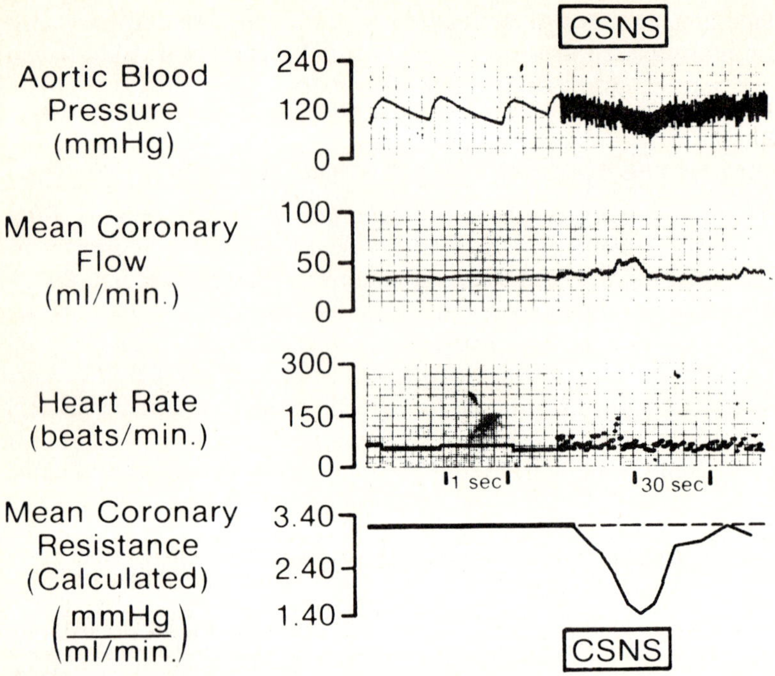

FIGURE 6-7
Effects of carotid sinus nerve stimulation (CSNS) in a conscious dog on coronary flow and resistance. Even though carotid sinus nerve stimulation decreased arterial pressure and presumably myocardial oxygen consumption, coronary dilation occurred. The decrease in coronary resistance is primarily mediated by withdrawal of sympathetic alpha-adrenergic tone to coronary vessels. (*Redrawn from data originally presented by SF Vatner et al* [*47*].)

augmented by atropine (Figure 6-7) [33]. This decrease in coronary resistance in response to sympathetic withdrawal will occur only if significant basal sympathetic tone is present. The level of tonic sympathetic tone in both dogs and in humans varies from near zero in the basal state to intense during maximal exercise [54–56]. Thus, the response of the coronary circulation to baroreceptor reflex activation is markedly influenced by the prevailing level of sympathetic tone.

Recently, Murray et al. [56a] have examined the effects of baroreceptor reflex activation on right ventricular coronary vascular resistance. The metabolic effects of baroreceptor reflex activation are less prominent in the right ventricle than in the left ventricle. Consequently, the adrenergic coronary constriction which accompanies baroreceptor reflex activation is more intense and sustained in the right ventricle than in the left ventricle. Murray et al. [56a] also demonstrated that right ventricular hypertrophy or right ventricular failure markedly attenuates right ventricular coronary vasoconstrictor responses to baroreflex activation.

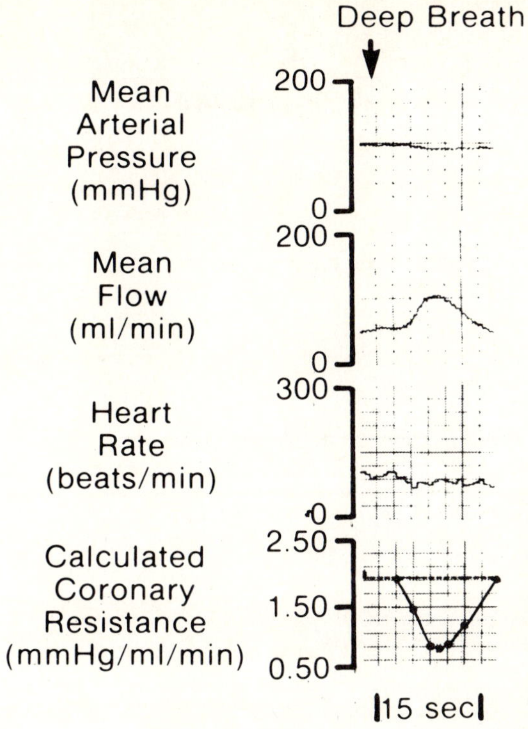

FIGURE 6-8
Effects of a spontaneous deep breath in a conscious dog on coronary flow (Mean Flow) and coronary vascular resistance. Spontaneous pulmonary inflation produced striking coronary dilation. The mechanism of this response has not been completely elucidated. (*Redrawn from data originally presented by SF Vatner and RJ McRitchie* [57].)

Pulmonary Inflation Reflex

Pulmonary inflation can produce marked coronary dilation (Figure 6-8) [57]. The afferent fibers of the reflex travel in the vagus nerve; the efferent response is mediated by the sympathetic nerves. Beta-receptor blockade has no effect on this reflex response; alpha-adrenergic blockade markedly attenuates the dilator response to pulmonary inflation [57]. Because coronary dilation associated with the pulmonary inflation reflex is mediated by withdrawal of sympathetic tone, it follows that the magnitude of the response is critically dependent on the level of sympathetic tone present at the time of stimulation (see above). The effects of the pulmonary inflation reflex on the coronary circulation are puzzling. The magnitude of this reflex response on coronary vascular tone is much greater than that observed with other reflex stimuli. Therefore, it is difficult to accept the notion that the intense coronary dilation that occurs with pulmonary inflation simply reflects sympathetic withdrawal. It should be recalled that in a normal resting dog adrenergic coronary vascular tone is negligible [55]. I suspect that other mechanisms in addition to sympathetic withdrawal must play a significant role in the pulmonary inflation reflex.

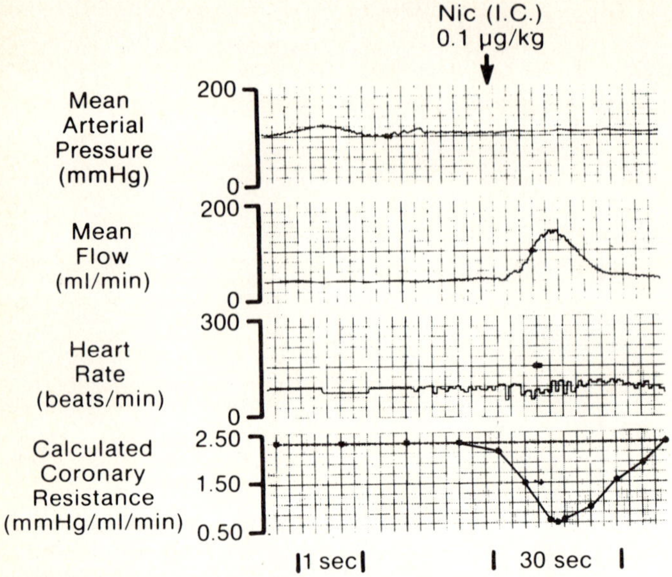

FIGURE 6-9
Effects of chemoreceptor activation in a conscious dog on coronary blood flow (Mean Flow) and coronary resistance. The chemoreceptor reflex was activated by intracarotid infusion of nicotine [Nic(I.C.)]. Activation of the chemoreceptor reflex produced net coronary dilation. Much of the coronary dilation results from the pulmonary inflation, which is stimulated by activation of the reflex. (*Redrawn from data originally presented by SF Vatner and RJ McRitchie* [57].)

Chemoreceptor Reflex

Under physiological conditions, the carotid chemoreceptor reflex is activated by hypoxia, hypercapnia, or acidosis [58]. Experimentally, the reflex can be elicited by injecting minute quantities of nicotine into the carotic artery [57,58]. Activation of the reflex with nicotine produces hypertension and tachycardia [58]. Consequently, one would expect an increase in cardiac metabolism and coronary dilation (Figure 6-9). Three neural effects are superimposed on the metabolic response. First, the chemoreceptor reflex stimulates the vagi, which results in coronary dilation that can be blocked by atropine [57,58]. Second, the reflex stimulates respiration, which activates the pulmonary inflation reflex and thus results in withdrawal of alpha-adrenergic tone to coronary vessels and coronary vasodilation [57]. Third, the chemoreceptor reflex causes an increase in sympathetic tone; under carefully controlled conditions, alpha-adrenergic coronary vasoconstriction has been demonstrated [57]. Recent evidence suggests that the latter component becomes manifest relatively late in the response. In the intact dog, these diverse influences are integrated. Because the initial response to activation of the chemoreceptor reflex is hyperventilation and because hyperinflation precedes major alterations in cardiac hemodynamics, activation of the chemoreceptor reflex first produces coronary dilation. Subsequently, as other components of the reflex are activated, the coronary dilation is attenuated and modest coronary constrictor influences become manifest.

The Bezold-Jarisch Reflex

This reflex, which produces bradycardia and hypotension, can be activated by intracoronary infusion of veratridine [59] or distention of afferent stretch receptors within the walls of the cardiac chambers. Activation of the reflex during alpha and beta blockade in paced heart produces coronary dilation that can be blocked with atropine. The significance of this reflex response is probably minimal in the intact coronary circulation.

EFFECTS OF CARDIAC DENERVATION

Prior to the first successful cardiac transplant in a patient, numerous experimental studies suggested that cardiac denervation did not have major adverse effects on the circulation [60-63]. An important study in this regard was performed by Donald at al. [61]. These investigators demonstrated that the racing time of greyhounds subjected to cardiac denervation was unchanged.

Clinical experience with patients who have received a cardiac transplant (totally denervated heart) indicates that cardiac function is not critically dependent on cardiac innervation [64]. Although the denervated heart cannot respond as quickly to various stressful stimuli as an innervated heart, circulating catecholamines and other humeral substances facilitate alterations in heart rate and myocardial contractility during exercise and other stresses. Taken together, these experimental and clinical observations support the notion that neural control of the coronary circulation is relatively insignificant under most conditions.

POTENTIAL CLINICAL SIGNIFICANCE OF NEURAL CONTROL MECHANISMS IN THE CORONARY CIRCULATION

The importance of neural control mechanisms is modulated to a large extent by the level of autonomic tone that prevails when a neurally mediated response occurs. Under basal conditions, sympathetic tone is minimal and vagal tone is relatively high [33,55]. During exercise, the opposite is the case. Although neural control mechanisms nave not been shown to play a critical role in regulating the normal coronary circulation, neural control could be important in disease states.

There is now convincing evidence that coronary spasm plays a significant role in several clinical syndromes that occur in patients with ischemic heart disease (see Chapter 12). The mechanism of spasm is unknown. In vitro studies by Yokoyama et al. [65] suggest that the vasconstrictor effects of alpha agonists are potentiated in atherosclerotic blood vessels.

Rosendorff et al. have shown in awake dogs that hypercholesterolemia sensitizes coronary vessels to the vasoconstrictor effects of norepinephrine [66]; however, Johannsen et al. [67], who studied anesthetized dogs, could not demonstrate that hypercholesterolemia augmented coronary responses to norepinephrine or other vasoconstrictors. In patients with coronary disease, exaggerated coronary vasoconstrictor response to sympathetic stimulation has been reported [68,69]. Thus, neural control mechanisms, alterations in adrenergic receptors, or circulating catecholamines could be involved in the pathogenesis of coronary spasm.

The importance of neural control mechanisms would be augmented if vasodilator responses to metabolic stimuli were blunted. Metabolically induced vasodilator responses are limited in patients with coronary obstructive disease and patients with cardiac hypertrophy (see Chapters 11 and 13). In these conditions, mild coronary constriction could produce a physiologically significant impairment in coronary blood flow.

Recent studies by Pasyk et al. [70] suggest that central neural control mechanisms have the potential to significantly alter coronary vascular resistance. Additional work in this area is needed.

Finally, hypertrophy of smooth muscle in the wall of arterioles could augment constrictor responses and limit dilation. Recent studies indicate that systemic hypertension causes hypertrophy of smooth muscle in coronary resistance vessels [71,72]. Thus, in patients with hypertension, neural control mechanisms could be particularly important.

Future studies may identify conditions under which the nerves play a critical role in the regulation of the coronary circulation.

REFERENCES

1 Gregg DE: *The Coronary Circulation in Health and Disease.* Philadelphia, Lea & Febiger, 1950.

2 Gregg DE, Fisher LC: Blood supply to the heart, in *Handbook of Physiology*, WF Hamilton (ed). Washington, DC, American Physiological Society, vol 2, sect 2 Circulation, chap 44, p 1517.

3 Friedman WF, Pool PE, Jacobowitz D, Seagren SC, Braunwald E: Sympathetic innervation of the developing rabbit heart. *Circ Res* 23: 25, 1968.

4 Dahlstrom A, Fuxe F, Mya-tu M, Zetterstrom BEM: Observations on adrenergic innervation of the dog heart. *Am J Physiol* 209: 689, 1965.

5 Malor R, Griffin CJ, Taylor S: Innervation of the blood vessels in guinea pig atria. *Cardiovasc Res* 7: 95, 1973.

6 Forbes MS, Rennels ML, Nelson E: Innervation of myocardial microcirculation; terminal autonomic axons associated with capillaries and postcapillary venules in mouse heart. *Am J Anat* 149: 71, 1977.

7 Woollard HH: Innervation of the heart. *J Anat* 60: 345, 1926.

8 Kent KM, Epstein SE, Cooper T, Jacobowitz DM: Cholinergic innervation of the canine and human ventricular conducting system: Anatomic and electrophysiologic correlations. *Circulation* 50: 948, 1974.

9 Klocke FJ, Kaiser GA, Ross J Jr, Braunwald E: An intrinsic adrenergic vasodilator mechanism in the coronary vascular bed of the dog. *Circ Res* 16: 376, 1965.

10 Zuberbuhler RC, Bohr DF: Responses of coronary smooth muscle to catecholamines. *Circ Res* 16: 431, 1965.

11 Pitt B, Elliot EC, Gregg DE: Adrenergic receptor activity in the coronary arteries of the unanesthetized dog. *Circ Res* 21: 75, 1967.

12 McRaven DR, Mark AL, Abboud FM, Mayer HE: Responses of coronary vessels to adrenergic stimuli. *J Clin Invest* 50: 773, 1971.

13 Andersson R, Holmberg S, Svedmyr N, Aberg G: Adrenergic α- and β-receptors in coronary vessels in man. *Acta Med Scand* 191: 241, 1972.

14 Gross GJ, Feigl EO: Analysis of coronary vascular beta receptors in situ. *Am J Physiol* 228: 1909, 1975.

15 Hamiton FN, Feigl EO: Coronary vascular sympathetic beta-receptor innervation. *Am J Physiol* 230: 1569, 1976.

16 Holtz J, Mayer E, Bassenge E: Demonstration of alpha-adrenergic coronary control in different layers of canine myocardium by regional myocardial sympathectomy. *Pflügers Arch* 372: 187, 1977.

17 Kelley KO, Feigl EO: Segmental α-receptor-mediated vasoconstriction in the canine coronary circulation. *Circ Res* 43: 908, 1978.

18 Orlick AE, Ricci DR, Alderman EL, Stinson EB, Harrison DC: Effects of alpha adrenergic blockade upon coronary hemodynamics. *J Clin Invest* 62: 459, 1978.

19 Vatner SF, Pagani M, Manders WT, Pasipoularides AD: Alpha adrenergic vasoconstriction and nitroglycerin vasodilation of large coronary arteries in the conscious dog. *J Clin Invest* 65: 5, 1980.

20 Ross G: Adrenergic responses of the coronary vessels. *Circ Res* 39: 461, 1976.

21 Feigl EO: Parasympathetic control of coronary blood flow in dogs. *Circ Res* 25: 509, 1969.

21a Cornish EJ, Miller RC: Comparison of the β-adrenoceptors in the myocardium and coronary vasculature of the kitten heart. *J Pharm Pharmac* 27: 23, 1975.

21b Johansson B: The β-adrenoceptors in the smooth muscle of pig coronary arteries. *European J Pharma* 24: 218, 1973.

21c Baron GD, Speden RN, Bohr DF: Beta-adrenergic receptors in coronary and skeletal muscle arteries. *Am J Physiol* 223: 878, 1972.

22 Mark AL, Abboud FM, Schmid PG, Heistad DD, Mayer HE: Differences in direct effects of adrenergic stimuli on coronary, cutaneous, and muscular vessels. *J Clin Invest* 51: 279, 1972.

23 Williams DO, Most AS: Responsiveness of the coronary circulation to brief vs sustained alpha-adrenergic stimulation. *Circulation* 63: 11, 1980.

24 Feigl EO: Sympathetic control of coronary circulation. *Circ Res* 20: 262, 1967.

25 Nayler WG, Carson V: Effect of stellate ganglion stimulation on myocardial blood flow, oxygen consumption, and cardiac efficiency during beta-adrenoceptor blockade. *Cardiovasc Res* 7: 22, 1973.

26 Feigl EO: Control of myocardial oxygen tension by sympathetic coronary vasoconstriction in the dog. *Circ Res* 37: 88, 1975.

27 Giudicelli J-F, Berdeaux A, Tato F, Garnier M: Left stellate stimulation: Regional myocardial flows and ischemic injury in dogs. *Am J Physiol* 239: H359, 1980.

28 Mark AL, Abboud FM, Schmid PG, Heistad DD, Mayer HE: Differences in direct effects of adrenergic stimuli on cornary, cutaneous and muscular vessels. *J Clin Invest* 51: 279, 1972.

29 Gerová M, Barta E, Gero J: Sympathetic control of major coronary artery diameter in the dog. *Circ Res* 44: 459, 1979.

30 Uchida Y, Ueda H: Non-uniform myocardial blood flow caused by stellate ganglion stimulation. *Japanese Heart J* 16: 162, 1975.

31 Breen DR, Mark AL, Marcus ML: Effects of cardiac sympathetic nerve stimulation on transmural distribution of myocardial blood flow in dogs. *Fed Proc* 36: 487, 1977.

31a Johanssen UJ, Mark AL, Marcus ML: Alpha-2 receptors modulate coronary responses to sympathetic nerve stimulation. *Circulation* (suppl II)66: 153, 1982.

31b Bassenge E, Holtz J, Sommer O, Saeed M: Vascular A_2-adrenoceptors mediate coronary constrictions induced by norepinephrine (NE) and by sympathetic nerve stimulation. *Circulation* (suppl II) 66: 153, 1982.

32 Feigl EO: Carotid sinus reflex control of coronary blood flow. *Circ Res* 23: 223, 1968.

33 Vatner SF, Franklin D, Van Citters RL, Braunwald E: Effects of carotid sinus nerve stimulation on the coronary circulation of the conscious dog. *Circ Res* 27: 11, 1970.

34 Domenech RJ, MacLellan PR: Transmural ventricular distribution of coronary blood flow during coronary $beta_2$-adrenergic receptor activation in dogs. *Circ Res* 46: 29, 1980.

35 Johannsen UJ, Mark AL, Marcus ML: Responses to cardiac sympathetic nerve stimulation during maximal coronary dilation produced by adenosine. *Circ Res* 50: 510, 1982.

36 Granata L, Olsson RA, Huvos A, Gregg DE: Coronary inflow and oxygen usage following cardiac sympathetic nerve stimulation in unanesthetized dogs. *Circ Res* 16: 114, 1965.

37 Mohrman DE, Feigl EO: Competition between sympathetic vasoconstriction and metabolic vasodilation in the canine coronary circulation. *Circ Res* 42: 79, 1978.

38 Buffington CW, Feigl EO: Adrenergic coronary vasoconstriction in the presence of coronary stenosis in the dog. *Circ Res* 48: 416, 1981.

39 Murray PA, Vatner SF: Alpha-adrenoceptor attenuation of the coronary vascular response to severe exercise in the conscious dog. *Circ Res* 45: 654, 1979.

40 Levy MN, Zieske H: Comparison of the cardiac effects of vagus nerve stimulation and of acetylcholine infusions. *Am J Physiol* 216: 890, 1969.

41 Blesa MI, Ross G: Cholinergic mechanisms on the heart and coronary circulation. *Br J Pharmac* 38: 93, 1970.

42 Gross GJ, Buck JD, Warltier DC: Transmural distribution of blood flow during activation of coronary muscarinic receptors. *Am J Physiol* 240: H941, 1981.

43 Daggett WM, Nugent GC, Carr PW, Powers PC, Hrada Y: Influence of vagal stimulation on ventricular contractility, O_2 consumption, and coronary flow. *Am J Physiol* 212: 8, 1967.

43a Cox D, Hintze T, Vatner SF: Effects of acetylcholine on large coronary vessels in conscious dogs. *Fed Proc* 40: 707, 1981.

44 Blinks JF: Field stimulation as a means of effecting the graded release of autonomic transmitters in isolated heart muscle. *J Pharmacol Exptl Therap* 151: 221, 1966.

45 De Geest H, Levy MN, Zieske H: Carotid chemoreceptor stimulation and ventricular performance. *Am J Physiol* 209: 564, 1965.

46 Levy MN, Martin PJ: Neural control of the heart, in *Handbook of Physiology*, RM Berne (ed). Bethesda, Maryland, American Physiological Society, 1979, vol 1, sect 2, The cardiovascular system, chap 16, p 581.

47 Vatner SF, Rutherford JD: Control of the myocardial contractile state by carotid chemo- and baroreceptor and pulmonary inflation reflexes in conscious dogs. *J Clin Invest* 61: 1593, 1978.

48 Vatner SHF, Braunwald E: Cardiovascular control mechanisms in the conscious state: Comparison of the effects of physiological and pharmacological stimuli in the presence and absense of general anesthesia. *N Engl J Med* 293: 970, 1975.

49 Heistad DD, Abboud FM, Mark AL, Schmid PG: Interaction of baroreceptor and chemoreceptor reflex: Modulation of the chemoreceptor reflex by changes in baroreceptor activity. *J Clin Invest* 53: 1226, 1974.

50 Berne RM, Rubio R: Coronary circulation, in *Handbook of Physiology*, RM Berne (ed). Bethesda, Maryland, American Physiological Society, 1979, vol 1, sect 2, The cardiovascular system, chap 25, p 873.

51 Abboud FM, Mark AL: Cardiac baroreceptors in circulatory control in humans, in *Cardiac Receptors*, R Hainsworth, C Kidd, RJ Linden (eds.) Cambridge, Cambridge University Press, 1979, p 437.

52 Feigl EO: Carotid sinus reflex control of coronary blood flow. *Circ Res* 23: 223, 1968.

53 Powell JR, Feigl EO: Carotid sinus reflex coronary vasoconstriction during controlled myocardial oxygen metabolism in the dog. *Circ Res* 44: 44, 1979.

54 Holtz J, Mayer E, Bassenge E: Demonstration of alpha-adrenergic coronary control in different layers of canine myocardium by regional myocardial sympathectomy. *Pflügers Arch* 372: 187, 1977.

55 Chilian WM, Boatwright RB, Tetsuro S, Griggs DM Jr: Evidence against significant resting sympathetic coronary vasoconstrictor tone in the conscious dog. *Circ Res* 49: 866, 1981.

56 Vatner SF, Pagani M: Cardiovascular adjustments to exercise: Hemodynamics and mechanisms. *Prog Cardiovasc Dis* 19: 91, 1976.

56a Murray PA, Vatner SF: Carotid sinus baroreceptor control of right coronary circulation in normal, hypertrophied, and failing right ventricles of conscious dogs. *Circ Res* 49: 1339, 1981.

57 Vatner SF, McRitchie RJ: Interaction of the chemoreflex and the pulmonary inflation reflex in the regulation of coronary circulation in conscious dogs. *Circ Res* 37: 644, 1975.

58 Hackett JG, Abboud FM, Mark AL, Schmid PG, Heistad DD: Coronary vascular responses to stimulation of chemoreceptors and baroreceptors: Evidence for reflex activation of vagal cholinergic innervation. *Circ Res* 31: 8, 1972.

59 Feigl EO: Reflex parasympathetic coronary vasodilation elicited from cardiac receptors in the dog. *Circ Res* 37: 175, 1975.

60 Cooper T, Willman VL, Hanlon CR: Drug responses of the transplanted heart. *Dis Chest* 45: 284, 1964.

61 Donald DE, Ferguson DA, Milburn SE: Effect of beta-adrenergic receptor blockade on racing performance of greyhounds with normal and with denervated hearts. *Circ Res* 22: 127, 1968.

62 Gregg DE, Khouri EM, Donald DE, Lowensohn HS, Paysk S: Coronary circulation in the conscious dog with cardiac neural ablation. *Circ Res* 31: 129, 1972.

63 Donald DE: Myocardial performance after excision of the extrinsic cardiac nerves in the dog. *Circ Res* 34: 417, 1974.

64 Stinson EB, Griepp RB, Schroeder JS, Shumway NE: Hemodynamic observations one and two years after cardiac transplantation in man. *Circulation* 45: 1183, 1972.

65 Yokoyama M, Goldman M, Henry PD: Supersensitivity of atherosclerotic arteries to ergonovine partially mediated by a serotonergic mechanism. *Circulation* 60: II-100, 1979.

66 Rosendorff C, Hoffman JLE, Verrier ED, Rouleau J, Boerboom LE: Cholesterol potentiates the coronary artery response to norepinephrine in anesthetized and conscious dogs. *Circ Res* 48: 320, 1981.

67 Johannsen UJ, Mark AL, Marcus ML, Armstrong ML: Effects of dietary hyperlipoproteinemia on coronary vascular responsiveness in vivo. *Circulation* 64 (suppl IV): 267, 1980.

68 Mudge GH Jr, Grossman W, Mills RM Jr, Lesch M, Braunwald E: Reflex increase in coronary vascular resistance in patients with ischemic heart disease. *N Engl J Med* 295: 1333, 1976.

69 Mudge GH Jr, Goldberg S, Gunther S, Mann T, Grossman W: Comparison of metabolic and vasoconstrictor stimuli on coronary vascular resistance in man. *Circulation* 59: 544, 1979.

70 Pasyk S, Walton J, Pitt B: Central opioid mediated coronary and systemic vasoconstriction in the conscious dog. *Circulation* 64 (suppl 4): 41, 1981.

71 Yamori Y, Mori C, Nishio T, Osshima A, Horie R, Ohtaka M, Soeda T, Saito M, Abe K, Nara Y, Nakao Y, Kihara M: Cardiac hypertrophy in early hypertension. *Am J Cardiol* 44: 964, 1979.

72 Hallback-Nordlander M, Noresson E, Thoren P: Hemodynamic consequences of left ventricular hypertrophy in spontaneously hypertensive rats. *Am J Cardiol* 44: 986, 1979.

CHAPTER **7**

MYOGENIC REGULATION OF CORONARY BLOOD FLOW

Myogenic regulation implies control of vascular tone by intrinsic mechanisms within the blood vessel wall. Specifically, a myogenic response occurs when application of force to vascular smooth muscle results in contraction and neural, humoral, and metabolic mechanisms are excluded. Although myogenic activity in veins was first noted by Jones in 1852 [1], the myogenic mechanism is often referred to as the *Bayliss reaction.* In 1902, Sir William Bayliss postulated that "the muscular coat of arteries reacts to increasing vascular pressure (by contracting)" [2]. Although this theory met with great skepticism during Bayliss' lifetime, in the last 25 years a large volume of experimental data has been reported that strongly supports the existence of a myogenic mechanism in various vascular beds [3].

EVIDENCE OF MYOGENIC MECHANISMS IN ISOLATED SMOOTH MUSCLE AND ISOLATED BLOOD VESSELS

When isolated smooth muscle strips from various organs [3], umbilical arteries [4,5], or portal veins [6] are subjected to quick or sustained stretch, contraction occurs (Figure 7-1). In the portal vein, the frequency of extracellular electrical spikes is closely correlated with mechanical contractions [7,8]. This suggests that stretch alters membrane properties of smooth muscle and the resulting depolarization facilitates muscle contraction.

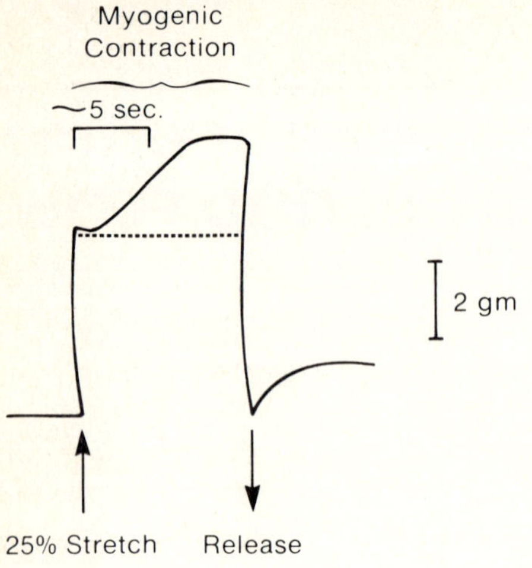

FIGURE 7-1
Myogenic contraction in an isolated ring of umbilical artery. A 25 percent stretch was applied to a ring of umbilical artery mounted in a myograph. The stretch was followed by significant contraction of the vascular ring. This active contraction response to stretch was presumably mediated by myogenic mechanisms. (*Redrawn from data originally presented by HV Sparks Jr.* [4].)

Recently, Duling et al. [9] have developed a preparation whereby microvessels 20 to 100 μm in diameter from brain, muscles, and hamster cheek pouch can be isolated and perfused. With this preparation, changes in intravascular pressure can be introduced and the vascular diameter measured. Such experiments have demonstrated that when intravascular pressure increases in microvessels, vascular diameter decreases (Figure 7-2). This type of response is best explained by postulating that an intrinsic vascular mechanism (myogenic tone) stimulates smooth muscle to respond to an increase in distending pressure by contracting.

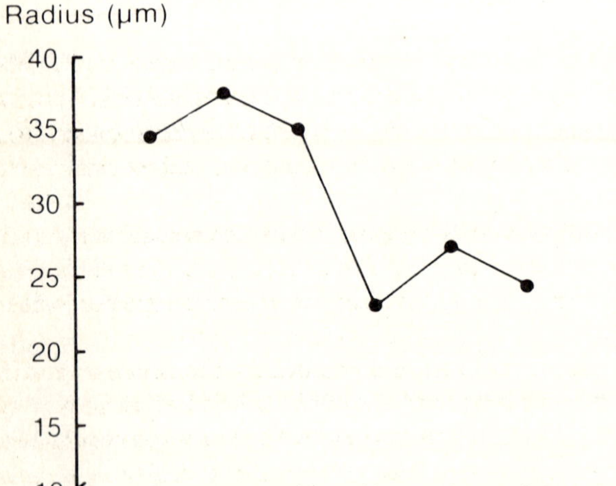

FIGURE 7-2
Effects of increasing intraluminal pressure on the radius of an isolated, perfused microvessel from the hamster cheek pouch. Increases in intraluminal pressure stimulated the vessel to constrict. This active contraction was almost certainly mediated by myogenic mechanisms. (*Redrawn from data originally presented by BR Duling et al* [9].)

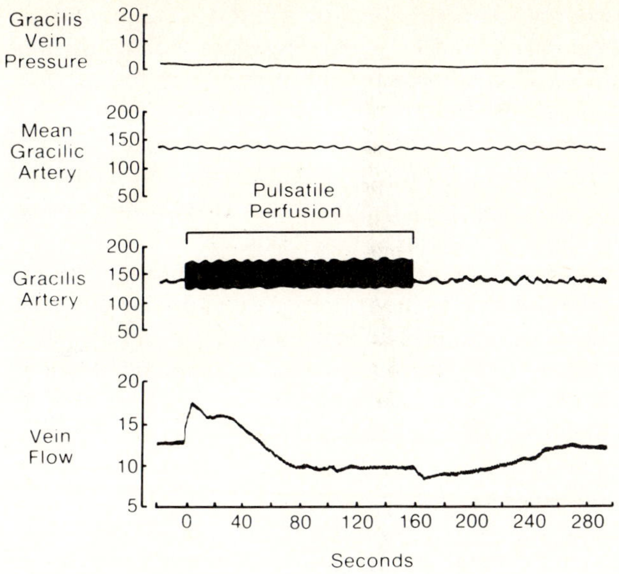

FIGURE 7-3
Effects of pulsatile and nonpulsatile perfusion on vascular resistance in the gracilis. During pulsatile perfusion, flow in the isolated perfused gracilis muscle decreased even though mean perfusion pressure and mean venous pressure remained constant. The data suggest that pulsatile distention of the gracilis artery produced vasoconstriction presumably mediated by myogenic mechanisms. (*Based on an experiment performed by BJ Lalone* [11]. *Redrawn from a figure presented by PC Johnson* [3].)

MYOGENIC RESPONSES OF BLOOD VESSELS STUDIED IN SITU

The vascular resistance in an isolated gracilis muscle increases if arterial perfusion is pulsatile rather than constant [10,11] (Figure 7-3). This occurs even though mean arterial and venous pressure are constant. Periodic distention of the vasculature could stimulate myogenic contraction and increase vascular resistance.

In the microvasculature of several organs [3], a sudden increase in pressure can cause individual capillaries to contract to the point of complete occlusion.

EVIDENCE OF MYOGENIC MECHANISMS IN THE VASCULATURE

Myogenic responses in the vasculature can manifest themselves in several ways. Sometimes the responses take the form of an increase in vasomotor frequency [12,13]. This is typically obeserved in venules and lymphatic channels. At other times, myogenic responses are characterized by steady or periodic contractions, which usually persist as long as a change in intravascular pressure is present [3,5,14]. This kind of response is typical of arterioles. The latency of the response is variable but can be as little as 0.5 s [3].

Many organs, including heart, kidney, skeletal muscle, and brain, exhibit autoregulation [15–18]. Over a range of perfusion pressures (usually 40 to 100 mmHg) flow remains constant. This autoregulatory response is probably mediated by metabolic and/or myogenic mechanisms. For a metabolic mechanism to be activated, a change in pressure would have to initially change the flow. If perfusion increased promptly in response to an augmentation in a driving pressure, a vasodilator metabolite could be washed out, vascular resistance would rise, and flow would return toward control. In the coronary circulation, step increases or decreases in pressure are associated with directionally similar changes in perfusion [17,19–21]. Within seconds, alterations in vascular resistance return flow toward the control level [17,19–21]. Thus, in the coronary circulation, autoregulation could be mediated by a metabolic mechanism. In theory, a myogenic mechanism could be activated without any initial fluctuation in flow rate.

The most convincing evidence that suggests myogenic mechanisms play a role in autoregulation comes from studies in which venous pressure is suddenly elevated. Under these conditions, flow decreases (metabolic mechanisms would favor dilation) and intravascular pressure rises (myogenic mechanisms would promote vascular constriction). In the liver, intestine, colon, and spleen, increases in venous pressure are associated with increased vascular resistance; i.e., myogenic mechanisms dominate [22–25].

Microvascular studies have shown that the responses of various classes of vessels within the vascular hierarchy to an increase in venous pressure are heterogenous. Baez et al. [14] demonstrated that a 15 mmHg increase in pressure in the ileocolic vein induced arterioles and precapillary sphincters to constrict intensely (greater than 70 percent decrease in diameter), metarterioles to constrict slightly (less than 20 percent decrease in diameter), and venules to dilate (6 percent increase in diameter) (Figure 7-4). *These data illustrate a fundamental concept: individual components of the microvascular network can respond in a diverse fashion to a common stimulus.*

EVIDENCE OF MYOGENIC MECHANISMS IN THE CORONARY CIRCULATION

A sudden change from pulsatile to pump perfusion of coronary vessels in association with a step change in pressure can produce transient undulations in vascular tone [26]. These responses could be manifestations of a myogenic mechanism. This interpretation, however, is speculative.

Bittar et al. [27] prevented pressure from falling distal to a coronary occlusion by perfusing the distal vascular segment with saline or plasma. Following release of the occlusion, the reactive hyperemic response was decreased by 25 percent. It is likely that washout of metabolites rather than elimination of a myogenic response was responsible for the attenuation of the reactive hyperemic response.

Effects of coronary sinus occlusion on coronary vascular resistance have also been examined. Mild increases in coronary venous pressure augment critical closing pressure, but the slope of the relationship between pressure and flow during a prolonged diastole is not changed [28]. Thus, this perturbation does not alter coronary vascular resistance. Although these studies are not comprehensive, the results suggest that the increase in intravascular force was not associated with vasoconstriction. Hence, no evidence of an active myogenic response was apparent.

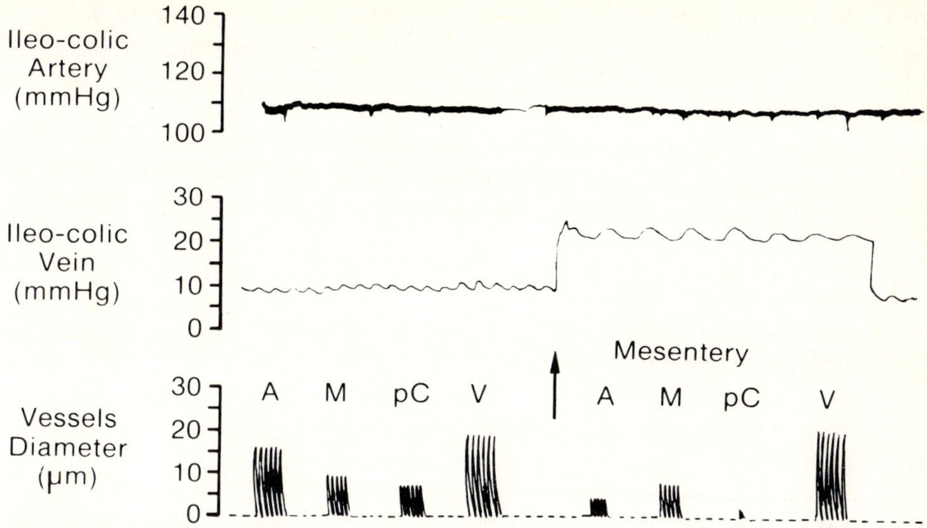

FIGURE 7-4
Effects of a step increase in venous pressure on the diameter of various segments of the microvasculature. A = arterioles; M = metarterioles; pC = precapillary sphincter; V = venule. In response to an increase in venous pressure, three segments of the microvasculature constricted (arterioles, metarterioles, and precapillary sphincters) and one segment dilated (venule). Constriction was presumably mediated by myogenic mechanisms. The data indicate that various segments of the microvasculature respond to a common stimulus in a heterogenous fashion. (*Redrawn from data originally presented by S Baez et al* [14].)

Studies by Giles and Wilcken [29] are often cited as evidence of a myogenic mechanism in the coronary circulation. These investigators noted that coronary occlusion for one cardiac cycle in dogs was followed by a reactive hyperemic response. We have noted similar responses in humans [30] (see Chapter 3). Giles and Wilcken reasoned that during these brief occlusions oxygen stores in the myocardium would prevent the development of ischemia. Hence, the dilator response was most likely myogenic. Recent studies suggest an alternative interpretation. Adenosine concentrations can rise significantly within one cardiac cycle [31]. Thus, increases in vasodilator metabolites stimulated by ischemia could explain the results of Giles and Wilcken without invoking a myogenic mechanism. Also, Schwartz et al. [32] have shown that if an inotropic stimulus (postextrasystolic potentiation) is applied in a single cardiac cycle, a decrease in coronary vascular resistance is apparent in the following cardiac cycle (refer to Figure 3-4). Thus, in less than one cardiac cycle, metabolic mechanisms can be activated. Also, recent studies concerning the response of the coronary circulation to 200 to 400 μm coronary occlusions, have concluded that a myogenic mechanism is not involved in the vascular response to transient coronary occlusion [33] (see Figure 3-11).

Finally, Saito et al. [34] have shown that intracoronary infusion of adenosine diaminase decreases the debt/repayment ratio following a transient coronary occlusion, but the peak flow immediately following release of the occlusion is unaltered. One interpretation of these data holds that the myogenic component of the response (peak flow following release of the occlusion) is not affected by adenosine, whereas the metabolic component of the response (debt/repayment ratio) is mediated in part by adenosine. This provocative interpretation is speculative.

Although these studies can be interpreted as demonstrating a myogenic mechanism in the coronary circulation, none is convincing.

DIFFICULTIES IN DEMONSTRATING MYOGENIC RESPONSES IN THE CORONARY CIRCULATION

There are three problems which have thus far prevented investigators from establishing the importance of myogenic control in the regulation of coronary vascular tone. First, in the heart, it is exceedingly difficult to exclude confounding mechanisms. Almost all approaches to altering the tramsmural force on coronary vessels simultaneously change cardiac metabolism, extravascular compressive forces, or both. Second, myogenic mechanisms have been demonstrated most convincingly in studies of the microvasculature. Methodological limitations currently prevent investigators from performing sophisticated studies of the microvasculature in the beating heart. Third, Johnson has suggested [3] that myogenic mechanisms are more readily demonstrable in tissues such as the abdominal viscera that have a high ratio of flow to oxidative metabolism. In contrast, in organs such as the heart, where blood flow more closely approximates metabolic needs, myogenic control may be difficult to demonstrate.

There is convincing evidence that myogenic mechanisms contribute importantly to blood flow regulation in several vascular beds [3]. *In the coronary circulation, the existence of myogenic control remains controversial.*

REFERENCES

1. Jones TW: Discovery that the veins of the bat's wing (which are furnished with valves) are endowed with rhythmical contractility and the onward flow of blood is accelerated by each contraction. *Physiol Trans* 1: 131, 1852.
2. Bayless WM: On the local reaction of the arterial wall to changes of internal pressure. *J Physio (London)* 28: 220, 1902.
3. Johnson PC: The myogenic response, in *Handbook of Physiology*, DF Bohr, AP Somlyo, HV Sparks, Jr (eds). American Physiological Society, Bethesda, Maryland, 1980, vol II, section 2, The cardiovascular system, p 409.
4. Sparks HV Jr: Effect of quick stretch on isolated vascular smooth muscle. *Circ Res* 15 (suppl 1): 254, 1964.
5. Davignon J, Lorenz RR, Shepherd JT: Response of human umbilical artery to changes in transmural pressure. *Am J Physiol* 209: 51, 1965.
6. Johansson B, Mellander S: Static and dynamic changes in the vascular myogenic response to passive changes in length as revealed by electrical and mechanical recordings from the rat portal vein. *Circ Res* 36: 76, 1975.

7 Axelsson J, Wahlström B, Johansson B, and Jonsson O: Influence of the ionic environment on spontaneous electrical and mechanical activity of the rat portal vein. *Circ Res* 21: 609, 1967.

8 Hermsmeyer K: Multiple sites in spontaneously active vascular muscle. *Circ Res* 33: 244, 1973

9 Duling BR, Gore RW, Dacey RG Jr, Damon DN: Methods for isolation, cannulation, and in vitro study of single microvessels. *Am J Physiol* 241: H108, 1981.

10 Mellander S, Arvidsson S: Possible 'dynamic' component in the myogenic vascular response related to pulse pressure distension. *Acta Physiol Scand* 90: 283, 1974.

11 LaLone BJ: *Local regulation of skeletal muscle blood vessels: Influence of pulse pressure and vasomotor tone* (PhD thesis). East Lansing, Michigan State University, 1975.

12 Wiederhielm CA: Effects of temperature and transmural pressure on contractile activity of vascular smooth muscle. *Bibl Anat* 9: 321,1967.

13 Hargens AR, Zweifach BW: Contractile stimuli in collecting lymph vessels. *Am J Physiol* 233: H57, 1977.

14 Baez S, Laidlaw Z, and Orkin LR: Responses of venous pressure elevation in the rat. *Blood Vessels* 11: 260, 1974.

15 Rothe CF, Nash FD, Thompson DE: Patterns in autoregulation of renal blood flow in the dog. *Am J Physiol* 220: 1621, 1971.

16 Rapela CE, Green HD: Autoregulation of canine cerebral blood flow. *Circ Res* 15 (suppl 1): 87, 1964.

17 Cross CE: Influence of coronary arterial pressure on coronary vasomotor tonus. *Circ Res* 15 (suppl 1): 87, 1964.

18 Jones RD, Berne RM: Local regulation of blood flow in skeletal muscle. *Circ Res* 15 (suppl 1): 30, 1964.

19 Berne RM: Cardiodynamics and the coronary circulation in hypothermia. *Ann NY Acad Sci* 80: 365, 1959.

20 Dole WP, Montville WJ, Bishop VS: Dependency of myocardial reactive hyperemia on coronary artery pressure in the dog. *Am J Physiol* 240: H709, 1981.

21 Mosher P, Ross J Jr, McFate PA, Shaw RF: Control of coronary blood flow by an autoregulatory mechanism. *Circ Res* 14: 250, 1964.

22 Johnson PC: Origin, localization, and homeostatic significance of autoregulation in the intestine. *Circ Res* 15 (suppl 1): 225, 1964.

23 Hanson KM, Johnson PC: Local control of hepatic arterial and portal venous flow in the dog. *Am J Physiol* 211: 712, 1966.

24 Hanson KM, Johnson PC: Pressure-flow relationships in isolated dog colon. *Am J Physiol* 212: 574, 1967.

25 Lutz J, Henrich H, Peiper V, Bauereisen E: Autoregulation and veno-vasomotoric reaction in the splenic circulation. *Pflüegers Arch European J Physiol* 313: 271, 1969.

26 Eng C, Kirk ES: A vascular waterfall mechanism (VWM) affecting coronary collaterals and ischemic myocardium (IM). *Circulation* 64 (suppl IV): 38, 1981.

27 Bittar N, Pauly TJ, Koke JR: Changes in ischemic coronary vasodilation produced by blood, plasma, and saline infusions. *Recent Adv Stud Cardiac Struct Metab* 10: 475, 1975.

28 Bellamy RF, Lowensohn HS, Ehrlich W, Baer RW: Effect of coronary sinus occlusion on coronary pressure-flow relations. *Am J Physiol* 239 (Heart Circ Physiol 8): H57, 1980.

29 Giles RW, Wilcken DEL: Reactive hyperemia in the dog heart. Evidence for a myogenic contribution. *Cardiovasc Res* 11: 64, 1977.

30 Marcus M, Wright C, Doty D, Eastham C, Laughlin D, Krumm P, Fastenow C, Brody

M: Measurements of coronary velocity and reactive hyperemia in the coronary circulation of humans. *Circ Res* 49: 877, 1981.

31 Thompson CI, Rubio R, Berne RM: Changes in adenosine and glycogen phosphorylase activity during the cardiac cycle. *Am J Physiol* 238: H389, 1980.

32 Schwartz GC, McHale PA, Greenfield JC Jr: Coronary vasodilation after a single ventricular extra-activation in the conscious dog. *Circ Res* 50: 28, 1982.

33 Schwartz GC, McHale PA, Greenfield JC Jr: Hyperemic response of the coronary circulation to brief diastolic occlusion in the conscious dog. *Circ Res* 50: 28, 1982.

34 Saito D, Steinhart CR, Nixon DG, Olsson RA: Intracoronary adenosine deaminase reduces canine myocardial reactive hyperemia. *Circ Res* 49: 1262, 1981.

CHAPTER **8**

HUMORAL CONTROL OF THE CORONARY CIRCULATION

Many substances that circulate in the blood or are released from tissues exert significant effects on coronary vascular resistance. Unfortunately, knowledge in this broad field is very limited. Less than a handful of the numerous endogenous substances that modulate coronary vasomotor tone (norepinephrine, epinephrine, adenosine, and acetylcholine) have been investigated intensively. Even for these compounds, many questions concerning their effects on the regulation of the coronary circulation remain unanswered.

To appreciate the effects of a vasoactive agent on the coronary circulation, the direct and indirect actions of the compound over a broad dose range should be elucidated. It is also important to know at which level(s) in the coronary bed the compound exerts its action, i.e., large vessels, small vessels, capillaries, etc. Ideally, the effects of physiological and pharmacologic concentrations of the compound should be explored. The action of the substance in various animal species, *especially humans,* should be ascertained. Finally, the action of the humoral agent should be determined under various physiological and pathological states, and specific interactions between various agents should be sought.

In most instances, the information available about a given vasoactive compound is circumscribed. In particular, very little is known about humoral regulation of the coronary circulation in humans. Often the effects of a pharmacologic dose of the humoral agent on total coronary flow in an anesthetized animal preparation constitutes all the available information.

The purpose of this chapter is to provide an overview of current knowledge concerning humoral regulation of the coronary circulation. The agents discussed constitute the principal endogenous compounds that have been shown to exert vasoactive effects in the coronary circulation.

CATECHOLAMINES

Epinephrine, norephinephrine, and dopamine are the only endogenous catecholamines [1]. Epinephrine is synthesized and stored in the adrenal medulla and other chromaffin tissues. Norepinephrine is synthesized and stored in postganglionic adrenergic neurons. Ten to twenty percent of the catecholamine content in the adrenal medulla is norepinephrine. Dopamine is the immediate precursor of norepinephrine. All three endogenous catecholamines are present in substantial concentrations in the central nervous system.

Catecholamines have a multitude of potent physiological effects [1]. These substances have direct effects on vascular smooth muscle, nonvascular smooth muscle, and the myocardium. The circulatory effects of catecholamines can activate various cardiac reflexes. In addition, catecholamines modulate metabolic responses such as glycogenolysis in liver and muscle and have direct effects on the central nervous system.

The catecholamines exert their effects by acting on five classes of receptors: $alpha_1$, $alpha_2$, $beta_1$, $beta_2$, and dopaminergic receptors [1]. Norepinephrine acts on alpha and beta receptors. Dopamine is the only endogenous catecholamine which interacts with dopaminergic as well as alpha and beta receptors.

Norepinephrine

Numerous studies which date back to 1914 have examined the effects of catecholamines on the coronary circulation [2–21]. When norepinephrine was infused for 1 to 3 min IV in awake dogs, at a dose (0.8 μm/kg/min) that increased mean arterial pressure by 50 percent, coronary blood flow increased by 33 percent [13]. With this dose of norepinephrine, heart rate decreased by 10 percent and the inotropic state of the heart was markedly enhanced (twofold increase at left ventricular *dp/dt*). Even though myocardial oxygen consumption increased under these conditions, calculated late diastolic coronary vascular resistance was augmented by 20 percent [13]. When heart rate was kept constant by ventricular pacing in conscious dogs, an IV bolus of norepinephrine (0.1 to 1.0 μg/kg) had a *biphasic effect* on mean diastolic coronary vascular resistance. During the first 20 to 30 s of infusion, metabolic influences predominated and coronary vascular resistance decreased by about 20 percent [14]. Subsequently, there was a sustained 30 percent increase in coronary vascular resistance (Figure 8-1) [14]. Coronary sinus pO_2 decreased slightly during intravenous infusions of norepinephrine [14]. Beta-receptor blockade with propranolol eliminated the initial coronary dilator

FIGURE 8-1
Effects of intravenous norepinephrine (NE) on the coronary circulation in awake dogs. Heart rate was kept constant by pacing. Norepinephrine had a biphasic response on coronary vascular resistance: (*a*) dilation followed by (*b*) constriction. (*Data originally presented by SF Vatner et al* [*14*].)

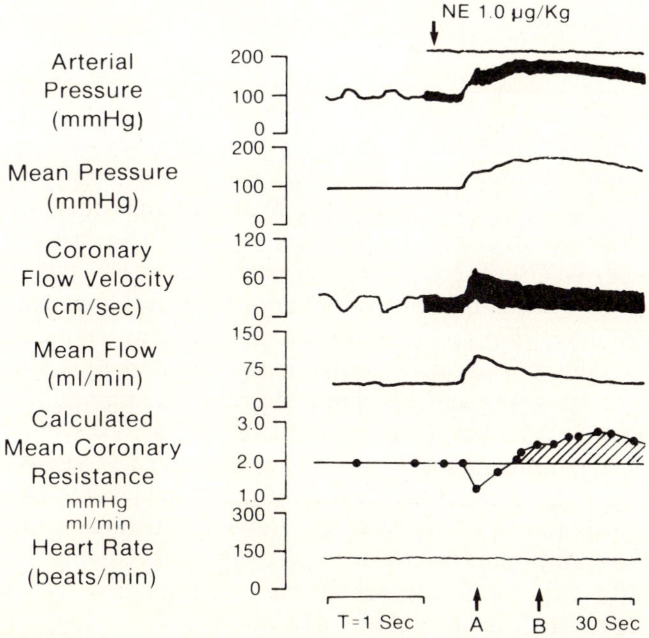

response to norepinephrine and augmented the late coronary constrictor response [14]. Alpha-receptor blockade with phentolamine had the opposite effect [14].

Although the coronary vasoconstrictor effects of norepinephrine are attenuated during hypoxemia in anesthetized dogs [15], in both anesthetized and awake dogs coronary vasoconstrictor effects of norepinephrine can be demonstrated during hypoxemia [15,16].

During beta blockade, norepinephrine infusion constricts both large and small coronary vessels [16]. In normally perfused myocardium, norepinephrine infusions increase flow more to the endocardial than to the epicardial third of the left ventricle [17].

Norepinephrine infusions increase flow through native collateral vessels because this vascular bed is extremely sensitive to increases in perfusion pressure [18]. Norepinephrine also increases flow via mature coronary collaterals [19].

When norepinephrine was infused in patients with normal coronary vessels and reasonably stable hemodynamics, a dose which increased mean aortic pressure by about 25 percent, increased myocardial oxygen consumption by about 20 percent and coronary blood flow (^{131}I-antipyrine method) by 15 percent [20]. Under these conditions, calculated coronary vascular resistance increased slightly. Intravenous infusion of norepinephrine, following coronary bypass surgery, increased mean arterial pressure and bypass graft flow by about 50 percent; hence, calculated coronary vascular resistance remained constant [21]. There is suggestive evidence that patients with coronary artery disease exhibit augmented coronary vasoconstriction in response to alpha-adrenergic stimulation [22].

Thus, in animals and humans, although norepinephrine increases myocardial oxygen consumption, it causes mild coronary vasoconstriction.

Epinephrine

Many investigators have studied the effects of epinephrine on coronary vascular resistance [2–12]. Intravenous infusions of epinephrine are associated with dose-related increases in myocardial contractility and heart rate [6,8–10,23–26]. The effects on arterial pressure are variable. Typically, with intravenous infusions of a modest dose of epinephrine (10 μg/min) diastolic pressure decreases slightly, systolic pressure increases modestly, and mean arterial pressure is unchanged [23]. The hemodynamic perturbations that accompany epinephrine infusions invariably increase myocardial oxygen consumption. Consequently, coronary blood flow increases markedly and coronary vascular resistance decreases substantially in response to moderate doses of intravenous epinephrine [6,8–10,25,26]. When 6 μg of epinephrine was administered intravenously as a bolus, a marked increase in coronary blood flow preceded the onset of tachycardia (Figure 8-2) [25,26]. Beta-receptor blockade with propranolol completely eliminates the coronary vasodilator effect of epinephrine and unmasks the mild coronary vasoconstrictor effects of this agent [6,8–10]. The vasoconstrictor effects of epinephrine can be blocked with an alpha blocker such as phentolamine [9,10].

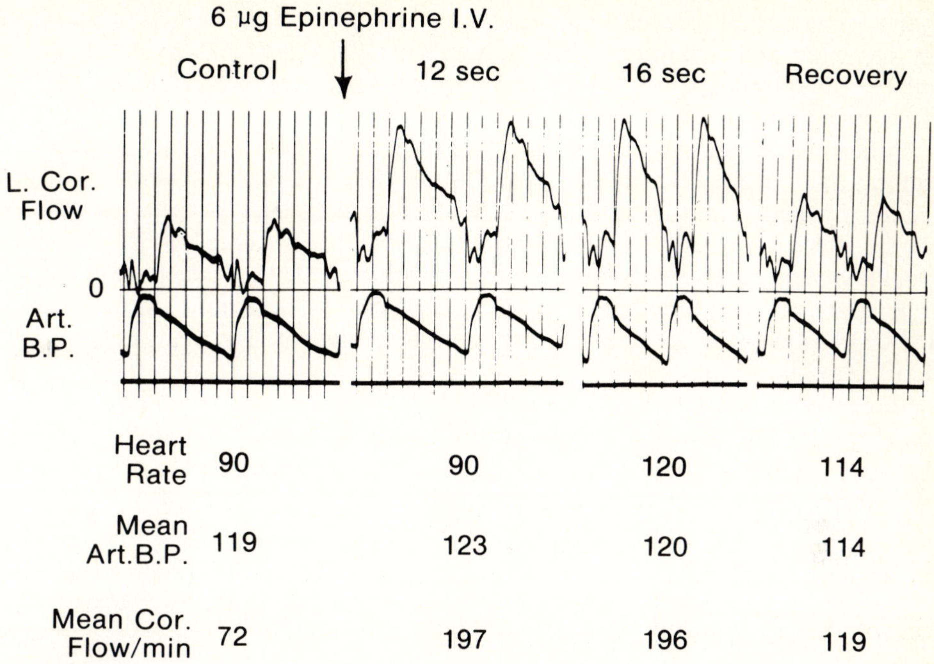

FIGURE 8-2
Effects of epinephrine on the coronary circulation. Intravenous (IV) epinephrine produced a marked increase in left coronary blood flow (L. Cor. Flow) which preceded changes in heart rate and arterial blood pressure (Art. B. P.) (*Modified from a figure originally presented by DE Gregg and LC Fisher* [26].)

Although the effect of epinephrine on flow though native collateral channels has not been reported, it is likely that the tachycardia unassociated with hypertension produced by epinephrine would adversely effect collateral flow (see Chapter 10).

In patients with normal coronary vessels and normal left ventricular function, small doses of epinephrine (1.5 to 3.5 μg/min IV) which increased heart rate by 10 percent increased coronary flow (^{85}Kr method) and myocardial oxygen consumption by about 30 percent and 20 percent, respectively. Calculated coronary vascular resistance decreased by 40 percent [27].

In summary, epinephrine produces net coronary vasodilation in animals and humans.

Dopamine

Dopamine has six actions which modulate coronary vascular resistance [28–38]: direct stimulation of beta$_1$ and alpha receptors, release of stored norepinephrine and consequently beta$_1$ and alpha stimulation, stimulation of myocardial metabolism secondary to alterations in hemodynamics, activation of the baroreceptor reflex secondary to induced changes in arterial pressure, excitation of dopaminergic receptors, and a complex interaction with acetylcholine [35]. Furthermore, the relative importance of these effects varies markedly with the concentration of dopamine in the blood [33,37].

Infusion of dopamine increases myocardial contractility and myocardial oxygen consumption in a dose-related fashion [28–35]. These effects are completely eliminated by beta blockade [28–36]. In conscious dogs and patients, dopamine causes tachycardia, which can be eliminated with beta blockade [28–35]. Effects of dopamine on heart rate are modified by activation of the baroreflex in association with increases in arterial pressure which accompany dopamine administration [28–35]. Systemic pressor effects of dopamine are augmented by beta or cholinergic blockade [35].

Bolus infusions of dopamine (4 to 40 μg/kg IV) in an intact dog with spontaneous cardiac rhythm caused a biphasic alteration in coronary vascular resistance, that is, mild transient coronary vasoconstriction followed by substantial coronary dilation [35]. Continuous infusions of dopamine cause persistent coronary dilation (Figure 8-3) [32]. If heart rate was held constant and beta and alpha receptors were blocked, the coronary dilator response to either bolus or continuous infusion of dopamine was produced which could be blocked with a specific dopaminergic blocker, haloperidol [35]. These studies clearly demonstrate the presence of dopaminergic receptors in the coronary vasculature. Recent studies also indicate the presence of a $dopamine_2$ receptor, which blocks the release of norepinephrine by sympathetic nerves [39].

Perfusion via native coronary collateral vessels is unaffected by doses of dopamine (10 μg/kg/min) that produce a 65 percent increase in left ventricular *dp/dt* [40]. When isoproterenol is administered in a dose that produces a similar increase in cardiac inotropy, perfusion via native collaterals falls significantly [40].

In normal myocardium, concentrations of dopamine which produce a 20 percent increase in mean left ventricular perfusion cause a 10 percent decrease in subendocardial/subepicardial perfusion ratio in the left ventricle [40].

When dopamine (5 to 10 μg/kg IV) was administered to relatively stable patients with normal coronary vessels 1 day following mitral valve replacement, heart rate and aortic pressure increased by 20 percent and 10 percent, respectively [41]. Under these conditions, myocardial oxygen consumption increased by 30 percent, coronary blood flow (^{131}I antipyrine method) increased by 25 percent, and calculated coronary vascular resistance decreased by 30 percent.

Although the effects of dopamine on the coronary circulation are complex, in the intact coronary circulation dopamine produces mild coronary vasodilation.

Effects of Endogenous Levels of Catecholamines on Regulation of the Coronary Circulation

Under basal conditions, sympathetic tone is minimal in normal animals and humans [42,43]. Consequently, it is reasonable to assume that under basal conditions, the effects of catecholamines on the coronary circulation are inconsequen-

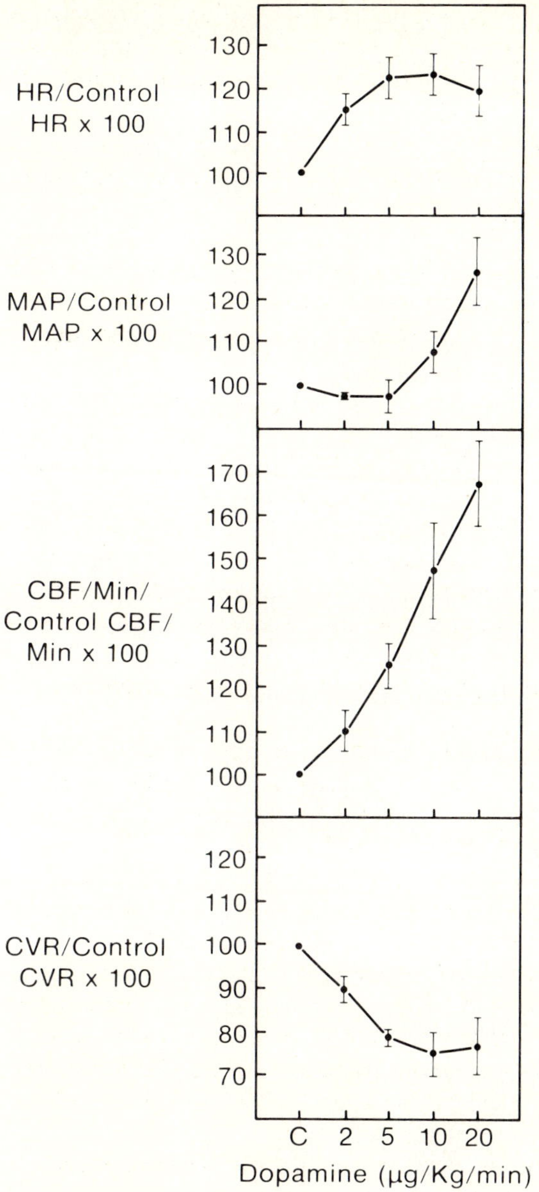

FIGURE 8-3
Effects of various doses of intravenous dopamine on heart rate (HR), mean arterial pressure (MAP), coronary blood flow (CBF), and coronary vascular resistance (CVR) in awake dogs. Dopamine produced marked coronary dilation. (*Based on data originally presented by FR Cobb et al [32].*)

tial. During stress, the opposite is true. Heart failure, acute myocardial infarction, myocardial ischemia, exercise, and excitement are all associated with increased circulating or neurally released catecholamines. Furthermore, the concentration of epinephrine and norepinephrine at active sites in the coronary circulation is sufficient to modulate coronary vascular resistance significantly (see Chapter 5).

The role of endogenous dopamine in the regulation of the coronary circulation remains to be defined.

Studies by Bevan et al. [44] and Hart et al. [45] indicate that sympathetic nerves have trophic effects on the vasculature in growing animals. The potential trophic effects of sympathetic nerves on coronary vessels remain to be elucidated.

Finally, hypercholesterolemia or atherosclerosis may accentuate the vasoactive effects of catecholamines on the coronary vasculature [46–48].

ANGIOTENSIN

Angiotensin II is the most potent pressor known. On a molar basis it has 40 times the vasoconstrictor activity of norepinephrine. Extensive studies of this peptide have been vigorously pursued for several decades [49–54]. Renin, an enzyme made and released by the kidney, catalyzes the conversion of a circulating $alpha_2$ globulin (angiotensinogen) into angiotensin I, a pharmacologically inert decapeptide. A converting enzyme transforms angiotensin I to the octapeptide angiotensin II. The effects of angiotensin II can be modified by saralasin, a competitive receptor antagonist of angiotensin II, and compounds which inhibit converting enzymes such as teprotide and captopril. Angiotensin II is hydrolyzed by aminopeptidase to a heptapeptide, angiotensin III, which is pharmacologically active. Sustained physiological effects of angiotensin II and III depend on continued formation of these peptides because their half-life in human blood is 2 to 4 min.

Since the initial discovery of angiotensin by Braun-Menendez et al. [55] and Page and Helmer [56] in 1940, investigators have uncovered many effects of angiotensin II which are of importance to circulatory control (see Table 8-1).

TABLE 8-1
DIRECT AND INDIRECT EFFECTS OF ANGIOTENSIN II

Central nervous system
Stimulates the area postrema (medullary vasomotor center)
Sympathetic nervous system
Stimulates sympathetic ganglia
Potentiates norepinephrine biosynthesis
Potentiates releases of norepinephrine from adrenergic nerve fibers
Releases catecholamines from the adrenal medulla
Inhibits norepinephrine uptake
Baroreflex activation
Prostaglandins
Stimulate prostaglandin synthesis in endothelial cells, smooth muscle cells, and perfused rabbit hearts
Release prostaglandins E_2 and F from the heart
Releases aldosterone
Direct potent constriction
Mild cardiac inotropic agent

Note: The cardiovascular effects of angiotensin I are described in detail in references 49 to 52.

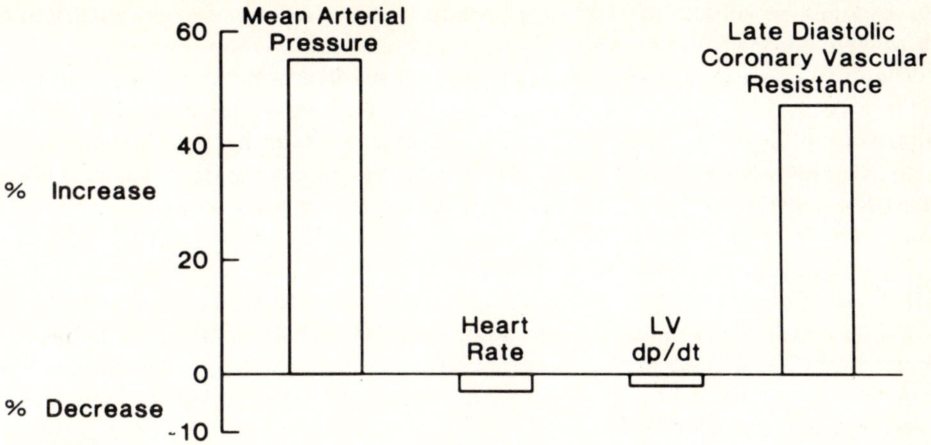

FIGURE 8-4
Effects of intravenous angiotensin on mean arterial pressure, heart rate, left ventricular (LV) *dp/dt*, and late diastolic coronary vascular resistance in awake dogs. Angiotensin produced significant coronary vasoconstriction. (*Based on data originally presented by GR Heyndrickx et al [66].*)

The effects of angiotensin on the coronary circulation have been the subject of many investigations [57–67]. All studies have concluded that angiotensin causes significant coronary vasoconstriction. For example, when angiotensin II was infused IV into awake dogs in doses that increased mean arterial pressure by 25 to 55 percent (0.02 to 0.25 g/kg/min), heart rate decreased by less than 5 percent, cardiac output decreased by 10 to 20 percent, and coronary blood flow increased by 10 percent [66]. Calculated late diastolic coronary vascular resistance increased by 47 percent (Figure 8-4). In anesthetized dogs, angiotensin II in a dose that increased mean arterial pressure by 50 percent increased myocardial oxygen consumption by a similar amount [59]. Oxygen extraction in the coronary bed increased slightly [59–61]. *Thus, even though angiotensin II significantly increases myocardial oxygen consumption, it produces net coronary vasoconstriction.*

The direct coronary vasoconstrictor effects of angiotensin II are attenuated in the intact coronary circulation by at least four mechanisms. First, angiotensin II increases systemic pressure and left ventricular wall stress. Second, it increases heart rate, probably via its effects on the sympathetic nervous system. This effect on heart rate is manifested by blunted bradycardia during hypertension, i.e., baroreflex-induced decreases in heart rate are attenuated. Third, angiotensin II has a mild positive cardiac inotropic effect. Increases in left ventricular wall stress, heart rate, and cardiac inotropy increase myocardial metabolism and produce coronary dilation, which offsets the direct coronary vasoconstriction of angiotensin II. Fourth, angiotensin II releases from the heart prostaglandins E_2 and F, which have coronary vasodilator properties [67]. When prostaglandin synthesis was inhibited with indomethacin, coronary constrictor responses to angiotensin II infusion were enhanced [67]. These indirect coronary vasodilator effects of angiotensin II provide an explanation for why this substance produces intense coronary vasoconstriction in isolated coronary vessels and only moderate vasoconstriction in vivo.

The vasoconstrictor effects of angiotensin II involve both large and small coronary vessels [64]. The transmural distribution of left ventricular perfusion is not altered by infusions of angiotensin II [67]. Studies by Gunther and Cannon indicate that angiotensin II increases coronary vascular resistance in vessels perfusing the right ventricle to a greater extent than coronary vessels that supply the left ventricle [67]. This differential response occurs because angiotensin II only slightly increases right ventricular pressure and the right ventricle may not produce sufficient prostaglandins to limit the direct coronary constrictor effects of angiotensin II.

When small intravenous doses of angiotensin II (2 to 6 μg/min) were administered to patients, myocardial oxygen extraction increased, myocardial oxygen consumption increased by 35 percent, and significant (22 percent) coronary vasoconstriction occurred [68].

Physiological Role of Angiotensin II in Modulating Coronary Vascular Resistance

In normal dogs, administration of an angiotensin antagonist (saralasin) or an inhibitor of converting enzyme (teprotide) has little effect on systemic or coronary vascular resistance [69]. In contrast, in sodium depleted dogs saralasin or teprotide significantly decreases systemic and coronary vascular resistance [69]. Thus, when circulating levels of angiotensin II are increased by conditions such as sodium depletion, heart failure, or high renin hypertension, it is likely that angiotensin II does exert a significant effect on coronary vascular resistance. The effects of endogenous levels of angiotensin II on the coronary circulation in patients with various disease states is a potentially important unexplored area.

VASOPRESSIN

Vasopressin, a peptide hormone formed in the supraoptic and paraventricular nuclei of the hypothalamus and stored and released by the posterior pituitary, promotes fluid balance by stimulating absorption of water by the collecting ducts in the kidney [70–72]. In so doing, the hormone contributes to the maintenance of normal arterial pressure. At concentrations that are manyfold greater than those needed to achieve maximal water reabsorption, vasopressin has direct vasoconstrictor effects [70–72].

Although the direct vascular effects of vasopressin have been known since 1895 [73], studies concerning the action of vasopressin on the coronary circulation have been performed only in the past 25 years [66,74–76]. Continuous intravenous infusion of vasopressin in conscious dogs at doses which increase mean arterial pressure by 55 percent decreased heart rate by about 33 percent and late diastolic coronary blood flow by 25 percent [66]. Calculated late diastolic coronary resistance increased by 140 percent (Figure 8-5) [66]. Even when heart rate was held constant, vasopressin increased late diastolic coronary vascular resistance sub-

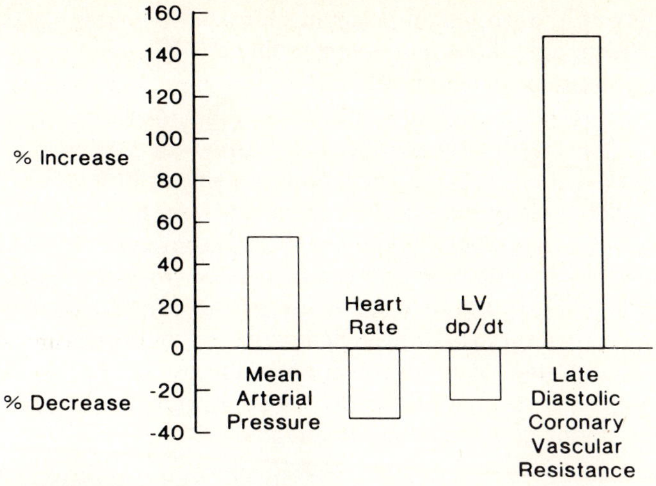

FIGURE 8-5
Effects of intravenous vasopressin on mean arterial pressure, heart rate, left ventricular (LV) *dp/dt*, and late diastolic coronary vascular resistance in awake dogs. Vasopressin produced striking coronary vasoconstriction. (*Based on data originally presented by GR Heyndrickx et al* [*66*].)

stantially [66]. The coronary vasoconstriction which occurs in response to vasopressin is associated with an increase in oxygen extraction by the myocardium [74]. Earlier studies suggested that decreases in coronary blood flow in response to vasopressin infusion might produce myocardial ischemia and impair left ventricular function [70–72]. Studies of lactate metabolism in hearts during vasopressin infusion do not support this contention [74]. The decreased left ventricular function that occurs with vasopressin infusion reflects the marked increase in afterload and a slight direct negative inotropic effect associated with infusion of the hormone.

The coronary vasoconstriction associated with infusions in antidiuretic hormone involve both large and small coronary vessels [75].

When anesthetized dogs are subjected to severe hemorrhagic shock (mean arterial pressure = 60 mmHg), doses of vasopressin which increase mean arterial pressure by 20 mmHg produce a twofold rise in coronary blood flow [76]. Thus, when coronary vessels are nearly maximally dilated by autoregulatory mechanisms (see Chapter 4), the pressor effects of vasopressin lead to increased myocardial perfusion.

Physiological Role of Vasopressin in the Regulation of the Coronary Circulation

Vasopressin affects myocardial perfusion indirectly by contributing to the maintenance of aortic pressure and cardiac output via its effects on extravascular fluid balance. Increased levels of vasopressin occur in many pathological states, including dehydration, hemorrhagic shock, and heart failure [70–72]. In addition, vasopressin may have a significant interaction with catecholamines [38]. Thus, the effects of vasopression on major determinants of coronary blood flow such as aortic driving pressure and heart rate influence coronary vasomotor tone.

The direct coronary vasoconstrictor effects of vasopressin are of little clinical significance because these effects occur only in the presence of very high levels of vasopressin [70–72,77]. Even when high circulating levels of vasopressin are present, activation of the baroreceptor reflex prevents vasopressin from producing large changes in arterial pressure [77]. Large doses of vasopressin are occasionally administered to patients in an effort to control hemorrhage from esophageal varices [70,71]. If excessive amounts of vasopressin are administered intravenously, cardiac catastrophies such as sudden death, severe hypertension, acute myocardial infarction, and angina can be precipitated [78].

CATIONS

Circulating cations have direct and indirect effects which can moderate coronary vascular resistance [79–85]. When cations are infused into a nonworking perfused heart, direct coronary vascular effects of these substances are manifest (Figure 8-6). In such a preparation, Na^+ has no effect, Ca^{2+} causes mild vasoconstriction, Mg^{2+} causes moderate vasodilation, and K^+ has a biphasic effect [82]. Small doses of intracoronary K^+ cause vasodilation, whereas larger doses produce coronary vasoconstriction.

Nonetheless, under physiological conditions the direct effects of these circulating cations do not contribute in a major way to the regulation of coronary vasomotor tone. Many homeostatic mechanisms in the body prevent broad fluctuations in the circulating levels of the cations. Consequently, major alterations in the circulating levels of these cations occur infrequently. Also, K^+, Ca^{2+}, and Mg^{2+} have significant effects on myocardial contractility and electrophysiological properties of myocardium. These effects can produce major alterations in cardiac metabolism and thereby indirectly alter coronary vascular resistance. For example, although Ca^{2+} infusions cause coronary constriction in a nonworking heart, in an unanesthetized dog Ca^{2+} infusion caused marked coronary dilation [83]. This occurred because the increase in ventricular contractility engendered increases myocardial metabolism and thereby decreases coronary vascular resistance. Local release of cations such as K^+ from the myocardium probably plays an insignificant role in modulating coronary vascular resistance (see Chapter 3).

In summary, in most instances circulating levels of cations probably do not significantly influence coronary vasomotor tone.

THYROID HORMONE

Triiodothyronine (T_3) and thyroxin (T_4) are the two biologically active hormones secreted by the thyroid gland [86]. The mechanism by which these hormones exert

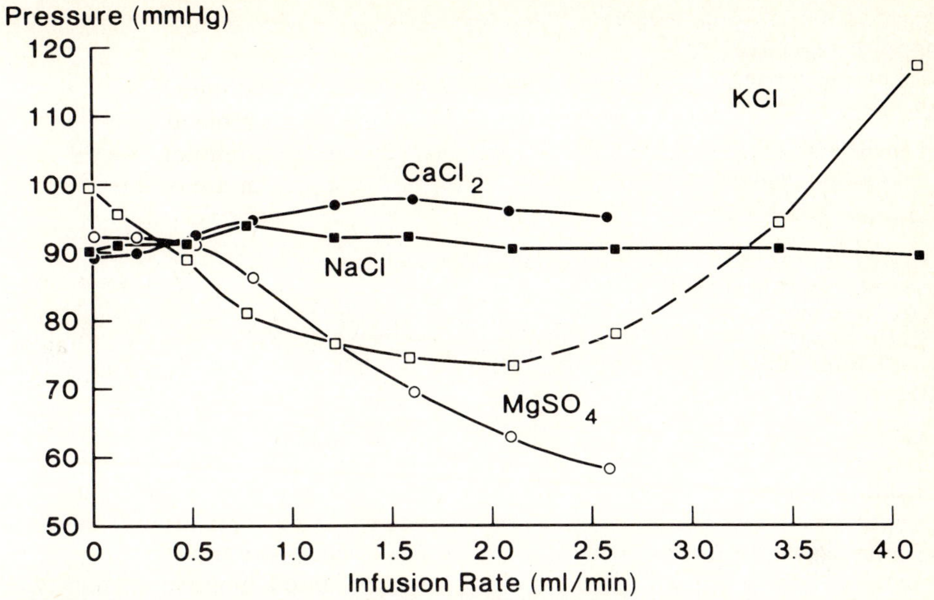

FIGURE 8-6
Effects of intracoronary infusions of various cations on coronary perfusion pressure (Pressure) in a nonworking heart perfused at constant flow. In such a preparation, changes in perfusion pressure reflect changes in coronary vascular resistance. Calcium chloride ($CaCl_2$) produced constriction, magnesium sulfate ($MgSO_4$) produced dilation, and potassium chloride (KCl) had a biphasic effect on coronary vascular resistance. NaCl = sodium chloride. Each milliliter of infusate contained an isotonic solution of the cation being tested. (*Based on data originally presented by JB Scott et al* [82].)

their potent effects remains controversial. It is likely that the actions of thyroid hormone are mediated by effects on cell membranes, mitochondria, ribosomes, and the cell nucleus [87]. The cardiovascular effects of thyroid hormone are preceded by a substantial latent period [88]. This observation is compatible with the hypothesis that the effects of thyroid hormone depend on the activation of synthetic processes.

Thyroid hormone has two prominent direct effects on the myocardium: it increases heart rate [89] and myocardial contractility [90–95]. In addition, thyroid hormone may directly stimulate myocardial metabolism by an effect on mitochondria [87]. These responses all promote a substantial increase in myocardial energy utilization [95]. In addition, prolonged administration of thyroid hormones produces substantial biventricular hypertrophy [96,97]. Total body metabolism and blood flow increase in response to excessive concentrations of thyroid hormone [98–100]. As a consequence, systemic vascular resistance and blood pressure decrease and cardiac output is substantially augmented [98–100]. The coronary circulation responds to these alterations by dilating, and consequently coronary blood flow increases markedly [98]. Thyroid hormone deficiency states have the opposite effect [101,102].

Thyroid hormone does not significantly alter the transmural distribution of coronary blood flow [103]. The effects of this hormone on large and small coronary vessels or on native or mature collateral vessels have not been reported.

Thus, thyroid hormone causes coronary dilation.

Indirect Effects of Thyroid Hormone Which May Influence the Coronary Circulation

Thyroid hormone has three indirect effects which may involve the coronary circulation: interactions with the sympathoadrenal system, modification of the atherosclerotic process, and stimulation of vascular growth.

For many years investigators have suggested that thyroid hormone potentiates the effects of catecholamines on the heart and the peripheral circulation [90]. In addition, thyroid hormone may modify the affinity and number of beta and alpha receptors in the myocardium [104]. The extent to which thyroid hormone interacts with the sympathoadrenal system is controversial. Present evidence favors either a very limited interaction or none at all [90].

In experimental animals, hypothyroidism accelerates and hyperthyroidism attenuates the atherogenic effects of hypercholesterolemia [102]. In addition, patients with long-term hypothyroidism have more coronary atherosclerosis than expected [105]. The interpretation of these effects is difficult because hypothyroidism augments two other factors, systemic pressure and serum cholesterol, which are atherogenic. The weight of evidence currently favors the notion that thyroid hormone deficiency accelerates coronary atherosclerosis [102].

Recent preliminary studies by Marcus et al. [106] suggest that coronary conductance is decreased in rat hearts that develop hypertrophy in response to chronic administration of large doses of thyroid hormone. These data suggest that thyroid hormone promotes growth of the coronary vascular bed.

Effects of Physiological Concentrations of Thyroid Hormone on the Regulation of the Coronary Circulation

Physiological concentrations of thyroid hormone have a very significant effect on the coronary circulation. This is clearly demonstrated by an examination of the coronary circulation before and after effective treatment of hyperthyroidism (Figure 8-7) [98]. When studies of euthyroid patients are compared to data obtained during the hyperthyroid state, a marked decrease in coronary blood flow and myocardial oxygen consumption and a substantial increment in coronary vascular resistance are noted. Because of the potent effects of thyroid hormone on the coronary circulation, many years ago thyroid ablation was used in the treatment of angina pectoris and congestive heart failure with reasonable success [102].

It is not clear that the effects of thyroid hormone on the sympathoadrenal system, the atherogenic process, or vascular growth are of clinical significance with regard to the coronary circulation.

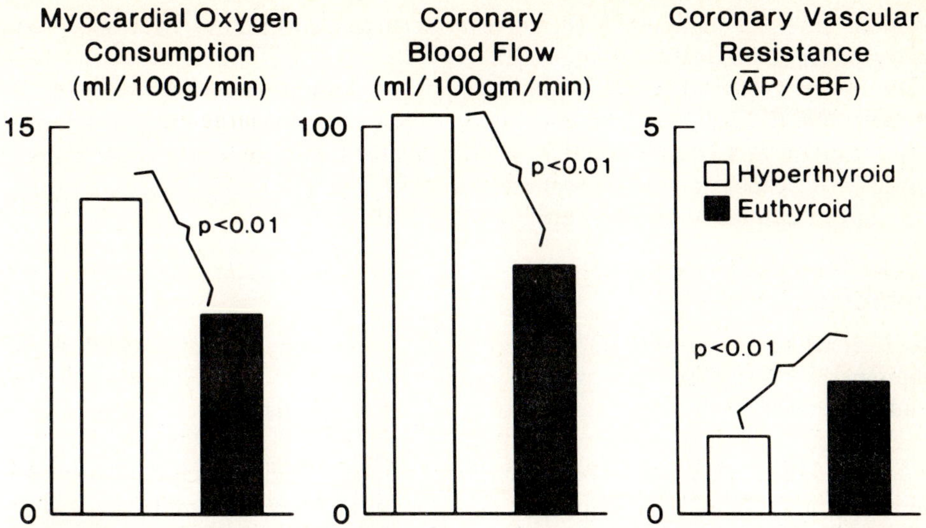

FIGURE 8-7
Effects of the treatment of hyperthyroidism on myocardial oxygen consumption, coronary blood flow, and coronary vascular resistance in patients. Following treatment of hyperthyroidism (euthyroid), myocardial oxygen consumption decreased, coronary blood flow decreased, and coronary vascular resistance increased significantly. AP = arterial pressure; CBF = coronary blood flow. (*Based on data originally presented by GG Rowe et al* [98].)

ADRENAL STEROIDS

The adrenal steroids (cortisol, aldosterone, etc.) have no direct effects on coronary vessels [106a]. However, these hormones play a major role in saltwater homeostasis, and thereby significantly modulate the level of systemic pressure. Hypertension is common in patients with excessive circulating levels of adrenal steroids. This relates in part to sodium retention. In addition, high blood renin levels are present in patients with Cushing's syndrome [107]. Systemic hypotension is one of the hallmarks of adrenal insufficiencies [106a].

Adrenal steroids alter coronary vascular resistance indirectly by modifying systemic arterial pressure.

GLUCAGON

The alpha cells of the pancreas manufacture and release glucagon, a single-chain polypeptide [108,109]. Physiological concentrations of this hormone direct the breakdown of fuels stored intracellularly [108,109].

Pharmacologic doses of glucagon have significant positive inotropic and chronotropic effects on the heart [110–116]. In addition, mean arterial pressure increases during glucagon infusion. As a consequence of these actions, the hormone increases myocardial oxygen consumption and coronary blood flow [113–116]. Calculated coronary vascular resistance decreases [113–116]. Studies in K^+ arrested, perfused hearts indicate that direct effects of glucagon on coronary vascular tone are negligible [115]. Physiological concentrations of glucagon have no significant cardiovascular effects [108,109].

In the late 1960s, large doses of intravenous glucagon were used in the treatment of patients with cardiac failure. The major attribute of glucagon was that it caused fewer cardiac arrhythmias than isoproterenol [114]. Because glucagon is not a particularly potent inotropic agent and can cause marked nausea and vomiting, it is no longer employed in the treatment of patients with cardiac disease.

ADENOSINE

Because adenosine is intimately involved in the synthesis and breakdown of high-energy phosphates, it is present in all living cells [117,118]. Adenosine can readily penetrate cell membranes and enter the interstitial or perivascular space [117,118].

Since 1929, the potent vasodilator properties of adenosine have been known [119]. In the coronary circulation, adenosine can produce maximal coronary dilation [120–124]. At intermediate doses, adenosine has greater vasodilator effects on coronary vessels in the subendocardial layers than the subepicardial layers of the left ventricle (Figure 8-8) [120]. At maximal doses, the effects of adenosine on the transmural distribution of perfusion in the left ventricle depend on extra-

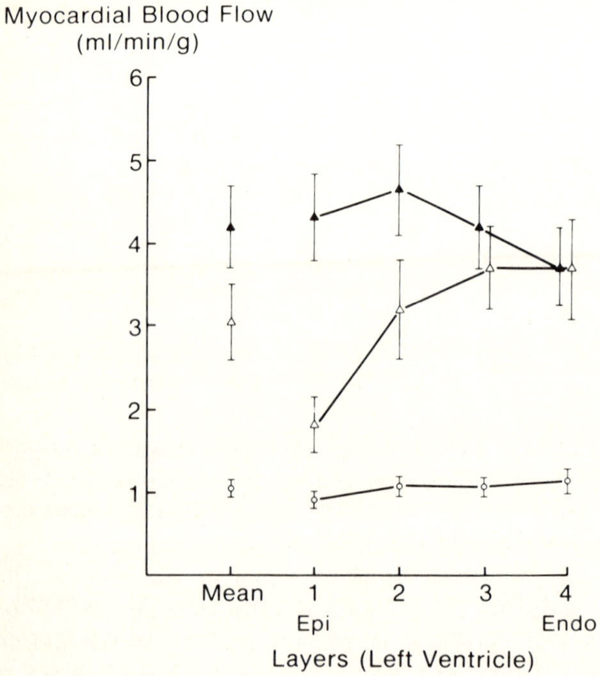

FIGURE 8-8
Effects of intravenous adenosine on myocardial blood flow in various layers of the left ventricle. Epi = epicardium; Endo = endocardium. Open circle = control; open triangle = intermediate dose of adenosine; solid triangle = maximal dose of adenosine. At the intermediate dose of adenosine, endocardial vessels dilated much more than epicardial vessels. During infusion of the maximal dose of adenosine, endocardial flow was less than epicardial flow. Adenosine increased myocardial blood flow more than fourfold. *(Modified from a figure originally presented by JC Rembert et al [120].)*

vascular compressive forces. If these forces were neutralized (nonbeating heart), the conductance of left ventricular subendocardial vessels would be substantially higher than that of subepicardial vessels [121,122]. This reflects the anatomic size of the coronary vascular bed in these two regions [122]. When extravascular compressive forces are present, the conductance of subendocardial coronary vessels in the left ventricle is less than that of subepicardial vessels during maximal dilation with adenosine [120,123,124]. This occurs because of the gradient of compressive forces across the wall of the left ventricle (see Chapter 4).

Although adenosine primarily relaxes small (less than 200 μm) coronary vessels, it also dilates large conduit coronary arteries [125a]. Harder et al. [125] have suggested that adenosine's differential effects on electrophysiological properties of smooth muscle in large and small coronary arteries account for this observation.

Studies which have meticulously excluded overlap perfusion have shown that adenosine decreases flow via native collaterals in the intact heart [126]. Mature collaterals dilate significantly in response to adenosine [127].

Physiological Effects of Adenosine on the Coronary Circulation

Berne and Rubio have recently summarized a large volume of experimental data which suggests that adenosine is the critical mediator that couples changes in myocardial metabolism to changes in coronary vascular resistance [117,118] (see Chapter 3).

ACETYLCHOLINE

Acetylcholine, the cholinergic neural transmitter, produces profound vasodilation in many vascular areas including the coronary bed. The effects of acetylcholine on the coronary circulation are discussed in detail in Chapter 5.

HISTAMINE

Histamine, which is formed by decarboxylation of the amino acid histidine, exerts a variety of actions including: smooth muscle contraction in the bronchi and gut, gastric secretion, stimulation of sensory nerve endings, and many potent effects on the cardiovascular system [128].

Most histamine is stored in mast cells and basophils [128]. The largest concentrations of histamine are present in the skin, intestinal mucosa, and lungs. Only small concentrations of histamine are present in the heart. Within the heart histamine is primarily present in the right atrium [128,129].

The cardiovascular effects of histamine are extensive (see Table 8-2). The development of specific H_1 and H_2 agonists and antagonists have permitted pharmacologists to determine the cardiovascular responses mediated by specific histamine receptors [128–135]. Although significant species differences are noted as

TABLE 8-2
CARDIOVASCULAR EFFECTS MEDIATED BY H_1 AND H_2 HISTAMINE RECEPTORS

	H_1 receptors	H_2 receptors	Net response
Heart rate	↓	↑↑	↑↑
Ventricular contractility		↑↑	↑↑
Atrial contractility	↑	–	↑
AV nodal transmission	↓	–	↑
Capillary dilation	↑	↑	↑↑
Capillary permeability	↑↑	±	↑↑
Systemic vascular resistance	↓↓	↓↓	↓↓↓↓
Pulmonary vascular resistance	↑	↓↓	↓
Coronary vascular resistance (direct)	↓↓	±↓	↓↓↓
Coronary vascular resistance (indirect)	↑	↓↓	↓↓

one ascends the zoological scale, large mammals such as dogs, sheep, monkeys, and humans elicit the cardiovascular responses to histamine listed in Table 8-2.

In sufficient doses, histamine can elicit near maximal coronary dilation (Figure 8-9) [133]. The coronary dilation is mediated by four mechanisms [129–135]. First, activation of H_1 and H_2 receptors produces direct coronary dilation. Second, histamine increases cardiac metabolism via its positive inotropic and chronotropic effects and, hence, produces indirect coronary dilation. Third, the systemic hypo-

FIGURE 8-9
Effects of an intracoronary injection of histamine on coronary blood flow (CBF). Histamine produced marked coronary dilation. Most of the coronary dilation was mediated by activation of H_1 histamine receptors. (*Modified from a figure originally presented by RW Giles et al* [*133*].)

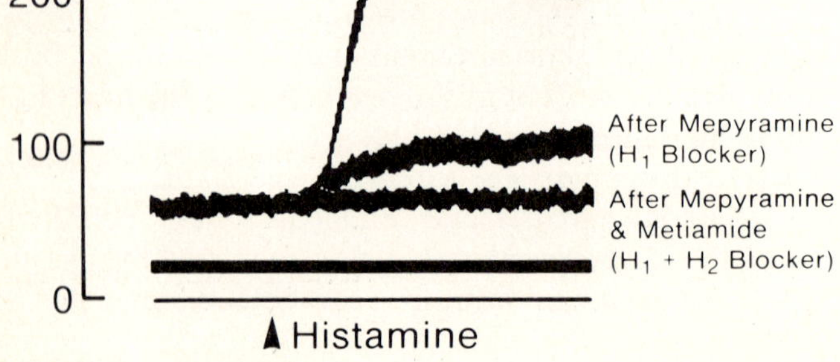

tension produced by histamine activates the baroreceptor reflex and autoregulatory influences. Fourth, histamine stimulates the release of catecholamines from sympathetic nerve endings, ganglia, and the adrenal medulla. All these effects would tend to increase coronary blood flow if systemic pressure were maintained.

No data are available concerning the effects of histamine on large and small coronary vessels, native and mature coronary collaterals, or the transmural or regional distribution of perfusion to the heart.

Physiological Effects of Histamine on the Coronary Circulation

Under normal conditions, histamine probably has no role in the regulation of the coronary circulation. Maximal coronary dilation in response to transient coronary occlusion is not attenuated if histamine receptors are blocked [133].

Massive histamine release can be triggered by an anaphylactic reaction [136–138] or various physical or chemical noxious agents [128,129]. Under such conditions, histamine could conceivably affect the coronary circulation. Under these circumstances, however, it is likely that the systemic effect of histamine, i.e., profound hypotension, would dominate the response of the coronary circulation.

No information is available concerning the direct effects of endogenous histamine on the coronary circulation in humans.

SEROTONIN

For about a century, physiologists have known that when blood is allowed to clot a vasoconstrictor material appears in the serum. Rapport et al. [139] prepared the vasoconstrictor substance in crystalline form and named it serotonin.

Serotonin, which is formed enzymatically from the amino acid tryptophane, is located primarily in the gastrointestinal tract. The other sites which contain appreciable amounts of this agent are the central nervous system and platelets. Serotonin ingested in the diet is quickly degraded by enzymes in the intestinal wall, liver, and lung [128].

The pharmacologic effects of serotonin, excluding the cardiovascular system, include: stimulation of smooth muscle in the gastrointestinal tract and uterus; alterations in gastric secretions; excitation of nerve endings; interactions with the autonomic nervous system at several levels, including sympathetic nerves, ganglia, and the adrenal medulla; and widespread effects in the central nervous system, where serotonin acts as a neurotransmitter [128,140,141].

The cardiovascular effects of serotonin are especially complex because in addition to potent direct effects on vascular tone, myocardial contractility and heart rate, serotonin activates reflex mechanisms by chemical stimulation as well as inducing hemodynamic perturbations [128,140,141]. These effects are thought to be responsible for the triphasic response of systemic arterial pressure (hypotension → hypertension → hypotension) to infusions of serotonin [128].

All studies that have examined the effects of serotonin on the coronary circulation have concluded that this agent acts as a dilator [142–145]. The coronary dilation associated with serotonin precedes other hemodynamic alterations and is associated with an increase in coronary sinus oxygen saturation and only a modest increase in myocardial oxygen consumption [143–145]. Thus, although serotonin does slightly increase myocardial oxygen consumption by its effects on heart rate, myocardial contractility, and stroke volume, most of the coronary dilation that occurs reflects the direct coronary dilator effects of serotonin. Recent studies indicate [146] that intracoronary infusion of serotonin constricts large coronary vessels even though total flow increases.

Although serotonin has potent pharmacologic actions in the cardiovascular system, endogenous serotonin acts primarily in the central nervous system and the gastrointestinal tract. Even in the presence of carcinoid syndrome, a state associated with high circulating levels of serotonin, competitive antagonists of serotonin have no detectable effects on the cardiovascular system.

KININS

The kinins are a group of peptides that possess an extraordinarily high degree of pharmacologic activity. The discovery of these agents began with the observation that human urine produced prolonged hypotension in the dog after intravenous injection [147].

It is now appreciated that the kinins consist of at least 12 separate peptides, 11 to 15 amino acids in length, which contain a similar nonapeptide sequence [147–149]. The plasma kinins which are best known are kalliden, a decapapeptide, and bradykinin, a nonapeptide. The kinins are present predominantly in the pancreas, intestine, colon, salivary glands, kidney, lymphs, and blood [147–149]. The synthesis and metabolism of these peptides have been described [147–149].

The noncardiovascular actions of the kinins involve blood coagulation, salt and water balance, sperm motility, cell proliferation, nerve-ending excitation, nonvascular smooth muscle contraction, autonomic central nervous system activation, and prostaglandin and histamine release [52,147–149].

The effects of kinins on the cardiovascular system are extensive [52,147,149]. Like histamine, the kinins increase vascular permeability in the microcirculation. The vasodilator effects of the kinins are 10-fold greater than those of histamine. However, because kinins cause venoconstriction and reflexly induce tachycardia, cardiac output rises following intravenous injection of bradykinin. Bradykinin has no direct effect on myocardial contractility.

In the coronary circulation, infusion of bradykinin (0.05 mg/kg IV over a period of 20 min) in anesthetized dogs was associated with a 50 percent increase in coronary blood flow and a similar decrease in coronary vascular resistance [150]. Heart rate increased twofold, and mean arterial pressure decreased by 25 percent [150]. Because coronary sinus oxygen saturation remained constant during bradykinin infusion, calculated myocardial oxygen increased significantly. Several recent studies indicate that the coronary dilator action of bradykinin may be partially mediated by prostaglandins [151,152].

Although the kinins have potent effects on the cardiovascular system, a recent extensive review in this area [149] concluded: "The fact remains, however, that 50 years since its [bradykinin] discovery, when it was considered to be a circulatory hormone involved in vascular regulation, its possible role in vascular physiology has not been established with any more certainty."

SUBSTANCE P

In 1931 VonEuler and Gaddum discovered a depressor substance in extracts of intestine [153]. This vasoactive agent (substance P) was isolated in pure form by Chang and Leeman [154] nearly 40 years later. Substance P is an undecapeptide which is primarily present in the intestine and brain [154,155]. Picamole quantities of substance P circulate in the blood [155].

The principal actions of substance P include contraction of longitudinal muscle in the gut, stimulation of salivary secretion, and a variety of effects on the central nervous system [155].

Studies of the circulation indicate that infusions of nanogram quantities of substance P dilate vessels to skin, muscle, intestine, liver, and fat. Total cardiac output increases and aortic pressure decreases slightly during substance P infusions. Substance P has no direct inotropic or chronotropic effects on the heart [155].

In the coronary bed, picamole quantities of substance P increase coronary blood flow twofold if coronary perfusion pressure is kept constant [156]. The coronary dilator effect persists for only a few minutes despite continued infusion of the agent, presumably because of marked tachyphylaxis [156]. The vasodepressor effects of substance P in other vascular beds do not exhibit tachyphylaxis [155].

Although substance P is a potent endogenous vasoactive agent, its role in the regulation of the circulation awaits definition.

VASOACTIVE INTESTINAL POLYPEPTIDE (VIP)

Vasoactive intestinal polypeptide was discovered in 1970 by Said and Mutt [157] and synthesized by Bodansky et al. in 1974 [158]. This peptide is structurally similar to glucagon and secretin [158]. Vasoactive intestinal polypeptide is present in large quantities in the gastrointestinal tract, pancreas, platelets, peripheral nerves, autonomic nerves, ganglia, and blood [159–161]. Vasoactive intestinal polypeptide is rapidly inactivated by the liver and has a plasma half-life of less than 1 min [159–161].

The pharmacologic actions of vasoactive intestinal polypeptide are widespread [159–161]. In the gastrointestinal tract, vasoactive intestinal polypeptide influences secretion, motility, blood flow, and secretion of other gastrointestinal hormones. Like glucagon, vasoactive intestinal polypeptide stimulates lipolysis and glycogenolysis.

In the central and peripheral nervous system, vasoactive intestinal polypeptide may act as the neurotransmitter or neuromodulator.

In the cardiovascular system, vasoactive intestinal polypeptide has positive inotropic effects on the heart and causes vasodilation in pulmonary and systemic blood vessels [159–161]. When 3.3 pmol/kg/min of vasoactive intestinal polypeptide was infused into normal volunteers, flushing occurred, mean arterial pressure decreased by 15 percent, and heart rate increased by 50 percent [162]. Animal studies suggest that in the coronary circulation vasoactive intestinal polypeptide causes dilation which is direct and not secondary to increases in cardiac metabolism [163].

The role of vasoactive intestinal polypeptide in circulatory control remains to be defined. In patients with cirrhosis or tumors which secrete vasoactive intestinal polypeptide it is possible that the high circulating levels of this agent present may influence the circulation [159–161].

PROSTAGLANDINS

In a recent review of this field [164], Moncada, Flower, and Vane noted, "The effects of prostaglandins and related products are awesome and bewildering."

At present, few substances command as much interest as the prostaglandins [164–167]. These compounds directly constrict and dilate coronary vessels and may mediate the vascular effects of other humoral substances and drugs. Furthermore, prostaglandins may act as the critical link that couples myocardial oxygen consumption to alterations in coronary vascular resistance. This section will focus on the effects of the prostaglandins on the coronary circulation.

Prostaglandins can be synthesized by all tissues in the body. The fundamental precursor, arachidonic acid, is derived from 20-carbon essential fatty acids. Arachidonic acid in coronary vessels can be transformed into the major classes of prostaglandins: A, B, C, D, E, F, G, H, I, and thromboxane A_2. Three of these classes—B, C, D—probably have little or no role in regulation of the coronary circulation. Prostaglandins G_2 and H_2 primarily serve as precursors to prostaglandins E, F, prostacycline (PGI_2), and thromboxane A_2. The prostaglandin A's are derived from prostaglandin B's. Recent studies indicate that PGI_2 is the major metabolite of prostaglandin synthesis in blood vessels [164–167].

The prostaglandins act primarily as local hormones. Circulating prostaglandins have minimal effects because pulmonary uptake (PGI_2, PGE_2, and $PGF_{2\alpha}$) or instability (PGI_2, PGE_2, $PGF_{2\alpha}$: 100-s half-life; thromboxane A_2: 30-s half-life) largely prevent these agents form accumulating in the blood stream [164–167].

Pharmacologic studies in a variety of animal preparations have shown that in vivo several prostaglandins (PGA_1, PGE_1, PGE_2, PGH_2, PGI_2) produce coronary dilation. The most potent coronary dilator in this class is PGI_2; the dominant coronary vasoconstrictor is thromboxane A_2 [164,167].

Potential Physiological Role of the Prostaglandins

Prostaglandins are released from the heart by a myriad of stimuli which have effects on the coronary circulation. These stimuli include myocardial ischemic hypoxia, adenine nucleotides, adrenergic nerve stimulation, bradykinin, angiotensin, mechanical stimulation, spontaneous coronary spasm, and alterations of myocardial metabolism [164–167]. Evidence that the prostaglandins mediate the vascular effects of these stimuli is steeped in controversy.

Table 3-1 lists the criteria that must be satisfied before one can state with confidence that a given substance modulates a specific vascular response, i.e., reactive hyperemia. In every instance, currently available data are not sufficient to state with certainty that prostaglandins play a critical role in mediating the response of the coronary circulation to any physiological stimulus. Often the results reported are applicable only to a specific species or a particular experimental preparation. Very few studies concerning the role of prostaglandins in regulation of the coronary circulation have been performed in awake, unanesthetized animals. Often the concentration of the prostaglandin administered is far in excess of the physiological range. Finally, very few studies in this field have been performed on humans.

Recently, attention has been focused on the concept that thromboxane A_2, a potent coronary vasoconstrictor, and prostacycline, a powerful vasodilator, may play key roles in regulating coronary vascular resistance. It has been postulated that these substances may be of great importance in the pathogenesis of coronary spasm or spontaneous intermittent decreases in coronary flow that occur in artificially stenosed coronary vessels [168–172]. A recent study by Robertson et al. [168] indicates that in patients with spontaneous coronary spasm increases in coronary sinus levels of thromboxane B_2 (an inactive hydration product of thromboxane A_2) do not precede episodes of coronary spasm.

In 1975, Alexander et al. [173] reported that inhibition of prostaglandin synthesis with indomethacin or meclophenamate decreased coronary flow by about 15 percent and attenuated the coronary reactive hyperemic response to 10- to 20-s coronary occlusions by two-thirds. These studies were done in a dog heart-lung preparation. Since then, four studies performed in more intact preparations have shown that inhibition of prostaglandin synthesis has little or no effect on basal coronary flow or vasodilator responses to transient coronary occlusions [174–177].

Although no detailed studies have been reported, exercise intolerance or manifestation of myocardial ischemia rarely occurs in patients who take aspirin and indomethacin in doses that should be large enough to totally inhibit prostaglandin synthesis. This suggests that prostaglandin and related products probably do not play a pivotal role in coupling changes in myocardial oxygen consumption to alterations in coronary vascular resistance.

Although numerous studies concerning the effects of prostaglandins in coronary blood flow have been performed, the role of this class of agents in mediating physiological or pharmacologic responses in the coronary circulation remains to be defined.

SUMMARY

Numerous humoral agents can alter coronary vascular resistance by direct and/or indirect effects on coronary vessels. It is of interest that only four humoral agents (norepinephrine, angiotensin, vasopressin, and thromboxane A_2) produce net coronary constriction. All others cause coronary dilation. The impact that all these substances have on the regulation of the coronary circulation is unknown. The general level of knowledge in this area, with the exception of the catecholamines, is woefully inadequate. Given the available information all one can say is that many of these humoral agents have potent vasoactive properties and that under physiological conditions several of them are present in sufficient concentrations to significantly modulate coronary vascular resistance.

REFERENCES

1 Weiner N: Norepinephrine, epinephrine, and the sympathetic amines: Catecholamines, in *The Pharmacological Basis of Therapeutics*, AG Gilman, LS Goodman, A Gilman (eds). London, Macmillan, 1980, chap 8.

2 Markwalder J, Starling EH: Note on some factors which determine blood flow through coronary circulation. *J Physiol* 47: 275, 1914.

3 Katz LN, Lindner E, Weinstein W, Abramson DI, Jochim K: Effects of various drugs on the coronary circulation of the denervated isolated heart of the dog and cat. *Arch Internat Pharmacodyn* 59: 399, 1938.

4 Berne RM: Effect of epinephrine and norepinephrine on coronary circulation. *Circ Res* 6: 644, 1958.

5 Hardin RA, Scott JB, Haddy FJ: Effect of epinephrine and norepinephrine on coronary vascular resistance in dogs. *Amer J Physiol* 201: 276, 1961.

6 Gall PG, Kattus AA, Kolin A, Ross G: Effects of adrenaline and noradrenaline on coronary blood flow before and after beta-adrenergic blockade. *Br J Pharmacol* 26: 713, 1966.

7 Klocke FJ, Kaiser GA, Ross J Jr, Braunwald E: Intrinsic adrenergic vasodilator mechanism in the coronary vascular bed of the dog. *Circ Res* 16: 376, 1965.

8 Pitt B, Elliot EC, Gregg DE: Adrenergic receptor activity in the coronary arteries of the unanesthetized dog. *Circ Res* 21: 75, 1967.

9 McRaven DR, Mark AL, Abboud FM, Mayer HE: Responses of coronary vessels to adrenergic stimuli. *J Clin Invest* 50: 773, 1971.

10 Mark AL, Abboud RM, Schmid PG, Heistad DD, Mayer HE: Differences in direct effects of adrenergic stimuli on coronary, cutaneous, and muscular vessels. *J Clin Invest* 51: 279, 1972.

11 Malindzak GS Jr, Van Dyke AH, Green HD, Meredith JH: Alpha and beta adrenergic receptors in the coronary vascular bed. *Arch Int Pharmacodyn* 197: 112, 1972.

12 Zuberbuhler R, Bohr DF: Responses of coronary smooth muscle to catecholamines. *Circ Res* 16: 431, 1965.

13 Vatner SF, McRitchie RJ, Maroko PR, Patrick TA, Braunwald E: Effects of catecholamines, exercise, and nitroglycerin on the normal and ischemic myocardium in conscious dogs. *J Clin Invest* 54: 563, 1974.

14 Vatner SF, Higgins CB, Braunwald E: Effects of norepinephrine on coronary circulation and left ventricular dynamics in the conscious dog. *Circ Res* 34: 812, 1974.

15 Heistad DD, Abboud FM, Mark AL, Schmid PG: Effect of hypoxemia on responses to norepinephrine and angiotensin in coronary and muscular vessels. *J Pharmacol Exp Thera* 193: 941, 1975.

16 Kelley KO, Feigl EO: Segmental alpha-receptor-mediated vasoconstriction in the canine coronary circulation. *Circ Res* 43: 908, 1978.

17 Dumont L, Lelorier J: Effect of norepinephrine on intramyocardial distribution of blood flow in normal and ischemic myocardium. *Can J Physiol Pharmacol* 55: 755, 1977.

18 Schaper W: Residual perfusion of acutely ischemic heart muscle, in *The Pathophysiology of Myocardial Perfusion.* Amsterdam, Elsevier/North-Holland Biomedical Press, 1979, chap 11, p. 345.

19 Schaper W, Wusten B: Collateral circulation, in *The Pathophysiology of Myocardial Perfusion.* Amsterdam, Elsevier/North-Holland Biomedical Press, 1979, chap 13, p 415.

20 Yurchak PM, Rolett EL, Cohen LS, Gorlin R: Effects of norepinephrine on the coronary circulation in man. *Circulation* 30: 180, 1964.

21 Greenfield JC Jr, Rembert JC, Young WG Jr, Oldham HN Jr, Alexander JA, Sabiston DC Jr: Studies of blood flow in aorta-to-coronary venous bypass grafts in man. *J Clin Invest* 51: 2724, 1972.

22 Mudge GH Jr, Grossman W, Mills RM Jr, Lesch M, Braunwald E: Reflex increase in coronary vascular resistance in patients with ischemic heart disease. *N Engl J Med* 295: 1333, 1976.

23 Goldenberg M, Aranow H Jr, Smith AA, Faber M: Pheochromocytoma and essential hypertensive vascular disease. *Arch Intern Med* 86: 823, 1950.

24 Allwood MJ, Cobbold AF, Ginsburg J: Peripheral vascular effects of noradrenaline, isopropylnoradrenaline and dopamine. *Br Med Bull* 19: 132, 1963.

25 Rayford CR, Huvos A, Khouri EM, Gregg DE: Some determinants of coronary flow in intact dogs. *Physiologist* 4: 92, 1961.

26 Gregg DE, Fisher LC: Blood supply to the heart, in *Handbook of Physiology*, WF Hamilton (ed). Washington, DC, American Physiological Society, 1963, sect 2, Circulation chap 44, p 1517.

27 Sullivan JM, Gorlin R: Effect of *l*-epinephrine on the coronary circulation in human subjects with and without coronary artery disease. *Circ Res* 21: 919, 1967.

28 Maxwell GM, Rowe GG, Castillo CA, Clifford JE, Afonso S, Crumpton CW: The effect of dopamine (3-hydroxytyramine) upon the systemic, pulmonary, and cardiac haemodynamics and metabolism of intact dog. *Arch Int Pharmacodyn Ther* 129: 62, 1960.

29 Brooks HL, Stein PD, Matson JL, Hyland JW: Dopamine-induced alterations in coronary hemodynamics in dogs. *Circ Res* 24: 699, 1969.

30 Nayler WG, McInnes JS, Carson V, Lowe TE: Effect of dopamine on coronary vascular resistance and myocardial function. *Cardiovascular Res* 5: 161, 1971.

31 Schuelke DM, Mark AL, Schmid PG, Eckstein JW: Coronary vasodilation produced by dopamine after adrenergic blockade. *J Pharmacol Exp Thera* 176: 320, 1971.

32 Cobb FR, McHale PA, Bache RJ, Greenfield JC Jr: Coronary and systemic hemodynamic effects of dopamine in the awake dog. *Am J Physiol* 222: 1355, 1972.

33 Goldberg LI: Cardiovascular and renal actions of dopamine: Potential clinical applications. *Pharmacol Rev* 24: 1, 1972.

34 McDonald RH Jr, Goldberg LI: Analysis of the cardiovascular effects of dopamine in the dog. *J Pharmacol Exp Ther* 140: 60, 1963.

35 Vatner SF, Millard RW, Higgins CB: Coronary and myocardial effects of dopamine in the conscious dog: Parasympatholytic augmentation of pressor and inotropic actions. *J Pharmacol Exp Thera* 187: 280, 1973.

36 Takenaka F, Morishita H: Possible mechanisms involved in the coronary vasodilator response to dopamine. *Arch Int Pharmacodyn* 222: 81, 1976.

37 Goldberg LI, Hsieh Y-Y, Resnekov L: Newer catecholamines for treatment of heart failure and shock: An update on dopamine and a first look at dobutamine. *Prog Cardiovasc Dis* 19: 327, 1977.

38 Vanhoutte PM, Verbeuren TJ, Webb RC: Local modulation of adrenergic neuroeffector interaction in the blood vessel wall. *Physiol Rev* 61: 151, 1981.

39 Goldberg L: Personal communication. University of Chicago, December 1981.

40 Vatner SF, Baig H: Importance of heart rate in determining the effects of sympathomimetic amines on regional myocardial function and blood flow in conscious dogs with acute myocardial ischemia. *Circ Res* 45: 793, 1979.

41 Mueller HS: Effects of dopamine on haemodynamics and myocardial energetics in man: Comparison with effects of isoprenaline and L-noradrenaline. *Resuscitation* 6: 179, 1978.

42 Chilian WM, Boatwright RB, Shoji T, Griggs DM Jr: Evidence against significant resting sympathetic coronary vasoconstrictor tone in the conscious dog. *Circ Res* 49: 866, 1981.

43 Marcus ML, Ehrhardt JC, Verani MS: Reproducibility and sensitivity of the exercise isotope ventriculogram. *Clin Res* 25: 556A, 1977.

44 Bevan RD: Effect of sympathetic denervation on smooth muscle cell proliferation in the growing rabbit ear artery. *Circ Res* 37: 14, 1975.

45 Hart MN, Heistad DD, Brody MJ: Effect of chronic hypertension and sympathetic denervation on wall/lumen ratio of cerebral vessels. *Hypertension* 2: 419, 1980.

46 Rosendorff C, Hoffman JEE, Verrier ED, Rouleau J, Boerboom LE: Cholesterol potentiates the coronary artery response to norepinephrine in anesthetized and conscious dogs. *Circ Res* 48: 320, 1981.

47 Yokoyama M, Goldman M, Henry PD: Supersensitivity of atherosclerotic rabbit arteries to α-adrenergic stimulation and ergonovine. *Circulation* 58: II-57, 1978.

48 Johannson UJ, Mark AL, Marcus ML, Armstrong ML: Effects of dietary hyperlipoproteinemia on coronary vascular responsiveness in vivo. *Circulation* 64(suppl IV): 1980.

49 Regoli D, Park WK, Rioux F: Pharmacology of angiotensin. *Pharmacol Rev* 26: 69, 1974.

50 Various authors: Symposium: The pharmacology of angiotensin antagonists. *Fed Proc* 35: 2486, 1976c.

51 Various authors: Symposium: Advances in our knowledge of the renin-angiotensin system. *Fed Proc* 36: 1753, 1977.

52 Douglas WW: Polypeptides – angiotensin, plasma, kinins, and others, in *The Phar-*

macological Basis of Therapeutics, AG Gilman, LS Goodman, A Gilman. London, Macmillan, 1980, chap 27, p 647.

53 Davis JO, Freeman RH: Mechanisms regulating renin release. *Physiol Rev* 56: 1976.

54 Ferrario CM, Gildenberg PL, McCubbin JW: Cardiovascular effects of angitensin mediated by the central nervous system. *Cir Res* 30: 257, 1972.

55 Braun-Menendez E, Fasciolo JC, Leloir LF, Munoz JM: The substance causing renal hypertension. *J Physiol* (London) 98: 283, 1940.

56 Page IH, Helmer OM: Angiotonin-activator, renin- and angiotonin-inhibitor and the mechanism of angiotonin tachyphylaxis in normal, hypertensive and nephrectomized animals. *J Exp Med* 71: 485, 1940.

57 Hill WHP, Andrus EC: Effects of renin and of angiotonin upon isolated perfused heart. *Proc Soc Exptl Biol Med* 44: 213, 1940.

58 Lorber V: The action of angiotonin on the completely isolated mammalian heart. *Am Heart J* 23: 37, 1942.

59 Fowler NO, Holmes JC: Coronary and myocardial actions of angiotensin. *Circ Res* 14: 191, 1964.

60 Douglas CR, Ponce/Zumino A, Ruiz-Petrich E, Puig F, Talesnik S: Effect of angiotensin upon coronary flow and oxygen consumption of the isolated heart of the cat. *Acta Physiol Lat Amer* 14: 161, 1967.

61 Meier M, Wirz E, Brunner H, Stamm W: Effects of norepinephrine and angiotensin II-amide on coronary flow and myocardial oxygen consumption in the cat. *Cardiologia* 47: 127, 1965.

62 Drimal J, Pavek K, Selecky FV: Primary and secondary effects of angiotensin on the coronary circulation. *Cardiologia* 54: 1, 1969.

63 Britton S, DiSalvo J: Effects of angiotensin I and angiotensin II on hindlimb and coronary vascular resistance. *Am J Physiol* 225: 1226, 1973.

64 Cohen MV, Kirk ES: Differential response of large and small coronary arteries to nitroglycerin and angiotensin. *Circ Res* 33: 445, 1973.

65 Heistad DD, Abboud FM, Mark AL, Schmid PG: Effect of hypoxemia on responses to norepinephrine and angiotensin in coronary and muscular vessels. *J Pharmacol Exp Thera* 193: 941, 1975.

66 Heyndrickx GR, Boettcher DH, Vatner SF: Effects of angiotensin, vasopressin, and methoxamine on cardiac function and blood flow distribution in conscious dogs. *Am J Physiol* 231: 1579, 1976.

67 Gunther S, Cannon PJ: Modulation of angiotensin II coronary vasoconstriction by cardiac prostaglandin synthesis. *Am J Physiol* 238: H895, 1980.

68 Mueller HS, Gregory JJ, Giannelli S Jr, Ayres SM: Systemic hemodynamic and myocardial metabolic effects of isoproterenol and angiotensin after open-heart surgery. *Circulation* 42: 491, 1970.

69 Liang C-S, Gavras H, Hood WB Jr: Renin-angiotensin system inhibition in conscious sodium-depleted dogs. *J Clin Invest* 61: 874, 1978.

70 Nakano J: Cardiovascular responses to neurohypophysial hormones, in *Handbook of Physiology*, RO Greep, EB Astwood (eds). Washington DC, American Physiological Society, 1974, vol 4, sect 7, Endocrinology, chap 15, p. 395.

71 Nakano J: Cardiovascular actions of vasopressin. *Jap Circ J* 37: 363, 1973.

72 Hays RM: Agents affecting the renal conservation of water, in *The Pharmacological Basis of Therapeutics*, AG Gilman, LS Goodman, A Gilman (eds). London, Macmillan, 1980, chap 37, p. 916.

73 Oliver G, Schäfer A: On the physiological action of extracts of pituitary body and certain other glandular organs. *J Physiol* (London) 18: 277, 1895.

74 Corliss RJ, McKenna DH, Sialer S, O'Brien GS, Rowe GG: Systemic and coronary hemodynamic effects of vasopressin. *Am J Med Sci* 256: 293, 1968.

75 West W, Guzman SV: Coronary dilation and constriction visualized by relative angiography. *Cir Res* 7: 527, 1959.

76 Ericsson BF: The effect of vasopressin on the coronary circulation in normovolemic and hypovolemic dogs. *Acta Chir Scand* 138: 235, 1972.

77 Pullan PT, Johnston WP, Anderson WP, Korner PI: Plasma vasopressin in blood pressure homeostasis and in experimental renal hypertension. *Am J Physiol* 239 (Heart Circ Physiol 8): H81, 1980.

78 Slotnik IL, Teigland JD: Cardiac accidents following vasopressin injection (pitressin). *JAMA* 146: 1126, 1951.

79 Katz LN, Lindner E: The action of excess Na^+, Ca^{++}, and K^+ on the coronary vessels. *Am J Physiol* 124: 155, 1938.

80 Bass P, Mazurkiewicz I, Melville KI: Effects of magnesium on coronary flow and heart action and its influence on the responses to adrenaline and noradrenaline. *Arch Int Pharmacodynther* 117: 9, 1958.

81 Katz LN, Lindner E: The action of excess NaCaK on the coronary vessels. *Am J Physiol* 124: 155, 1938.

82 Scott JB, Frohlich ED, Hardin RA, Haddy FJ: Na^+, K^+, Ca^{++}, and Mg^{++} action on coronary vascular resistance in the dog heart. *Am J Physiol* 201: 1095, 1961.

83 Pitt B, Sugishita Y, Gregg DE: Coronary hemodynamic effects of calcium in the unanesthetized dog. *Am J Physiol* 216: 1456, 1969.

84 Brace RA, Anderson DK, Chen W-T, Scott JB, Haddy FJ: Local effects of hypokalemia on coronary resistance and myocardial contractile force. *Am J Physiol* 227: 590, 1974.

85 Murray PA, Sparks HV: The mechanism of K^+-induced vasodilation of the coronary vascular bed of the dog. *Cir Res* 42: 35, 1978.

86 Haynes RC Jr, Murad F: Thyroid and antithyroid drugs, in *The Pharmacological Basis of Therapeutics*, AG Gilman, LS Goodman, A Gilman (eds). London, Macmillan, 1980, chap 60, pp 1397–1419.

87 Shambaugh GE III: Chemistry and actions of thyroid hormone, biologic and cellular effects, in *The Thyroid*, SG Werner, SH Ingbar (eds). New York, Harper & Row, 1978, chap 7, p. 115.

88 Skelton CL, Karch FE, Wildenthal K: Lack of acute effects of thyroid hormones on myocardial contractility. *Am J Physiol* 224 (4): 957, 1973.

89 Markowitz C, Yater WM: Response of explanted cardiac muscle to thyroxine. *Am J Physiol* 100: 162, 1932.

90 Skelton CL, Sonnenblick EH: Cardiovascular system, in *Hyperthyroidism*, SC Werner, SH Ingbar (eds). New York, Harper & Row, 1978, chap 36, p. 688.

91 Buccino RA, Spann JF Jr, Pool PE, et al: Influence of thyroid state on the intrinsic contractile properties and energy stores of the myocardium. *J Clin Invest* 46: 1669, 1967.

92 Murayama M, Goodkind MJ: Effect of thyroid hormone on the frequency-force relationship of atrial myocardium from the guinea pig. *Circ Res* 23: 743, 1968.

93 Amidi M, Leon DF, deGroot WJ, et al: Effect of the thyroid state on myocardial contractility and ventricular ejection rate in man. *Circulation* 38: 229, 1968.

94 Skelton CL, Sonnenblick EH: Heterogeneity of contractile function in cardiac

hypertrophy. *Circ Res* (suppl 34 & 35): 83, 1974.

95 Skelton CL, Pool PE, Seagren SC, Braunwald E: Mechanochemistry of cardiac muscle. Part V. Influence of thyroid state on energy utilization. *J Clin Invest* 50: 463, 1971.

96 Beznak M, Marcsan A, Fournier T: Cardiovascular effects of thyroxine treatment in normal rats. *Can J Biochem Physiol* 40: 1647, 1962.

97 Cohen J, Aroesty JM, Rosenfeld MG: Determinants of thyroxine-induced cardiac hypertrophy in mice. *Circ Res* 18: 388, 1965.

98 Rowe GG, Huston JH, Weinstein AB, Tuchman H, Brown JF, Crumpton CW: The hemodynamics of thyrotoxicosis in man with special reference to coronary blood flow and myocardial oxygen metabolism. *J Clin Invest* 35: 272, 1956.

99 Graettinger JS, Muenster JJ, Selverstone LA, Campbell JA: A correlation of clinical and hemodynamic studies in patients with hyperthyroidism with and without congestive heart failure. *J Clin Invest* 38: 1316, 1959.

100 deGroot WJ, Leonard JJ: Hyperthyroidism as a high cardiac output state. *Am Heart J* 79: 265, 1970.

101 Graettinger JS, Muenster JJ, Checchia CS, Grissom RL, Campbell JA: A correlation of clinical and hemodynamic studies in patients with hypothyroidism. *J Clin Invest* 37: 502, 1958.

102 Skelton CL, Sonnenblick EH: Cardiovascular system in hypothyroidism, *The Thyroid,* SC Werner, SH Ingbar (eds). New York, Harper & Row, 1978, chap 46, p 861.

103 White C: Personal communication. University of Iowa, December 1981.

104 Williams LT, Lefkowitz RJ, Watanabe AM, et al: Thyroid hormone regulation of β-adrenergic receptor number. *J Biol Chem* 252: 2787, 1977.

105 Steinberg AD: Myxedema and coronary artery disease–a comparative autopsy study. *Ann Intern Med* 68: 338, 1968.

106 Marcus ML, Chilian WM, Wangler RD, Peres KG, Tomanek RJ: Does the stimulus producing hypertrophy alter the interaction between the coronary vascular bed and myocardial mass? *Fed Proc* 41: 1097, 1982.

106a Haynes RC Jr, Murad F: Adrenocorticotropic hormone; Adrenocortical steroids and their synthetic analogs; Inhibitors of adrenocortical steroid biosynthesis, in *The Pharmacological Basis of Therapeutics,* AG Gilman, LS Goodman, A Gilman (eds). London, Macmillan, 1980, chap 63, pp 1466–1496.

107 Krakoff L, Nicolis G, Amsel B: Pathogenesis of hypertension in Cushing's syndrome. *Am J Med* 58: 216, 1975.

108 Unger RH, Orci L: Physiology and pathophysiology of glucagon. *Physiol Rev* 56: 779, 1976.

109 Larner J: Insulin and oral hypoglycemic drugs; Glucagon, in *The Pharmacological Basis of Therapeutics,* AG Gilman, LS Goodman, A Gilman (eds). London, Macmillan, 1980, chap 64, pp 1497–1523.

110 Farah A, Tuttle R: Studies on the pharmacology of glucagon. *J Pharmacol Exp Ther* 129: 49, 1960.

111 Reagan TJ, Lehan PH, Henneman DH, Behar A, Hellems HK: Myocardial metabolic and contractile response to glucagon and epinephrine. *J Lab Clin Med* 63: 638, 1964.

112 Glick G, Parmley WW, Wechsler AS, Sonnenblick EH: Glucagon: Its enhancement of cardiac performance in the cat and dog and persistence of its inotropic action despite beta-receptor blockade with propranolol. *Circ Res* 22: 789, 1968.

113 Luchesi BR: Cardiac actions of glucagon. *Circ Res* 22: 777, 1968.

114 Parmley WW, Glick G, Sonnenblick EH: Cardiovascular effects of glucagon in man. *New Eng J Med* 279: 12, 1968.

115 Moir TW, Nayler WG: Coronary vascular effects of glucagon in the isolated dog heart. *Circ Res* 26: 29, 1970.

116 Goldschlager N, Robin E, Cowan CM, Leb G, Bing RJ: The effect of glucagon on the coronary circulation in man. *Circulation* 40: 829, 1969.

117 Berne RM, Rubio R: Coronary circulation, in *Handbook of Physiology*. Bethesda, Maryland, American Physiological Society, 1979, vol 1, sect 2, The cardiovascular system, chap 25, p 873.

118 Berne RM: The role of adenosine in the regulation of coronary blood flow. *Circ Res* 47: 807, 1980.

119 Drury AN, Szent-Gyorgyi A: The physiological activity of adenine compounds with special reference to their action upon the mammalian heart. *J Physiol* (London) 68: 213, 1929.

120 Rembert JC, Boyd LM, Watkinson WP, Greenfield JC Jr: Effect of adenosine on transmural myocardial blood flow distribution in the awake dog. *Am J Physiol* 239: H7, 1980.

121 Verrier ED, Baer RW, Hickey RF, Vlahakes GJ, Hoffman JIE: Transmural pressure-flow relations during diastole in the canine left ventricle. *Circulation* 62 (suppl 3): 62, 1980.

122 Wusten B, Buss DD, Deist H, Schaper W: Dilatory capacity of the coronary circulation and its correlation to the arterial vasculature in the canine left ventricle. *Basic Res Cardiol* 72: 636, 1977.

123 Mueller TM, Marcus ML, Kerber RE, Young YA, Barnes RW, Abboud FM: Effect of renal hypertension and left ventricular hypertrophy on the coronary circulation in dogs. *Circ Res* 42: 543, 1978.

124 Bache RJ, Vrobel TR, Arentzen CE, Ring WS: Effect of maximal coronary vasodilation on transmural myocardial perfusion during tachycardia in dogs with left ventricular hypertrophy. *Circ Res* 49: 742, 1981.

125 Harder DR, Belardinelli L, Sperelakis N, et al: Differential effects of adenosine and nitroglycerin on the action potentials of large and small coronary arteries. *Circ Res* 44: 176, 1979.

125a Hintz TH, Vatner SF: Adenosine and dipyridimole dilate large coronary arteries in the conscious dog. *Circulation* (suppl II): 143, 1982.

126 Patterson RE, Kirk ES: Apparent improvement in canine collateral myocardial blood flow during vasodilation depends on criteria used to identify ischemic myocardium. *Circ Res* 47: 108, 1980.

127 Schaper W: *The Collateral Circulation of the Heart*. Amsterdam, North-Holland, 1971.

128 Douglas WW: Histamine and 5-hydroxytryptamine (serotonin) and their antagonists, in *The Pharmacological Basis of Therapeutics*, AG Gilman, LS Goodman, A Gilman (eds). London, Macmillan, 1980, chap 26, pp 609–646.

129 Owen DAA: Histamine receptors in the cardiovascular system. *Gen Pharmac* 8: 141, 1977.

130 Reinhardt D, Wiemann HM, Schumann HJ: Effects of the H_1-antagonist promethazine and the H_2-antagonist burimamide on chronotropic, inotropic and coronary vascular responses to histamine in isolated perfused guinea-pig hearts. *Agents and Actions*, vol 6/6, Basel, Birkhauser Berlag, 1976.

131 Black JW, Duncan WAM, Durant CJ, Ganellin CR, Parsons EM: Definition and antagonism of histamine H_2-receptors. *Nature* 236: 385, 1972.

132 Altura BM, Halevy S: Recent developments of the histamine problem: Pharmacological actions. Cardiovascular actions of histamines, in *Histamine II and Anti-Histaminics*, MR Silva (ed). Berlin, Springer-Verlag, 1978.

133 Giles RW, Heise G, Wilcken DEL: Histamine receptors in the coronary circulation of the dog. Effects of mepyramine and metiamide on responses to histamine infusions. *Circ Res* 40: 542, 1977.

134 Woods JR Jr, Brinkman CR III, Dandavino A, Murayama K, Assali NS: Action of histamine and H_1 and H_2 blockers on the cardiopulmonary circulation. *Am J Physiol* 232: H73-H78, 1977.

135 Zavecz JH, Levi R: Histamine-induced negative inotropism. Mediation by H_1-receptors. *J Pharmacol Exp Thera* 206: 274, 1978.

136 Feigen GA, Prager DJ: Experimental cardiac anaphylaxis. Physiologic, pharmacologic and biochemical aspects of immune reactions in the isolated heart. *Am J Cardiol* 24: 474, 1969.

137 Levi R: Effects of exogenous and immunologically released histamine on the isolated heart: A quantitative comparison. *J Pharmacol Exp Thera* 182: 227, 1972.

138 Capurro N, Levi R: The heart as a target organ in systemic allergic reactions. Comparison of cardiac anaphylaxis in vivo and in vitro. *Circ Res* 36: 520, 1975.

139 Rapport MM, Green AA, Page IH: Serum vasoconstrictor (serotonin). IV. Isolation and characterization. *J Biol Chem* 176: 1243, 1948.

140 Garattini S, Valzelli L: *Serotonin*. Amsterdam, Elsevier, 1965.

141 Erspamer V: Peripheral physiological and pharmacological actions of indolealkylamines. I. Acute toxicity of indolealkylamines, in *5-Hydroxytryptamine and Related Indolealkylamines*. New York, Springer-Verlag, 1966, chap 7.

142 Schofield BM, Walker JM: Perfusion of the coronary arteries of the dog. *J Physiol* 122: 489, 1953.

143 Griggs DM Jr, Case RB: Effect of serotonin on coronary vascular resistance and myocardial oxygen consumption. *Circulation* 22: 758, 1960.

144 Maxwell GM, Castillo CA, Clifford JE, Crumpton CW, Rowe GG: Effect of serotonin (5-hydroxytryptamine) on the systemic and coronary vascular bed of the dog. *Am J Physiol* 197: 736, 1959.

145 Rowe GG, Skoda A, Castillo CA, Kyle JC, Leicht TR, Crumpton CW: Systemic and coronary hemodynamic effects of an amine oxidase inhibitor and of serotonin. *Clin Pharm Thera* 4: 467, 1965.

146 Bove AA, Dewey JD: Mediators of epicardial coronary artery vasoactivity in the intact dog. *Fed Proc* 41: 1528, 1982.

147 Schachter M: Kallikreins and kinins. *Physiol Rev* 49: 510, 1969.

148 McGiff JC, Nasjletti A: Symposium: Kinins, renal function and blood pressure regulation. *Fed Proc* 35: 172, 1975.

149 Schachter M, Barton S: Kallikreins (kininogenases) and kinins, in *Endocrinology*, LJ deGroot et al (eds). New York, Grune & Stratton, vol 3, chap 136, pp 1699–1709.

150 Maxwell GM, Elliot RB, Kneebone GM: Effects of bradykinin on the systemic and coronary vascular bed of the intact dog. *Circ Res* X: 359, 1962.

151 Needleman P, Marshall GR, Sobel BE: Hormone interactions in the isolated rabbit heart. Synthesis and coronary vasomotor effects of prostaglandins, angiotensin, and bradykinin. *Circ Res* 37: 802, 1975.

152 Regoli D, Barabe J, Therialult B: Does indomethacin antagonize the effects of peptides and other agents on the coronary circulation of rabbit isolated hearts? *Can J Physiol Pharmacol* 55: 307, 1977.

153 Euler US von, Gaddum JH: An unidentified depressor substance in certain tissue

extracts. *J Physiol* 72: 74, 1931.
154 Chang MM, Leeman SE: Isolation of a sialogogic peptide from bovine hypothalamic tissue and its characterization as substance P. *J Biol Chem* 245: 4784, 1970.
155 Bury RW, Mashford ML: Substance P: Its pharmacology and physiological roles. *Aust J Esp Biol Med Sci* 55: 671, 1977.
156 Losay J, Mroz EA, Treagear GW, Leeman SE, Gamble WJ: Action of substance P on the coronary blood flow in the isolated dog heart, in *Substance P*, US von Euler, B Pernow (eds). New York, Raven Press, 1976.
157 Said SI, Mutt V: Polypeptide with broad biological activity: Isolation from small intestine. *Science* 169: 1217, 1970.
158 Bodanszky M, Klausner YS, Yang Lin C, Mutt V, Said SI: Synthesis of the vasoactive intestinal peptide (VIP). *J Am Chem Soc* 96: 4973, 1974.
159 Said SI: Vasoactive intestinal polypeptide (VIP) current status, in *Gastrointestinal Hormones. A Symposium*, JC Thompson (ed). Austin, University of Texas Press, 1975.
160 Said SI: VIP: Overview in *Gut Hormones*, SR Bloom (ed). Edinburgh, Churchill Livingstone, 1978, chap 73, p 465.
161 Said SI: Vasoactive intestinal polypeptide (VIP) as a neural peptide, in *Gut Peptides, Secretion, Function and Clinical Aspects*, A Miyoshi (ed). Tokyo, Kodansha Ltd, 1979.
162 Domschke S, Domschke W, Bloom SR, Mitznegg P, Mitchell S, Lux G, Strunz U, Demling L: Pharmacokinetics and pharmacodynamics of VIP in man, in *Gut Hormones*, SR Bloom (ed). London, Churchill Livingstone, 1978, chap 75, p 475.
163 Yoshida T, Geumei AM, Schmitt RJ, Said SI: Vasoactive intestinal peptide: A potent coronary vasodilator, abstracted. *Fed Proc* 33: 378, 1974.
164 Moncada S, Flower RJ, Vane JR: Prostaglandins, prostacyclin, and thromboxane A_2, in *The Pharmacological Basis of Therapeutics*, New York, Macmillan, 1980, chap 28, pp 668–681.
165 Needleman P, Kaley G: Cardiac and coronary prostaglandin synthesis and function. *N Engl J Med* 298: 1122, 1978.
166 Sivakoff M, Pure E, Hsueh W, Needleman P: Prostaglandins and the heart. *Fed Proc* 38: 78, 1979.
167 Dusting GJ, Moncada S, Vane JR: Prostaglandins, their intermediates and precursors: Cardiovascular actions and regulatory roles in normal and abnormal circulatory systems. *Prog Cardiovas Dis* 21: 405, 1979.
168 Robertson RM, Robertson D, Roberts LJ, Maas RL, FitzGerald GA, Friesinger GC, Oates JA: Thromboxane A_2 in vasotonic angina pectoris. *N Engl J Med* 304: 998, 1981.
169 Kuzuya T, Tada M, Inoue M, et al: Increased levels of thromboxane A_2 in peripheral and coronary circulation in patients with angina pectoris. *Am J Cardiol* 45: 454, 1980.
170 Folts JD, Crowell EB Jr, Rowe GG: Platelet aggregation in partially obstructed vessels and its elimination with aspirin. *Circulation* 54: 365, 1976.
171 Uchida Y, Yoshimoto N, Murao S: Prostaglandin E_2 and epinephrine participate in cyclical reduction of coronary blood pressure and flow. *Jpn Heart J* 19(2): 281, 1978.
172 Esumi K, Tada M, Kuzuya T, Ohmori M, Matsuda H, Inoue M, Abe H, Uchida Y, Murao S: Thromboxane A_2 and prostaglandin I_2 in canine circulation during transient myocardial ischemia. *Circulation* 64 (suppl IV): 266, 1981.
173 Alexander RW, Kent KM, Pisano JJ, et al: Regulation of postocclusive hyperemia by

endogenously synthesized prostaglandins in the dog heart. *J Clin Invest* 55: 1174, 1975.

174 Owen TL, Ehrhart IC, Weidner WJ, et al: Effects of indomethacin on local blood flow regulation in canine heart and kidney. *Proc Soc Exp Biol Med* 149: 871, 1975.

175 Hintze TH, Kaley G: Prostaglandins in the control of blood flow in the canine myocardium. *Circ Res* 40: 313, 1977.

176 Giles RW, Wilcken DEL: Reactive hyperaemia in the dog heart: Inter-relations between adenosine, ATP, and aminophylline and the effect of indomethacin. *Cardiovasc Res* 11: 113, 1977.

177 Block AJ, Feinberg H, Herbaczynska-Cedro K, et al: Anoxia-induced release of prostaglandins in rabbit isolated hearts. *Circ Res* 36: 34, 1975.

PART **FOUR**

EFFECTS OF DISEASE PROCESSES ON THE CORONARY CIRCULATION

CHAPTER 9

EFFECTS OF CORONARY OCCLUSION ON MYOCARDIAL PERFUSION

Myocardial infarction is the scourge of western humanity in our age. Ischemic heart disease is the leading cause of death and the most prominent cause of disability in the United States; hence, it is understandable that an enormous effort has been directed toward improving our understanding of this problem. In the past two decades, substantial progress in this area has been made. This chapter will review those aspects of myocardial infarction that are closely related to myocardial perfusion.

INFARCT-RISK RELATIONSHIP

When a coronary artery is suddenly occluded, the principal determinants of the size of the resulting infarction are the size of the perfusion field that has been occluded and the level of residual perfusion within this risk zone [1–4]. In the absence of a stimulus which promotes the growth of collateral vessels (see Chapter 10), collateral flow is primarily dependent on genetic, geometric, and hemodynamic factors. For many years it was assumed that the size of the risk zone could be accurately predicted from the site of coronary occlusion. It is now generally acknowledged that this assumption is false. One cannot estimate the perfusion field of a coronary vessel from the epicardial surface distribution of the vessel. In dogs, when a coronary artery is occluded at a specific site, the size of the resulting infarction is extremely variable (Figure 9-1) [5–9b]. This variability is primarily related to two factors. First, when a major coronary vessel is occluded, if the perfusion field of the vessel determined by coronary stereoangiography involves less than 18 percent of left ventricular mass, no infarction occurs (Figure 9-1) [5–9b]. Small risk zones probably do not develop necrosis because collateral flow to such zones is relatively abundant. Collateral vessels enter an ischemic zone from its periphery. Consequently, small risk zones, which have a larger circumference-to-area ratio than larger risk zones, have greater collateral flow per gram (see Chapter 10). Second, if the risk zone is defined by postmortem coronary stereoangiography, within the zone the amount of tissue that develops necrosis is variable (Figure 9-1) [5–9b]. This occurs because severe perfusion deficits develop only in the central portion of a large risk zone defined by stereoangiography [9]. The peripheral zone is perfused by collateral flow or composed in part of interdigitating tissue perfused by adjacent, unoccluded vessels (overlap flow).

It has not been established that in other animal species infarct-risk relationships are similar to those described in the dog. However, one clinical study suggests that

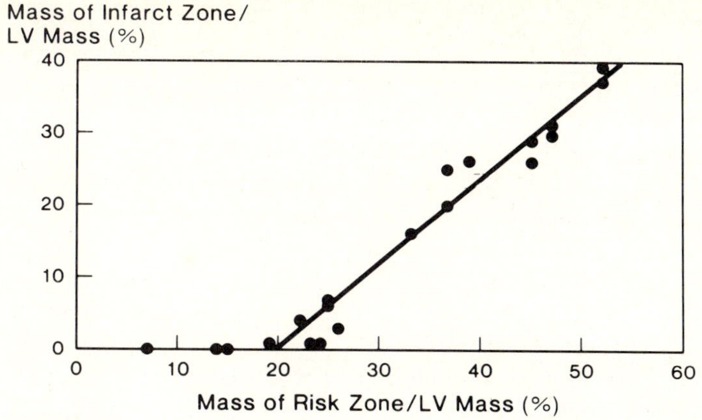

FIGURE 9-1
Relationship between the risk zone and the infarct zone in dogs. In this study, occlusion of the circumflex coronary artery at a constant location (just distal to the first marginal branch of the circumflex) was associated with a risk zone that varied widely in size. When the risk zone involved less than 18 percent of left ventricular (LV) mass, no infarction was evident 2 days following coronary occlusion. When the risk zone was greater than 18 percent of left ventricular mass, there was a linear relationship between the size of the risk zone and the infarct zone. Each dot on this graph represents data obtained from one dog. (*From S Koyanagi et al* [9].)

the infarct-risk relationship in patients does closely resemble that which has been observed in the dog [10].

Recent studies by Koyanagi et al. [9] indicate that the infarct-risk relationship for the entire left ventricle is a composite of several infarct-risk relationships specific to various layers of the left ventricle (see Figure 9-2). Furthermore, at least one intervention—hypertension and left ventricular hypertrophy—shifts the total infarct-risk relationship primarily by altering the infarct-risk relationship in the midwall of the left ventricle [11]. Thus, in studies assessing the effects of interventions that may alter infarct size, it may be worthwhile to examine both global and regional (layer-by-layer) infarct-risk relationships.

The concept that infarct size must be related to the perfusion field of the occluded vessel has major implications for research studies concerning interventions that may alter infarct size.

Since the early 1970s, many prominent investigators, following the lead of Eugene Braunwald, have published numerous studies in which the effects of interventions on infarct size have been assessed [12–14]. These studies have stimulated substantial interest in this area. Unfortunately, in most of these studies, infarct size was not expressed in relation to the size of the risk zone, the experimental preparation was an anesthetized open-chest dog, and usually the number of animals employed in each subgroup was less than 15. Often the presumed size of the ischemic zone was dependent on electrocardiographic data or infarct size

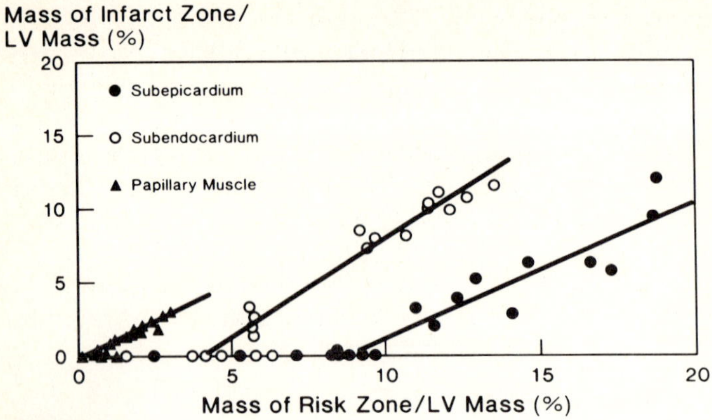

FIGURE 9-2
Relationship between the size of the risk zone and the size of the infarct zone in specific layers of the left ventricular (LV) myocardium. The infarct-risk relationship was steeper in the subendocardium and papillary muscle regions than in the subepicardium. Thus, the infarct-risk relationship for the entire left ventricle is a composite of several infarct-risk relationships specific to various layers of the left ventricle. (*From S Koyanagi et al* [9].)

was based on serial measurements of creatine kinase in the blood. Because of these serious deficiencies, both the qualitative and the quantitative aspects of the differences reported should be interpreted with great caution.

Virtually all clinical trials that have been reported concerning the effects of interventions on infarct size have not estimated the size of the risk zone [14]. In addition, the methods used to assess infarct size in clinical studies have been very crude (see below). Thus, it follows that interpretations of the results of these clinical trials should be guarded. Unfortunately, all ongoing large clinical trials concerning interventions that may limit infarct size have similar deficiencies in their design.

The influence of the infarct-risk relationship on the outcome of studies aimed at evaluating interventions that modify infarct size can be reckoned with in two ways: (1) direct determination of the infarct-risk relationship in every patient or animal studied and (2) use of very large randomized treatment groups (n = greater than 50) in which the site of coronary occlusion is constant. In clinical studies only the first approach is practical, provided that techniques for assessing the infarct-risk relationship in humans are developed. If the infarct-risk relationship is ignored, it is likely that the quantitative aspects of the results obtained in intervention trials will be open to serious question.

Methods of Determining Infarct-Risk Relationships in Animals

The size of an infarction is best determined with pathological techniques (gross pathology, histology, ultrastructure, and various special stains such as nitrotetrozolium blue) [15–20]. The best method for determining the risk zone in animals remains controversial. The general approaches for estimating the size of the risk zone are briefly summarized below.

Postmortem Coronary Stereoangiography This approach, initially introduced by Schaper [2,4], involves analysis of postmortem arteriograms of the whole heart and multiple transverse slices of the left ventricle. The coronary vessels are perfused post mortem at a pressure 10 to 30 mmHg higher than mean systemic pressure with a barium-gelatin mixture which solidifies in the vessels within minutes following injection (refer to Figure 1-5). The transmural perfusion field of the occluded vessel (the *anatomic risk zone*) can be accurately determined from the slice angiograms even if collateral vessels are present (Figure 9-3). By superimposing a diagram of the slice angiograms on the corresponding tissue slice, the relationship between the geometry of the infarcted zone and risk zone can be

FIGURE 9-3
Method of defining the risk and infarct zones using postmortem coronary angiography. (*a*) Ventricular slice from which the zone of infarction can be traced. (*b*) Slice arteriogram which is used to outline the perfusion field of the occluded vessel. Dotted lines in (*b*) represent the boundaries of the perfusion field of the occluded vessel. (*c*) Diagram of the ventricular slice in which the infarct and risk areas are superimposed.

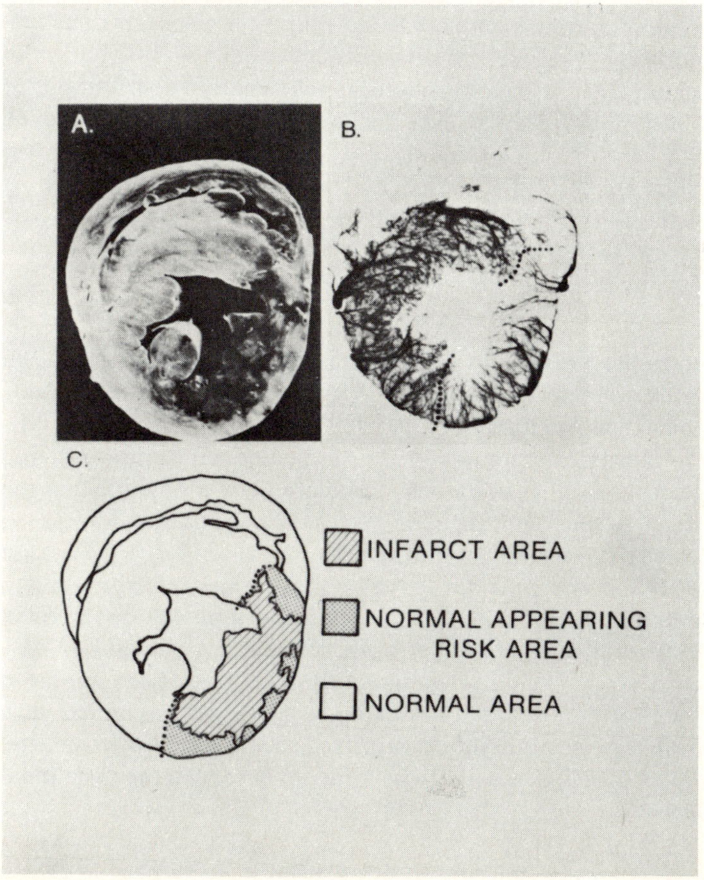

ascertained. The total size of the infarcted and risk zones for the entire heart can be calculated by using an approach similar to Simpson's rule. The reproducibility of this method in our laboratory is excellent (plus or minus 2 percent for the risk region; plus or minus 1 percent for the infarcted zone) [9]. There are three problems with this method: the normal-appearing risk zone contains about 10 percent necrotic tissue; the infarcted zone contains about 10 percent normal tissue; and the noninfarcted risk zone is perfused largely by overlap flow [9,20a]. Overlap flow is delivered to a presumably ischemic zone by unoccluded vessels which interdigitate in the perfusion field of the occluded vessels. The major advantage of postmortem coronary stereoangiography is that the risk zone can be determined days after coronary occlusion. This facilitates studies in chronically instrumented awake animals.

Perfusion of the Occluded Vessel This approach is accomplished by cannulating the occluded vessel immediately distal to the point of occlusion and perfusing the area with an indicator at systemic pressure. This can be done when the animal is alive or immediately post mortem. This is another method of defining the anatomic risk zone. Best results are obtained by utilizing an indicator that is confined to the arterial circulation, such as labeled microspheres or various colored batches of Microfil [21]. The risk zone is identified from the distribution of the indicator in ventricular slices with color photographs (Microfil distribution) or autoradiography (labeled microspheres). The location of the risk zone can be defined accurately with a resolution of less than 0.5 mm. This method has two limitations: (1) the results are best if the occluded zone is perfused within hours of coronary occlusion and (2) the possibility that the size of the risk zone post occlusion will be different from the preocclusion risk zone cannot be excluded because of the no-reflow phenomenon.

Perfusion of Nonoccluded Vessels A negative image of the risk zone can be obtained by perfusing the nonoccluded vessels with an indicator [22]. Ideally, such an indicator (carbon black; technetium 99m–labeled albumin microspheres; Microfil) should remain in the arterial circulation. The indicator can be administered at any time following coronary occlusion. With this method, it is possible that the risk zone being measured, a *functional risk zone*, varies with the time following the onset of occlusion or may conceivably be altered by an intervention. Because collateral channels can deliver the indicator to the risk zone, steps must be taken to prevent this. Simultaneous perfusion of the occluded and nonoccluded beds at systemic pressure with the indicator in the perfusate of the nonoccluded bed only eliminates coronary collaterals. The disadvantages of this technique are similar to those noted for perfusion of the occluded vessel alone. Some studies which have utilized this method have reported that infarct size exceeds the size of the risk zone [22]. Such a result implies that the anatomic risk zone must exceed the functional risk zone being defined.

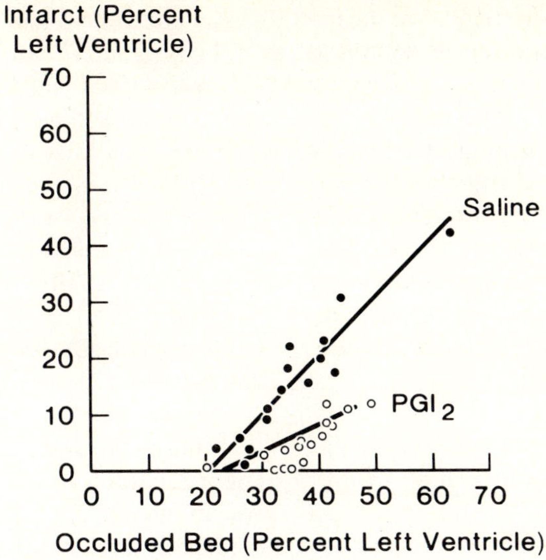

FIGURE 9-4
Effects of an intravenous infusion of the prostaglandin PGI_2 on the infarct-risk relationship in dogs. Infusion of PGI_2 shifted the intercept of the infarct-risk relationship to the right and decreased the slope of the infarct-risk relationship. Thus, PGI_2 decreased infarct size over a wide range of risk areas. (*Redrawn from data originally presented by BI Jugdutt et al* [7].)

When these various approaches to assessing the size of the risk zone are employed, the angiographic method and perfusion of the occluded vessel defines an "anatomic risk zone," and the perfusion of the nonoccluded vessels identifies a "functional risk zone." With both approaches it is possible to demonstrate a close relationship between the size of the risk zone and the resulting infarction ($r = 0.9$) [4–10,20a,22]. Invariably, the functional risk zone is smaller than the anatomic risk zone. With each of these approaches it is possible to demonstrate that certain interventions limit or expand the infarct area (Figure 9-4) [2,4–8,11,22].

Prediction of Infarction on the Basis of Measurements of Perfusion Studies by Rivas et al. [22a] indicate that the perfusion of myocardium served by a vessel which has been suddenly occluded can be utilized to predict the extent of myocardial necrosis. These results have been confirmed by Marcus et al. [22b] and Mueller et al. [22d]. Studies of Rivas et al. have shown that the subendocardium develops more extensive necrosis than the subepicardium for any given perfusion deficit. Furthermore, interventions can shift this relationship [22c]. Although this approach is promising, it is expensive and time-consuming to determine percent of necrosis in multiple tissue blocks. Furthermore, the system is somewhat artificial because the segments with perfusions in the intermediate range must contain a variable percentage of severely ischemic and normally perfused myocardium.

Methods of Defining the Risk Zone in Patients

No method of defining the risk zone in patients has gained wide acceptance. Several possible approaches are briefly described here.

The anatomic size of the perfusion field of an occluded vessel could be determined by coronary angiography performed within hours following infarction when the site of occlusion can be normally demonstrated. Negative images which may define the functional size of the risk zone can be obtained by injecting an indicator that will primarily enter normally perfused myocardium. Potential indicators include thallium 201, $^{13}NH_4$, and ^{11}C palmitate [23–25]. It also may be possible to define the risk zone with contrast-enhanced computer x-ray tomographic images of the heart or studies which employ nuclear magnetic resonance [26–27]. A recent study has employed intracoronary injections of thallium 201 to define the risk zone with reasonable success [23].

With these approaches, entrance of the indicator into the anatomic risk zone via collaterals is not prevented and quantification is poor unless the distribution of the indicator is shown in a tomographic format.

Future studies directed at the efficacy of interventions which may alter infarct size should determine the size of the risk zone in every patient included in the study. If this variable and the site of coronary occlusion are unknown, clinical studies will have to randomize treatments in huge numbers of patients in the hope of minimizing the confounding effects of these critical variables.

EFFECTS OF CORONARY OCCLUSION ON REGIONAL MYOCARDIAL PERFUSION IN THE LEFT VENTRICLE

Immediately following sudden coronary occlusion, perfusion in the center of the occluded zone usually decreases to 1 to 15 percent of the control flow. The perfusion of tissue in the occluded bed is species dependent. In goats, pigs, and primates perfusion in the occluded bed is often less than 5 percent of control [28–31]. This reflects the paucity of native collateral channels in these species. In dogs, perfusion to tissue supplied by an occluded vessel is usually 5 to 15 percent of control [3–9]. In addition, because collaterals enter from the periphery, collateral flow per gram will be less in large ischemic areas (see Chapter 10). Thallium 201 scintigrams in patients with acute myocardial infarction suggest that perfusion to the myocardium served by the occluded vessel is profoundly decreased [23].

The transmural distribution of perfusion in a segment of myocardium in the perfusion field of an occluded vessel is usually altered. The anatomic distribution of the occluded vessel and native collaterals, as well as the transmural distribution of extravascular compressive forces, are the primary factors that determine transmural flow and distribution to the myocardium by an occluded vessel. In the dog [4–9] and probably in humans [10] the subendocardial flow deficit is more intense than the subepicardial flow deficit. In goats, pigs, and baboons, the transmural distribution of the perfusion deficit is nearly uniform [28–31].

The effects of occlusion of vessels that supply the right ventricle on right ventricular perfusion have not been extensively examined. One preliminary study indicates that such coronary occlusions in the dog have highly variable effects on right ventricular perfusion [32].

THE BORDER ZONE IN EVOLVING MYOCARDIAL INFARCTION

Prior to the 1970s it was commonly held that following coronary occlusion a large "border zone" of intermediate ischemia surrounded the central area of necrosis. It was suggested that this border zone represented potentially salvageable myocardium. In the past decade, determining the existence, size, and location of the border zone has become a subject plagued by controversy and confusion. The controversy has arisen mainly because of technical limitations of the methods applied to this question. Much of the confusion stems from the ill-defined terminology which permeates many studies in the area.

Terminology Related to the Border Zone Controversy

In an excellent review concerning the border zone, Hearse and Yellon [33] have clearly defined the terminology often used in this research area. The key terms and their definitions are listed below.

1 Reversible injury A state whereby the myocardium, depressed because of severe ischemia, can return to normal metabolic and contractile function following restoration of normal perfusion. The state has definite time limits, following which irreversible injury will supervene. *Example:* tissue perfused by a vessel that has been occluded less than 5 min.

2 Jeopardized tissue Chronic suboptimal perfusion of a segment of myocardium. Often contractile function is depressed or lost but cell viability is maintained. This situation can persist for a long time interval. *Example:* tissue perfused by a compromised collateral circulation.

3 Condemned tissue Myocardium that has experienced injury which was initially reversible but has progressed to a point where deterioration to irreversibility and cell death is inevitable. *Example:* center of a severely ischemic zone following 30 min of complete coronary occlusion.

4 Zone of change A tissue area which is transitional from predominantly normal to predominantly abnormal based on measurements of regional perfusion, metabolism, or electrophysiological characteristics. This is an analytic phenomenon. *The width of this zone is determined by the spatial resolution of the analytic technique being applied.* Within this zone of change sharp interfaces, or border zones, are located if they exist.

5 Border zone tissue A spatially defined zone of intermediate, reversible injury. The presence of sharp interfaces between abnormal and normal tissue would suggest that such a border zone is exceedingly small or nonexistent. *A true gradient of abnormality free of technical artifacts would support the existence of a border zone.*

6 Salvageable tissue Reversibly injured, jeopardized or border tissue that can be returned to normal structure and function. In addition, some tissue elements in the zone of change are salvageable.

Whenever the above terms are employed, three dimensions should be considered: (1) the lateral extent of the zone, (2) the transmural distribution of the involved tissue, and (3) temporal considerations–the duration that a given state has existed. All three dimensions will influence the transition of tissue from one state to another, i.e., irreversible injury to condemned tissue.

If the definitions of these terms set forth by Hearse and Yellon gain wide acceptance, much of the confusion concerning the border zone will be eliminated.

Interdigitation of the Coronary Vasculature

In the myocardium, there is considerable interdigitation of the coronary vasculature at the macroscopic and microscopic levels (refer to Figure 1-2). If this interdigitation is ignored, zones of change are created which can be easily mistaken for border zones. Such errors frequently occur when the spatial resolution of the analytic technique (wall motion abnormalities; epicardial ST segment maps) is greater than 0.5 to 1.0 cm. Because the interdigitation of the coronary vasculature is indisputable, this variable must be carefully considered in future studies concerning the effects of coronary occlusion upon perfusion of the myocardium. Furthermore, it is fruitless to seek a border zone unless the analytic technique employed has a spatial resolution of less than 1 to 2 mm.

Methods of Delineating Gradients between Ischemic and Nonischemic Myocardium

Ten methodological approaches have been used to assess the size and location of gradients between severely ischemic and normally perfused myocardium (see Table 9-1). The conclusions of studies aimed at defining these gradients usually reflect the spatial resolution of the technique employed. Studies which have used approaches with superb (0.1 mm) spatial resolution such as NAD-NADH fluorescence [34,35], Microfil perfusion [21], microspectrophotometric determinations of regional oxygen consumption [36], and histology [37,38] have concluded that in

TABLE 9-1
METHODS EMPLOYED TO ASSESS THE EXTENT OF THE BORDER ZONE

Distribution of cyanosis on the surface of the heart
Multiple oxygen electrodes
NADH fluorescence photography
Structural analysis (gross pathology, histology, ultrastructure)
Histochemistry
Biochemical markers (tissue levels of ATP, CP, etc.)
Regional perfusion
Regional electrograms
Regional wall motion
Regional oxygen consumption

the dog the width of the gradient varies between 30 μm and 0.1 mm. In contrast, studies which have employed techniques with relatively poor spatial resolution (0.5 to 10 cm), such as epicardial electrograms [39,40], wall motion studies [41], and oxygen electrodes [42]—have concluded that in the dog the width of the gradient is greater than 5 to 10 mm.

My view is that the width of the gradient at the lateral border between severely ischemic and normally perfused myocardium is less than 1 mm in the dog.

Dynamic Nature of a Salvageable Zone of Myocardium within the Risk Area

Even if one assumes that following coronary occlusion there is a sharp interface (less than 0.1 mm) between normally perfused and severely ischemic myocardium, several factors would modulate the process whereby a reversibly damaged myocardial segment is transformed into a zone of infarction. The following factors significantly affect this transition.

1 Immediate compensatory mechanisms Immediately following the onset of severe ischemia, the myocardium can consume its meager stores of oxygen, begin to utilize stored glycogen and ATP, and terminate active contraction (see Chapter 3). These mechanisms will conserve the meager energy supplies available and markedly decrease energy requirements. In effect, this prolongs the transition phase from reversible injury to myocardial necrosis.

2 Coronary collateral flow In dogs coronary collateral channels can deliver about 5 to 15 percent of normal perfusion to the ischemic zone under favorable conditions. The extent and the initial distribution of the perfusion delivered by the

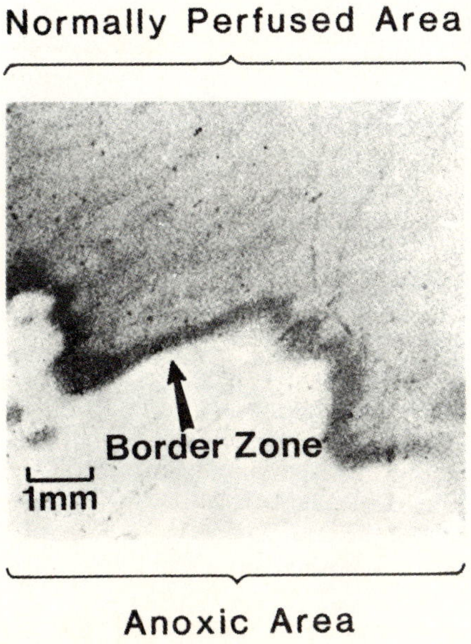

FIGURE 9-5
NAD-NADH fluorescence micrograph obtained from a segment of myocardium near the border zone of the perfusion field of an occluded coronary artery. The dark area at the top of the figure represents the anoxic zone (fluorescent positive); and the light area at the bottom of the figure is the normally perfused area of myocardium. In the photomicrograph; the border zone between the anoxic and the normally perfused zones is narrow (0.2 mm) and discrete. (*Modified from a figure originally presented by MB Simson et al* [35].)

native collateral channels is determined by genetic, geometric, and hemodynamic factors. For reasons that are not understood, as time proceeds and subendocardial segments become necrotic, available collateral flow is directed toward the surviving subepicardium [4,43]. Following coronary occlusion, mature collaterals in dogs and humans can deliver sufficient flow to prevent myocardial infarction and maintain myocardial function (see Chapter 10).

3 Myocardial oxygen consumption Schaper has shown that the level of myocardial consumption at the onset of coronary occlusion has a profound effect on the amount of reversibly injured myocardium that is transformed into necrotic tissue (Figure 9-6) [4]. In addition, it is possible that increases in myocardial oxygen consumption following the onset of coronary occlusion hasten the transition from reversible injury to necrosis. The latter point is controversial [4,12–14].

4 Transmural gradients In normal myocardium, wall stress and myocardial oxygen consumption are greater in the subendocardium than in the subepicardium (Chapters 3 and 4). If this transmural gradient persists following coronary occlusion (an unproven postulate) the subepicardium should progress more slowly than the subendocardium from reversible injury to necrosis. In addition, extravascular compressive forces which impede coronary collateral flow are greater in

FIGURE 9-6
Effects of myocardial oxygen consumption (MVO_2, ml/min/100 g), coronary collateral blood flow (coll flow, ml/min/100 g), and duration of coronary occlusion (occlusion time) on infarct size expressed as a percentage of the perfusion area. The myocardial oxygen consumption prior to coronary occlusion has a marked effect on the size of the resulting infarction. The smallest infarcts occur if myocardial oxygen consumption is low and coronary collateral flow is relatively high. Also, the duration of occlusion plays a major role in determining infarct size. All three of these factors (myocardial oxygen consumption; coronary collateral flow; and duration of occlusion) interact to determine infarct size in dogs subjected to experimental coronary occlusion. Permanent = 48 h of coronary occlusion. (*From W Schaper* [4].)

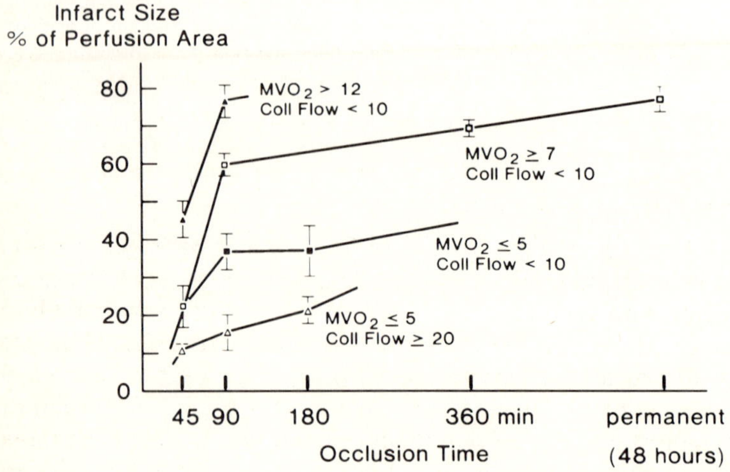

the subendocardial layers of the left ventricle. As a consequence, in myocardium distal to the occluded vessel, subendocardial flow is usually significantly less than subepicardial flow. In view of these considerations, it is not surprising that in dogs and in humans the wave of cell death following coronary occlusion [10,15] proceeds from subendocardium to subepicardium. From the standpoint of salvage of myocardium, the midwall and subepicardium of a transmural segment of ischemic cardiac muscle may be thought of as a border zone.

5 Hemodynamic state Because hemodynamics markedly affect myocardial oxygen consumption and extravascular compressive forces on coronary collateral channels (see below), adverse factors such as hypotension, tachycardia, and increased left ventricular filling pressure hasten the progress of the wave of cell death following coronary occlusion.

6 Rate constants of biochemical processes Following coronary occlusion, the rate at which high energy phosphates are utilized, glycogen is consumed, and autolytic processes progress is probably influenced by diffusion, active transport, and other metabolic phenomena [33]. The rate constants of these biochemical reactions probably affect the duration of the process whereby injured cells are transformed into necrotic cells.

In the aggregate, the factors described above contribute to the temporal dimension that can modify the rate at which cell necrosis develops following the onset of severe myocardial ischemia. *This temporal dimension is probably the most important aspect of the border zone controversy* because it is only in this dimension that there exists the potential salvage of a significant amount of jeopardized tissue.

Quantitative Significance of the Lateral Border Zone

Recently, Hearse and Yellon [33] developed a model to predict the quantitative effects of border zones on infarct size. The model suggests that if the width of the lateral borders zone is less than 1 mm it is too small to be of any functional significance. Assuming a lateral border zone width of less than 1 mm, the mass of the zone would average less than 10 percent of the size of the involved area over the full range of infarct sizes. The dimensions of the border zone or salvageable zone in the *transmural dimension* remain to be defined.

Limitations of Currently Available Studies

The vast majority of data pertaining to the border zone controversy have been obtained by suddenly occluding a previously normal coronary vessel in a healthy mongrel dog. Patients who sustain acute myocardial infarction frequently have multivessel coronary disease, and the occluded vessel responsible for the infarction was partially obstructed for many years prior to the time of occlusion. Consequently, extrapolation of currently available animal studies to the clinical arena may not be appropriate. It is of paramount importance to define the transmural, lateral, and temporal dimensions of the salvageable zone of myocardium following coronary occlusion in patients with ischemic heart disease. Without this information therapeutic approaches for limiting infarct size in patients will remain empirical. Results of clinical trials which do not assess the risk zone in each patient will probably be inconclusive or negative.

HEMODYNAMIC PATTERNS THAT FREQUENTLY ACCOMPANY SUDDEN CORONARY OCCLUSION

Hemodynamic abnormalities that accompany sudden coronary occlusion are determined by neural mechanisms, cardiac rhythm, and the size of the ischemic or infarcted zone.

Neural Mechanisms

The effects of neural mechanisms on hemodynamics are most clearly manifest when the size of the ischemic zone is modest and sinus rhythm is present. Three common patterns are observed.

In patients, coronary occlusion causes chest pain and often a "feeling of impending doom." Central neural mechanisms are activated and the "fight or flight" response occurs. This is characterized by tachycardia, increased peripheral vascular resistance, increased arterial pressure, and tachypnea. These hemodynamic abnormalities adversely affect ischemic myocardium (increased extravascular compressive forces on the coronary collateral circulation and increased cardiac metabolism) but augment the function of normally perfused cardiac muscle. Even in the absence of excessive anxiety, sudden coronary occlusion usually produces mild tachycardia and a variable alteration in peripheral vascular resistance [44]. The increase in heart rate that accompanies sudden coronary occlusion in awake dogs averages 34 beats per minute and occurs within 8 to 10 s following coronary occlusion. The chronotropic response to sudden coronary occlusion is abolished by baroreceptor denervation and beta blockade [44].

Sudden occlusion of the circumflex coronary artery in the dog produces dyskinesia in the posterior inferior wall of the left ventricle. This stimulates stretch receptors which are primarily located in this region of the left ventricle [45,46]. Vagal afferents transmit this information to the brain. In anesthetized barodenervated dogs, dyskinesia of the inferior posterior wall of the left ventricle elicits a response characterized by relative bradycardia and peripheral vasodilation. These responses are the result of efferent vagal stimulation and withdrawal of sympathetic tone. Although bradycardia should decrease cardiac metabolism (favorable effect), severe bradycardia can contribute to arterial hypotension. Decreases in arterial pressure regardless of the mechanism responsible adversely affect perfusion to the ischemic zone. Occlusion of the left anterior descending coronary artery in anesthetized barodenervated dogs produces tachycardia and peripheral vasoconstriction. This hemodynamic response reflects the relative paucity of stretch receptors in the anterior wall of the left ventricle [45,46]. Recent studies in humans with coronary spasm indicate that severe ischemia in the inferior wall secondary to spasm of the right coronary artery is associated with sinus bradycardia, whereas ischemia of the anterior wall of the left ventricle (spasm of the left anterior descending coronary artery) is accompanied by tachycardia [47].

In the intact organism, the neural mechanisms described above can be elicited simultaneously. The hemodynamic pattern which emerges following sudden coronary occlusion is an integrated response to these diverse inputs.

Cardiac Rhythm Disturbance

A large variety of cardiac rhythm disturbances often occur following coronary occlusion. The ventricular arrhythmias are unrelated to the site of infarction and can occur with infarctions of any size. Bradyarrhythmias, particularly heartblock, depend on the site of infarction. Such rhythm disturbances primarily occur with septal or inferior wall infarction. Supraventricular tachycardias occur mainly when superimposed cardiac failure has produced atrial distention.

Tachyarrhythmias have devastating effects on the coronary collateral circulation. These arrythmias increase cardiac metabolism and extravascular compressive forces (per unit time). In addition, diastolic time per minute decreases and arterial pressure often declines. These adverse effects can markedly decrease perfusion to the ischemic zone and thereby extend the size of an infarction. For this reason, when excessive tachycardia occurs in the presence of acute myocardial infarction, it should be promptly terminated.

Bradyarrhythmias adversely affect the coronary collateral circulation if diastolic ventricular pressure increases or arterial pressure falls significantly. These hemodynamic abnormalities usually do not occur unless heart rate is less than 45 to 50 beats per minute. Bradyarrhythmias can be easily reversed by atropine or pacing.

Size of the Ischemic/Infarcted Zone

In patients, when 40 percent of the mass of the left ventricle undergoes infarction [48], adequate arterial pressure can no longer be maintained. Cardiogenic shock supervenes, and death occurs within hours. Large infarcts which involve less than 40 percent of left ventricular mass produce cardiac failure with adequate systemic pressure. If the myocardial infarction is large, hyperfunction of the noninfarcted segments is demonstrable [49]. This compensatory response will increase cardiac metabolism and perfusion to the hypercontractile segments. Infarctions which involve less than 20 percent of the circumference of the left ventricle usually do not produce major hemodynamic abnormalities [50].

Heart failure and cardiogenic shock profoundly impair function of the coronary collateral circulation. The perfusion of the myocardium subserved by coronary collateral vessels is critically dependent on arterial driving pressure (arterial driving pressure equals aortic pressure minus left ventricular diastolic pressure). Heart failure increases left ventricular diastolic pressure and shock decreases aortic pressure. Consequently, during cardiogenic shock, arterial driving pressure is remarkably diminished and perfusion via the coronary collateral circulation is strikingly reduced. In patients with hypotension or shock secondary to coronary occlusion, every effort should be made to improve arterial driving pressure with either mechanical or pharmacologic means.

Because the coronary collateral circulation is critically affected by alterations in arterial driving pressure and extravascular compressive forces, hemodynamic abnormalities which adversely affect these parameters should be promptly corrected in patients with acute myocardial infarction.

THE NO-REFLOW PHENOMENON

In the mid-1960s and the early 1970s, it was noted that restoration of flow to a previously ischemic area in the kidney, brain, or heart was not followed by homogeneous tissue reperfusion [51–55]. Subsequently, the effects of reperfusion in the heart were described in greater detail [4,56–63]. Following occlusion of a coronary artery for less than 20 min, restoration of the flow is usually associated with marked hyperemia in the previously ischemic region (Figure 9-7). This hyperemic response may persist for 30 min or longer [4,62]. With coronary occlusions that last about 40 min, reopening of the occluded vessel restores perfusion to the affected zone but hyperemia is minimal or absent (Figure 9-7) [4,56–61,63]. Following release of a prolonged occlusion (greater than 90 min), perfusion of the involved zone is heterogeneous and average flow to the area is much less than normal (no reflow) (Figure 9-7). This entire sequence of events is most dramatic in myocardial segments within the involved zone that have the lowest collateral flows

FIGURE 9-7
A schematic diagram which relates perfusion following release of a coronary occlusion to the duration of the occlusion prior to reperfusion. Release of a 30-min occlusion is followed by prolonged hyperemic response in a subendocardial layer of the left ventricle in the perfusion field of the occluded vessel. Release of a 120-min coronary occlusion is followed by no reflow; i.e., following release of the occlusion, perfusion to the involved zone of subendocardium does not return to the flow in the adjacent normal areas. The more vulnerable subendocardium proceeds through this cycle of events at shorter occlusion times than the subepicardium, which is more resistant to the adverse effects of coronary occlusion.

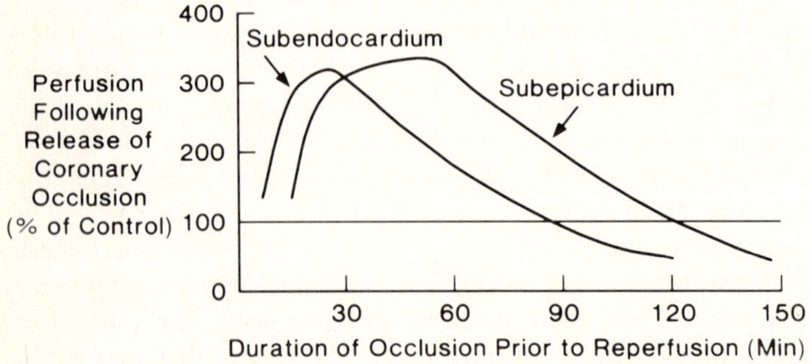

during occlusion [4,56–63]. Hence, subendocardial segments are more involved than subepicardial segments; also, the subendocardial segments progress through this cycle at a faster pace than do the subepicardial segments. Consequently, at one time reperfusion of the ischemic zone could be associated with hyperemia of the subepicardium and hypoperfusion of the subendocardium [62]. Invariably, regions of myocardium which demonstrate no reflow are irreversibly damaged [4,61,62]. Even areas which demonstrate prolonged hyperemia following reperfusion are often found to be necrotic on subsequent examination [4,62].

No reflow is an epiphenomenon of minimal importance to the pathogenesis of the myocardial infarction. No reflow follows irreversible tissue damage—it does not precede it. The notion that no reflow extends the size of a myocardial infarction is not supported by available data [4,61,62]. Typically, the no-reflow zone in the area of myocardial infarction is surrounded by a necrotic zone that can be reperfused.

Mechanisms of No Reflow

Many factors contribute to the no-reflow phenomenon, including loss of vasomotor tone [4], capillary compression by swollen myocytes [56–58], direct capillary damage [56–58,61], and occlusion of capillaries by packed cells surrounded by fibrin plugs and white blood cells [56–58,61]. No reflow is a late manifestation of severe damage to the microvasculature. Capillaries are more resistant to the damaging effects of ischemia than are myocytes because the oxygen requirements of endothelium are modest compared to that of myocytes and the capillaries are closest to the oxygen supply. Therefore, if ischemia is sufficiently severe to limit reflow, the myocytes are no longer viable. Another late manifestation of microvascular damage is hemorrhage [64–67a]. If blood flow is restored to damaged microvessels in the myocardium, gross abnormalities in capillary permeability will permit large numbers of red cells to traverse the walls of damaged capillaries and enter the tissue. Consequently, the infarction will become hemorrhagic.

Hemodynamic Consequences of Reperfusion

When a normal vessel in an anesthetized dog is occluded for more than several minutes, and subsequently flow is restored, within seconds ventricular arrhythmias often develop and culminate in ventricular fibrillation [68,69]. When an occluded vessel in a patient with acute myocardial infarction is reopened with intracoronary streptokinase, severe life-threatening arrhythmias are infrequently observed (Chapter 20). The explanation for these differences is probably related to the protocol employed and possibly to the condition of the occluded vessel. When coronary occlusions are released after several hours in awake dogs, lethal ventricular arrhythmias are uncommon. Another point of consideration is that in animal studies the reperfused vessel is usually normal, whereas in patients the reperfused vessel almost invariably contains a high-grade atherosclerotic obstructive lesion. The results of a preliminary study in dogs [70] which involved perfusion of an occluded artery with a superimposed stenosis indicate that in this situation reperfusion is not associated with lethal ventricular arrhythmias.

Attenuation of the No-Reflow Phenomenon

Because no reflow follows irreversible tissue injury, interventions which delay or limit ischemic tissue damage may attenuate the no-reflow phenomenon. Hyperosmotic agents such as mannitol are effective under some conditions in this regard [57].

INTERVENTIONS THAT MAY LIMIT INFARCT SIZE: ANIMAL STUDIES

The possibility that the consequences of permanent coronary occlusion could be modified with a pharmacologic or mechanical intervention has encouraged many investigators to assess the efficacy of various approaches to altering infarct size [12–14]. The methods employed in early animal studies (ST segment maps or measurements of blood levels of creatine kinase) were less than ideal, and hence interpretation of results of these earlier studies must be guarded. Recently, more vigorous approaches which have expressed infarct size as a percentage of the area at risk have demonstrated that a variety of interventions can modify infarct size [4,5,7,8,22]. These animal studies are encouraging. The most important questions in this area that remain unanswered are listed below.

Effects of Elapsed Time Following Coronary Occlusion

Patients usually do not seek medical attention until hours after the initial symptoms of myocardial infarction. In many communities, the median delay time between the onset of symptoms of myocardial infarction and hospitalization is 3 to 6 h [71,71a]. The length of this delay is crucial because animal studies suggest that the transition from reversible injury to cell death in ischemic myocardium occurs in minutes to hours [4,15–19,61–63,66–67a]. Thus, if an intervention is efficacious only if applied within minutes of coronary occlusion, it may have little practical value. The effects of elapsed time following coronary occlusion on therapeutic efficacy of an intervention have been infrequently examined. Two studies suggest that counterpulsation [72] and hyaluronidase [73] can limit infarct size even if they are applied 3 to 6 h post occlusion. Unfortunately, the conclusions of these studies rely heavily on epicardial ST segment maps. Studies of this type should be pursued with the more rigorous experimental techniques which are currently available.

Duration of a Therapeutic Intervention

Following coronary occlusion, major changes in coronary collateral perfusion depend on the transformation of tiny native collateral vessels into larger vascular channels. This process involves acute dilation and cellular proliferation of native collateral channels. Although some dilation may occur promptly [73a], the cellular growth cycle for coronary collateral vessels has a time constant of about 20 to 24 h (see Chapter 10). Thus, it seems likely that once a therapeutic intervention aimed at limiting infarct size is instituted, unless perfusion by the occluded vessel can be restored the agent should probably be administered for several days. The optimal duration for administration of agents which may alter infarct size has not been determined. One recent study has clearly shown that it is possible for a therapeutic agent to delay the progression of myocardial necrosis for hours without altering ultimate infarct size [73b]. Hence, brief acute studies can easily provide misleading results. In most experimental studies reported thus far, the therapeutic agent has been administered for only a few hours following the onset of sudden coronary occlusion. Studies aimed at determining the optimal duration that therapeutic intervention should be administered should be encouraged.

Effects of Coexistent Disease

The majority of patients who sustain their first myocardial infarction have multivessel coronary disease [74,75]. The presence of multiple coronary obstructions could stimulate the development of coronary collaterals (a positive effect) or limit the ability of native collaterals to increase flow to an ischemic zone by jeopardizing the supply channel (a negative effect). In addition, superimposed heart failure or the presence of impaired coronary reserve secondary to coexistent hypertensive heart disease could modify the efficacy of interventions that may alter infarct size (see Chapters 10 and 13). Because coexistent heart disease is common in patients who suffer acute myocardial infarction, this area deserves additional attention. One study by Koyanagi [11] suggests that hypertension and left ventricular hypertrophy adversely affect the complications of sudden coronary occlusion (see Chapter 13).

Functional Status of Salvaged Myocardium

Even if an intervention reduces infarct size by 20 to 30 percent, it is possible that the salvaged tissue will have deleterious effects on long-term survival. For example, islands or peninsulas of salvaged cells in the subepicardium may contribute very little to global left ventricular performance. At the same time, such foci could contribute to electrical heterogeneity of the jeopardized zone and promote the genesis of lethal arrhythmias. Several recent studies have examined the functional state of salvaged myocardium [76,76b]. The data indicate that the salvaged tissue regains some function and responds to inotropic stimulation but that recovery takes weeks and is far from complete.

Efficacy of Various Interventions That May Alter Infarct Size Following Reperfusion

Most previous studies concerned with interventions that may limit infarct size have been designed to test the efficacy of such approaches assuming that the occluded vessel responsible for the infarction could not be reopened. Recent clinical studies with intracoronary steptokinase indicate that the occluded coronary vessel responsible for infarction can be reopened (see Chapter 20). It is possible that metabolic support specifically tailored to assist reversibly damaged myocardium may be of considerable value under such circumstances. Preliminary results with AICAR [77] and pyruvate [78] are particularly promising. This is a relatively new area of investigation which should be vigorously pursued.

Although a large number of studies concerning the effects of infarct interventions and infarct size have been reported, much remains to be done. *To date, no studies have been performed that clearly show that an intervention applied under realistic conditions (2 to 6 h following coronary occlusion) in a clinically relevant animal model (awake preparation with a chronic multivessel disease) would salvage myocardium of sufficient mass and functional capacity to significantly enhance long-term survival.*

INTERVENTIONS THAT MAY LIMIT INFARCT SIZE: PATIENT STUDIES

Limited studies concerning the efficacy of several agents which may limit infarct size in humans have been reported. Most of the interventions tested—beta blockade [79–82], nitrates [83,84], hyaluronidase [85], glucose-insulin-potassium [86,87], intraaortic balloon counterpulsation [88], reperfusion [23,89], and treatment of hypertension [90]—have had a favorable effect on some indirect index of infarct size. The only intervention examined which yielded a net negative result was corticosteroids [91,92]. Repeated administration of high doses of steroids immediately following acute myocardial infarction does not decrease the release of creatine kinase and may predispose to ventricular rupture.

Thus far, the clinical trials reported have had four major problems: (1) the study groups have been relatively small (n = less than 100 per group); (2) no attempt has been made to assess the size of the area at risk in each patient; (3) methods of estimating infarct size in humans are relatively crude; and (4) if myocardium was salvaged, the functional importance of preserved tissue has not been assessed. Because of these serious limitations the interpretation of these clinical results should be guarded.

METHODS OF ESTIMATING INFARCT SIZE IN HUMANS

Because of the critical importance of measurements of infarct size in humans, the general methods that have been employed will be briefly reviewed.

Electrocardiographic Approaches

Alterations in ST segment elevation or QRS morphology have been used extensively to estimate infarct size [14]. There are numerous reasons why this approach is not quantitative. First, surface electrocardiographic recordings are dependent on the shape and composition of the torso (volume conductor) and the location of the involved zone [93]. Second, ST segment elevation does not reflect the extent of subendocardial ischemia or infarction (Figure 9-8) [94–97]. Third, electrophysiologists have argued that the theoretical basis for assuming that surface electrocardiographic recordings can assess infarct size has many deficiencies [93]. *Although electrocardiographic abnormalities are of qualitative value in assessing the presence or absence of an infarction in patients, it is unreasonable to assume that this approach will provide an accurate estimate of infarct size.*

Enzyme Release

The release of creatine kinase from infarcted myocardium has been used to estimate infarct size for about a decade [98]. In animals, a linear relationship

FIGURE 9-8
Relationship between epicardial ST segment elevation and transmural coronary blood flow in dogs subjected to sudden coronary occlusion. It is obvious that ST segment elevation is a poor predictor of the extent of transmural myocardial ischemia. (*Redrawn from data originally presented by HJ Smith et al* [95].)

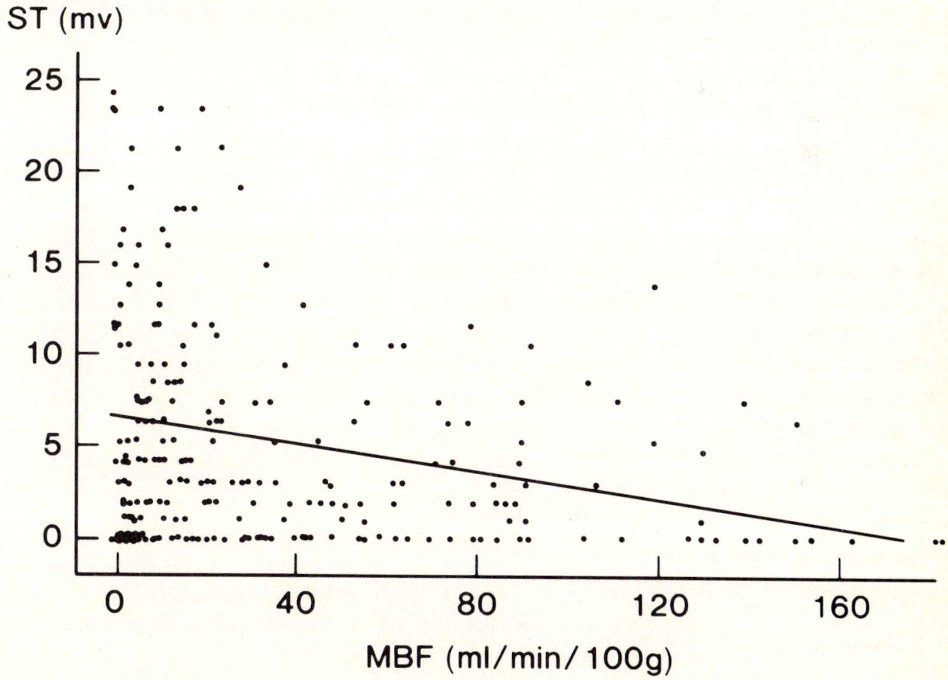

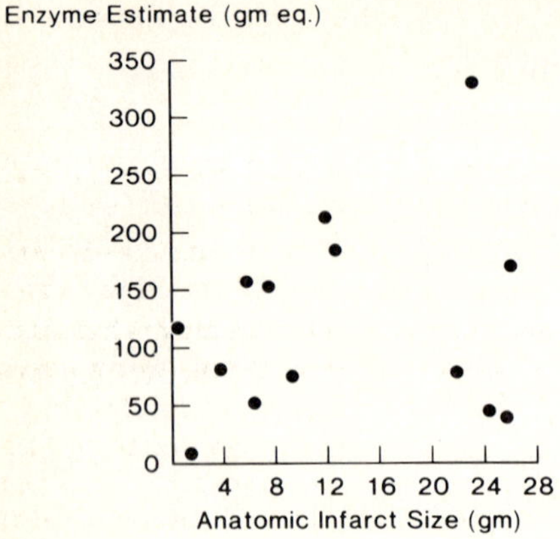

FIGURE 9-9
Relationship between estimates of infarct size from serial measurements of creatine kinase concentrations in the blood (CK clearance) and infarct size determined with pathological techniques. These studies were performed by permanently occluding a single coronary artery in dogs. If one considers only small infarcts (i.e., 12 g or less), there is a reasonable correlation between CK clearance curve estimates of infarct size and infarct size measured pathologically. When a wide range of infarct sizes are considered, it is clear that CK clearance curves cannot be used to accurately estimate infarct size. (*Redrawn from data originally presented by CR Roe et al* [*100*].)

between infarct size and creatine kinase clearance curves in plasma exists over a small range of infarct sizes [98,99]. However, when a large range of infarct sizes was examined in dogs and humans, the relationship between creatine kinase release and infarct size was poor (Figure 9-9) [99–100a]. Small and large infarcts yielded creatine kinase curves that were remarkably similar. A variable amount of creatine kinase is inactivated as the released enzyme is transported via cardiac lymphatics to the venous circulation [101,102]. Most current methods measure only enzymatically active creatine kinase [103]. Also, the analysis of the creatine kinase clearance curves cannot determine if the enzyme was released from a right or left ventricular infarction. Perfusion of the infarcted zone markedly alters the amount of enzyme released into the blood. Reperfusion increases release [104], whereas infarct extension produced by more proximal coronary occlusion of a vessel that was occluded distally actually decreases enzyme release [105]. Finally, the peak of the plasma creatine kinase curve occurs at a variable time—5 to 10 h—after infarction. Unfortunately, infarct size estimates are based on the area under the clearance curve beyond the peak. Thus, any intervention being tested cannot be administered until 5 to 10 h after infarction if the dependent variable infarct size is assessed by creatine kinase clearance curves. By this time, most reversibly damaged myocardium is probably necrotic.

In my view, the numerous problems with creatine kinase estimates of infarct sizes severely undermine the usefulness of this technique in quantitative studies of infarct size in humans.

Technetium 99m–Pyrophosphate Scintigrams

Technetium 99m–pyrophosphate is a bone-scanning agent with an affinity for acutely necrotic myocardium [106–107]. After the intravenous injection of technetium 99m-pyrophosphate, the distribution of the radionuclide detected with a gamma camera correlates roughly with the size of anterior transmural myocardial infarction [109,110]. This technique can localize the site of infarction with reasonable precision. However, with conventional imaging techniques the transmural extent of inferior infarction cannot be determined [111]. Also, the size of subendocardial infarcts is difficult to estimate with technetium-phosphate scintigrams [111]. The analysis of tomographic technetium 99m-pyrophosphate scintigrams may provide an accurate method of assessing infarct size [112,113].

Wall Motion Studies

Wall motion abnormalities in patients with acute myocardial infarction have been assessed by two-dimensional, or M-mode, echocardiography, contrast ventriculograms, and radionuclide ventriculograms [41]. None of these methods can accurately assess the transmural extent of infarction, and all of them overestimate the size of infarctions [41]. This occurs because a segment of normally perfused myocardium that separates the dyskinetic ischemic zone from the bulk of the normal zone is tethered and therefore contracts in an abnormal fashion [114]. This abnormally contracting well-perfused myocardium cannot be differentiated from abnormally contracting necrotic myocardium.

Thus, all four approaches to estimating infarct size in humans—electrocardiographic techniques, enzyme release, technetium 99m-pyrophosphate scintigrams, and wall motion studies—have major deficiencies. None of these procedures provides a precise enough estimate of the mass of infarcted tissue to be clinically useful.

New Approaches

Several relatively new approaches may provide an accurate means of estimating infarct size in humans. These approaches include tomographic scintigrams with various radionuclides, computed tomography with enhancement techniques, nuclear magnetic resonance methods, and tissue characterization with echocardiographic techniques. All of these methods are in the early stages of development.

Studies directed toward developing practical approaches to limiting infarct size in patients are of great importance. Despite the many problems noted above, there is reason to believe that continued research in this area will eventually yield useful methods of salvaging reversibly injured myocardium in patients.

REFERENCES

1 Spateholz W: Die Arterien der Herzwand, Hirzel, Leipzig, 1924.

2 Schaper W, Remysen P, Xhonneux R: The size of myocardial infarction after experimental coronary artery ligation. *Z Kreislaufforsh* 58: 904, 1969.

3 Schaper W: *The Collateral Circulation of the Heart*. Amsterdam, North-Holland Publishing, 1971.

4 Schaper W: Residual perfusion of acutely ischemic heart muscle, in *The Pathophysiology of Myocardial Perfusion*, W Schaper (ed). Amsterdam, Elsevier, North-Holland Biomedical Press, 1979.

5 Jugdutt BI, Hutchins GM, Bulkley BH, Becker LC: Salvage of ischemic myocardium by ibuprofen during infarction in the conscious dog. *Am J Cardiol* 46: 74, 1980.

6 Jugdutt BI, Hutchins GM, Bulkley BH, Becker LC: Myocardial infarction in the conscious dog: Three-dimensional mapping of infarct, collateral flow and region at risk. *Circulation* 60: 1141, 1979.

7 Jugdutt BI, Hutchins GM, Bulkley BH, Becker LC: Dissimilar effects of prostacyclin, prostaglandin E_1, and prostaglandin E_2 on myocardial infarct size after coronary occlusion in conscious dogs. *Circ Res* 49: 685, 1981.

8 Jugdutt BI, Hutchins GM, Bulkley BH, Pitt B, Becker LC: Effect of indomethacin on collateral blood flow and infarct size in the conscious dog. *Circulation* 59: 734, 1979.

9 Koyanagi S, Eastham CL, Harrison DG, Marcus ML: Transmural variation in the relationship between myocardial infarct size and risk area. *Am J Physiol* 242: H867, 1982.

9a Lowe JE, Reimer KA, Jennings RB: Experimental infarct size as a function of the amount of myocardium at risk. *Am J Pathol* 90: 363, 1978.

9b Reimer KA, Ideker RE, Jennings RB: Effect of coronary occlusion site on ischaemic bed size and collateral blood flow in dogs. *Cardiovasc Res* 15: 668, 1981.

10 Lee JT, Ideker RE, Reimer KA: Myocardial infarct size and location in relation to the coronary vascular bed at risk in man. *Circulation* 64: 526, 1981.

11 Koyanagi S, Eastham CL, Harrison DG, Marcus ML: Increased size of myocardial infarction in dogs with chronic hypertension and left ventricular hypertrophy. *Circ Res* 50: 55, 1982.

12 Kloner RA, Braunwald E: Observations on experimental myocardial ischemia. *Cardiovasc Res* 14: 371, 1980.

13 Braunwald E, Maroko PR: Protection of the ischemic myocardium, in *The Pathophysiology of Myocardial Perfusion*, W Schaper (ed). Amsterdam, Elsevier, North-Holland Biomedical Press, 1979.

14 Braunwald E, Sobel BE: Coronary blood flow and myocardial ischemia in *Heart Disease, A Textbook of Cardiovascular Medicine*, Philadelphia, Saunders, 1980, vol 2, p 1279.

15 Reimer KA, Jennings RB: The "wave front phenomenon" of myocardial ischemic cell death. II. Transmural progression of necrosis within the framework of ischemic bed size (myocardium at risk) and collateral flow. *Lab Invest* 40: 633, 1979.

16 Lie JT, Pairolero PC, Holley KE, Titus JL: Macroscopic enzyme-mapping verification of large homogeneous experimental myocardial infarcts of predictable size and location in dogs. *J Thorac Cardiovasc Surg* 69: 599, 1975.

17 Schaper J, Mulch J, Winkler B, Schaper W: Ultrastructural, functional, and biochemical criteria for estimation of reversibility of ischemic injury: A study of the effects of global ischemia on the isolated dog heart. *J Mol Cell Cardiol* 11: 521, 1979.

18 Jennings RB, Baum JG, Herdson PB: Fine structural changes in myocardial ischemic injury. *Arch Path* 79: 135, 1965.

19 Jennings RB, Sommers H, Smyth GA, Flack HA, Linn H: Myocardial necrosis induced by temporary occlusion of a coronary artery in the dog. *Arch Path* 70: 68, 1960.

20 Nachlas MM, Shnitka TK: Macroscopic identification of early myocardial infarcts by alterations in dehydrogenase activity. *Am J Pathol*, 42: 379, 1963.

20a Harrison DG, Koyanagi S, Alden B, Marcus ML: Role of overlap perfusion in survival of non-infarcted risk zone following coronary occlusion. *Fed Proc* 40: 602, 1981.

21 Factor SM, Okun EM, Kirk ES: The histological lateral border of acute canine myocardial infarction. *Circ Res* 48: 640, 1981.

22 DeBoer LWV, Strauss HW, Kloner RA, Rude RE, Davis RF, Maroko PR, Braunwald E: Autoradiographic method for measuring the ischemic myocardium at risk:

The effects of verapamil on infarct size following experimental coronary artery occlusion. *Proc Natl Acad Sci* 77: 6119, 1980.

22a Rivas F, Cobb F, Bache RJ, Greenfield JC Jr: Relationship between blood flow to ischemic regions and extent of myocardial infarction: Serial measurement of blood flow to ischemic regions in dogs. *Circ Res* 38: 439, 1976.

22b Marcus ML, Tomanek RJ, Ehrhardt JC, Kerber RE, Brown DD, Abboud FM: Relationships between myocardial perfusion, myocardial necrosis, and 99m technetium pyrophosphate uptake in dogs subjected to sudden coronary occlusion. *Circulation* 54: 647, 1976.

22c Pantely, GA, Oyama A, Metcalfe L, Maralee S, Welch JE: Improvement in the relationship between flow to ischemic myocardium and the extent of necrosis with glycolytic intermediates that decrease blood oxygen affinity in dogs. *Circ Res* 49: 395, 1981.

22d Mueller TM, Tomanek RJ, Kerber RE, Marcus ML: Myocardial infarction in dogs with chronic hypertension and left ventricular hypertrophy. *Am J Physiol* 239: H731, 1980.

23 Markis JE, Malagold M, Parker JA, Silverman KJ, Barry WH, Als AV, Paulin S, Grossman W, Braunwald E: Myocardial salvage after intracoronary thrombolysis with streptokinase in acute myocardial infarction: Assessment by intracoronary thallium-201. *N Engl J Med* 305: 777, 1981.

24 Schelbert HR, Phelps ME, Hoffman EJ, Huang SC, Selin CE, Kuhl DE: Regional myocardial perfusion assessed with N-13 labeled ammonia and positron emission computerized axial tomography. *Am J Cardiol* 43: 209, 1979.

25 Ter-Pogossian MM, Klein MS, Markham J, Roberts R, Sobel BE: Regional assessment of myocardial metabolic integrity in vivo by positron-emission tomography with ^{11}C-labeled palmitate. *Circulation* 61: 242, 1980.

26 Skiöldebrand CG, Lipton MJ, Redington RW, Berninger WH, Wallace A, Carlsson E: Myocardial infarction in dogs, demonstrated by non-enhanced computed tomography. *Acta Radiologica* 22: 1, 1981.

27 Buonanno FS, Pykett IL, Brady TJ, Vielma J, Goldman MR, Hinshaw WS, Pohost GM, Kistler JP: Detection and evolution of experimental ischemic infarction by nuclear magnetic resonance imaging. *Circulation* 64: 19, 1981.

28 Vastesaeger MM, van der Straeten PP, Friart J, Candaele G, Ghys A, Bernard M: Les anastomoses intercoronariennes telles qu'elles apparaissent a la coronarographie post-mortem. *Acta Cardiol* 12: 365, 1957.

29 Most AS, Williams DO, Millard RW: Acute coronary occlusion in the pig: Effect of nitroglycerin on regional myocardial blood flow. *Am J Cardiol* 42: 947, 1978.

30 Lubbe WF, Persach M, Pretorius R, Brynell KJJ, Opie LH: Distribution of myocardial blood flow before and after coronary artery ligation in the baboon: Relation to early ventricular fibrillation. *Cardiovasc Res* 8: 478, 1974.

31 Grayson J, Irvine M: Myocardial infarction in the monkey: Studies on the collateral circulation after acute coronary occlusion. *Cardiovasc Res* 2: 170, 1968.

32 Schaper W, Sass S: Right ventricular infarct size and collateral blood flow following occlusion of the right coronary artery in the dog. *Circulation* 64: 118, 1981.

33 Hearse DJ, Yellon DM: The "border zone" in evolving myocardial infarction: Controversy or confusion? *Am J Cardiol* 47: 1321, 1981.

34 Barlow CH, Chance B: Ischemic areas in perfused rat hearts: Measurement by NADH fluorescence photography. *Science* 10: 193, 1976.

35 Simson MB, Harden W, Barlow CH, Harken AH: Visualization of the distance between perfusion and anoxia along an ischemic border. *Circulation* 60: 1151, 1979.

36 Weiss HR: Effect of coronary artery occlusion on regional arterial and venous O_2 saturation, O_2 extraction, blood flow, and O_2 consumption in the dog heart. *Circ Res* 47: 400, 1980.

37 Janse MJ, Cinca J, Morena H, et al: The "border zone" in myocardial ischemia: An electrophysiological, metabolic and histochemical correlation in the pig heart. *Circ Res* 44: 576, 1979.

38 Factor SM, Sonnenblick EH, Kirk ES: The histologic border zone of acute myocardial infarction–islands or peninsuals. *Am J Pathol* 92: 111, 1978.

39 Braunwald E, Marok PR, Libby P: Reduction of infarct size following coronary occlusion. *Circ Res* 35: 192, 1974.

40 Maroko PR, Kjekshus JK, Sobel BE, et al: Factors influencing infarct size following experimental coronary artery occlusions. *Circulation* 43: 67, 1971.

41 Falsetti HL, Marcus ML, Kerber RE, Skorton DJ: Quantification of myocardial ischemia and infarction by left ventricular imaging. *Circulation* 63: 747, 1981.

42 Sayen JJ, Sheldon WF, Horwitz O, et al: Studies of coronary disease in the experimental animal. II. Polarographic determinations of local oxygen availability in the dog's left ventricle during coronary occlusion and pure oxygen breathing. *J Clin Invest* 30: 932, 1952.

43 Hirzel HO, Nelson GR, Sonnenblick EH, Kirk ES: Redistribution of collateral blood flow from necrotic to surviving myocardium following coronary occlusion in the dog. *Circ Res* 39: 214, 1976.

44 Peterson DF, Kaspar RL, Bishop VS: Reflex tachycardia due to temporary coronary occlusion in the conscious dog. *Circ Res* 32: 652, 1973.

45 Felder RB, Thames MD: Interaction between cardiac receptors and sinoaortic baroreceptors in the control of efferent cardiac sympathetic nerve activity during myocardial ischemia in dogs. *Circ Res* 45: 728, 1979.

46 Thames MD, Klopfenstein HS, Abboud FM, Mark AL, Walker JL: Preferential distribution of inhibitory cardiac receptors with vagal afferents to the inferoposterior wall of the left ventricle activated during coronary occlusion in the dog. *Circ Res* 43: 512, 1978.

47 Perez-Gomez F, DeDios RM, Rey J, Aguado AG: Prinzmetal's angina: Reflex cardiovascular response during episode of pain. *Brit Heart J* 42: 81, 1979.

48 Page DL, Caulfield JB, Kastor JA, DeSanctis RW, Sanders CA: Myocardial changes associated with cardiogenic shock. *N Engl J Med* 285: 133, 1971.

49 Kerber RE, Marcus ML, Wilson R, Ehrhardt J, Abboud FM: Effects of acute coronary occlusion on the motion and perfusion of the normal and ischemic interventricular septum. *Circulation* 54: 928, 1976.

50 Bleifeld W, Mathey D, Hanrath P, Buss H, Effert S: Infarct size estimated from serial serum creatine phosphokinase in relation to left ventricular hemodynamics. *Circulation* 55: 3, 1977.

51 Krug A, DE Rochemont WM, Korb G: Blood supply of the myocardium after temporary coronary occlusion. *Circ Res* 19: 57, 1966.

52 Majno G, Ames A III, Chaing J, Wright RL: No reflow after cerebral ischemia. *Lancet* 2: 569, 1978.

53 Ames A III, Wright RL, Kowada M, Thurston JM, Majno G: Cerebral ischemia, Part 2 (the no-reflow phenomenon). *Am J Pathol* 52: 437, 1968.

54 Summers WK, Jamison RL: The no reflow phenomenon in renal ischemia. *Lab Invest* 25: 635, 1971.

55 Flores J, DiBona DR, Beck CH, Leaf A: The role of cell swelling in ischemic renal damage and the protective effect of hypertonic solute. *J Clin Invest* 51: 118, 1972.

56 Kloner RA, Ganote CE, Jennings RB: The "no-reflow" phenomenon after temporary coronary occlusion in the dog. *J Clin Invest* 54: 1496, 1974.

57 Willerson JT, Powell WJ Jr, Guiney TE, Stark J, Sanders CA, Leaf A: Improvement in myocardial function and coronary blood flow in ischemic myocardium after mannitol. *J Clin Invest* 51: 2989, 1972.

58 Leaf A: Cell swelling: A factor in ischemic tissue injury. *Circulation* 48: 455, 1973.

59 Camilleri JP, Joseph D, Fabian JN, Deloche A, Schlumberger M, Relland J, Carpentier A: Microcirculatory changes following early reperfusion in experimental myocardial infarction. *Virchows Arch* (Pathol Anat) 369: 315, 1976.

60 Deloche A, Fabiani JN, Camilleri JP, Relland J, Joseph D, Carpentier A, Dubost CA: The effect of coronary artery reperfusion on the extent of myocardial infarction. *Am Heart J* 93: 358, 1977.

61 Kloner RA, Rude RE, Carlson N, Maroko PR, DeBoer LWV, Braunwald E: Ultrastructural evidence of microvascular damage and myocardial cell injury after coronary artery occlusion: Which comes first? *Circulation* 62: 945, 1980.

62 Cobb FR, Bache RJ, Rivas F, Greenfield JC Jr: Local effects of acute cellular injury on regional myocardial blood flow. *J Clin Invest* 57: 1359, 1976.

63 Willerson JT, Watson JT, Hutton I, Templeton GH, Fixler DE: Reduced myocardial reflow and increased coronary vascular resistance following prolonged myocardial ischemia in the dog. *Circ Res* 36: 771, 1975.

64 Capone RJ, Most AS: Myocardial hemorrhage after coronary reperfusion in pigs. *Am Heart J* 96: 295, 1975.

65 Bresnahan GF, Roberts R, Shell WE, Ross J Jr, Sobel BE: Deleterious effects due to hemorrhage after myocardial reperfusion. *Am J Cardiol* 33: 82, 1974.

66 Ginks WR, Sybers HD, Maroko PR, Covell JW, Sobel BE, Ross JJ: Coronary artery reperfusion, Part 2 (reduction of myocardial infarct size at 1 week after the coronary occlusion). *J Clin Invest* 51: 2717, 1972.

67 Maroko PR, Libby P, Ginks WR, Bloor CM, Shell WE, Sobel BE, Ross J Jr: Coronary artery reperfusion, Part 1 (early effects on local myocardial function and the extent of myocardial necrosis). *J Clin Invest* 51: 2710, 1972.

67a Khalafbeigui F, Becker LC, Hutchins GM, Bulkley BH: Time course of necrosis after coronary artery occlusion in the conscious dog. *Circulation* 64 (suppl IV): 98, 1981.

68 Lang T, Corday E, Gold H, Meerbaum S, Rubins S, Costantini C, Hirose S, Osher J, Rosen V: Consequences of reperfusion after coronary occlusion: Effects on hemodynamic and regional myocardial metabolic function. *Am J Cardiol* 33: 69, 1974.

69 Baughman KL, Maroko PR, Vatner SF: Effects of coronary reperfusion on myocardial infarct size and survival in conscious dogs. *Circulation* 63: 317, 1981.

70 Sheehan FH, Epstein SE: Determinants of arrhythmic death due to coronary spasm: Pre-existing coronary stenosis reduces risk of VF following release of coronary occlusion. *Circulation* 62: 145, 1980.

71 Hackett TP Cassem NH: Factors contributing to delay in responding to the signs and symptoms of acute myocardial infarction. *Am J Cardiol* 25: 651, 1969.

71a Simon AB, Feinleib M, Thompson HK Jr: Components of delay in the prehospital phase of acute myocardial infarction. *Am J Cardiol* 30: 476, 1972.

72 Maroko PR, Bernstein EF, Libby P, DeLaria GA, Covell JW, Ross J Jr, Braunwald E: Effects of intraortic balloon counter pulsation on the severity of myocardial ischemic injury following acute coronary occlusion: Counterpulsation and myocardial injury. *Circulation* 45: 1150, 1972.

73 Hillis LD, Maroko PR, Braunwald F, Fishbein MC: The influence of the time interval between coronary artery occlusion and the administration of hyaluronidase on salvage of ischemic myocardium in dogs. *Circ Res* 41: 26, 1977.

73a Marcus ML, Kerber RE, Ehrhardt J, Abboud FM: Effects of time on volume and distribution of coronary collateral flow. *Am J Physiol* 230, 1976.

73b Chambers DE, Yellon DM, Hearse DJ, Downey JM: Flurbiprofen may limit infarct size 6 but not 24 hours following coronary occlusion in the dog. *Fed Proc* 82: 1531, 1982.

74 DeWood MA, Spores J, Notske R, et al: Prevalence of total coronary occlusion during the early hours of transmural myocardial infarction. *N Engl J Med* 303: 897, 1980.

75 Phillips SJ, Kougtahworn C, Zeff RH, et al: Emergency coronary artery revascularization: a possible therapy for acute myocardial infarction. *Circulation* 60: 241, 1979.

76 Kloner RA, DeBoer LWV, Darsee JR, Ingwall JS, Braunwald E: Recovery from prolonged abnormalities of canine myocardium salvaged from ischemic necrosis by coronary reperfusion. *Proc Natl Acad Sci USA*, 78: 7152, 1981.

76a Blumenthal DS, Becker LC, Bulkley BH, Hutching GM, Weisfeldt ML, Garrison JB, Jenkins R, Weiss JL: Impaired function of "salvaged" myocardium. *Clin Res* 29: 178a, 1981.

76b Lavallee M, Cox D, Vatner SF: Time required for myocardial function salvaged by coronary artery reperfusion to respond appropriately to stress. *Clin Res* 30: 483a, 1982.

77 Sabina RL, Kernstine K, Holmes EW, Swain JL: Expansion of cardiac and skeletal muscle nucleotide pools by infusion of the nucleotide precursor 5-aminoimidazole-4-carboxamide riboside (AICAR). *Circulation* 64:275, 1981.

78 Regitz V, Azumi T, Hartmut S, Schaper W: Infarct size reduction by pyruvate-biochemical mechanism. *Circulation* 62: 242, 1980.

79 Peter T, Norris RM, Clarke ED, Heng MK, Singh BN, Williams B, Howell DR, Ambler PK: Reduction of enzyme levels by propranolol after acute myocardial infarction. *Circulation* 57: 1091, 1978.

80 Pelides LJ, Reid DS, Thomas M, Shillingford JP: Inhibition by β-blockade of the ST segment elevation after acute myocardial infarction in man. *Cardiovasc Res* 6: 295, 1972.

81 Maroko PR, Kloner RA, Gold HK, Braunwald E: Propranolol in acute myocardial infarction: Experimental and clinical considerations, in *Beta-Adrenergic Blockade—A New Era in Cardio-vascular Medicine*, E. Braunwald (ed). New York, Excerpta Medica, 1978, p 154.

82 Gold HK, Leinbach RC, Maroko PR: Propranolol-induced reduction of signs of ischemic injury during acute myocardial infarction. *Am J Cardiol* 38: 689, 1976.

83 Borer JS, Redwood DR, Levitt B, Cagin N, Bianchi C, Vallin H, Epstein SE: Reduction in myocardial ischemia with nitroglycerin or nitroglycerin plus phenylephrine administered during acute myocardial infarction. *N Engl J Med* 293: 1008, 1975.

84 Come PC, Flaherty JT, Baird MG, Rouleau JR, Weisfeldt ML, Greene HL, Becker L, Pitt B: Reversal by phenylephrine of the beneficial effects of intravenous nitroglycerin in patients with acute myocardial infarction. *N Engl J Med* 293: 1004, 1975.

85 Maroko PR, Hillis LD, Muller JE, Tavazzi L, Heyndrickz GR, Ray M, Chiariello M, Distante A, Askenazi J, Salerno J, Carpentier J, Reshetnaya NI, Radvany P, Libby P, Raabe DS, Chazov EI, Bobba P, Braunwald E: Favorable effects of hyaluronidase on electrocardiographic evidence of necrosis in patients with acute myocardial infarction. *N Engl J Med* 65: 93, 1979.

86 Russel RO Jr, Rogers WJ, Mantle JA, McDaniel HG, Rackley CE: Glucose-insulin-potassium, free fatty acids and acute myocardial infarction in man. *Circulation* 53: 207, 1975.

87 Heng MK, Norris RM, Singh BN, Barratt-Boyes C: Effects of glucose and glucose-insulin-potassium on haemodynamics and enzyme release after acute myocardial infarction. *Brit Heart J* 39: 748, 1977.

88 Leinbach RC, Gold HK, Harper RW, Buckley MJ, Austen WG: Early intraaortic balloon pumping for anterior myocardial infarction without shock. *Circulation* 58: 204, 1978.

89 Reduto LA, Smalling RW, Freund GC, Gould KL: Intracoronary infusion of streptokinase in patients with acute myocardial infarction: Effects of reperfusion on left ventricular performance. *Am J Cardiol* 48: 403, 1981.

90 Shell WE, Sobel BE: Protection of jeopardized ischemic myocardium by reduction of ventricular afterload. *N Engl J Med* 291: 481, 1974.

91 Roberts R, DeMello V, Sobel BE: Deleterious effects of methylprednisolone in patients with myocardial infarction. *Circulation* 53: 204, 1976.

92 Bulkley BH, Roberts WC: Steroid therapy during acute myocardial infarction: A cause of delayed healing and of ventricular aneurysm. *Am J Med* 56: 244, 1974.

93 Holland RP, Brooks H: Precordial and epicardial surface potentials during myocardial ischemia in the pig: A theoretical and experimental analysis of the TQ and ST segments. *Circ Res* 37: 471, 1975.

94 Kjekshus JK, Maroko PR, Sobel BE: Distribution of myocardial injury and its relation to epicardial ST-segment changes after coronary artery occlusion in the dog. *Cardiovasc Res* 6: 490, 1972.

95 Smith HJ, Singh BN, Norris RM, Murray JB, Hurley PJ: Changes in myocardial blood flow and S-T segment elevation following coronary artery occlusion in dogs. *Circ Res* 36: 697, 1975.

96 Cohen MV, Kirk ES: Reduction of epicardial S-T segment elevation following increased myocardial ischemia: Experimental and theoretical demonstration (abstr). *Clin Res* 22: 269A, 1974.

97 Irvin RG, Cobb FR: Relationship between epicardial ST-segment elevation, regional myocardial blood flow, and extent of myocardial infarction in awake dogs. *Circulation* 55: 825, 1977.

98 Shell WE, Kjekshus JK, Sobel BE: Quantitative assessment of the extent of myocardial infarction in the conscious dog by means of analysis of serial changes in serum creatine phosphokinase activity. *J Clin Invest* 50: 2614, 1971.

99 Swain JL, Cobb FR, McHale PA, Roe CR: Nonlinear relationship between creatine kinase estimates and histologic extent of infarction in conscious dogs: Effects of regional myocardial blood flow. *Circulation* 62: 1239, 1980.

100 Roe CR, Cobb FR, Starmer CF: The relationship between enzymatic and histologic estimates of the extent of myocardial infarction in conscious dogs with permanent coronary occlusion. *Circulation* 55: 438, 1977.

100a Grande P, Fischer Hansen B, Christiansen, C, Naestoft J: Estimation of acute myocardial infarct size in man by serum CK-MB measurements. *Circulation* 62: 756, 1982.

101 Malmberg P: Time course of enzyme escape via heart lymph following myocardial infarction in the dog. *Scand J Clin Invest* 30: 405, 1972.

102 Clark GE, Robinson AK, Gnepp DR, Roberts R, Sobel BE: Effects of lymphatic transport of enzyme on plasma creatine kinase time-activity curves after myocardial infarction in dogs. *Circ Res* 43: 162, 1978.

103 Roberts R, Henry PD, Sobel BE: An improved basis for enzymatic estimation of infarct size. *Circulation* 52: 743, 1975.

104 Vatner SF, Baig H, Manders WT, Maroko PR: Effects of coronary artery reperfusion on myocardial infarct size calculated from creatine kinase. *J Clin Invest* 61: 1048, 1978.

105 Cobb FR, Irvin RG, Hagerty RC, Roe CC: Effect of extension of infarction on serial CK activity. *Circulation* 60: 145, 1979.

106 Bonte FJ, Parkey RW, Graham KD, Moore J, Stokely EM: A new method for radionuclide imaging of myocardial infarcts. *Radiology* 110: 473, 1974.

107 Willerson JT, Parkey RW, Bonte FJ, Meyer SL, Atkins JM, Stokely EM: Technetium stannous pyrophosphate myocardial scintigrams in patients with chest pain of varying etiology. *Circulation* 51: 1046, 1975.

108 Marcus ML, Go RT, Ehrhardt JC, Van Kirk OC: Clinical applications of ^{99m}Tc-PYP infarct scintigrams, in *Progress in Nuclear Medicine*, A Donath, AN Serafini (eds). Basel, Karger, 1980, vol 6, p 18.

109 Botvinick EH, Shames D, Lappin H, Tyberg JV, Townsend R, Parmley WW: Noninvasive quantitation of myocardial infarction with technetium-99m pyrophosphate. *Circulation* 52: 909, 1975.

110 Stokely EM, Buja LM, Lewis SE, Parkey RW, Bonte FJ, Harris RA, Willerson JT: Measurement of acute myocardial infarcts in dogs with ^{99}m Tc-stannous pyrophosphate scintigrams. *J Nucl Med* 17: 1, 1975.

111 Willerson JT, Parkey RW, Harris RA, Bonte FJ, Stokely EM, Buja LM: Sizing acute myocardial infarction utilizing technetium stannous pyrophosphate myocardial scintigrams in dogs and man. *Clin Res* 23: 214a, 1975.

112 Singh M, Berggren MJ, Gustafson DE, Dewanjee MK, Bahn RC, Ritman EL: Emission-computed tomography and its application to imaging of acute myocardial infarction in intact dogs using Tc-99m pyrophosphate. *J Nucl Med* 20: 50, 1979.

113 Lewis M, Buja LM, Saffer S, Mishelevich D, Stokely EM, Lewis S, Parkey R, Bonte F, Willerson J: Experimental infarct sizing using computer processing and a three-dimensional model. *Science* 197: 167, 1977.

114 Kerber RE, Marcus ML, Ehrhardt J, Wilson R, Abboud FM: Correlation between echocardiographically demonstrated segmental dyskinesis and regional myocardial perfusion. *Circulation* 52: 1097, 1975.

CHAPTER **10**

THE CORONARY COLLATERAL CIRCULATION

In animals and humans, vascular channels link large coronary arteries to one another. These connecting channels are called coronary collaterals. Although coronary collaterals were first described by Lower in 1669 [1], their existence and functional significance remained controversial for over 250 years [2]. In 1924, post-mortem injection studies by Spalteholz [3] documented the existence of coronary collaterals in dog hearts. Similar studies performed in human hearts by Fulton [4] left little doubt concerning the existence of coronary collateral vessels. Preexisting or native coronary collaterals are small and few in number. Ischemia, however, can stimulate these coronary collaterals to develop into a major vascular network that can modify the effects of coronary occlusive disease. Since Schaper published a classic treatise on the coronary collateral circulation in 1971 [2], a substantial amount of new knowledge concerning the coronary collateral circulation has been acquired.

ANATOMIC FEATURES OF THE CORONARY COLLATERAL CIRCULATION

In the dog, native or preexisting collateral vessels are tiny thin-walled conduits. Mautz and Gregg [5] described them as "overstretched arterioles." Histologically, these vessels are composed of an endothelial lining and a fibrous tunic [2]. The elastic tissue is often scanty but sometimes forms a continuous elastic lamina. The smooth muscle cells are either isolated or organized into one or two smooth muscle layers. In dogs, these native collaterals are primarily found in the epicardium and within the ventricular septum [2,6].

Schaper has shown that the density of the epicardial collaterals in the dog is about 10 vessels per centimeter squared; average internal diameter is about 40 μm [2]. Native collateral vessels greater than 100 μm in diameter are rarely observed in the dog. The total cross-sectional area of the native collateral circulation is minute compared to the normal coronary vasculature.

Schaper was the first to demonstrate [2,7–12] that native coronary collaterals undergo a remarkable transformation in response to myocardial ischemia. This process can be divided into several distinct stages.

The *initial stage* of the transformation, following the onset of coronary occlusion, involves passive widening and damage to the native collateral channels. The internal elastic lamina is ruptured, and its fragments are displaced toward the media. The vessel wall becomes leaky, as evidenced by the passage of cellular blood components through the vascular wall. Recent studies by Schaper et al. [12,13] indicate that monocytes in particular migrate into the vascular wall. These cells may participate in the transformation process. In addition, in this early stage, perivascular inflammation occurs. This is indicated by the presence of polymorphonuclear leukocytes in the vascular wall.

In the *subacute stage* (1 to 2 weeks), the perivascular infiltration subsides and the vessel is transformed into a much larger channel with a relatively thin wall. This "vascular growth" is facilitated by mitotic division of all three cell types–endothelial cells, smooth muscle cells, and fibroblasts–in the vessel wall. Initially, the newly formed smooth muscle cells in the vascular wall are poorly organized. Over many weeks these smooth muscle cells in the vascular wall will arrange themselves into circular and longitudinal layers. DNA replication in vascular smooth muscle begins immediately following the onset of ischemia. Because a single synthetic cycle of the cells which constitute the vascular wall takes 20 to 22 h [2,12], it takes about 1 day for collateral channels to grow significantly following the onset of an intense ischemic stimulus.

During these initial phases, the lumen of the native vascular channel increases about eightfold (40 μm to 320 μm internal diameter). The wall of this "overstretched vessel" is not sufficiently thick to maintain normal wall stress. In the ensuing weeks, the arterial wall thickens by continued cellular proliferation and synthesis of elastin and collagen. By 6 months following coronary occlusion, the "remodeled native collateral vessel" resembles a normal coronary artery of similar size.

In a series of studies, Schaper and colleagues [2,7–12] have assessed the growth rate of coronary collateral vessels in dogs following gradual coronary constriction. Cell division within the wall of the collateral vessel following infusion of H_3 thymidine to label DNA was measured by autoradiography. Changes in lumen size and wall thickness were assessed with histological techniques. The results of these classic studies are shown in Figures 10-1 through 10-3. These studies have been confirmed [14–16] by others.

Several features of a transformed coronary collateral differentiate it from a normal coronary artery of similar size [2,12]. First, there are small defects in the internal elastic lamina. This may contribute to the tortuosity of coronary collaterals. Second, the extent of adrenergic innervation in the vessel is substantially reduced. Third, some vessels demonstrate "overshoot repair." This is manifest by subintimal proliferation of smooth muscle, which in the extreme can cause near obliteration of the vascular lumen. The transformation of native collaterals to mature collaterals evolves over many months and is essentially complete 1 year following coronary occlusion. The functional capacity of these collateral channels is near maximal 4 weeks following coronary occlusion (Figure 10-4).

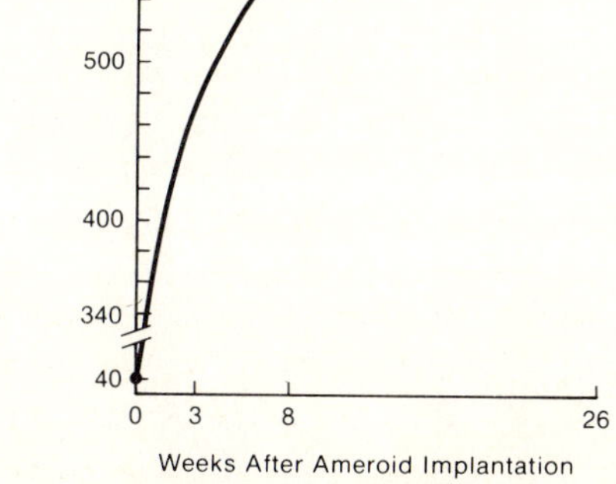

FIGURE 10-1
Alterations in the internal diameter of coronary collateral vessels following progressive coronary occlusion with an implanted Ameroid constrictor. Within 8 weeks of Ameroid implantation, the diameter of coronary collateral vessels increases almost 15-fold. *(Based on data originally presented by W Schaper* [2].*)*

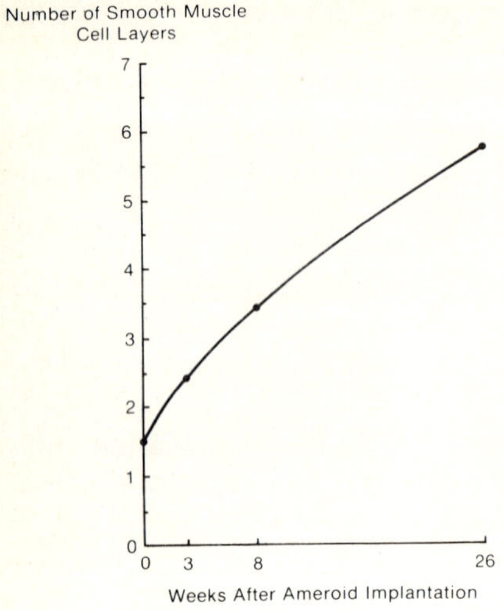

FIGURE 10-2
Alterations in the number of smooth muscle cell layers following progressive coronary occlusion with an implanted Ameroid constrictor. The increase in wall thickness in these stimulated collateral channels progresses at a slower rate than the increase in internal diameter (see Figure 10-1). As a consequence, at 8 weeks following Ameroid implantation, the stimulated collateral vessels are relatively thin walled. (*Based on data originally presented by W Schaper* [2].)

METHODS OF ASSESSING COLLATERAL FUNCTION

The classic approach to the measurement of coronary collateral flow is to insert a small cannula into the coronary vessel just beyond the site of occlusion and measure retrograde flow by timed volume collection and retrograde or peripheral coronary pressure. This method was extensively used by Gregg and his coworkers

FIGURE 10-3
Changes in the number of nuclei in the wall of collateral vessels following coronary occlusion with an Ameroid constrictor. Over an 8-week period, the number of nuclei in the wall of the collateral vessels increased tenfold. (*Based on data originally presented by W Shaper* [2].)

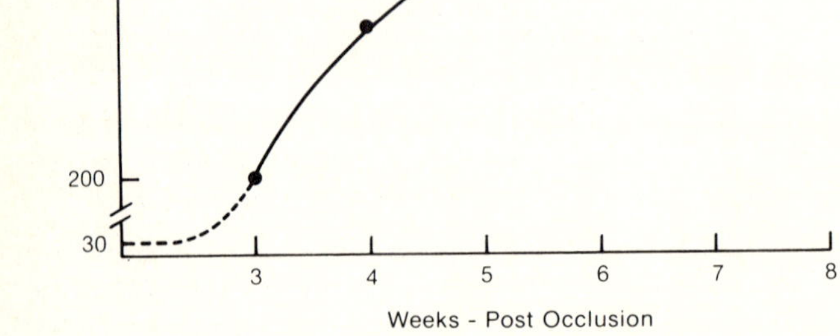

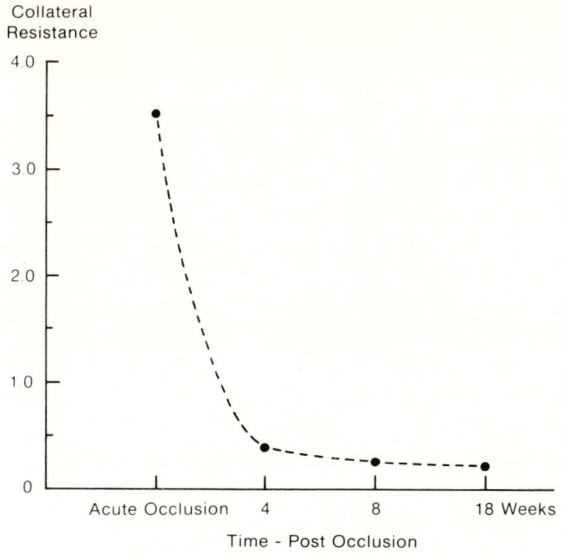

FIGURE 10-4
Effects of time following Ameroid implantation on minimal collateral resistance. When acute coronary occlusion is produced, the resistance of native collateral vessels is almost 10 times greater than the resistance in stimulated collaterals months after Ameroid implantation. The rate at which changes in resistance occur in these stimulated collaterals reflects the rate of dilation of the collateral channels (see Figure 10-1). (*Based on data originally presented by W Schaper* [2].)

[17–23]. There are five major deficiencies with this approach. First, some flow inevitably escapes anterograde and ideally should be blocked by peripheral embolization [24]. Second, blood from a collateral dependent zone which passes through microvascular channels and terminates distal to a significant source of resistance cannot be diverted in a retrograde fashion [25]. Third, collecting retrograde flow against atmospheric pressure–i.e., no resistance–almost certainly introduces an artifact into the measurement [26]. Fourth, Schaper has shown that peripheral coronary pressure and flow provide a *usable index of collateral development* only in the presence of maximal vasodilation and carefully controlled extravascular coronary resistance [2,12]. Finally, retrograde flow and peripheral coronary pressure do not allow the investigator to assess the transmural distribution of coronary collateral perfusion.

The net effect of these methodological deficiencies is that retrograde coronary flow seriously underestimates coronary collateral blood flow [24,25]. Although measurements of retrograde collateral flow and peripheral coronary pressure have allowed investigators to make important contributions to our conceptual understanding of the coronary circulation [17–23], this approach has been replaced by more quantitative methods.

Microspheres or diffusible indicators can be used to assess coronary collateral flow [12,27,28]. With either technique it is critically important to separate "true collateral flow" from "overlap flow." Overlap flow is blood delivered to the vicinity of the occluded zone by nonoccluded vessels which interdigitate with the occluded vessels both macroscopically and microscopically (see Chapters 1, 2, and 9). Failure to distinguish overlap flow from collateral flow yields results which are uninterpretable. This is a common error. When microspheres are used to assess collateral flow and overlap flow is excluded, the regional distribution of coronary collateral flow can be readily determined.

In an isolated, blood perfused heart, collateral flow can be assessed by simultaneous measurement of anterograde and retrograde flow in all major coronary vessels with electromagnetic flow meters and timed venous collection [6,16,29]. Maximal coronary dilation can be achieved with infusion of a potent coronary dilator and extravascular compressive forces can be controlled. This method permits the investigator to determine collateral resistance between the four major coronary vascular arteries in the dog [6,16,29]. It would be worthwhile to compare this method of measuring coronary collateral flow with the microsphere approach.

Methods of assessing coronary collateral flow in animals are reasonably precise. In contrast, approaches to measuring coronary collateral flow in patients are remarkably crude. This is an area of research which should receive additional attention.

METHODS OF STIMULATING THE GROWTH OF CORONARY COLLATERAL VESSELS

There are four approaches presently used to stimulate the growth of coronary collateral channels: Ameroid constrictors, fixed stenosis, intermittent coronary occlusion, and certain types of cardiac stress.

In 1957, Litvak et al. [30] demonstrated that if a hygroscopic plastic material (Ameroid), enclosed in a steel ring to prevent outward swelling, was placed snugly around a coronary vessel, over 8 weeks the plastic would expland and coronary occlusion would occur. Schaper [2,12] has demonstrated that three factors are responsible for coronary occlusion: (1) swelling of the Ameroid material decreases the coronary lumen by about 60 percent, (2) sterile inflammation in response to the plastic material causes fibrosis and additional coronary constriction, and (3) severe luminal stenosis promotes complete obstruction by platelet plugs or thrombi [2,13]. With the Ameroid technique, coronary occlusion occurs within 8 weeks in 95 percent of dogs with implanted constrictors (Figure 10-5). When this technique is carefully applied, about 60 to 70 percent of dogs experience complete coronary occlusion without myocardial infarction [2].

Fixed obstructive rings of Teflon, which do not generate sterile inflammatory reactions, will promote coronary collateral growth if the narrowing produced by the ring decreases coronary diameter by 80 percent or more [12].

Franklin et al. [31] recently demonstrated that repeated 2- to 5-min periods of coronary occlusion in dogs will stimulate the functional capacity of coronary collateral vessels.

Finally, the decreased oxygen supply to the myocardium secondary to severe anemia [32,33] can increase the capacity of the coronary collateral circulation. Zoll et al. [34] noted that "native collaterals" are increased in severely hypertrophied hearts. The functional significance of this observation is unknown.

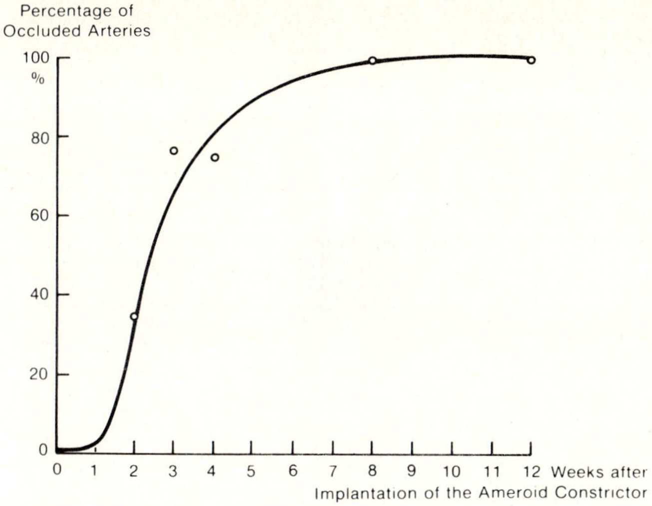

FIGURE 10-5
Time course of coronary occlusion following Ameroid implantation. Eight weeks following Ameroid implantation, greater than 90 percent of vessels are totally occluded. *(Based on data originally presentd by W Schaper* [2].*)*

FUNCTIONAL CAPACITY OF CORONARY COLLATERALS

Because coronary collaterals can undergo vast developmental changes in response to certain stimuli, any discussion of their functional capacity must separate native or preexisting collaterals from those in various stages of development.

Native or Immature Collaterals

In the dog, if extravascular compressive forces are minimized, the resistance through native collateral channels in the left ventricle has been reported to be 12 to 40 times greater than the resistance through normal coronary vessels (Figure 10-6) [2,6,16,35,36]. Under in situ conditions, when normal extravascular compressive forces are present, the effective resistance through native collateral channels has been reported to be much higher, i.e., 60 to 80 times greater than minimal resistance through normal coronary vessels (Figure 10-6) [13,36,36a].

Investigations which have employed the microsphere technique to measure collateral flow have suggested that flow to an ischemic zone delivered via native collaterals can approach 30 to 50 percent of the flow delivered to normally perfused myocardium [37–41]. This implies that the resistance through native collaterals in the beating dog heart is only two or three times greater than the resistance through normal channels.

Why is it that estimates of native collateral resistance in the dog vary over such a broad range? The answer lies in a methodologic problem. In the dog, there is

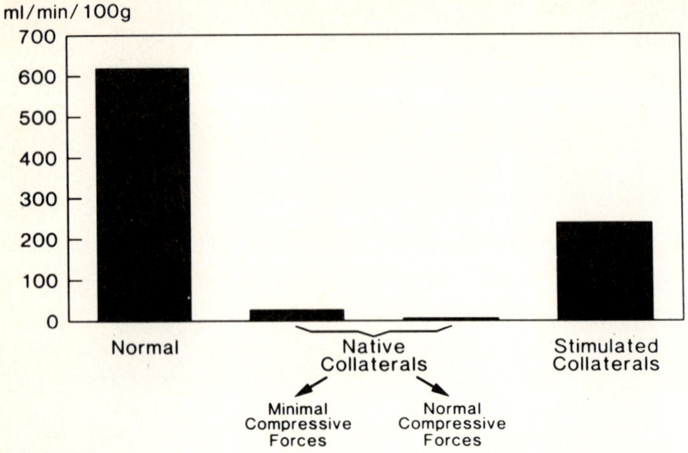

FIGURE 10-6
Coronary flow during maximal coronary dilation in normal coronary vessels (normal), native collaterals, and mature stimulated collaterals. All flows were measured at a coronary perfusion pressure at 100 mmHg. The data emphasize the minimal capacity of native collaterals. The maximal flow that can be delivered by mature stimulated collaterals is less than half of that which can be delivered by normal collateral channels. (*Based on data originally presented by W Schaper* [*12*].)

extensive macroscopic and microscopic interdigitation of the vascular territories of individual vessels (see Chapters 1, 2, and 9). Consequently, if tissue samples are obtained from the presumed ischemic zone, they almost invariably include a mixture of normally perfused and ischemic tissue. A tissue sample which contains 50 percent normal and 50 percent ischemic tissue would have a flow which is about one-half of the mean flow rate to the normal zone. Because "twinkling" of the coronary microvasculature can cause flow in the normal myocardium to decrease transiently to 50 percent below the mean value [42,43], segments of tissue obtained from the ischemic region that have flows greater than 50 percent of mean flow to the normal area are often assumed to contain only normally perfused tissue. When heterogeneous tissue sampling is eliminated [12,36,44], flow through native collateral channels in the dog obtained with microspheres indicates that collateral resistance is 10 to 50 times greater than normal coronary vascular resistance.

Whenever collateral flow is assessed with microspheres or a similar technique, unless heterogeneous tissue sampling is carefully eliminated, the data are uninterpretable.

Developing Collaterals

Immediately following the onset of sustained myocardial ischemia, the tiny thin-walled native collateral channels undergo a process which will eventually transform them into medium-sized coronary arteries. This transformation process is not completed until 6 to 12 months after the onset of ischemia [2,12]. Anatomic studies indicate that dilation progresses at a much faster pace than restructuring of the vascular wall (Figure 1-3). Consequently, near maximal functional capacity of these transformed vessels is realized long before the structural remodeling is completed. Studies in dogs from the laboratories of Schaper, Gregg, and Scheel [2,12,23,35,36] have indicated that within 4 weeks the functional capacity of coronary collateral vessels is about 90 percent of maximal capacity to be achieved many months following coronary occlusion (Figure 10-4).

WHAT IS THE PROXIMATE STIMULUS THAT PROMOTES COLLATERAL GROWTH?

Three types of factors are responsible for vascular growth: mechanical, chemical, and hereditary.

Mechanical stimuli that act on coronary collaterals include intravascular pressure, blood velocity, viscous drag, and tangential wall stress. Schaper reasoned that the first three are unlikely to play a meaningful role in collateral development [2]. In contrast, changes in tangential wall stress (tangential wall stress = pressure × radius ÷ wall thickness) in developing collaterals show a striking parallelism with the growth rate of these channels. Collateral growth is maximal during the first few weeks following coronary occlusion and then continues at a slower pace for months after normal tissue perfusion is restored. Scheel and coworkers [45] have developed a model which suggests that changes in wall stress in a developing collateral vessel exhibit a similar time course. Other features also favor the notion that tangential wall stress is a critical determinant of coronary collateral growth. Tangential wall stress is the only mechanical factor that exerts its influence on the entire vascular wall. Restructuring of the collateral vessel continues until the wall-to-lumen ratio reaches a value which returns predicted wall stress to normal. Also, growth processes in other organs such as the heart [46] appear to be regulated in part by alterations in wall stress. Although a cause and effect relationship between tangential wall stress and collateral growth has not been established, it is likely that wall stress plays a major role in mediating the growth of developing coronary collateral channels.

Chemical mediation probably influences collateral growth in two ways. First, hypoxia almost certainly initiates intense dilation of native coronary collateral channels and thus starts the process of vascular transformation. Hypoxia, produced by any of several mechanisms (coronary occlusion, partial obstruction, or severe anemia), can initiate this process. Unknown chemical substances probably contribute to sustained growth of coronary collaterals. Although collaterals grow primarily toward the ischemic zone, following coronary occlusion growth occurs in all directions [6,35]. Furthermore, the vascular growth involves both venous and arterial channels [12]. Finally, substances which promote angiogenesis in organs other than the heart have been identified [47,48]. *These observations are best reconciled by assuming that a diffusible substance may contribute to the growth of coronary collateral channels.*

Hereditary factors also affect the growth pattern of coronary collaterals. De novo appearance of coronary collaterals does not occur. Native collaterals are transformed into larger vessels. Present data suggest that native collaterals are more abundant in the dog than in the pig, baboon, or goat (see Chapter 9).

Finally, coronary occlusion produces inflammation of overstretched native collateral vessels, and the inflammatory process may stimulate angiogenesis [2,12].

FACTORS THAT MODULATE THE GROWTH AND FUNCTIONAL CAPACITY OF CORONARY COLLATERAL VESSELS

A large number of studies have been directed toward identifying exogenous stimuli that may modulate the growth of collateral coronary vessels. At present, only three factors—severity of coronary stenosis, exercise training, and anemia—have been shown to promote the growth of coronary collaterals.

Schaper has recently demonstrated that, in the dog, growth of coronary collateral vessels is not stimulated until a coronary stenosis which causes an 80 percent reduction in the cross-sectional area of a coronary vessel is produced [12]. The conductance of coronary collaterals produced by such a stenosis is much less than that observed in chronic collaterals produced by gradual coronary occlusion (Figure 10-7) [12]. In patients, coronary collaterals do not develop until a proximal stenosis of about 80 to 90 percent is present [49]. Hence, the severity of coronary obstruction is a critical determinant of the growth of coronary collateral channels.

Although physical exercise produces many favorable effects on the circulation, in the absence of a severe coronary stenosis or coronary occlusion, relatively intense prolonged exercise in dogs and pigs does not affect the native coronary collateral circulation [6,50–51a].

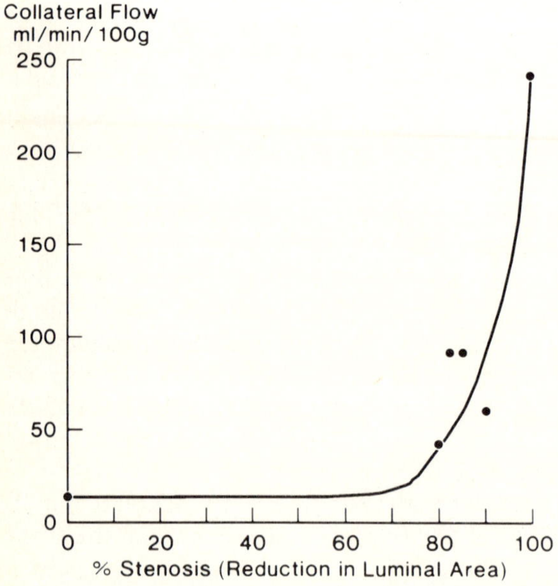

FIGURE 10-7
Maximal flow that can be delivered via mature or stimulated collaterals that developed as a consequence of a coronary stenosis. The data indicate that a coronary stenosis in a dog does not stimulate collateral growth unless the stenosis decreases luminal area by about 80 percent. Furthermore, the collateral growth stimulated by a stenosis (80 to 90 percent decrease in luminal area) is much less than that which occurs in response to complete coronary occlusion. (*Based on data originally presented by W Schaper* [*12*].)

Many studies have examined the effects of exercise training on the growth of coronary collaterals in dogs with either coronary stenosis or occlusion [6,12, 52–57a]. The results of these investigations have been inconsistent. Although two studies have reported that exercise promotes collateral development [6,52], most studies suggest that exercise training has a negligible effect on the coronary collateral circulation [12,53–57a].

The effects of anemia on coronary collateral growth have been examined by Eckstein [32] and Scheel and coworkers [33]. The results of both studies indicate that severe anemia tends to promote the growth of coronary collateral vessels.

The effects of many drugs (nitrates, lidoflazine, dipyridamole, calcium blockers, beta blockers), hormones (corticosteroids, growth hormones), and cholesterol on the functional capacity of native coronary collaterals have been examined and in the main no positive results have been found [58]. In 1979, Schaper wrote, "I know of no pharmacologic agent that has been conclusively shown to increase conductance of preexistent collaterals in the normal heart" [58]. In addition, no pharmacologic agent has been shown to augment the growth of coronary collaterals in response to myocardial ischemia.

Mature coronary collaterals are invested with a normal muscular coat. These vessels are responsive to the same stimuli that modulate coronary vascular tone in normal coronary arteries, with the possible exception of adrenergic control.

FUNCTIONAL CHARACTERISTICS OF MATURE COLLATERALS

Many studies [6,12,23,35–36a,53–57,59,59a] have indicated that a well-developed mature collateral circulation in the dog has a minimal vascular resistance which is two to four times greater than normal (Figure 10-6). Under resting conditions, this impairment in vascular reserve is concealed. Perfusion of the normal and collateral-dependent regions of myocardium are identical (see Figure 10-8). During stress, however, the impaired vasodilator reserve of collateral-dependent areas can be demonstrated. During maximal vasodilation, tachycardia (heart rate = 200 beats per minute) impairs perfusion of the inner layers in collateral-dependent zones, whereas in normally perfused myocardium these abnormalities do not occur [12,60]. Also, during maximal vasodilation, factors which increase extravascular compressive forces (left ventricular diastolic pressure, left ventricular systolic pressure, increased inotropic state) impair perfusion in the subendocardial layers of collateral-dependent zones to a greater extent than that which occurs in normally perfused zones [12]. During moderate exercise, mature collaterals can provide normal perfusion to the myocardium (see Figure 10-8) [59,59a]. In contrast, during intense free-ranging exercise, myocardial dysfunction in collateral-dependent zones occurs [61]. Thus, although mature collateral coronary vessels in the dog possess substantial vasodilator capacity, myocardial ischemia can develop during intense stress.

There are several additional features of the mature coronary collateral circulation which warrant comment. The size of the collateral-dependent zone affects the adequacy of collateral perfusion. Because collateral vessels arise from the periph-

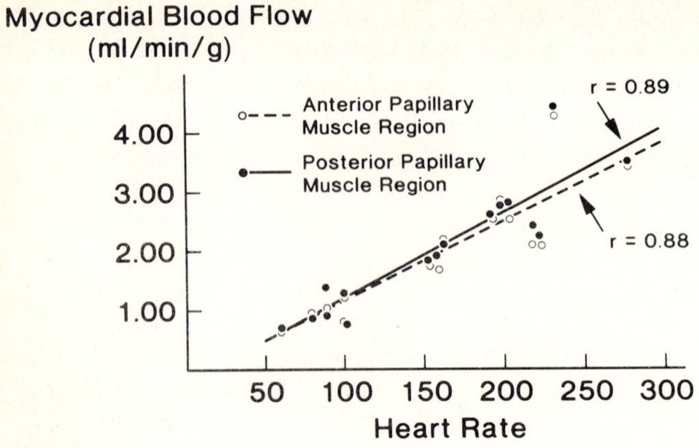

FIGURE 10-8
Effects of exercise on myocardial blood flow in a normally perfused area of the left ventricle (anterior papillary muscle region) and a collateral-dependent area of the left ventricle (posterior papillary muscle region). The collateral circulation to the posterior papillary muscle was stimulated to develop by gradual occlusion of the circumflex coronary artery with an implanted Ameroid constrictor months prior to the exercise study. The data indicate that the blood flow to the two regions was equal during exercise to heart rates of almost 300 beats per minute. In almost all the animals studied, the maximal flow rates achieved were less than 3 ml/g/min. During exercise, mean arterial pressure increases. Hence, at a flow of 3 ml/g/min and an increase in mean arterial pressure, calculated coronary vascular resistance would probably be twofold greater than minimal coronary vascular resistance that can be achieved in the dog. The decrease in coronary vascular resistance achieved in this exercise study is about equal to the maximal capacity of coronary collateral vessels to dilate (see Figure 10-6). Thus, the data in Figure 10-6 and this figure are consistent. *(Based on data originally presented by PR Lambert et al* [59].*)*

ery of the occluded zone, geometric considerations dictate that large areas will have fewer collaterals per square centimeter than small arees [36a]. Under some conditions, collateral vessels can facilitate coronary steal [12,62]. Recent studies suggest that partially developed collaterals may dilate significantly during the first 5 min following coronary occlusion [62a]. Finally, if a single normal vessel provides perfusion to a large collateral-dependent zone, the vasodilator reserve in the normally perfused zone will be mildly impaired [12]. The explanation for this latter phenomenon is not clear.

DISAPPEARANCE AND REAPPEARANCE OF CORONARY COLLATERALS

In 1971, Khouri, Gregg, and McGranahan demonstrated that complete relief of coronary occlusion led to the rapid disappearance of functional evidence of coronary collaterals [21]. When the reopened vessel was occluded 3 months later, within 60 min the collateral circulation was functioning as if it had never been disturbed. Thus, disappearance and reemergence of coronary collaterals can occur rapidly. The recent introduction of balloon angioplasty should stimulate interest in this phenomenon (see Chapter 19).

CORONARY COLLATERALS IN HUMANS

The mature coronary collateral circulation in the dog is capable of providing normal perfusion to the myocardium under many conditions. In contrast, several clinical studies have suggested that coronary collaterals in patients are of little importance [63–69]. Various investigators have concluded that coronary collaterals in patients do not "preserve ventricular function," "alter the clinical manifestations of coronary disease," or "prevent sudden death" [63,69]. If these claims are taken at face value, one must conclude that the functional capacity of the collateral coronary circulation in humans is far inferior to that of the dog. Gorlin summarized his views concerning the coronary collateral circualtion in humans as follows: "In the last analysis, coronary collaterals in man are more an indication of severe myocardial ischemia than a sign of biological 'compensation' for a perfusion deficit" [69]. In my opinion, a clear understanding of the potential value of the collateral circulation in humans has been clouded by clinical studies which have many weaknesses in their methodology and design. The key problems with most clinical studies are briefly reviewed below.

Rate of Collateral Development

Studies in dogs have demonstrated that maximal development of coronary collaterals occurs if a coronary vessel is completely occluded over a period of weeks or months. In patients, the rate at which coronary occlusion occurs is unknown. Recent clinical studies suggest that coronary occlusion often occurs acutely—when a thrombus suddenly occludes a partially obstructed coronary vessel [70,71]. Unfortunately, investigators who have studied the coronary collateral circulation in humans have often combined results obtained in patients with partial and complete coronary occlusion [63–69]. The interpretation of such data is exceedingly difficult.

Patient Selection

Patients with coronary disease who come to the attention of cardiologists and cardiac surgeons are likely to have clinical symptoms which may be related to inadequate coronary collaterals. Patients with excellent collateral function may remain asymptomatic, and hence they have little chance of being included in clinical studies. Consequently, it is inevitable that clinical study groups will be heavily weighted with patients that have relatively inadequate coronary collaterals [71a].

Coexistent Disease

Patients with ischemic heart disease often have two concomitant problems—multivessel obstructions and myocardial infarction—which make it difficult to assess the functional capacity of coronary collaterals. Both of these conditions will tend to decrease the functional capacity of coronary collaterals. Most clinical studies have not subgrouped patients on the basis of these variables [63–69]. This further confounds the interpretaton of the data obtained.

Methods of Evaluating the Coronary Collateral Circulation in Humans

Sophisticated methods of evaluating coronary collateral channels cannot be used in patients. The most commonly applied clinical method—angiographic assessment of coronary collaterals—is remarkably poor. Coronary collaterals less than 100 to 200 μm are not detectable by angiography. Animal studies indicate that the angiographic assessment of collaterals is unrelated to the functional capacity of these vascular channels [2,12]. However, clinical studies indicate that patients with "large as opposed to small collaterals" have high peripheral coronary pressure and retrograde flow in the diseased coronary vessels served by the collateral channels [72,73].

Indirect approaches to assessing the functional capacity of coronary collaterals such as clinical symptoms and exercise electrocardiography are of limited value because multivessel coronary disease often clouds the interpretation of such studies.

In a few studies, a more direct index of the functional capacity of coronary collaterals has been obtained. Such indices include measurements of peripheral coronary pressure [72–74], retrograde coronary flow [72–74], or tissue perfusion measured by isotope clearance [75–77]. These studies concluded that flow delivered by collaterals to jeopardized zones is less than normal. In these studies, the confounding effect of coexistent infarction was usually not excluded and the maximal dilator capacity of coronary collateral channels was not assessed.

In summary, the four major problems with clinical studies—unknown rate of coronary collateral development, patient selection, coexistent disease, and methodological limitations—make it difficult to appreciate the potential functional capacity of coronary collateral vessels in humans. In addition, misinterpretation of collected data has led to the commonly held notion that coronary collaterals are of little significance in patients. I believe this notion is incorrect.

FUNCTIONAL CAPACITY OF CORONARY COLLATERALS IN HUMANS

What is the evidence that coronary collaterals are of value to patients with ischemic heart disease?

It is well known that a small percentage of patients with total occlusion of a major coronary vessel maintain normal ventricular function at rest and demonstrate no evidence of myocardial infarction. In rare instances, total oclusion of the left main coronary artery is unassociated with evidence of infarction or any abnormality in the function of the left ventricle at rest [78]. This could not occur unless collateral channels provided substantial flow to the myocardium subserved by the occluded vessel.

A carefully designed study by Schwarz et al. [49,79] examined myocardial structure and function in patients with an *occluded* vessel with and without angiographically apparent coronary collaterals. The myocardial segment served by occluded vessels with well-developed coronary collaterals had less fibrosis and better contractile function than segments in the distribution of noncollateralized occluded vessels (see Figures 10-9 and 10-10). Similar results have been reported by Levin [80].

Three studies have utilized thallium 201 perfusion scintigrams during exercise to assess the functional significance of coronary collaterals in patients [81–83]. Patients who had angiographically detectable collaterals to a noninfarcted area in the perfusion field of an occluded vessel usually did not exhibit decreases in thallium 201 uptake during exercise. This suggests that the collateral vessels maintained adequate perfusion to the jeopardized zone both with rest and during exercise. These studies support the notion that coronary collaterals can prevent or limit abnor-

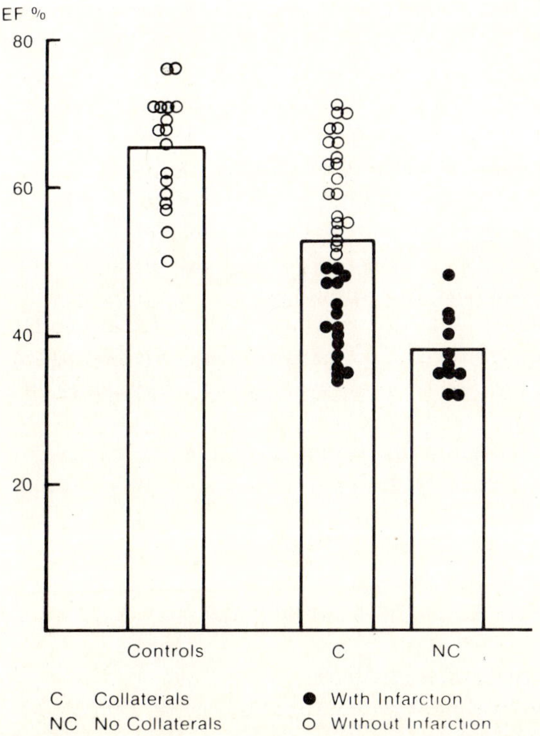

FIGURE 10-9
Left ventricular function in three patient groups: normal controls; patients with total coronary occlusion of one vessel and angiographically apparent coronary collaterals (C); and patients with total coronary occlusion and no angiographically apparent coronary collateral vessels (NC). Myocardial infarction was less frequent and myocardial function was better preserved in patients with angiographically apparent coronary collaterals vs. those that did not have such collateral vessels. The data suggest that in patients coronary collaterals can preserve left ventricular function and decrease the incidence of myocardial infarction. *(Based on data originally presented by F Schwarz et al* [79].)

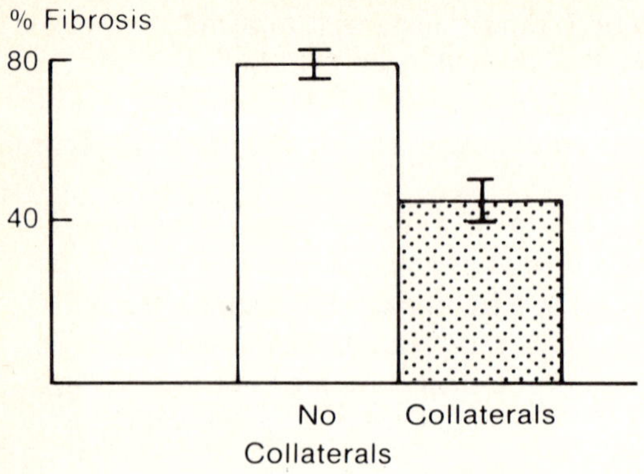

FIGURE 10-10
Percent of fibrous tissue in myocardial biopsies obtained from patients with complete coronary occlusion in the presence or absence of angiographically apparent coronary collateral vessels. The biopsies, obtained at the time of cardiac surgery, were from the myocardial perfusion field of the occluded coronary vessel. Fibrosis was less prominent in patients with coronary collateral vessels apparent at the time of coronary angiography. (*Based on data originally presented by F Schwarz et al* [79].)

malities in myocardial perfusion during exercise. Because thallium 201 scintigrams are relatively insensitive and do not provide a quantitative index of transmural myocardial perfusion, these studies do not prove that coronary collaterals restore myocardial perfusion during exercise to normal.

Thus, considerable evidence indicates that coronary collaterals in humans can preserve myocardial structure and function in the presence of total occlusion of a major coronary vessel.

Although coronary collaterals in humans can preserve resting myocardial function, the limited capacity of coronary collaterals in humans becomes manifest in the presence of moderate stress [49,79]. Schwarz et al. have shown that during pacing, regional wall motion deteriorates in myocardial segments perfused by collateral channels [49,79]. Finally, unpublished data from my laboratory suggests that the vascular reserve of coronary collateral-dependent zones assessed by the Doppler technique at the time of open heart surgery is diminished.

A few studies have assessed the effects of exercise on collateral function in patients [84–91]. In general, these studies have not demonstrated that this intervention improves collateral function. The clinical improvement observed (decreased angina) can be attributed to exercise conditioning.

In the aggregate, these studies suggest that the capacity of the coronary collateral circulation in humans is limited. *However, coronary collaterals in humans can supply sufficient oxygen to the myocardium to preserve myocardial structure and resting myocardial function.*

Many important questions concerning the functional capacity of coronary collaterals in humans remain to be answered. Research in this area should be strongly encouraged.

REFERENCES

1 Lower R: *Tractus de Corde.* Amsterdam, Elsevier, 1669.
2 Schaper W: *The Collateral Circulation of the Heart.* New York, Elsevier, 1971.
3 Spalteholz W: *Die Arterien des Herzwand.* Leipzig, Hirzel, 1924.

4 Fulton WFM: *The Coronary Arteries*. Springfield, Ill, Charles C Thomas, 1965.

5 Mautz FR, Gregg DE: Dynamics of collateral circulation following chronic occlusion of coronary arteries. *Proc Soc Exp Biol Med* 36: 797, 1937.

6 Scheel KW, Ingram LA, Wilson JL: Effects of exercise on the coronary and collateral vasculature of beagles with and without coronary occlusion. *Circ Res* 48: 523, 1981.

7 Schaper W: Collateral circulation in the canine coronary system. Thesis, Faculty of Medicine, University of Leuven, Belgium, 1967.

8 Schaper W,Vandesteene R: The rate of growth of interarterial anastomoses in chronic coronary artery occlusion, in *Life Sciences*, Oxford, England, Pergamon Press, 1967, vol 6, p 1673.

9 Schaper W, Schaper J, Xhonneux R, Vandesteene R: Morphology of intercoronary anastomoses in chronic coronary artery occlusion. *Cardiovasc Res* 3: 315, 1969.

10 De Brabander M, Schaper W: Quantitative histology of the canine coronary collateral circulation in localized myocardial ischemia, in *Life Sciences*, Oxford, England, Pergamon Press, 1971, vol 10, p 857.

11 Schaper W, De Brabander M, Lewi P: DNA synthesis and mitoses in coronary collateral vessels of the dog. *Circ Res* 28: 671, 1971.

12 Schaper W, Wusten B: Collateral circulation, in *The Pathophysiology of Myocardial Perfusion*, W Schaper (ed). Amsterdam, Elsevier, North-Holland Biomedical Press, 1979, chap 13.

13 Schaper J,König R, Franz D, Schaper W: The endothelial surface of growing coronary collateral arteries. *Virchows Arch* 370: 193, 1976.

14 Verheyen A, Xhonneux R, Borgers M, Reneman RS: Cell proliferation in developing coronary collaterals and the influence of lidoflazine on this process. *J Mol Cell Cardiol* 8: 53, 1976.

15 Yabe Y,Takahashi T, Yoshimura S, Tsuzuku A, Fujii, K, Kashiwakura Y, Tanaka H, Morita H, Koike M: A study of cell proliferation kinetics of coronary collateral vessels and myocardial muscles in the ischemic heart in dog. *Jap Circ J* 38: 154, 1974.

16 Scheel KW, Galindez TA, Cook B, Rodriguez RJ, Ingram LA: Changes in coronary and collateral flows and adequacy of perfusion in the dog following one and three months of circumflex occlusion. *Circ Res* 39: 654, 1976.

17 Gregg DE, Thornton JJ, Mautz FR: The magnitude, adequacy and source of the collateral blood flow and pressure in chronically chronically occluded coronary arteries. *Am J Physiol* 127: 161, 1939.

18 Gregg DE: *Coronary Circulation in Health and Disease*. Philadelphia, Lea & Febiger, 1950.

19 Kattus AA, Gregg DE: Some determinants of coronary collateral flow in the open-chest dog. *Circ Res* 7:628, 1959.

20 Elliot EC, Bloor CM, Jones EL, Mitchell WJ, Gregg DE: Effect of controlled coronary occlusion on collateral circulation in conscious dogs. *Am J Physiol* 220: 857, 1971.

21 Khouri EM, Gregg DE, McGranahan GM Jr: Regression and reappearance of coronary collaterals. *Am J Physiol* 220: 655, 1971.

22 Elliot EC, Jones EL, Bloor CM, Leon AS, Gregg DE: Day-to-day changes in coronary hemodynamics secondary to constriction of circumflex branch of left coronary artery in conscious dogs. *Circ Res* 22: 237, 1968.

23 Gregg DE: The natural history of coronary collateral development. *Circ Res* 35: 335, 1974.

24 Shulz FW, Raff WK, Meyer U, Lochner W: Messung der Kollateral-durchblutung am Hundeherzen mit Hilfe der selektiven Embolisierung eines Coronargefasses. *Pflügers Arch ges Physiol* 341: 243, 1973.

25 Downey HF, Crystal GJ, Bashour FA: Functional significance of microvascular collateral anastomoses after chronic coronary artery occlusion. *Microvasc Res* 21: 212, 1981.

26 Eckstein RW: The ineffectiveness of cortisone on functional coronary interarterial anastomoses. *Circ Res* 2: 466, 1954.

27 Cibulski AA, Lehan PH, Timmis HH: Retrograde flow technique vs. Krypton-85 clearance technique for estimation of myocardial collaterals. *Am J Physiol* 223: 1081, 1972.

28 Levy MN, Imperial ES, Zieske H Jr: Collateral blood flow to the myocardium as determined by the clearance of $Rb^{86}Cl$. *Circ Res* 9: 1035, 1961.

29 Scheel KW, Banet M, Ott C, Lehan PH: A quantitative approach to collateral and antegrade flows after coronary occlusion. *Am J Physiol* 222: 687, 1972.

30 Litvak J, Siderides LE, Vineberg AM: The experimental production of coronary artery insufficiency and occlusion. *Am Heart J* 53: 505, 1957.

31 Franklin D, McKown D, McKown M, Hartley J, Caldwell M: Development and regression of coronary collaterals induced by repeated, reversible ischemia in dogs. *Fed Proc* 3: 603, 1981.

32 Eckstein RW: Development of interarterial coronary anastomoses by chronic anemia; disappearance following correction of anemia. *Circ Res* 3: 306, 1955.

33 Scheel KW, Brody DA, Ingram LA, Keller F: Effects of chronic anemia on the coronary and coronary collateral vasculature in dogs. *Circ Res* 38: 553, 1976.

34 Zoll PM, Wessler S, Schlesinger MJ: Interarterial coronary anastomoses in the human heart, with particular reference to anemic and relative cardiac anoxia. *Circulation* 4: 797, 1951.

35 Scheel KW, Rodriguez RJ, Ingram LA: Directional coronary collateral growth with chronic circumflex occlusion in the dog. *Circ Res* 40: 384, 1977.

36 Schaper W, Flameng W, Winkler B, Wüsten B, Türschmann W, Neugebauer G, Carl M: Quantification of collateral resistance in acute and chronic experimental coronary occlusion in the dog. *Circ Res* 39: 371, 1976.

36a Schaper W: Residual perfusion of acutely ischemic heart muscle, in *The Pathophysiology of Myocardial Perfusion*, W Schaper (ed). Amsterdam, Elsevier, North-Holland Biomedical Press, 1979, chap 11.

37 Marcus ML, Kerber RE, Ehrhardt J, Abboud FM: Three dimensional geometry of acutely ischemic myocardium. *Circulation* 52: 254, 1975.

38 Marcus ML, Kerber RE, Ehrhardt J, Abboud FM: Effects of time on volume and distribution of coronary collateral flow. *Am J Physiol* 230: 279, 1976.

39 Becker LC, Ferreira R, Thomas M: Mapping of left ventricular blood flow with radioactive microspheres in experimental coronary artery occlusion. *Cardiovasc Res* 7: 391, 1973.

40 Becker LC, Pitt B: Collateral blood flow in conscious dogs with chronic coronary artery occlusion. *Am J Physiol* 221: 1507, 1971.

41 Hearse DJ, Yellon DM: The "Border Zone" in evolving myocardial infarction: Controversy or confusion? *Am J Cardiol* 47: 1321, 1981.

42 Falsetti HL, Carroll RJ, Marcus ML: Temporal heterogeneity of myocardial blood flow. *Circulation* 52: 848, 1975.

43 Sestier FJ, Mildenberger RR, Klassen GA: Role of autoregulation in spatial and temporal perfusion heterogenity in canine myocardium. *Am J Physiol* 235: 464, 1978.

44 Hirzel HO, Sonnenblick EH, Kirk ES: Absence of a lateral border zone of intermediate creatine phosphokinase depletion surrounding a central infarct 24 hours after acute coronary occlusion in the dog. *Circ Res* 41: 673, 1977.

45 Scheel KW, Fitzgerald EM, Martin RO, Larsen RA: The possible role of mechanical stresses on coronary collateral development during gradual coronary occlusion, in *The Pathophysiology of Myocardial Perfusion*, W Schaper (ed). Amsterdam, Elsevier North-Holland Biomedical Press, 1979, chap 15.

46 Sasayama S, Ross J, Franklin D, Bloor CM, Bishop S, Dilley RB: Adaptations of the left ventricle to chronic pressure overload. *Circ Res* 38: 172, 1976.

47 Folkman J, Merler E, Abernathy C, Williams G: Isolation of a tumor factor responsible for angiogenesis. *J Exper Med* 133: 275, 1971.

48 Cuttino JT Jr, Bartrum RJ Jr, Hollenberg NK, Abrams HL: Collateral vessel formation: Isolation of a transferable factor promoting a vascular response. *Basic Res Cardiol* 70: 568, 1975.

49 Schwarz F: Correlation between the degree of coronary artery obstruction and myocardial dysfunction, in *The Pathophysiology of Myocardial Perfusion*, W Schaper (ed). Amsterdam, Elsevier North-Holland Biomedical Press, 1979, chap 10.

50 Cohen MV, Yipintsoi T, Malhotra A, Penpargkul S, Scheuer J: Effect of exercise on collateral development in dogs with normal coronary arteries. *J Appl Physiol* 45: 797, 1978.

51 Sanders TM, White FC, Bloor CM: Effects of exercise on myocardial perfusion, in *The Pathophysiology of Myocardial Perfusion*, W Schaper (ed). Amsterdam, Elsevier North-Holland Biomedical Press, 1979, chap. 17.

51a Scheuer J: Effects of physical training on myocardial vascularity and perfusion. *Circulation* 66: 491, 1982.

52 Eckstein RW: Effect of exercise and coronary artery narrowing on coronary collateral circulation. *Circ Res* 5: 230, 1957.

53 Heaton WH, Marr KC, Capurio NL, Goldstein RE, Epstein SE: Beneficial effect of physical training on blood flow to myocardium perfused by chronic collaterals in the exercising dog. *Circulation* 57: 575, 1978.

54 Schaper W: Influence of physical exercise on coronary collateral blood flow in chronic experimental two-vessel occlusion. *Circulation* 65: 905, 1982.

55 Schaper W: Influence of physical exercise on myocardial perfusion, in *The Pathophysiology of Myocardial Perfusion*, W Schaper (ed). Amsterdam, Elsevier North-Holland Biomedical Press, 1979, chap 16.

56 Cohen MV, Yipintsoi T, Scheuer J: Exercise training stimulates coronary collateral development. *Circulation* 62: 232, 1980.

57 Neill WA, Oxendine JM: Exercise can promote coronary collateral development without improving perfusion of ischemic myocardium. *Circulation* 60: 1513, 1979.

57a Kaplinsky E, Hood WB Jr, McCathy B, McCombs L, Lown B: Effects of physical training in dogs with coronary artery ligation. *Circulation* 37: 556, 1968.

58 Schaper W: Effect of drugs on collateral circulation, in *The Pathophysiology of Myocardial Perfusion*, W Schaper (ed). Amsterdam, Elsevier North-Holland Biomedical Press, 1979.

59 Lambert PR, Hess DS, Bache RJ: Effect of exercise on perfusion of collateral-dependent myocardium in dogs with chronic coronary artery occlusion. *J Clin Invest* 59: 1, 1977.

59a Fedor JM, Rembert JC, McIntosh DM, Greenfield JC Jr: Effects of exercise- and pacing-induced tachycardia on coronary collateral flow in the awake dog. *Circ Res* 46: 214, 1980.

60 Pasyk S, Flamengo W, Wüsten B, Schaper W: Influence of tachycardia on regional myocardial flow in chronic experimental coronary occlusion. *Basic Res Cardiol* 71: 243, 1976.

61 Kumada T, Gallagher KP, Buttler A, White F, Kemper WS, Ross J: Comparison of post-pacing and exercise induced myocardial dysfunction during collateral development in conscious dogs. *Circulation* 65: 1178, 1982.

62 Schaper W, Lewi P, Flemeng W, Gijpen L: Myocardial steal produced by coronary vasodilation in chronic coronary artery occlusion. *Basic Res Cardiol* 68: 3, 1973.

62a Fedor JM, Brazzamano S, Rembert JC, Greenfield JC Jr: Coronary collateral vascular conductance in awake dogs. *Fed Proc* 41: 1530, 1982.

63 Helfant RH, Pantel SV, Gorlin R: Functional importance of the human coronary collateral circulation. *New Eng J Med* 284: 1277, 1971.

64 Helfant RH, Kemp HG, Gorlin R: Coronary atherosclerosis, coronary collaterals, and their relation to cardiac function. *Ann Int Med* 73: 189, 1970.

65 Bodenheimer MM, Banka VS, Hermann GA, Trout RG, Pasdar H, Helfant RH: The effect of severity of coronary artery obstructive disease and the coronary collateral circulation on local histopathologic and electrographic observations in man. *Am J Med* 63: 93, 1977.

66 Carrol RJ, Verani MS, Falsetti HL: The effect of collateral circulation on segmental left ventricular contraction. *Circulation* 50: 709, 1974.

67 Lavine P, Filip Z, Hajmi M, Kimbiris D, Segal BL, Linhart JW: Clinical and hemodynamic evaluation of coronary collateral vessels in coronary artery disease. *Am Heart J* 87: 343, 1974.

68 Helfant R: The coronary collateral circulation. *Ann Int Med* 77: 995, 1972.

69 Gorlin R: Coronary collaterals, in *Coronary Artery Disease.* Philadelphia, Saunders, 1976, chap 4.

70 DeWood MA, Spores J, Notske R, et al: Prevalence of total coronary occlusion during the early hours of transmural myocardial infarction. *N Eng J Med* 303: 897, 1980.

71 Phillips J, Kongtahworn C, Zeff R, Benson M, Iannone L, Brown T, Gordon DF: Emergency coronary artery revascularization: A possible therapy for acute myocardial infarction. *Circulation* 60: 241, 1979.

71a Gregg DE, Patterson RE: Functional importance of the coronary collaterals. *New Eng J Med* 303: 1404, 1980.

72 Goldstein RE, Stinson EB, Scherer JL, Seningen RP, Grehl TM, Epstein SE: Intraoperative coronary collateral function in patients with coronary occlusive disease: Nitroglygerin responsiveness and angiographic correlation. *Circulation* 49: 298, 1974.

73 Goldstein RE, Michaelis LL, Morrow AG, Epstein E: Coronary collateral function in patients without occlusive coronary artery disease. *Circulation* 51: 118, 1975.

74 Parker FB, Jr, Neville JF Jr, Hanson EL, Webb WR: Retrograde and antegrade pressures and flows in preinfarction syndrome. *Circulation* (suppl 2) 49 & 50: 122, 1974.

75 Smith SC, Gorlin R, Herman MV, Taylor WJ, Collins JJ Jr: Myocardial blood flow in man: Effects of coronary collateral circulation and coronary artery bypass surgery. *J Clin Invest* 51: 2556, 1972.

76 Cannon PJ, Weiss MB, Casarella WJ: Studies of regional myocardial blood flow: Results in patients with left anterior descending coronary artery disease. *Semin Nucl Med* 6: 279, 1976.

77 Arani DT, Greene DG, Bunnell IL, Smith G, Klocke FJ: Simultaneous quantitation of collateral flow and adjacent left ventricular flow in patients with left anterior descending occlusion. *Circulation* 64(suppl 4): 117, 1981.

78 Frye R, Gurah GM, Chesebro JH, Ritman EL: Complete occlusion of the left main coronary artery and the importance of coronary collateral circulation. *Mayo Clinic Proc* 52: 742, 1977.

79 Schwarz F, Flameng W, Ensslen R, Sesto M, Thormann J: Effect of collaterals on left ventricular function at rest and during stress. *Am Heart J* 95: 570, 1978.

80 Levin DC: Pathways and functional significance of the coronary collateral circulation. *Circulation* 50: 831, 1974.

81 Rigo P, Becker LC, Griffith LSC, Alderson PO, Bailey IK, Pitt B, Burow RD, Wagner HN Jr: Influence of coronary collateral vessels on the results of thallium^{201} myocardial stress imaging. *Am J Cardiol* 44: 452, 1979.

82 Eng C, Patterson RE, Horowitz SF, Halgash DA, Pichard AD, Midwall J, Herman MV, Gorlin R: Coronary collateral function during exercise. *Circulation* 66: 309, 1982.

83 Kolibash AJ, Bush CA, Wepsic RA, Schroeder DP, Tetalman MR, Lewis RP: Coronary collateral vessels: Spectrum of physiologic capabilities with respect to providing rest and stress myocardial perfusion, maintainance of left ventricular function and protection against infarction. *Am J Cardiol* 50: 230, 1982.

84 Ferguson RJ, Cote P, Gauthier P, Bourassa MG: Changes in exercise coronary sinus blood flow with training in patients with angina pectoris. *Circulation* 58: 41, 1978.

85 Nolewajka AJ, Kostuk WJ, Rechnitzer PA, Cunningham DA: Exercise and human collaterization: An angiographic and scintigraphic assessment. *Circulation* 60: 114, 1979.

86 Sim DN, Neill WA: Investigation of the physiological basis for increased exercise threshold for angina pectoris after physical conditioning. *J Clin Invest* 54: 763, 1974.

87 Kennedy CC, Spiekerman RE, Lindsay MI Jr, Mankin HT, Frye RL, McCallister BD: One-year graduated exercise program for men with angina pectoris. Evaluation by physiologic studies and coronary arteriography. *Mayo Clin Proc* 51: 231, 1976.

88 Ferguson RJ, Petitclerc R, Choquette G, Chaniotis L, Gauthier P, Huot R, Allard C, Jankowski L, Campeau L: Effect of physical training on treadmill exercise capacity, collateral circulation and progression of coronary disease. *Am J Cardiol* 34:764, 1974.

89 Barmeyer J: Physical activity and coronary collateral development. *Adv Cardiol* 18: 104, 1976.

90 Verani MS, Hartung GH, Hoepfel-Harris J, Welton DE, Pratt CM, Miller RR: Effects of exercise training on left ventricular performance and myocardial perfusion in patients with coronary artery disease. *Am J Cardiol* 47: 797, 1981.

91 Froelicher V, Jensen D, Atwood JE, McKirnan MD, Gerber K, Slutsky R, Battler A, Ashburn W, Ross J Jr: Cardiac rehabilitation: Evidence for improvement in myocardial perfusion and function. *Arch Phys Med Rehabil* 61: 517, 1980.

CHAPTER **11**

PHYSIOLOGICAL EFFECTS OF A CORONARY STENOSIS

Atherosclerosis, the most important of the diseases that affect the coronary circulation, manifests itself primarily by producing vascular obstruction. As the atherosclerotic plaque enlarges within the vessel wall, the vascular lumen is progressively compromised. Atherosclerotic obstructions are most prominent in proximal segments of epicardial coronary vessels and at the point of major bifurcations [1,2]. Angiographically, atherosclerotic lesions in patients appear to be segmental–frequently confined to a short segment of a proximal coronary vessel. Isolated obstructive disease in secondary branches is very uncommon [3]. In patients, the most common pathological finding is diffuse vessel involvement with superimposed segmental obstruction of greater severity [4].

The clinical manifestations of coronary heart disease (angina, myocardial dysfunction, arrhythmias, acute myocardial infarction, sudden death) depend in large part on the severity and distribution of the obstructive coronary lesions. Consequently, a major effort has been put forth to define the factors that determine the physiological significance of coronary stenosis in animal models and in patients.

FACTORS THAT DETERMINE THE PHYSIOLOGICAL SIGNIFICANCE OF A CORONARY STENOSIS

Carefully designed and executed studies in animals provide a remarkably precise quantitative description of the factors that determine the physiological significance of a coronary stenosis. The major determinants are discussed in detail below.

Percent Narrowing and Absolute Lesion Diameter

Many years ago, studies by Shipley and Gregg [5] predicted that resting coronary flow would not decline unless a large decrease in luminal area of a coronary artery occurred. Later studies by Khouri et al [6] demonstrated that progressive coronary obstruction diminished coronary reserve in a systematic manner. More recently, detailed studies by many investigators have precisely defined the effects of progressive stenosis on resting and maximal flow in the coronary vessels of animals (Figure 11-1) [7–20]. It has been generally concluded that in normal dogs, maximal coronary flow begins to decline when percent diameter stenosis in a short coronary segment is greater than 45 percent. Resting flow is unaffected until percent diameter stenosis exceeds 80 to 90 percent. Unfortunately, cardiologists and cardiac surgeons have extended this data to clinical situations. Thus, it is often said that the physiological severity of a coronary lesion can be predicted by measuring percent diameter stenosis of a coronary lesion defined by a single angiographic projection. When this is done, two assumptions are accepted: (1) the lesion is symmetrical, and (2) the vascular segment immediately proximal and distal to the stenotic segment is normal. *In patients, both assumptions are often invalid* (Figures 11-2 and 11-3) [4,21–23]. Furthermore, the variability of disease in the proximal and distal segments and unpredictable lesion geometry contribute greatly to the poor correlation between percent diameter stenosis and the physiological significance of a given obstruction in patients [24].

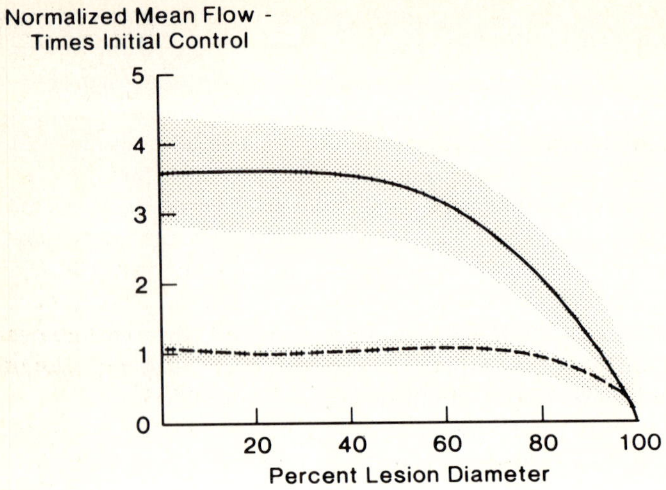

FIGURE 11-1 Relationship between resting (*dashed line*) and maximal coronary blood flow (*solid line*) and percent diameter stenosis in a dog. Progressive coronary stenosis was achieved by progressively narrowing a short segment of a proximal coronary artery. Resting coronary blood flow did not change until coronary diameter stenosis exceeded 90 percent. Maximal coronary blood flow began to decrease when percent diameter stenosis exceeded 50 percent. *(Modified from an illustration originally presented by KL Gould et al* [8].*)*

Length (Stenoses in Series)

At intermediate levels of coronary obstruction (less than 90 percent decrease in vessel diameter), the length of the narrowed segment has a moderate effect on the physiologic significance of the obstruction [9,13,16]. This is most dramatic when very short obstructions are compared to long ones (see Figure 11-4*a* and *b*). The length of the coronary obstruction is often given little consideration by physicians who interpret coronary arteriograms.

Multiple discrete obstructions in a single vessel occur frequently in patients with coronary disease. Several investigators have shown that the adverse effects of these serial lesions on maximal coronary flow cannot be predicted by "simple addition" (Figure 11-5) [8,16]. In the clinical setting the importance of these serial lesions is exceedingly difficult to assess.

Entrance and Exit Effects

In a narrowed vascular segment, blood velocity (kinetic energy) increases and pressure (static energy) decreases in accordance with the Bernoulli principle. If the entrance and exit from the narrowed segment were very gradual, the conversion of static and dynamic energy components would occur without major net energy loss. However, in the coronary circulation, the entrance and exit angles associated with obstructive lesions are relatively abrupt. Hence, when the fluid column enters the narrowed segment or emerges from it, substantial energy losses occur. The most important site of energy loss is at the exit of a stenosis. At this point, separation of the fluid column occurs. This creates vortices or turbulence at the boundaries of the fluid column which in turn are associated with striking energy losses (Figure

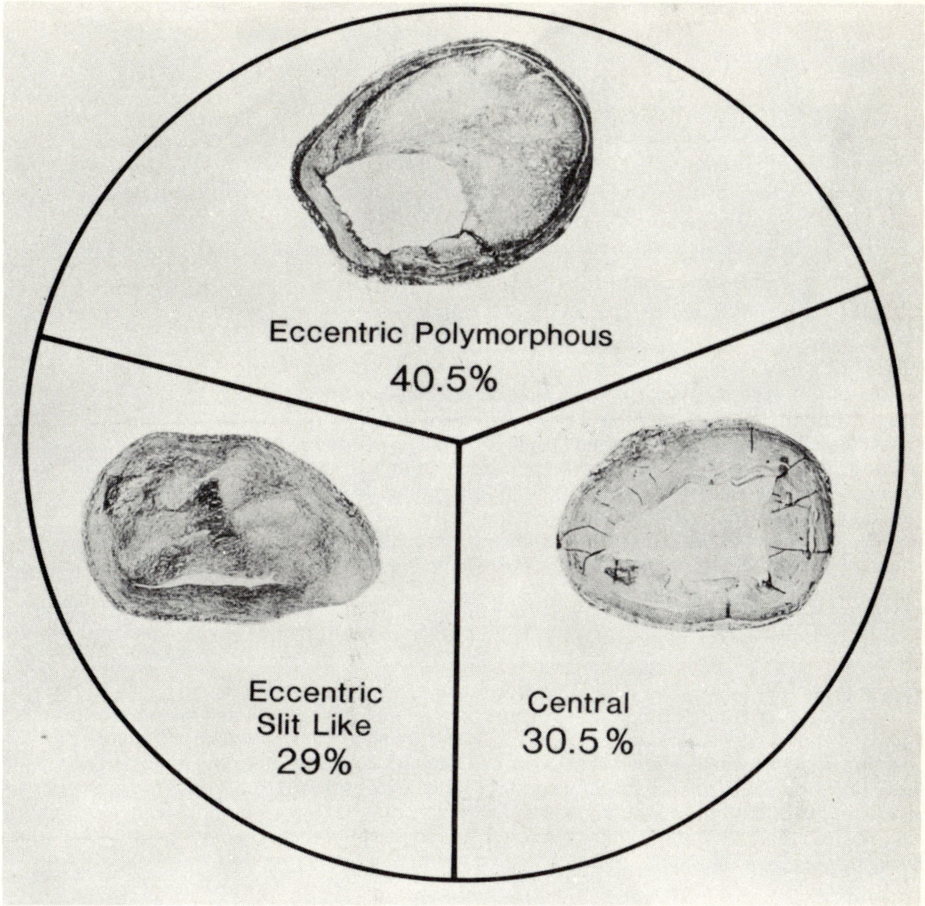

FIGURE 11-2
Frequency of various shapes of coronary obstructive lesions encountered in patients with atherosclerotic cardiovascular disease. The lesion shapes were classified into three general categories—eccentric polymorphous, eccentric slitlike, and central—by analyzing histological sections of undistended coronary vessels. The majority of coronary obstructive lesions encountered were either eccentric polymorphous or eccentric slitlike. The histological sections in each segment of the pie diagram are representative of the shape classification. The percent age values in the pie diagram indicate the frequency with which these various shapes were encountered in a large series of coronary arteries examined. Because most coronary lesions have complex geometry, it is unlikely that the cross-sectional area of these obstructions could be predicted from a single projection of a coronary arteriogram. (*Based on data presented originally by Z Vlodaver and JE Edwards* [23].)

11-6) [10,25–27]. The separation losses are particularly exaggerated when blood flow velocity is increased. This is so because classic fluid dynamic theory suggests that frictional losses across a stenotic segment increase as a function of blood flow velocity, whereas separation losses increase as a function of the blood flow velocity squared (see Figure 11-6).

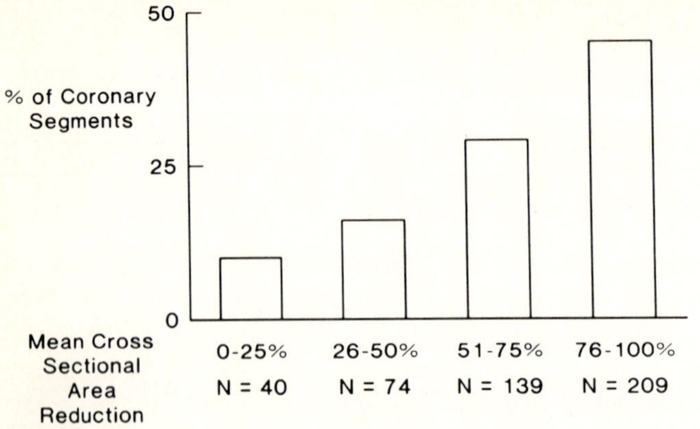

FIGURE 11-3
Percent of coronary segments with various degrees of reduction in their mean cross-sectional area. These data were obtained by analyzing serial histological sections (1-mm intervals) obtained from undistended coronary arteries which contained at least one severely obstructive lesion. Only 40 of the 462 segments examined had less than 25 percent reduction in their cross-sectional area. The data strongly suggest that coronary atherosclerosis in humans is a diffuse disease which involves the entire coronary vessel. (*Based on data originally presented by EN Arnett et al* [4].)

FIGURE 11-4
Effects of the length of a coronary obstruction on the relationship between the percent stenosis and percent of maximal coronary blood flow. Progressive coronary obstruction was produced in dogs and maximal coronary blood flow was achieved by inducing a maximal coronary reactive hyperemic response. (*a*) Short and (*b*) long occluders were utilized. These data indicate that the length of the coronary obstructive lesion contributes to the hemodynamic significance of the obstruction, particularly when percent stenosis is in the immediate range (20–60 percent stenosis). (*Redrawn from data originally presented by GC Freisinger and WS Hillis* [13].)

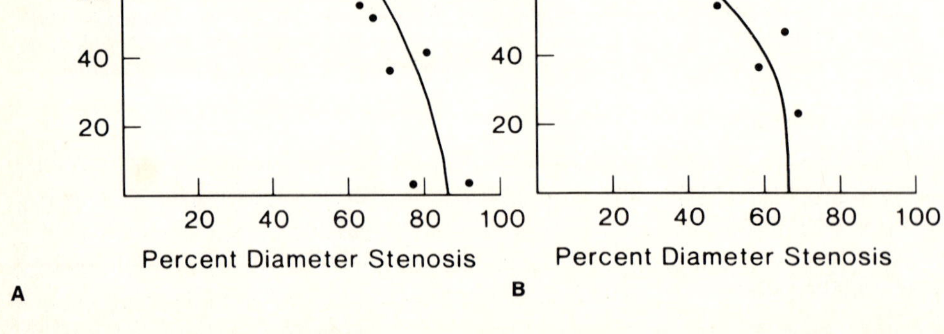

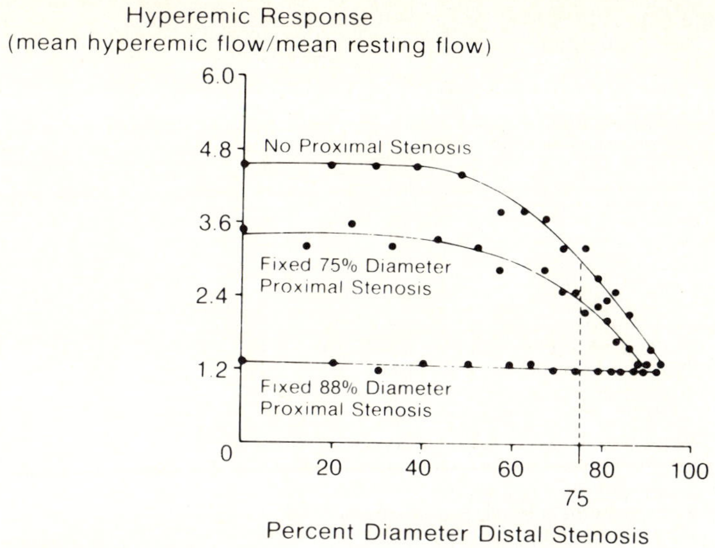

FIGURE 11-5
Effects of stenoses in series on maximal coronary blood flow (hyperemic response). No proximal stenosis means only the effects of a distal stenosis of varying severity are shown. Fixed 75 percent diameter proximal stenosis means studies depict the effects of a fixed 75 percent diameter proximal stenosis plus a distal stenosis of variable severity. Fixed 88 percent diameter proximal stenosis means studies depict the effects of a fixed 88 percent diameter proximal stenosis plus a distal stenosis of variable severity. Note that a distal stenosis did not increase the severity of a proximal 75 percent stenosis until the distal stenosis decreased vessel diameter about 60 percent. These studies emphasize that serial obstructions have a complex effect on the physiological significance of coronary obstructive lesions. (*Based on data originally presented by KL Gould et al* [7].)

Blood Flow Velocity

Blood flow velocity and stenosis pressure gradient are related in an exponential fashion (Figure 11-7) [10,18,26]. Thus, the resistance across a stenotic segment is critically dependent on blood flow velocity. As a consequence, hemodynamic perturbations which increase diastolic coronary blood flow velocity are frequently associated with clinical manifestations of myocardial ischemia in patients with coronary stenosis.

Inertia and Friction

Because the pressure gradient across a stenosis can be predicted with reasonable accuracy if inertial factors are disregarded [10], this factor is probably of little importance to the physiological significance of a coronary obstruction. Energy losses across a stenosis do depend in part on frictional losses in the stenotic segment [10,18,26]. Such losses can be predicted by the Poiseuille relationship:

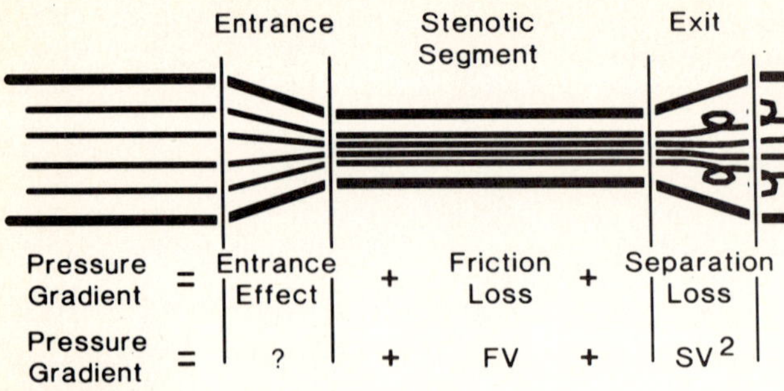

FIGURE 11-6
Sources of energy loss across a stenosis. The three segments of the stenosis which contribute to the pressure gradient across the lesion are entrance effects, friction losses in the stenotic segment, and separation losses at the exit of the stenosis. Equations that have been developed to predict pressure gradients across a stenosis ignore entrance effects, multiply friction losses by blood flow velocity, and multiply separation losses by blood flow velocity squared. The formulation indicates that separation losses become progressively more important as blood velocity increases. V = blood velocity; F = friction loss (1° depends on Poiseuille relationship; S = separation losses (° depends on exit geometry).

The relative contribution of friction losses across a stenotic segment varies with blood flow velocity (see Figure 11-6) [10,18,26].

Formulations for Predicting the Physiological Significance of a Stenosis

Young et al. [26] have developed a formula which accurately predicts the gradient across a stenosis with carefully defined geometry (see Figure 11-8). Gould has indicated that this general formulation requires an additional term to account for changes in stenosis geometry that occur in the presence of coronary dilation [10,11]. These mathematical expressions, which have been validated in vivo, demonstrate that the relative contribution of various factors that determine the stenosis gradient are well understood. The problem at hand is to apply this basic knowledge in the clinical arena.

Although the formula described by Young et al. [26] is complex, in essence there are two and potentially three factors that determine the pressure gradient across a stenosis: entrance effects, drag effects (frictional losses), and separation of the fluid column at the exit of the obstruction. The drag effects are dependent on the parameters included in the Poiseuille equation. The separation of the fluid column depends on geometric factors.

DYNAMIC NATURE OF A CORONARY STENOSIS

For many years it has been assumed that the diameter of a stenotic coronary segment was fixed. Studies by Gould [10,11], Schwartz et al. [19], Santamore [20]

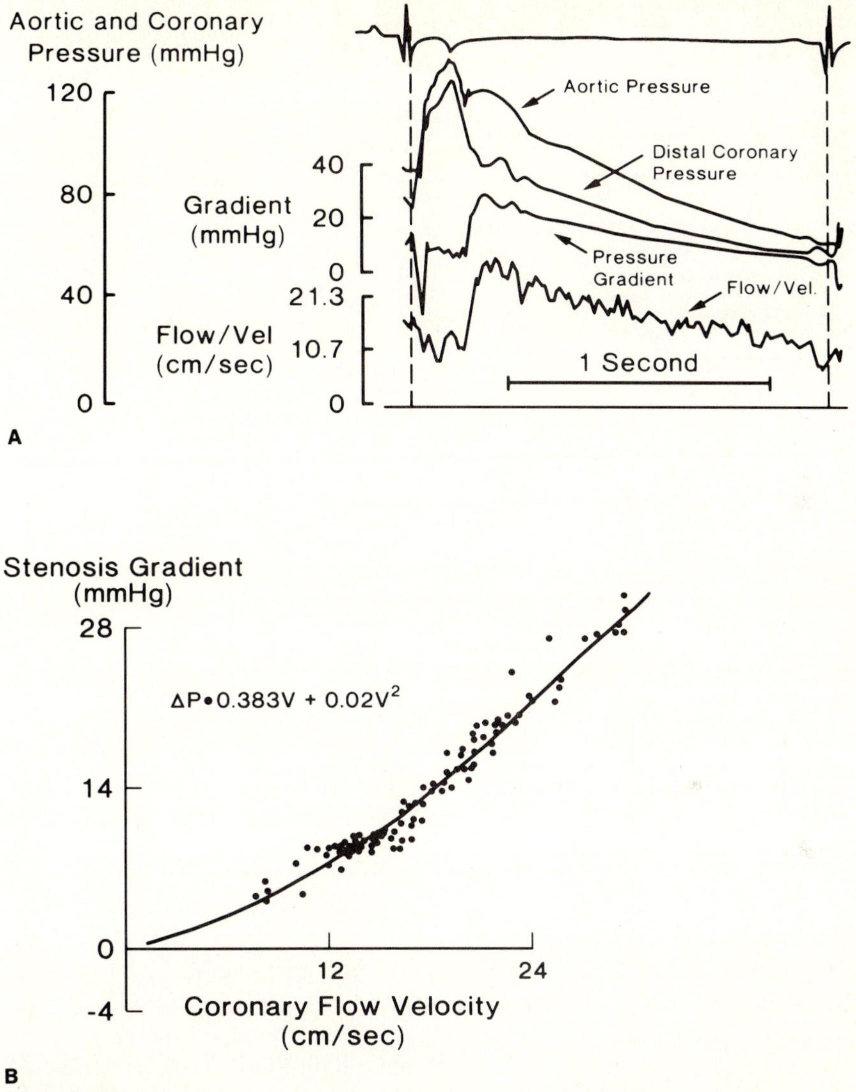

FIGURE 11-7
(*a*) Phasic aortic pressure, distal coronary pressure beyond a coronary obstruction, the gradient between aortic pressure and distal coronary pressure, and coronary blood flow velocity measured simultaneously in a dog. Data from one cardiac cycle are illustrated. Note that the magnitude of the gradient between aortic pressure and distal coronary pressure is directly related to coronary blood flow velocity. (*b*) Stenosis gradient is plotted as a function of coronary blood flow velocity. The data plotted are based upon pressure gradient and coronary blood flow velocity data illustrated in (*a*). The pressure gradient across the stenosis can be predicted by the equation which multiplies the friction loss term (0.383) times blood flow velocity and the separation loss term (0.02) times the velocity squared. (*Modified from data originally presented by KL Gould* [*10*].)

$$\Delta p = \frac{K_v \mu}{D} U + \frac{K_t}{2}\left(\frac{A_0}{A_1} - 1\right)^2 \rho |U| U + K_\mu \rho L \frac{dU}{dt}$$

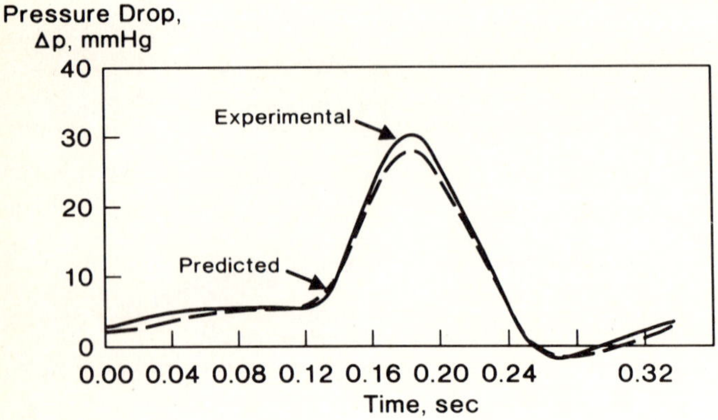

FIGURE 11-8
Pressure gradient across a femoral arterial stenosis in a dog during a cardiac cycle. The solid line is the measured gradient and the dashed line is the predicted gradient. The predicted gradient was derived from the formula shown above. The close relationship between the experimentally measured and predicted pressure gradient suggests that the formula employed to predict the pressure gradient is valid. p = pressure gradient; D = diameter of the unobstructed vessel; A_0 = area of the unobstructed vessel; A_1 = minimum area of the stenosis; K_ν, K_t, K_μ = experimentally determined coefficients; U = instantaneous velocity in the unobstructed vessel; L = length over which the pressure drop is measured; ρ = fluid density. (*Based on data originally presented by DF Young et al* [26].)

and Brown et al. [20a] suggest that this concept is incorrect. Various types of experimentally produced and clinically encountered stenoses demonstrate dynamic behavior in response to various interventions. Schwartz et al. [19] and Santamore [20] have postulated that decreases in distending pressure foster collapse of the stenotic segment and consequently stenosis resistance is considerably increased. Direct angiographic measurements of the stenotic coronary segment during coronary dilation do not support this hypothesis [20a,20b]. Gould [10,11,20b] and Brown et al. [20a] have shown convincing data which indicate that the normal vascular segments distal to a stenotic segment dilate with increases in flow and administration of nitrates. In addition, in many stenotic vascular segments, a portion of the vascular wall is uninvolved by the atheroma. If this relatively normal segment of the wall were responsive to vasomotor stimuli, this might give the illusion on an angiogram that the diseased portion of the vessel was responsive to dilator or constrictor stimuli. Thus, several mechanisms could contribute to alterations in stenosis geometry which in turn could change the physiological significance of a coronary obstruction.

Coronary obstructions produced by atherosclerosis are not fixed. The narrowed segment dilates in response to nitroglycerin [20a,28]. In susceptible patients, stenotic segments can constrict intensely following infusion of ergonovine [29].

Thus, both experimental and clinical coronary stenoses are responsive to vasomotor stimuli and to physical forces such as intravascular distending pressure. Although the magnitude of these changes in stenosis dimensions have not been precisely defined under many conditions, it is likely that dynamic alterations in the geometry of coronary stenotic segments contribute to the clinical manifestations of ischemic heart disease.

CLINICAL APPROACHES TO DETERMINING STENOSIS SEVERITY

In the animal laboratory, a coronary stenosis can be characterized precisely by simultaneous measurements of flow and stenosis gradient throughout the cardiac cycle coupled with a quantitative angiographic evaluation of stenosis geometry. In patients, these techniques cannot be applied on a routine basis. Consequently, clinicians have used a variety of indirect approaches to assess the severity of coronary stenoses in patients with coronary obstruction.

Clinical Symptoms

For years, clinicians believed that physiologically significant coronary obstructions were associated with the classic symptom of ischemic heart disease—angina pectoris. Although many patients with significant coronary obstructions have various anginal syndromes, it is now generally held that there is only a weak correlation between the severity of coronary obstructive disease and the severity of angina pectoris [30]. Furthermore, 25 percent of patients who die from severe coronary disease have never experienced any chest discomfort prior to the day of their demise [31]. At least 10 percent of patients with a classic history of exertional angina have no evidence of coronary obstructive disease [32]. Thus, angina pectoris is not a sensitive or specific indicator of physiologically significant coronary obstructive disease.

Graded Exercise Electrocardiography

Arthur Master was one of the early investigators to note that the ST segment depression on the electrocardiogram during exercise frequently occurred in patients with significant coronary heart disease [33]. Unfortunately, many confounding factors (drugs, prior infarction, cardiac hypertrophy, conduction disturbances, etc.) interfere with the use of exercise-induced ST segment depression to assess the functional significance of coronary obstructions [34]. The sensitivity and specificity of ST segment depression as an indicator of coronary heart disease is limited [34]. In addition, ST segment depression does not localize the obstructed vascular segment.

Perfusion Scintigrams

During coronary dilation induced by treadmill exercise [35–37] or intravenous dipyridamole [38], the concentration of thallium 201 is diminished in myocardial segments perfused by coronary vessels with significant obstructive lesions. In addition, the subsequent clearance of thallium 201 from the myocardium is delayed in myocardial segments served by severely obstructive vessels [39]. Thallium 201 perfusion scintigrams are more sensitive and specific for detecting coronary artery disease than electrocardiograms obtained during graded-treadmill exercise tests [39]. With perfusion scintigrams the location of perfusion defects can be used to predict the coronary vessel that is obstructed.

Thallium 201 perfusion scintigrams have several limitations, however, in defining the functional significance of individual coronary obstructions: (1) sensitivity of the technique is limited by inherent problems associated with the use of a low-energy gamma camera [40]; (2) certain regions of the myocardium which are far removed from the camera, such as the posterior wall of the left ventricle, are difficult to evaluate [39]; (3) because relative rather than absolute differences in thallium 201 concentration are measured, the perfusion scintigram can be normal if severe obstruction is present in all coronary vessels [35–39]; (4) thallium 201 scintigrams in a significant number of patients with multivessel obstructions demonstrate only one perfusion defect [35–39]; and (5) myocardial fibrosis due to any cause will markedly decrease thallium 201 accumulation [39]. In spite of these limitations, a segmental thallium 201 perfusion defect usually implies that the affected myocardium is either infarcted or perfused by a coronary vessel with a hemodynamically significant obstruction.

Other types of perfusion scintigrams which employ positron-emitting radionuclides and tomographic images may eventually provide a precise method of determining the physiological significance of coronary obstructions in patients [41].

Ventricular Wall Motion Studies during Rest and Exercise

Various methods of assessing segmental left ventricular wall motion during rest and exercise (contrast ventriculograms, radionuclide ventriculograms, and echocardiograms) have been used to determine the functional significance of coronary obstructions [42]. Patients who have normal left ventricular function at rest and develop significant segmental wall motion abnormalities during stress usually have coronary disease [43]. Unfortunately, the sensitivity of these techniques in patients with single vessel disease [44] is limited. In patients with multivessel coronary disease, exercise is often associated with only one segmental wall motion abnormality. This occurs because angina, which develops during the exercise procedure, limits the intensity of exertion, and hence only the most significant coronary obstruction is associated with a wall motion abnormality. Furthermore, in most cardiac imaging laboratories, exercise wall motion studies are only obtained in one projection. Nonetheless, under carefully defined conditions it may be possible to determine the physiological significance of coronary obstructions by studying segmental ventricular wall motion during stress.

Coronary Arteriography

The coronary arteriogram is the "gold standard" to which all other methods designed to assess the physiological significance of coronary stenoses in humans are compared. Recent studies suggest that this gold standard has many deficiencies. Many studies have confirmed that marked inter- and intraobserver variability exists in the interpretation of the coronary arteriogram [45–48]. Zir et al. [48] reported that four experienced angiographers agreed about the significance of a proximal or midleft anterior descending lesion in only 13 of 20 angiograms. When compared to pathological studies, even "majority opinion angiography" has shown that an incorrect interpretation is likely to be accepted half of the time [4,45]. Although disagreement is greater when analyzing distal segments, 35 to 40 percent error rates occur when analyzing proximal or midleft anterior descending lesions [46]. Detre et al. [47] reported intraobserver agreement among 22 experienced angiographers on two ciné viewings to range from 9 to 72 percent.

Other factors also interfere with accurate determination of coronary obstructive lesions. Overlapping vessels can introduce substantial error unless multiple angulated views are taken [49]. The amount of collateral flow to an obstructed segment may influence the estimation of distal vessel caliber [50]. Uniform diffuse narrowing may produce underestimation of luminal obstruction [4,51]. Spontaneous or catheter-induced coronary spasm may exaggerate abnormalities by causing greater coronary dilation of the normal than the obstructed vascular segments [52]. Lesion eccentricity and asymmetry also contribute to the difficulties associated with the interpretation of coronary arteriograms. Several studies [4,21–23] have examined the eccentricity of coronary luminal obstructions in patients. Although these studies did not examine the shape of coronary lesions distended by normal intraluminal pressures, the data do suggest that asymmetrical eccentric lesions are not rare. The luminal area of an asymmetric lesion cannot be accurately estimated unless multiple views at widely different angles are analyzed quantitatively. In clinical practice this is rarely done. Hence, estimates of the severity of luminal obstruction are only rough approximations.

At present, the coronary arteriogram is the only diagnostic approach which allows one to determine precisely the location of coronary obstructions in all major coronary vessels. *Unfortunately, the coronary arteriogram cannot accurately assess the physiological significance of coronary obstructions of intermediate severity (10 to 90 percent diameter narrowing)* [24].

Measurements of Stenosis Pressure Gradient

Pressure distal to a coronary stenosis can be measured by passing a very small arterial catheter beyond the coronary obstruction [53], thereby measuring the gradient across the lesion. As noted above, the pressure gradient across an obstruction is proportional to the physiological significance of the coronary lesion. There are several reasons why measurements of the stenosis pressure gradient in patients are of dubious value: (1) the superimposed obstruction due to the trans-stenosis catheter is a major confounding variable; (2) the pressure gradient is dependent upon the velocity of flow in the vessel [10,18,26]; and (3) there is undoubtedly a risk associated with such a catheterization procedure. Stenosis pressure gradients are routinely measured during coronary angioplasty procedures [53]. In this instance, however, the small risk associated with measuring the stenosis gradient is overshadowed by the potential benefit associated with the dilation of the obstructing lesion.

None of the clinical approaches cited above allows one to define precisely the physiological significance of the coronary obstructive lesion preoperatively. Methods that will allow quantitative assessment of the physiological significance of coronary obstructions in humans are needed.

PHYSIOLOGICAL ASSESSMENT OF THE SEVERITY OF A CORONARY STENOSIS AT THE TIME OF CARDIAC SURGERY

Since 1979, my colleagues and I have obtained coronary reactive hyperemic responses in individual coronary vessels at cardiac surgery in an effort to assess the physiological significance of coronary obstructive lesions [24,54–57]. These studies are based on the premise that obstructive lesions that are physiologically significant should decrease vasodilator reserve [5–20]. Our measurements of coronary reactive hyperemia were obtained at surgery prior to cardiopulmonary bypass.

In our studies, phasic coronary blood flow velocity was measured with a single-crystal, pulsed Doppler probe (see Figure 2-3). The ultrasonic crystal was placed in a small (3 to 4 mm diameter) silastic cup which is coupled to the epicardial coronary vessel being studied by applying a few millimeters of negative pressure to the cup. Thus, no coronary dissection is required.

Animal studies have shown that changes in coronary blood flow velocity measured with the Doppler probe are closely related to changes in coronary flow under a wide variety of conditions [55]. A 20-s coronary occlusion produces intense myocardial ischemia. When the coronary occlusion is released, normal perfusion pressure is restored and flow increases markedly (see Chapter 3). The quantitative characteristics of the reactive hyperemic response can be used to characterize the intensity of the vasodilation (Figure 3-15). Thus, studies in patients with normal coronary vessels perfusing a normal ventricle have defined the range of coronary dilator responses observed in normal humans (Figure 3-15) [55].

Comparisons of Coronary Reactive Hyperemic Responses and Conventional Coronary Angiography

We have compared maximal coronary reactive hyperemic responses to the angiographic appearance of coronary stenoses in a large series of patients [24,54–57]. To illustrate our results, three representative cases will be discussed and then group data will be presented.

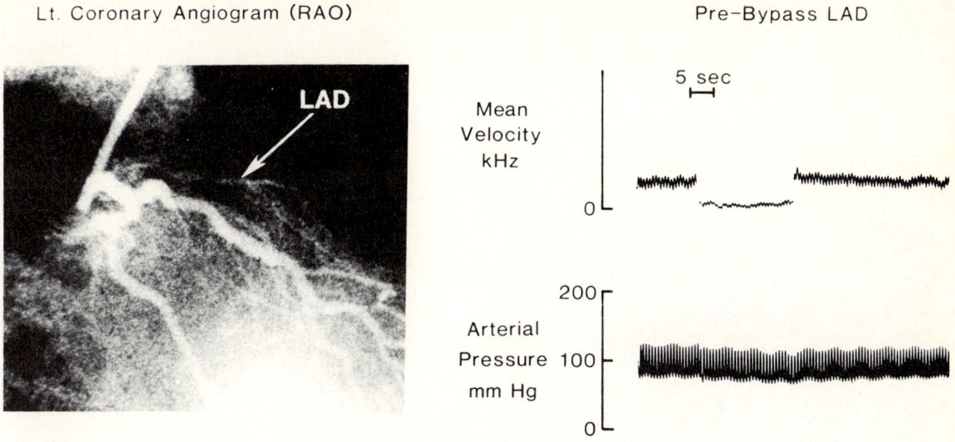

FIGURE 11-9
Relationship between angiographic anatomy and physiological function. The coronary arteriogram shown on the left demonstrates that the left anterior descending coronary artery is severely obstructed. The right side of this figure shows a recording of mean coronary artery blood flow velocity in the left anterior descending coronary artery, obtained in the operating room prior to cardiopulmonary bypass. The coronary reactive hyperemic response was severely blunted. This suggests that the vasodilator reserve of the left anterior descending coronary artery was minimal. During the coronary reactive hyperemic response, arterial pressure remained stable. In this example, the anatomic and physiological data are concordant; i.e., severe angiographic obstruction was associated with striking physiological abnormality. *(From C Wright et al [56].)*

Case 1 Figure 11-9 illustrates our observations in the patient with almost total obstruction of the left anterior descending coronary artery. Following a 20-s coronary occlusion of this vessel there was essentially no reactive hyperemic response. Thus, in this instance, severe proximal obstruction markedly limited the dilator response of the obstructed vascular segment.

Case 2 In this case we assessed the vasodilator capacity of a vessel that appeared to have minimal evidence of obstruction by angiography (Figure 11-11). Following a 20-s coronary occlusion of the left anterior descending coronary artery, the reactive hyperemic response was markedly impaired (peak-to-resting velocity ratio = 1.5; repayment/debt ratio = 0.2). This suggests that a so-called insignificant obstruction detected by coronary angiography can produce a severe hemodynamic impairment. Following the placement of the vein-bypass graft in the left anterior descending coronary artery distal to the point of apparent obstruction, the vasodilator capacity of the left anterior descending coronary artery was restored toward normal, as evidenced by an improved reactive hyperemic response in the immediate postoperative period.

Case 3 Figure 11-10 illustrates our results in a patient with an obstruction in the left anterior descending coronary artery. The obstruction was thought to be physiologically significant by the coronary angiographer who performed the car-

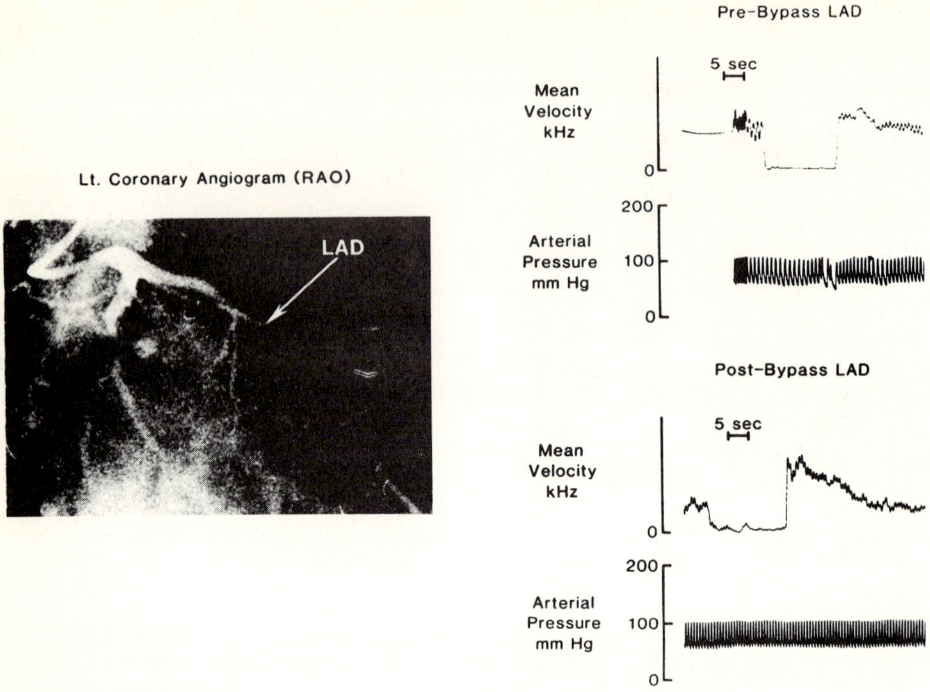

FIGURE 11-10
Relationship between angiographic anatomy and physiological function. (*Left*) Coronary arteriogram showing severe obstruction in the proximal circumflex artery and only questionable obstruction of the left anterior descending coronary artery. (*Right*) A recording of mean coronary blood flow velocity in the left anterior descending coronary artery before, during, and following release of a 20-s coronary occlusion. The coronary reactive hyperemic response is severely blunted. This suggests that the vasodilator reserve of the left anterior descending coronary artery was severely compromised. The left anterior descending coronary artery was bypassed. Postbypass recordings of mean coronary blood flow velocity in the left anterior descending coronary artery distal to the point of graft insertion indicated that, following occlusion of the proximal left anterior descending and the graft for 20 s, the reactive hyperemic response was much improved compared to the preoperative study. The data suggest that a significant proximal obstruction in the left anterior descending coronary artery was effectively bypassed. During the coronary reactive hyperemic studies, arterial pressure and heart rate were stable. In this example, the anatomic and physiological data are discordant; i.e., an apparent minimal angiographic abnormality in the left anterior descending artery was associated with a severe physiological abnormality. (*From C Wright et al* [*56*].)

diac catheterization. Following a 20-s coronary occlusion, the reactive hyperemic response in this vessel was normal (peak-to-resting velocity ratio = 7.1; repayment/debt ratio = 3.9). In this instance, an apparently significant coronary obstruction was associated with no impairment in coronary vasodilator reserve.

The last two cases are presented to emphasize the difficulties involved in judging the physiological significance of many coronary obstructions by visual analysis of the coronary arteriogram.

Many investigators working with experimental animals and model systems

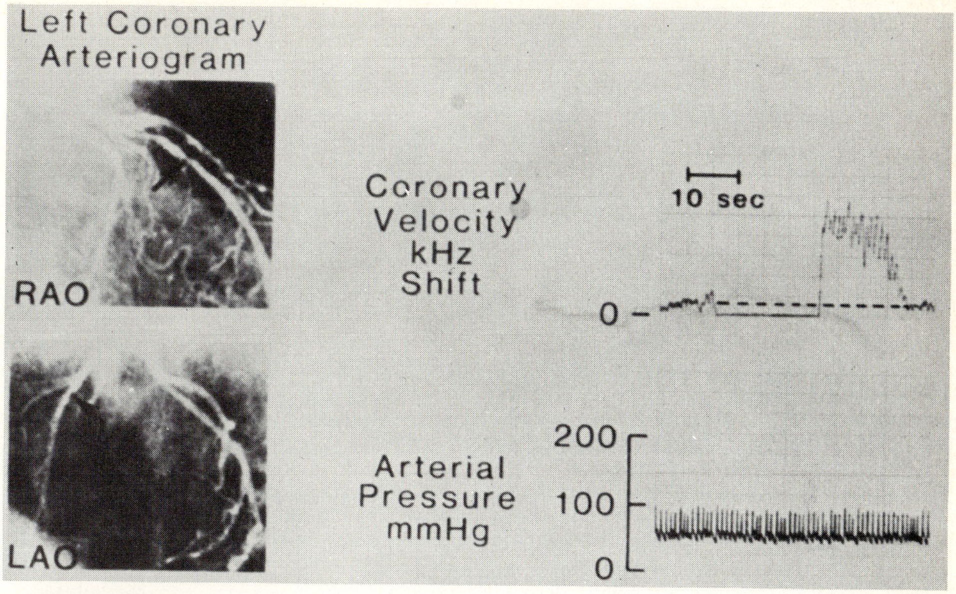

FIGURE 11-11
Relationship between angiographic anatomy and physiological function. The coronary arteriograms demonstrate what appears to be a significant obstruction of the proximal left anterior descending coronary artery in both the right and left anterial oblique projections. (Right) A recording of mean coronary blood flow velocity in the obstructed left anterior descending coronary artery before, during, and following release of a 20-s coronary occlusion. The coronary reactive hyperemic response in the left anterior descending coronary artery was normal. This suggests that the vasodilator reserve of this vessel was normal. During the coronary reactive hyperemic response, arterial pressure remained stable. In this example, the anatomic and physiological data are again discordant; i.e., an apparent severe angiographic obstruction was associated with no physiological limitation. (*From CB Wright et al* [57].)

have demonstrated that coronary obstructions of increasing severity progressively limit maximal coronary dilator responses in a very orderly way [6–20]. We have recently performed similar experiments in patients [24,54–57]. The y-axis point (Figure 11-12) was determined by obtaining reactive hyperemic responses following a 20-s coronary occlusion and measuring the peak-to-resting velocity ratio. The x-axis point (Figure 11-12) was obtained by measuring the percent stenosis with micrometers on an arteriogram of the vessel being examined. Maximum percent narrowing of the obstruction in question was determined from analysis of the patient's coronary arteriogram. Patients were excluded from this study if the coronary arteriogram was not of excellent quality, if visible coronary collaterals were present, or if the patient had evidence of cardiac hypertrophy.

In patients there was not an "orderly relationship" between the severity of the coronary stenosis estimated from visual analysis of a coronary arteriogram and the maximal vasodilator capacity of the vessel measured with our Doppler system

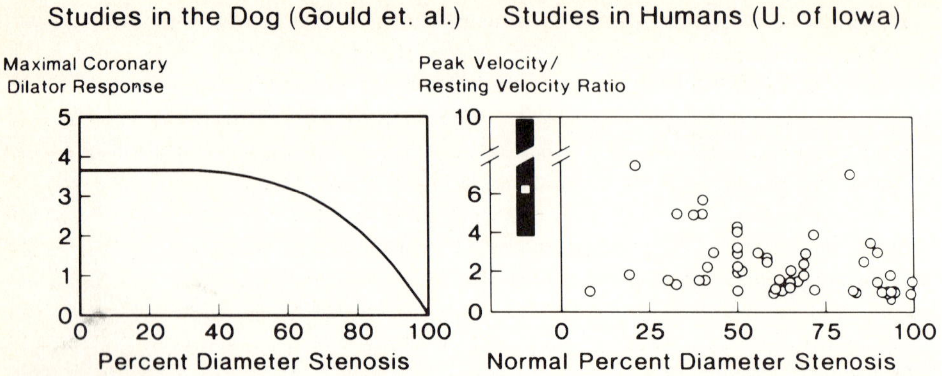

FIGURE 11-12
Relationship between maximal coronary flow or blood flow velocity and percent stenosis in an experimental study (*left*) and a clinical study (*right*). The experimental animal study is described in detail in Figure 11-1. To achieve maximal coronary blood flow velocity in the clinical study, the coronary vessel being examined was occluded for 20 s and then the occlusion was released. Maximal coronary blood flow was expressed as a ratio of peak velocity following release of the occlusion and resting velocity. The percent stenosis of the vessel being examined was measured with calipers from the angiographic projection that showed the lesion to be most severe. The range of normal responses in humans is shown by the black bar. Each open circle represents a study in one patient. Although there was an orderly relationship between percent stenosis and maximal coronary flow in the experimental study (*left*) this was not the case in the clinical study. See text for additional discussion. (*The clinical studies are based on data originally reported by C Wright et al* [24].)

(Figure 11-12). The 20 patients that we studied who had severe coronary obstructions (greater than 90 percent diameter narrowing) all had markedly impaired coronary reactive hyperemic responses (peak-to-resting velocity ratio = 1.4; debt area/repayment area ratio = 0.6). However, with coronary obstructions of intermediate severity (10 to 90 percent diameter narrowing) the correlation between the severity of the coronary stenosis and the vasodilator capacity of the vessel was poor ($r = 0.1$).

These studies emphasize a critical problem in clinical cardiology: Although the coronary arteriogram can determine the location of obstructions in all major coronary vessels, conventional analysis of the arteriogram does not yield a precise assessment of the physiological significance of coronary obstructions of intermediate severity.

Comparisons with Quantitative Computer-Based Coronary Angiography

One explanation for the poor correlation between coronary vasodilator capacity and percent diameter narrowing of coronary vessels is that the conventional analysis of the coronary arteriogram is crude. This deficiency could contribute a great deal of variability to the relationship between the severity of a stenosis determined by conventional arteriography and the physiological significance of the coronary obstruction. To improve the analysis of the coronary arteriogram we have employed a sophisticated analytic system initially described by Brown et al. [58] for analyzing coronary arteriograms.

Description of Quantitative Computer-Based Coronary Angiography Ciné coronary arteriograms obtained at 90° angles are projected on a 52–67 cm^2 screen. The frames selected for analysis are high-quality angiograms that clearly demonstrate the obstructed vascular segment. Films in which overlapping vessels obscure the borders of the obstructed vascular segment are excluded. In addition, patients with angiographically apparent coronary collaterals or cardiac hypertrophy are not included. The film pairs (90° projections) analyzed are selected from a similar point in the cardiac cycle. The projected angiograms of the vascular segment to be analyzed are traced manually three times. The *xy* coordinates of the lesion in both planes are noted. Also, the coronary catheter is traced. The information concerning the three-dimensional location of the coronary segment, the coronary catheter, and data describing the magnification and distortion characteristics of the x-ray system are utilized to calculate the absolute dimensions of the vascular segment containing the obstruction. Results of studies with a brass coronary artery model indicate that, with the model placed anywhere in the x-ray field, the dimensions of a simulated vessel can be determined with an accuracy of ± 1 percent. The traced images are digitized, and then a computer program developed by Brown et al. [58] is used to perform the necessary calculations (Figure 11-13). The final result reported is the average obtained from the analysis of three pairs of tracings of the vascular segment being studied.

FIGURE 11-13
Analysis of a coronary arteriogram with computer-based coronary angiography. The lesion being studied is traced in two orthogonal projections—left anterior oblique (LAO) and right anterior oblique (RAO). The computer program realigns the vascular segments and corrects the tracings for magnification and distortion errors introduced by the x-ray system. The program then calculates diameter and area of the proximal vascular segment, diameter and area of the distal vascular segment, and minimal diameter and area of the vascular segment at its narrowest point, as well as percent area stenosis of the lesion. Sten = stenosis; min = minimal cross-sectional area of the stenosis. (*Courtesy of David Harrison, Assistant Professor of Medicine, University of Iowa.*)

Vessel	Proximal	Distal	Minimum	Sten.
LAO (mm)	2.693	2.710	0.310	88.5%
RAO (mm)	2.813	2.449	0.380	85.6%
AREA (mm2)	5.950	5.212	0.107	98.1%

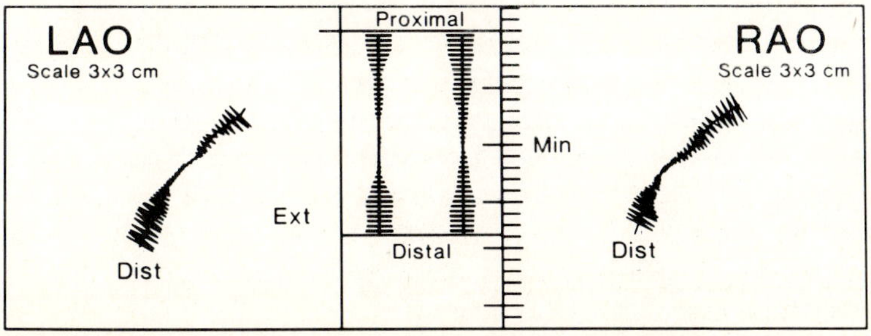

Studies by Brown et al. [58] have shown that with this system repeated determinations of percent area stenosis and minimal cross-sectional area of various portions of the coronary vascular segment vary by 2 percent and 0.1 mm, respectively. Similar results have been achieved by Harrison [54] and Kelley and Gould [59]. In addition, experimental measurements [59] in dogs have validated the formulations employed by Brown et al. [58] to compute stenosis resistance.

The major advantages of the computer-based analysis of the coronary arteriogram are (1) reproducibility is excellent, and (2) both absolute and relative lumen cross-sectional areas can be estimated (Figure 11-14). In contrast, with conventional visual analysis of the coronary arteriogram, reproducibility is poor [45–49] and only relative diameter measurements are available. Such relative measurements are particularly deficient in the presence of diffuse arterial disease.

Correlations between Computer-Based Coronary Angiography and Physiological Studies In a series of 26 patients, Harrison et al. [54] examined the ability of computer-based analysis of coronary arteriograms to predict the functional significance of coronary obstructons. The studies were limited to isolated proximal obstructions of the left anterior descending coronary artery. Furthermore, patients were excluded from this series if the left anterior descending vessel was unusually small, as evidenced by termination of the vessel proximal to the left ventricular apex. In each patient the arteriogram was of superior quality. At cardiac surgery, the quantitative characteristics of coronary reactive hyperemia in the left anterior descending coronary artery following a 20-s coronary occlusion were determined.

The data relating percent area stenosis and peak-to-resting velocity ratio are shown in Figure 11-15. The relationship between percent area stenosis and

FIGURE 11-14
Effects of a 50 percent stenosis in a normal vessel (*left*) and a vessel with diffuse obstructive disease *right*). In the normal vessel, the obstructive lesion decreases the cross-sectional area CSA of the vessel at its narrowest point to 4.9 mm^2. In the diseased vessel, the obstructive lesion decreases the CSA at the narrowest point to 1.43 mm^2. Pathological studies indicate that coronary disease is often a diffuse process which involves the entire length of a coronary artery (see Figure 11-2). As a consequence, percent stenosis is an inadequate approach to assessing the severity of coronary obstructive disease in patients with a coronary atherosclerosis.

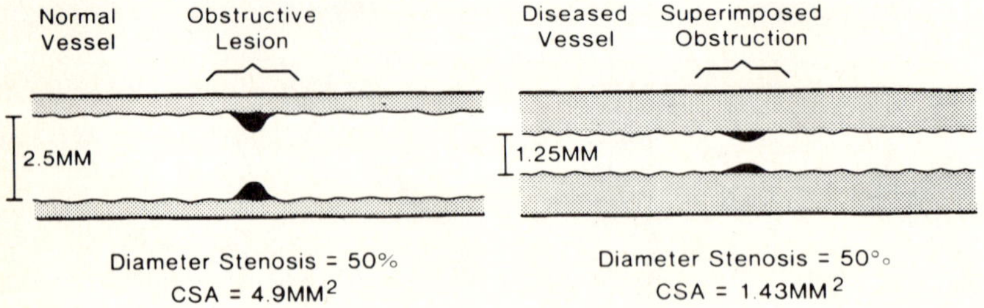

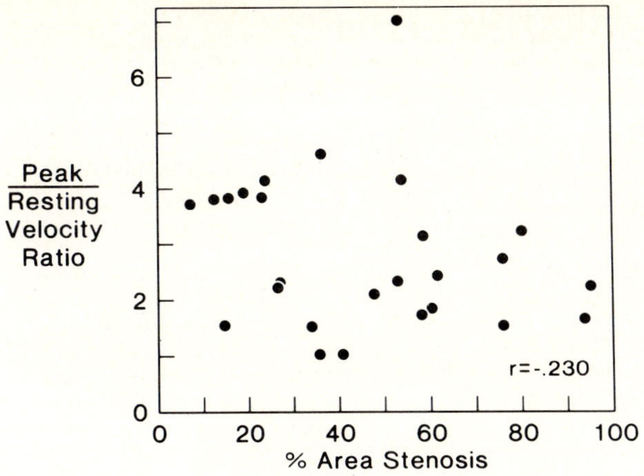

FIGURE 11-15
Relationship between percent area stenosis and the peak-to-resting velocity ratio following release of a 20-s coronary occlusion in patients with a single proximal left anterior descending coronary artery. Percent area stenosis was determined by computer-based coronary angiography. The poor relationship between percent area stenosis and the vasodilator reserve (peak-to-resting velocity ratio) of the vessels being examined is obvious. (*Based on data originally presented by DG Harrison et al* [*54*].)

peak-to-resting velocity ratio was poor ($r = 0.23$). Thus, the percent diameter stenosis assessed by conventional analysis of the coronary arteriogram or percent area stenosis assessed by computer-based coronary angiography does not accurately predict the effects of a coronary stenosis on coronary vasodilator capacity.

For the entire patient group, the relationship between minimal cross-sectional area of the lesion and peak-to-resting velocity ratio was much better ($r = 0.79$) than that noted for percent area stenosis. Previous experimental studies have emphasized the importance of minimal cross-sectional area as opposed to percent coronary stenosis when determining the physiological significance of obstructive lesions [10,26,58–61].

Effects of the Daughter Branching Pattern on the Importance of a Given Coronary Obstruction When the absolute dimensions of the narrowed vascular segment are calculated, the functional significance of the lesion must be related to the expected normal cross-sectional area of the vessel at the point of obstruction. The normal cross-sectional area of any vessel is determined in part by its position in the vascular hierarchy. When a vessel branches, the sum of the diameter cubed of the two daughter branches is equal to the diameter cubed of the mother vessel (Figure 11-16) [62]. Hence, when a large vessel gives rise to a major branch, the cross-sectional area of the main vessel distal to the branch point is significantly less than its cross-sectional area proximal to the branch point. The left anterior descending coronary artery in humans usually gives rise to one to four large diagonal branches and one or two large perforating arteries (see Chapter 1). The other branches of the left anterior descending coronary artery are relatively small.

Because of the daughter branching effect on vessel caliber, Harrison et al. [54] divided their patients with left anterior descending coronary obstructions into two

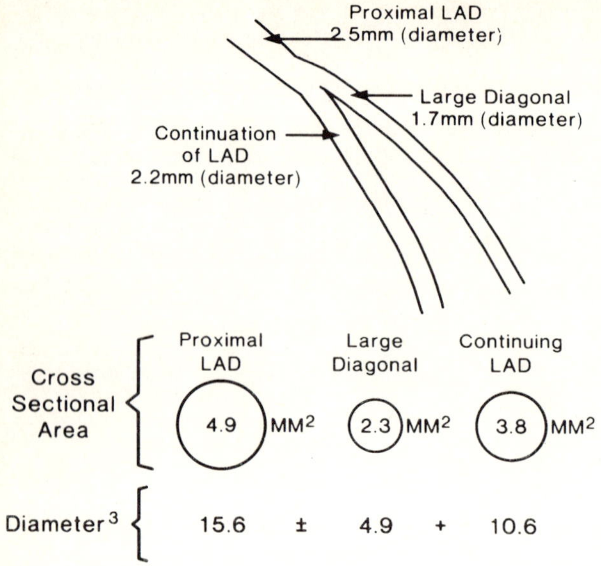

FIGURE 11-16
Anatomic relationship between a parent vessel and its daughter branches. Whenever a parent vessel gives rise to daughter branches, the parent vessel distal to the takeoff of the daughter branches would be smaller than it was proximal to the takeoff of these branch vessels. The sum of the areas of the branch vessels will be greater than the area of the parent vessel prior of the point of bifurcation. The diameter to the third power of the parent vessel will equal the sum of the diameter cubed of the daughter vessels. Because of this relationship between the parent vessel and the daughter branches, when absolute cross-sectional area is measured, one must pay great attention to the vascular distribution pattern.

groups: patients in whom the obstructive lesion occurred proximal to the takeoff of the first large diagonal branch and patients in whom the obstructive lesion occurred distal to this branch. This is a simple method of trying to normalize for expected vessel caliber. Our experience with lesions beyond the first diagonal is limited. In patients with lesions proximal to the first diagonal, the relationship between minimal cross-sectional area of the lesion and coronary vasodilator capacity was remarkably good (Figures 11-17 and 11-18). *This data suggests that one parameter–minimal cross-sectional area of the lesion–which can be measurd only with computer-based coronary angiography can predict the coronary vasodilator capacity of obstructed vessels in patients. At present, no other approach to assessing the physiological significance of the coronary obstructions of intermediate severity preoperatively is available.*

LIMITATIONS OF CURRENT PHYSIOLOGIC STUDIES

The studies of Harrison et al. [54] are very provocative. They challenge the widely held notion that the physiological significance of a coronary stenosis of intermediate severity can be assessed by conventional analysis of the coronary arteriogram. The finding of Wright et al. [24] and Harrison et al. [54] concerning the poor relationship between percent stenosis and the physiological effects of a coronary obstruction reflect three often-neglected considerations concerning the evaluation of coronary stenoses in patients. First, coronary obstructive lesions are often asymmetrical and eccentric [4,21–23]; hence, maximal percent stenosis in one angiographic projection will not accurately predict the severity of the

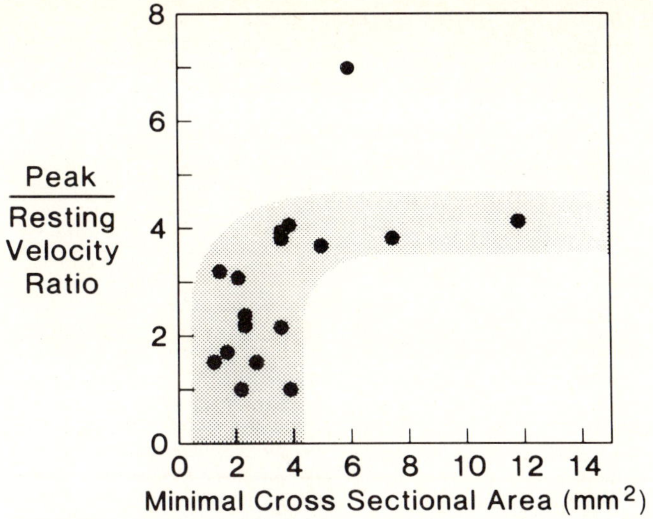

FIGURE 11-17
Relationship between the peak-to-resting velocity ratio following a 20-s coronary occlusion and a minimal cross-sectional area of the coronary obstructive lesion. In this study, only patients with a single left anterior descending obstruction proximal to the takeoff of any diagonal branches were included. This was done to minimize variation in expected vessel diameter if no atherosclerotic disease was present. With the constraints noted above, a minimal cross-sectional area of the coronary obstructive lesion could predict the physiological significance of the coronary obstruction with a reasonable degree of accuracy. This approach is far superior to utilizing percent stenosis measurements. (*Based on data reported by DG Harrison et al* [54].)

obstruction. Second, the vascular segments proximal and distal to an apparent segmental coronary obstruction are usually not free of significant atherosclerotic obstructions (Figures 11-2 and 11-3) [4,51]. As a consequence, percent stenosis measurements will underestimate the severity of coronary obstructions. Third, alterations in vasomotor tone of the stenotic segment or the vascular segments proximal or distal to it [28,29,52] contribute to the difficulty of assessing the severity of the obstruction from an angiogram. Each of these three factors contribute variability to the relationship between percent diameter or area stenosis and the coronary vasodilator capacity of the given vascular segment. With coronary obstructions of intermediate severity, the aggregate variability related to these three factors and intra- and interobserver errors in interpretation of the angiograms [45–49] are so large that there appears to be no significant relationship between percent narrowing and maximal dilator responses.

There are four considerations which could potentially threaten the validity of the conclusions of the studies presented by Wright et al. [24] and Harrison et al. [53]. Although these considerations are unlikely to explain the results obtained they should be mentioned.

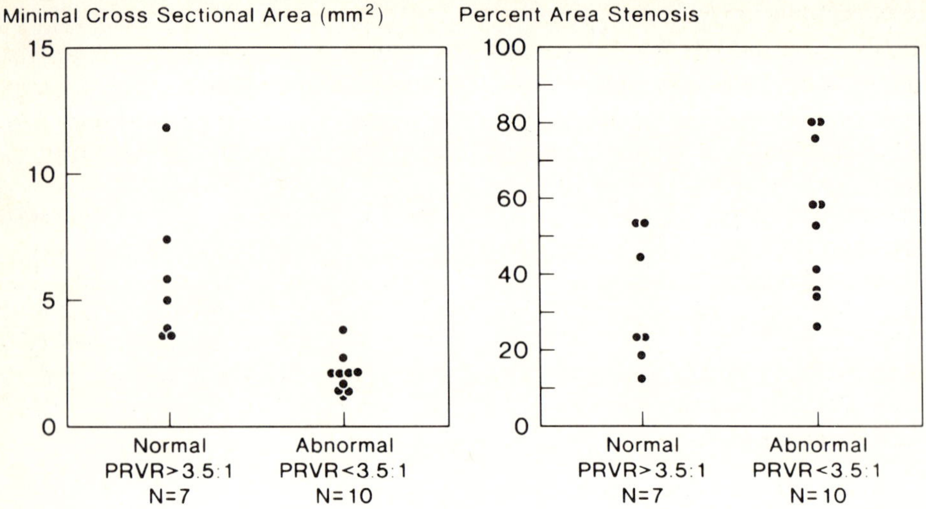

FIGURE 11-18
(*Left*) Effectiveness of minimal cross-sectional and (*right*) percent area stenosis in separating patients with normal and abnormal hyperemic responses. In our experience a peak-to-resting velocity ratio (PRVR) of 3.5:1 following the release of a 20-s occlusion is the lower limit of normal. Separation of abnormal and normal reactive hyperemic responses was best accomplished when minimal cross-sectional area is used as a criterion. (*Based on data reported by DG Harrison et al* [*54*].)

Relative-Absolute Flow

When a Doppler probe is applied to a vessel, the angle between the blood column and the ultrasonic crystal is not precisely known and the diameter of the vessel is usually not measured. Hence, absolute flow cannot be assessed (see Chapter 2). Because of this deficiency in the studies of Wright et al. [24] and Harrison et al. [54] estimates of coronary vasodilator capacity were based on the ratio between peak and resting blood flow velocity following a 20-s coronary occlusion. In essence, it was assumed that resting flow was in the physiological range. This assumption is reasonable because (1) the hemodynamic determinants of myocardial oxygen consumption in the left ventricles of the control and coronary disease patients studied were similar and in the normal physiological range (heart rate = 80 ± 10 beats per minute, aortic pressure = 70 ± 15 mmHg, and left atrial pressure = 11 ± 2 mmHg); hence, coronary blood flow in these patient groups should be similar and in the in the normal range; (2) the primary anesthetic employed (halothane) decreases resting coronary blood flow in a relatively consistent manner and does not alter the transmural distribution of coronary flow [63]; and (3) direct measurements of coronary blood flow under these conditions have demonstrated that coronary flow is in the physiological range [64]. Finally, control (normal vessels) and experimental measurements (obstructed vessels) are obtained under similar conditions. Thus, it is unlikely that the poor relationship between percent diameter or area stenosis of a coronary lesion and the peak-to-resting velocity ratio of the reactive hyperemic response can be explained by marked variations in the level of resting coronary blood flow.

Coronary Collaterals

When a coronary vessel is occluded, the myocardium served by the vessel will become intensely ischemic unless a well-developed coronary collateral circulation is present (see Chapter 10). In the studies of Wright et al. [24] and Harrison et al. [54] it was assumed that undetected collaterals did not prevent the development of ischemia when coronary occlusions were performed to assess the coronary reactive hyperemic response. This assumption was reasonable because patients with angiographically visible collaterals were excluded from the study. Furthermore, significant collaterals develop only when a coronary stenosis is severe (see Chapter 10). In the studies of Wright et al. [24] and Harrison et al. [54] only the patients with coronary stenosis of intermediate severity showed a poor correlation between percent stenosis and the coronary reactive hyperemic response. It is unlikely that many of these patients have well-developed coronary collaterals that were undetected by angiography.

Cardiac Hypertrophy and Scar

Many studies have shown that coronary reserve is markedly decreased in patients with cardiac hypertrophy (see Chapter 13). Also, it is possible that myocardial segments that are largely fibrotic may respond to a transient interruption in coronary flow in an unusual manner. To eliminate these potential sources of variability, Wright et al. [24] and Harrison et al. [54], excluded from their studies patients with segmental wall motion abnormalities suggesting previous myocardial infarction or patients with cardiac hypertrophy.

Variable Coronary Vasomotor Tone

The studies of Wright et al. [24] and Harrison et al. [54] assume that coronary vasomotor tone at the time of coronary angiography and cardiac surgery were similar. At coronary angiography, patients routinely received sublingual nitroglycerin to diminish the likelihood of coronary spasm. In addition, none of the patients included in the study had obvious evidence of spasm on the angiogram. At surgery, we have never observed evidence of coronary spasm. Following coronary occlusion, coronary blood flow velocity always returns to the control level. Although it is unlikely that intermittent coronary spasm contributed a great deal of variability to our studies, it is possible that less dramatic changes in coronary vasomotor tone did contribute to the variability we observed between physiological and anatomic evidence of coronary obstruction.

FUTURE APPROACHES TO ESTIMATING THE SEVERITY OF CORONARY STENOSIS IN HUMANS

Intraoperative assessment of coronary stenosis will be improved by measurements of absolute rather than relative coronary flow or velocity. This may be possible with a gated Doppler currently being developed at the University of Iowa. With this device integrated, mean coronary velocity and coronary diameter can be measured simultaneously, and thus flow can be calculated if the angle between the ultrasonic crystal and the blood column can be precisely determined. The recent development of a single-fiber laser Doppler may permit cardiologists to directly measure coronary blood flow velocity proximal and distal to a coronary obstruction [64a].

Demonstrating that a coronary occlusion produces intense ischemia will also be helpful. This can be done by measuring segmental wall thickening with a specially designed echocardiographic transducer [65]. In the absence of functionally important coronary collaterals, transient coronary occlusion is associated with transient wall thinning. Thus, this approach would eliminate the possibility of unsuspected coronary collaterals which could prevent transient coronary occlusion from producing intense myocardial ischemia and hence stimulating coronary dilation.

The preoperative assessment of coronary stenosis would also be improved by computer-based coronary angiography that employs an algorithm that has been validated in patients. Other techniques for measuring coronary blood flow (computed x-ray tomography, tomographic scintigrams of positron-emitting radionuclides) (see Chapter 2) also show considerable promise.

The development of a clinically applicable method that can be employed preoperatively to assess the physiological significance of coronary obstruction in individual coronary vessels is of paramount importance. Such measurements will almost certainly improve the quality of care extended to patients with chronic obstructive coronary disease.

REFERENCES

1 Gensini GG: Coronary arteriography, in *Heart Disease: A Textbook in Cardiovascular Medicine*. E Braunwald (ed). Philadelphia, Saunders, 1980, vol 1, p 308.

2 Baroldi G, Scomazzoni G: Stenosing-occlusive arterio-atherosclerotic lesions of the principal extramural branches, in *Coronary Circulation in the Normal and the Pathologic Heart*. Washington, Armed Forces Institute of Pathology, Office of the Surgeon General, 1967, chap 11.

3 Iskandrian AS, Klein BL, Segal BL, Kimbiris D, Bemis CE: Coronary artery disease confined to secondary branches of the left coronary system. *Clin Cardiol* 4: 130, 1981.

4 Arnett EN, Isner JM, Redwood DR, Kent DM, Baker WP, Ackerstein H, Roberts WC: Coronary artery narrowing in coronary heart disease: Comparison of cineangiographic and necropsy findings. *Ann Int Med* 91: 350, 1979.

5 Shipley RE, Gregg DE: The effect of external constriction of a blood vessel on blood flow. *Amer J Physiol* 141: 289, 1944.

6 Khouri EM, Gregg DE, Lowensohn HS: Flow in the major branches of the left coronary artery during experimental coronary insufficiency in the unanesthetized dog. *Circ Res* 23: 99, 1968.

7 Gould KL, Lipscomb K, Hamilton GW: Physiologic basis for assessing critical coronary stenosis. *Am J Cardiol* 33: 87, 1974.

8 Gould KL, Lipscomb K: Effects of coronary stenoses on coronary flow reserve and resistance. *Am J Cardiol* 34: 48, 1974.

9 Gould KL, Lipscomb K, Calvert C: Compensatory changes of the distal coronary

vascular bed during progressive coronary constricton. *Am J Physiol* 222: 705, 1975.
10 Gould KL: Pressure-flow characteristics of coronary stenoses in unsedated dogs at rest and during coronary vasodilation. *Circ Res* 43: 245, 1978.
11 Gould KL: Dynamic coronary stenosis. *Am J Cardiol* 45: 286, 1980.
12 Elzinga WE, Skinner DB: Hemodynamic characteristics of critical stenosis in canine coronary arteries. *J Thorac Cardiovasc Surg* 69: 217, 1975.
13 Fresinger GC, Hillis WS: Reactive hyperemia: An index to coronary arterial narrowing. *Am Heart J* 92: 737, 1976.
14 Folts JD, Gallagher K, Rowe GG: Hemodynamic effects of controlled degrees of coronary artery stenosis in short-term and long-term studies in dogs. *J Thorac Cardiovasc Surg* 73: 722, 1977.
15 Gallagher KP, Folts JD, Rowe GG: Comparison of coronary arteriograms with direct measurements of stenosed coronary arteries in dogs. *Am Heart J* 95: 338, 1978.
16 Feldman RL, Nichols WW, Pepine CJ, Conti CR: Hemodynamic effects of long and multiple coronary arterial narrowings. *Chest* 74: 280, 1978.
17 Feldman RL, Nichols WW, Pepine CJ, Conti CR: Hemodynamic significance of the length of a coronary arterial narrowing. *Am J Cardiol* 41: 865, 1978.
18 Mates RE, Gupta RL, Bell AC, Klocke FJ: Fluid dynamics of coronary artery stenosis. *Circ Res* 42: 152, 1978.
19 Schwartz JS, Caryle PF, Cohn JN: Effect of dilation of the distal coronary bed on flow and resistance in severely stenotic coronary arteries in the dog. *Am J Cardiol* 43: 219, 1979.
20 Santamore WP, Walinsky P: Altered coronary flow responses to vasoactive drugs due to coronary arterial stenosis in the dog. *Am J Cardiol* 45: 276, 1980.
20a Brown BG, Petersen RB, Pierce CD, Bolson EL, Dodge HT: *Dynamics of Human Coronary Stenosis: Interactions Among Stenosis Flow, Distending Pressure and Vasomotor Tone.* Baltimore, Urban & Schwarzenberg, 1982.
20b Gould, KL, Kelley KO: Physiological significance of coronary flow velocity and changing stenosis geometry during coronary vasodilation in awake dogs. *Circ Res* 50: 695, 1982.
21 Hort W: Anatomy and pathology of the human coronary circulation, in *The Pathophysiology of Myocardial Perfusion*, W Schaper (ed). New York, Elsevier, 1979, chap 8, p 247.
22 Schaper W: Personal communication. Max Planck Institute, Bad Naheim, West Germany.
23 Vlodaver Z, Edwards JE: Pathology of coronary atherosclerosis. *Prog Cardiovasc Dis* 14: 256, 1971.
24 Wright C, White C, Furda J, Doty D, Eastham C, Laughlin D, Marcus M: Can the coronary arteriogram predict the functional significance of a coronary stenosis? *Circulation* 62: 214, 1980.
25 Yongchareon W, Young DF: Initiation of turbulence in models of arterial stenoses. *J Biomechanics* 12: 185, 1979.
26 Young DF, Cholvin NR, Roth AC: Pressure drop across artificially induced stenoses in the femoral arteries of dogs. *Circ Res* 36: 735, 1975.
27 Clark C: The propagation of turbulence produced by a stenosis. *J Biomechanics* 13: 591, 1980.
28 Doerner TC, Brown GB, Bolson E, Frimer M, Dodge HT: Vasodilatory effects of nitroglycerine and nitroprusside in coronary arteries—a comparative analysis (abstr). *Am J Cardiol* 43: 416, 1979.
29 Heupler FA, Proudfit WL, Razavi M, Shirey EK, Greenstreet R, Sheldon WC: Er-

gonovine maleate provocative test for coronary arterial spasm. *Am J Cardiol* 41: 631, 1978.

30 Proudfit WL, Shirey EK, Sones FM Jr: Selective cine coronary arteriography: Correlation with clinical findings in 1,000 patients. *Circulation* 33: 901, 1966.

31 Kuller LH, Lilienfeld A, Fisher R: An epidemiologic study of sudden and unexpected deaths in adults. *Medicine* 48: 341, 1968.

32 Kemp HG, Vokonas PS, Cohn PF, Gorlin R: The anginal syndrome associated with normal coronary arteriograms: Report of a six year experience. *Am J Med* 54: 735, 1973.

33 Master AM, Friedman R, Dack S: The electrocardiogram after standard exercise as a functional test of the heart. *Am Heart J* 24: 777, 1942.

34 Weiner DA, Ryan TJ, McCabe CH, Kennedy JW, Schloss M, Tristani F, Chaitman BR, Fisher LD: Correlations among history of angina, ST-segment response and prevalence of coronary-artery disease in the coronary artery surgery study (CASS). *N Eng J Med* 301: 230, 1979.

35 Bailey IK, Come PC, Kelly DT, Burow RD, Griffith LSC, Strauss HW, Pitt B: Thallium-201 myocardial perfusion imaging in aortic valve stenosis *Am J Cardiol* 40: 889, 1977.

36 Ritchie JL, Trobaugh GB, Hamilton GW, Gould KL, Narahara KA, Murray JA, Williams DL: Myocardial imaging with thallium-201 at rest and during exercise. Comparison with coronary arteriography and resting and stress electrocardiography. *Circulation* 56: 66, 1977.

37 Verani MS, Marcus ML, Razzak MA, Ehrhardt JC: Sensitivity and specificity of thallium-201 exercise perfusion scintigrams in the diagnosis of coronary artery disease. *J Nucl Med* 19: 773, 1978.

38 Gould KL: Non-invasive assessment of coronary stenosis by myocardial perfusion imaging during pharmacologic coronary vasodilation. I. Physiological basis and experimental validation. *Am J Cardiol* 41: 267, 1978.

39 Pohost GM, Alpert NM, Ingwall JS, Strauss HW: Thallium redistribution: Mechanism and clinical utility. *Sem Nucl Med* 10: 70, 1980.

40 Mueller TM, Marcus ML, Ehrhardt JC, Chaudhuri T, Abboud FM: Limitations of thallium–201 myocardial perfusion scintigrams. *Circulation* 54: 640, 1970.

41 Gould KL, Schelbert HR, Phelps ME, Hoffman EJ: Noninvasive assessment of coronary stenoses with myocardial perfusion imaging during pharmacologic coronary vasodilation. *Am J Cardiol* 43: 200, 1979.

42 Falsetti HL, Marcus ML, Kerber RE, Skorton DJ: Quantification of myocardial ischemia and infarction by left ventricle imaging (editorial). *Circulation* 63: 747, 1981.

43 Borer JS, Bacharach SL, Green MV, Kent KM, Epstein SE, Johnston GS: Real-time radionuclide cineangiography in the noninvasive evaluation of global and regional left ventricular function at rest and during exercise in patients with coronary artery disease. *N Eng J Med* 296: 839, 1977.

44 Gibbons RJ, Lee KL, Cobb FR, Coleman RE, Jones RH: Ejection fraction response to exercise in patients with chest pain, coronary artery disease and normal resting ventricular function. *Circulation* 66: 643, 1982.

45 Galbraith JE, Murphy ML, De Soyza: Coronary angiogram interpretation. *JAMA* 240: 2053, 1978.

46 DeRouen TA, Murray JA, Owen W: Variability in the analysis of coronary arteriograms. *Circulation* 55: 2, 1977.

47 Detre KM, Wright E, Murphy ML, Takaro T: Observer agreement in evaluating coronary angiograms. *Circulation* 52: 979, 1975.

48 Zir LM, Miller SW, Dinsmore RE, Gilbert JP, Hawthorne JW: Interobserver variability in coronary angiography. *Circulation* 53: 4, 1976.

49 Aldridge HE, McLoughlin MJ, Taylor KW: Improved diagnosis in coronary cinearteriography with routine use of 100° oblique views and cranial and caudal angulations. Comparison with standard oblique views in 100 patients. *Am J Cardiol* 36: 468, 1975.

50 Levin DC, Baltaxe HA, Sos TA: Potential sources of error in coronary arteriography. II. In interpretation of the study. *Am J Roentgenol* 124: 386, 1975.

51 Schwartz JN, Kong Y, Hackell DB, Bartel AG: Comparison of angiographic and postmortem findings in patients with coronary artery disease. *Am J Cardiol* 36: 174, 1975.

52 Feldman RL, Pepine CJ, Curry RC, Conti CR: A case against the routine use of nitroglycerin prior to coronary angiography. *Brit Heart J* 40: 992, 1978.

53 Gruentzig AR, Senning A, Siegenthaler WE: Nonoperative dilation of coronary-artery stenosis. *N Eng J Med* 301: 61, 1979.

54 Harrison DG, White CW, Hiratzka LF, Wright CB, Doty DB, Miller MR, Eastham CL, Marcus ML: Can the significance of a coronary stenosis be predicted by quantitative coronary angiography? *Circulation* 64: 160, 1981.

55 Marcus M, Wright C, Doty D, Eastham C, Laughlin D, Krumm P, Fastenow C, Brody M: Measurements of coronary velocity and reactive hyperemia in the coronary circulation of humans. *Circ Res* 49: 877, 1981.

56 Wright C, Doty D, Eastham C, Laughlin D, Marcus M: A method for assessing the physiologic significance of coronary obstructions in man at cardiac surgery. *Circulation* 62: 111, 1980.

57 Wright CB, Doty DB, Eastham CL, Marcus ML: Measurements of coronary reactive hyperemia with a Doppler probe: An intraoperative guide to hemodynamically significant lesions. *J Thorac Cardiovasc Surg* 80: 888, 1980.

58 Brown BG, Bolson E, Frimer M, Dodge HT: Quantitative coronary arteriography. Estimation of dimensions, hemodynamic resistance, and atheroma mass of coronary artery lesions using the arteriogram and and digital computation. *Circulation* 55: 2, 1977.

59 Kelley K, Gould L: Validation of computerized quantitative coronary angiography. *Circulation* 64: 107, 1981.

60 Lipscomb K, Hooten S: Effect of stenotic dimensions and blood flow on the hemodynamic significance of model coronary arterial stenoses. *Am J Cardiol* 42: 781, 1978.

61 McMahon MM, Brown BG, Cukingnan R, Rolett EL, Bolson E, Frimer M, Dodge HT: Quantitative coronary angiography: Measurement of the "critical" stenosis in patients with unstable angina and single vessel disease without collaterals. *Circulation* 60: 1, 1979.

62 Hutchins GM, Miner MM, Boitnott JK: Vessel caliber and branch-angle of human coronary artery branch-points. *Circulation* 36: 572, 1976.

63 Eastham CL, Moyers JR, Carter JG, Brooks LA, Marcus ML: Effects of halothane on the coronary circulation. *Circulation* 64: 120, 1981.

64 Moyers J: Personal communication. Department of Anesthesiology, University of Iowa, June 1982.

64a Kilpatrick D, Linderer T, Sievers RE, Tyberg JV: Measurement of coronary sinus blood flow by fiber-optic laser Doppler anemometry. *Am J Physiol* 242: H1111, 1982.

65 Likoff M, Peichek N, Macoviak J, Harken A, Sutton MST, Muhammed A, Plappert T, Kastor JA: High frequency epicardial echo mapping of segmental myocardial performance at multiple sites on right and left ventricles. *Am J Cardiol* 47: 403, 1981.

CHAPTER **12**

EFFECTS OF CORONARY SPASM ON THE CORONARY CIRCULATION

For almost 200 years it was assumed that the primary cause of angina pectoris was fixed atherosclerotic obstructions in epicardial coronary arteries. Although Osler suggested that spasm of large coronary vessels might cause angina pectoris [1], this hypothesis was discarded because pathological studies strongly supported the notion that obstructive coronary disease was the primary culprit [2]. Prinzmetal et al. [3] revived interest in coronary spasm in 1959 by describing the clinical syndrome of "variant angina": Afflicted patients had angina pectoris at rest in association with ST segment elevation on their electrocardiogram. Prinzmetal et al. [3] postulated that this syndrome was caused by spasm of large coronary arteries. Since then, a large volume of data has firmly established the importance of coronary spasm in the pathogenesis of angina pectoris [4–10].

EVIDENCE OF CORONARY SPASM IN HUMANS

Four types of studies—hemodynamic, angiographic, scintigraphic, and metabolic—provide independent evidence of coronary spasms in humans.

Hemodynamic Studies

A small percentage of all patients with angina pectoris present with the syndrome of variant angina originally described by Prinzmetal [6–10]. Typically these patients have severe substernal chest pain at rest associated with ST segment elevation on the electrocardiogram. The episodes may occur at rest or during activity and are usually not associated with evidence of myocardial necrosis. In most patients, the pain and electrocardiographic abnormalities are ameliorated with sublingual nitroglycerin. Classically, these patients have normal exercise tolerance and a normal electrocardiographic response to intense treadmill exercise.

Pain at rest can occur in patients with fixed coronary obstruction if undetected changes in hemodynamics (tachycardia and/or hypertension) precede the onset of pain [11–11b]. Under such conditions, myocardial ischemia occurs because limited coronary vasodilator capacity cannot accommodate an increase in myocardial oxygen consumption. In this group of patients, spasm is not the cause of angina at rest.

In contrast, elegant studies by Maeri et al. [5] have shown that the following sequence (Figure 12-1) of events occurs at the onset of coronary spasm: stable hemodynamics, ST depression, a modest decrease in left ventricular *dp/dt*, ST segment elevation on the electrocardiogram followed by a consistent rise in left ventricular end diastolic pressure, and a modest fall in systolic arterial pressure. Mild tachycardia and hypertension often follow the onset of chest pain. This chain of events is compatible with the hypothesis that coronary spasm was the primary event. The early hemodynamic changes reflect a decrease in ventricular contractility secondary to myocardial ischemia. The later hemodynamic events reflect activation of the autonomic nervous system in response to chest pain.

Although these hemodynamic observations do not definitively demonstrate the existence of coronary spasm, they are very suggestive. Such studies stimulated investigators to provide more direct proof for the existence of coronary spasm.

Angiographic Studies

In 1962, Gensini et al. [12] provided the first angiographic evidence of spasm of a major coronary vessel in a patient with variant angina. Since 1972, numerous investigators have reported the presence of spontaneous spasm of major coronary vessels in patients with a clinical syndrome of variant angina (see Figure 12-2) [4,5,7–8,13–20]. Spasm may occur in any major coronary vessel and may be focal or diffuse. In 60 percent of patients spasm occurs just distal to a fixed obstructive lesion [20a]. Typically, the luminal diameter of the spastic segment decreases by greater than 75 percent. Total occlusion is not uncommon. Spasm of the right coronary artery is usually associated with bradycardia and hypotension [21]. When the left anterior descending coronary artery develops spasm, tachycardia often occurs [4,5,7–9]. The differential effects of right and left coronary spasm on heart rate and blood pressure may be related to the preferential distribution of stretch receptors in the inferior wall of the left ventricle [22,23]. As a consequence

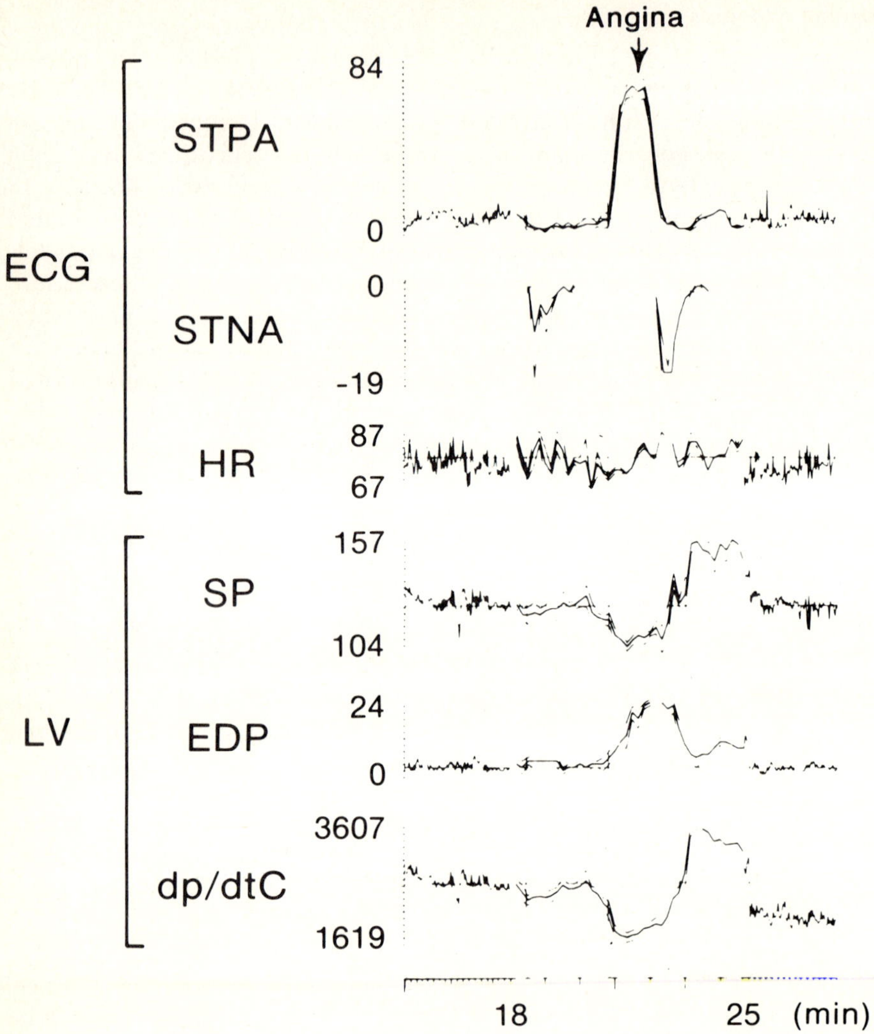

FIGURE 12-1
Electrocardiographic and hemodynamic recordings before, during, and following an episode of spontaneous coronary spasm. STPA = ST segment positive area (values above 0 indicate ST segment elevation); STNA = ST segment negative area (values below 0 indicate ST segment depression); HR = heart rate in beats per minute; SP = systolic left ventricular pressure in mm Hg; EDP = left ventricular end-diastolic pressure in mmHg; dp/dtC = the first derivative of the rise in the left ventricular pressure during systole. Prior to the onset of angina, coronary spasm is associated with ST segment elevation and a decrease in left ventricular function manifested by a decrease in left ventricular systolic pressure, *dp/dt*, and a rise in end-diastolic pressure. With the onset of angina, a slight increase in heart rate occurs. Subsequently there is improvement in left ventricular function and a decrease in ST elevation, followed by ST depression. This suggests that the coronary spasm abated spontaneously. (*Modified from original data reported by A Maseri et al* [5].)

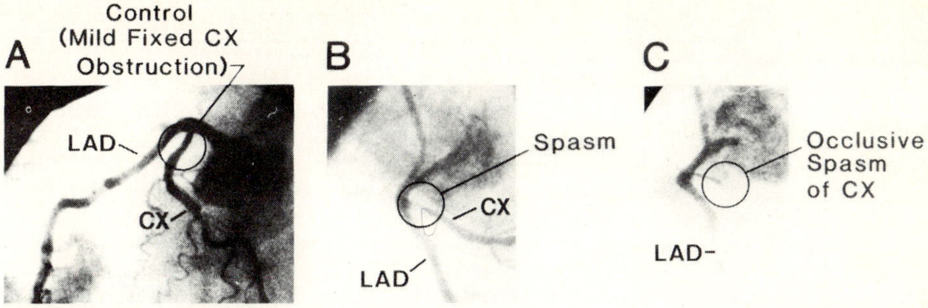

FIGURE 12-2
A coronary arteriogram in a patient with spontaneous spasm of the circumflex coronary artery. (*a*) Normal coronary angiogram with the exception of a minor degree of narrowing in the proximal circumflex coronary artery. (*b*) Significant coronary vasoconstriction involving the proximal circumflex coronary artery. (*c*) Obliterative coronary spasm of the circumflex coronary artery. Spasm was subsequently relieved by the administration of sublingual nitroglycerin. *(Study performed by JM Kioschos, Associate Professor of Medicine, University of Iowa.)*

of spasm, global left ventricular hemodynamics often deteriorate [4,5,9,16–19]. The spastic coronary segment either relaxes spontaneously within a few minutes or dilation occurs in response to administration of nitroglycerin [4,5,7–9,12,16–19]. Rarely, prolonged coronary spasm produces acute myocardial infarction [3–5, 9,10,17,24–26].

Perfusion Scintigrams

If thallium 201 is injected intravenously during an episode of intense coronary spasm, scintigrams obtained subsequently demonstrate a perfusion defect in the zone perfused by the spastic vessel [5,19,27,28]. In the same patient, when spasm is not present, thallium 201 perfusion scintigrams demonstrate normal distribution of coronary blood flow.

These perfusion studies indicate that intense coronary spasm is associated with a striking decrease in regional myocardial perfusion.

Metabolic Studies

Studies which have measured coronary blood flow during a spontaneous episode of coronary spasm have noted that a decrease in flow precedes the onset of angina (Figure 12-3) [27]. Two studies [29,30] have examined several metabolic indices of ischemia (coronary sinus oxygen saturation, lactate extraction or production, pH, and pCO_2) during spontaneous [29] or provoked [30] coronary spasm. Electrocardiographic evidence of spontaneous spasm is preceded by a decrease in coronary oxygen saturation. This change in coronary sinus oxygen saturation also precedes the hemodynamic abnormalities characteristic of coronary spasm (Figure 12-3). Both spontaneous and provoked coronary spasm are associated with myocardial

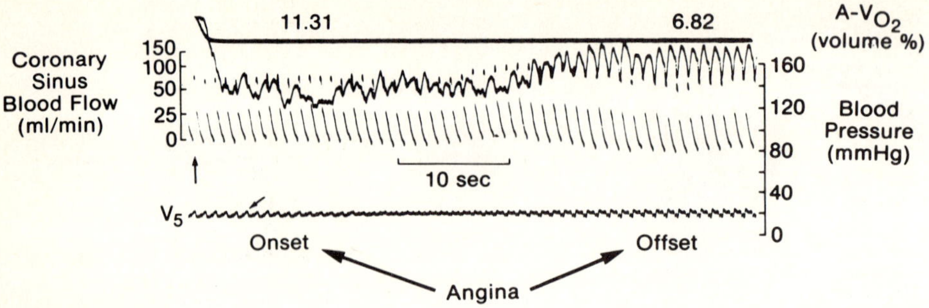

FIGURE 12-3
Measurement of coronary sinus blood flow (thermodilution technique) during an episode of spontaneous coronary spasm. Just preceding the onset of angina, coronary flow decreased and the arterial venous oxygen difference (A-V_{O_2}) across the coronary bed increased. Because these alterations in coronary hemodynamics were not associated with a change in blood pressure or heart rate, it is likely that the change in coronary hemodynamics was the result of spasm of one or more major vessels that drain into the coronary sinus. When coronary hemodynamics returned to control, angina abated. Volume percent = blood oxygen content in volumes percent. (*Modified from data originally presented by RC Curry et al* [30].)

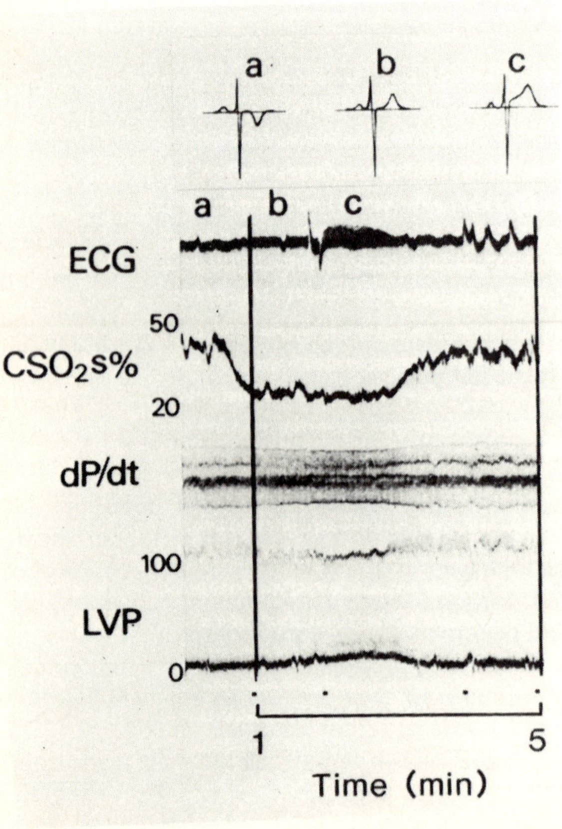

FIGURE 12-4
Continuous measurements of the electrocardiogram (ECG), coronary sinus oxygen saturation ($CSO_2s\%$), left ventricular *dp/dt*, and left ventricular pressure in mmHg before and during an episode of spontaneous coronary spasm. Angina was preceded by a decrease in coronary sinus oxygen saturation, left ventricular *dp/dt*, and left ventricular pressure. This sequence of events suggests that the primary event leading to the onset of angina was coronary spasm. (*Modified from data originally presented by S Chierchia et al* [29].)

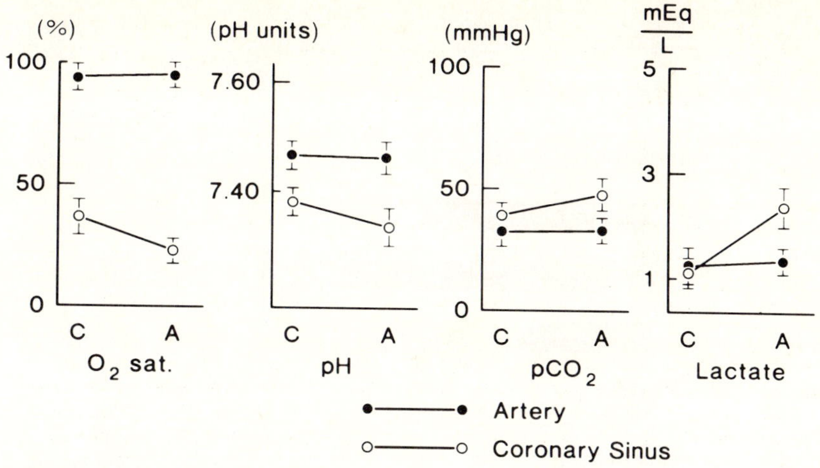

FIGURE 12-5
Metabolic abnormalities associated with ergonovine-induced coronary spasm. C = control; A = angina secondary to ergonovine-induced coronary spasm. Angina secondary to coronary spasm was associated with a decrease in both coronary sinus oxygen saturation and pH and an increase in both coronary sinus pCO_2 and lactate. These metabolic indices indicate that coronary spasm was associated with myocardial ischemia. (*Redrawn from data originally presented by RC Curry et al* [*30*].)

lactate production (Figure 12-4) [29,30]. In association with lactate production, coronary sinus pH decreased and pCO_2 increased (Figure 12-5) [29].

These metabolic studies strongly support the notion that coronary spasm is associated with significant myocardial ischemia.

In summary, hemodynamic, angiographic, scintigraphic, and metabolic studies have firmly established that intense spasm of major coronary vessels occurs in humans and produces marked myocardial ischemia. The frequency of these abnormalities in patients with various clinical syndromes associated with coronary heart disease is less well established. The early experience of Maseri et al. [5] in Italy suggested that in 10 percent of patients admitted to the hospital with anginal pain spontaneous coronary spasm contributed significantly to the pathogenesis of their symptoms. More recently, Bertrand et al. [20a] have reported that provocative testing with methylergonovine will elicit evidence of focal coronary spasm in 38 percent of patients who experience angina at rest and 20 percent of patients who have suffered a recent transmural myocardial infarction (Figure 12-6). Recent experience of Maseri and Chierchia in England suggests that 45 percent of patients with anginal syndromes have coronary spasm which can be provoked with ergonovine infusion (see below).

APPROACHES TO PROVOKING CORONARY SPASM

Because coronary spasm can occur spontaneously, stimuli which have been reported to provoke it should be carefully scrutinized.

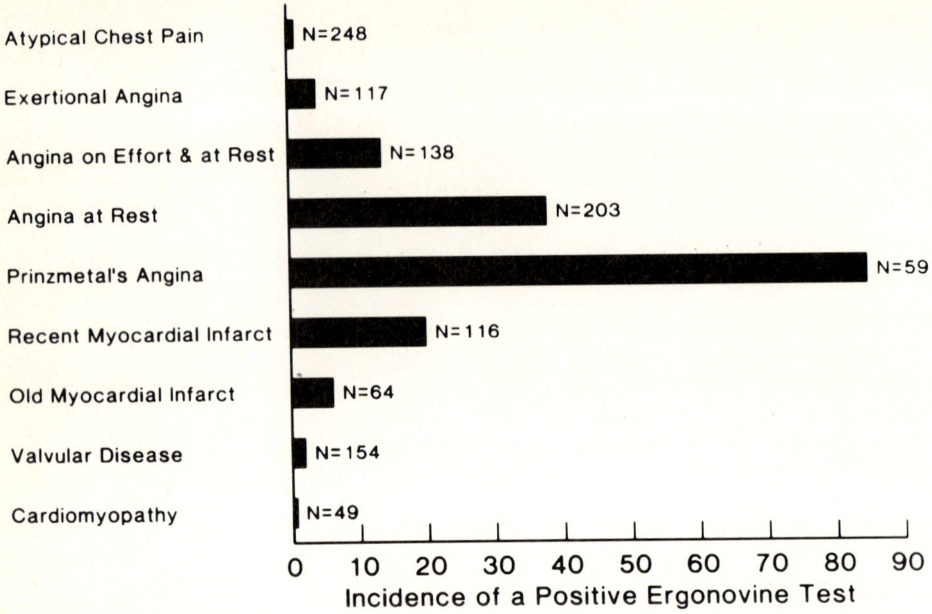

FIGURE 12-6
Incidence of provokable coronary spasm (IV methylergonovine 0.4 mg) in various patient groups. In each clinical group, patients with normal coronary vessels and fixed obstructive lesions are included. Recent myocardial infarct = transmural myocardial infarction within 6 weeks of the ergonovine tests; old myocardial infarct = transmural myocardial infarction occurred more than 6 weeks prior to the ergonovine test. *(Data presented are based on studies reported by ME Bertrand et al* [20a].)

Two types of mechanically induced coronary spasm occur. The mechanical irritation of a coronary vessel that occurs in the course of coronary angiography occasionally produces spasm [31–34]. Although this "catheter-induced spasm" can complicate the interpretation of coronary angiograms, it plays no role in the pathogenesis of angina pectoris. Catheter-induced spasm is rarely associated with electrocardiographic or hemodynamic evidence of myocardial ischemia or chest discomfort [31–34]. Furthermore, the presence of catheter-induced spasm does not identify a subset of patients who are likely to have spontaneous spasm or spasm inducible by ergonovine infusion [20a].

The coronary spasm that results from mechanical irritation of a coronary vessel during coronary angioplasty has different clinical features from that which occurs in the course of coronary angiography. When coronary spasm occurs during angioplasty it is often severe and associated with chest pain and hemodynamic and electrocardiographic evidence of severe myocardial ischemia. This type of spasm occasionally cannot be relieved by nitrates. In this situation, the "spasm" that occurs may be indistinguishable from coronary dissection or occlusion of the involved vessel. Furthermore, spasm and dissection may occur simultaneously during the course of coronary angioplasty.

Many reports indicate that adrenergic stimuli can provoke coronary spasm in susceptible patients [35–39]. Reflex or pharmacologic stimulation of alpha receptors in coronary vessels occasionally provoke intense vasoconstriction of the large coronary vessels. In some studies, the administration of an alpha-blocking agent prevented recurrences of coronary spasm [37]. Recent work by Maseri and Chierchia suggests that the cold pressor test—a stimulus that evokes intense sympathetic activity—is only 25 percent as effective as intravenous ergonovine in provoking coronary spasm in susceptible patients.

A variety of other compounds and conditions have been reported to produce spasm, including methacholine [40], alcohol [41], alkalosis [42], exercise [43,44], epinephrine [36], propranolol [36], coronary bypass surgery [45], and acute myocardial infarction [46]. The relative importance of these stimuli in the pathogenesis of coronary spasm remains to be defined.

In discussing the ergonovine test, it is important to recognize that the presence or absence of fixed coronary obstructive disease affects the safety, sensitivity, and specificity of this diagnostic procedure.

The ergonovine test has proven to be the most effective method of provoking coronary spasm in susceptible patients [5,7,8,47–52]. The mechanism by which ergonovine produces spasm is uncertain. The ergot alkaloids in general have alpha agonist activity. However, it is notable that the alpha agonist activity of ergonovine is particularly weak. Nonetheless, in vitro studies suggest that part of the vasoconstriction produced by ergonovine is mediated by activation of alpha receptors [53b]. Ergonovine also stimulates serotonergic receptors [53,53a]. In vitro studies suggest that serotonergic receptors may be particularly abundant in atherosclerotic vessels [53b]. Studies in isolated arteries suggest that the constriction produced by ergonovine can be partially prevented by a serotonin antagonist [53b–53d].

The intravenous infusion of ergonovine to provoke coronary spasm was first suggested by Stein [53e]. This approach was reintroduced by Schroeder et al. in 1977 [47].

The ergonovine infusion test has proven to be reasonably safe in patients with normal coronary vessels or mild obstructive coronary disease. In a collected series of 862 patients who underwent testing with ergonovine and coronary angiography, no deaths occurred [8]. Nonetheless, deaths, myocardial infarction, and life-threatening arrhythmias have occurred during ergonovine infusion tests [20a,53f,53g]. In many cardiac catheterization laboratories, including the one at the University of Iowa, ergonovine is considered unsafe in patients with severe obstructive coronary disease [20a].

In one study, following an appropriate dose of intravenous ergonovine 98 percent of patients (110 of 112) with the classical features of variant angina ST segment elevation associated with substernal chest pain at rest developed localized coronary spasm in a coronary vessel concordant with the localization of the electrocardiographic abnormality [8]. In another clinical series [20a] 50 of 59 patients (85 percent) with variant angina developed focal coronary spasm. It should be emphasized that most of these patients had normal coronary vessels or only mild fixed coronary obstructive lesions. Thus, in this patient subgroup, the ergonovine test had a sensitivity of 85 to 98 percent for detecting the presence of coronary spasm in patients with clinical evidence of variant angina.

In patients *without spasm* ergonovine produces mild diffuse coronary narrowing (about 18 percent decrease in coronary diameter) [49]. Patients with no clinical history of angina, however, rarely have coronary spasm following intravenous ergonovine [48]. In a series of patients reported by Heupler et al. [48], no patient (n = 15) with normal coronary arteries and a negative history of angina had a positive ergonovine test. Furthermore, of 63 patients with atypical chest pain and normal or mild coronary lesions, none developed spasm in response to ergonovine infusion [8]. In another series [20a], methylergonovine induced focal coronary spasm in about 1 percent of 397 patients with normal coronary vessels and various cardiac syndromes including atypical chest pain (n = 221), cardiomyopathy (n = 44), and valvular heart disease (n = 32) (Figure 12-6). Thus, in patients with normal coronary vessels and no clinical history suggestive of coronary spasm, the ergonovine test has a high degree of specificity.

Although ergonovine infusion is reasonably safe in patients with normal or near normal coronary vessels, this diagnostic procedure is less safe in patients with severe, fixed, coronary obstructions. In a recent review based on data compiled from many clinical studies, Meyers [53f] noted that potentially significant complications from ergonovine tests occurred in 8 percent of 257 patients with spasm and normal coronary arteries; important complications occurred in 23 percent of 87 patients with spasm superimposed on fixed coronary obstructive disease. In a large series of ergonovine tests reported by Bertrand et al. [20a], 5 percent of 134 patients with provokable spasm experienced potentially life-threatening arrhythmias. In this clinical series, no irreversible complications occurred.

Ergonovine infusion is a highly sensitive and specific method of demonstrating evidence of coronary spasm in susceptible patients with normal or near normal coronary arteries. In contrast, the sensitivity and specificity of ergonovine testing in patients with severe fixed coronary obstructions has not been so well defined. As a consequence of these problems, the diagnosis of superimposed spasm in patients with severe, fixed coronary obstructions often remains uncertain.

METHODS OF RELIEVING CORONARY SPASM

Nitroglycerin, administered by any route (sublingual, intravenous, or intracoronary) is very effective in relieving coronary spasm regardless of the stimulus that provoked the coronary constriction [3–10]. Coronary relaxation in spastic vascular segments usually occurs within seconds following parenteral administration of nitroglycerin. Nitrates can also prevent ergonovine from provoking coronary spasm [52].

Several calcium blocking agents–nifedipine [54], verapamil [55], diltiazem [56], and perhexiline [57]–are very useful in relieving coronary spasm or preventing its recurrence. These agents can be administered intravenously, via the buccal mucosa or orally. One large clinical study has shown that greater than 90 percent, of patients with variant angina who received oral nifedipine experienced a marked decrease in the frequency of their anginal attacks [54].

A few clinical studies suggest that the administration of a beta blocker, such as propranolol, may be ineffective [58] or may actually potentiate coronary spasm [59] in susceptible patients. Although it is tempting to attribute this to unrestrained alpha constriction of coronary vessels, this hypothesis is unproven. The vasoconstrictor effects of alpha-adenergic stimulation on normal coronary vessels are modest (see Chapter 5).

Two features of coronary spasm have brought this clinical entity to the forefront of clinical cardiology: a sensitive and specific provocative test (ergonovine) and an effective therapeutic regimen (nitroglycerin and calcium-blocking agents).

MECHANISMS OF CORONARY SPASM

Any proposed mechanism of coronary spasm must provide an explanation for the following important clinical features of this disease:

1 Spasm is intermittent and unassociated with any obvious external stimulus, such as an increase in myocardial oxygen demand or a marked change in autonomic tone.

2 Spasm involves selected coronary vascular segments. In most patients coronary spasm occurs in one vascular segment. Adjacent coronary vessels with similar angiographic anatomy remain unaffected by the disease process.

3 The coronary constriction associated with the coronary spasm is *intense*. Potent endogenous coronary vasoconstrictors such as angiotensin, vasopressin, and thromboxane produce only mild to moderate coronary vasoconstriction in vivo when they are administered in doses that are clinically relevant.

4 Only a small percentage of patients with atherosclerotic coronary disease have a clinically obvious form of coronary spasm. Presumably, spasm of lesser severity or frequency occurs in a larger percentage of patients with coronary artery disease.

5 Two time-related phenomena affect the clinical presentation of patients with coronary spasm. First, during any given day, spontaneous spasm tends to occur more frequently in the evening and in the early morning hours. Second, patients with coronary spasm exhibit substantial spontaneous variations over a time span of days, weeks, and months in the intensity and frequency of their episodes of coronary spasm. Maseri has noted that when patients with coronary spasm have ergonovine tests on two separate occasions, the dose of ergonovine needed to provoke spasm may vary by tenfold or more between the two studies.

At present, the mechanism of coronary spasm has not been established. Furthermore, there is no in vivo animal model which even vaguely resembles this disease entity. Many mechanisms have been suggested that may contribute to the pathogenesis of coronary spasm. These include increases in adrenergic tone [36–38], release of thromboxane [60], and platelet aggregates [61].

Provocative studies relevant to the potential mechanisms of coronary spasm have emanated from the laboratory of Phillip Henry [53b,62,63]. These studies and others in isolated vessels have shown that hypercholesterolemia or diet-induced atherosclerosis can dramatically shift the dose response relationships of vasoconstrictors to the left [53b,53c,62,63]. Henry has postulated that alterations in the lipid composition of vascular endothelium may allow fat-soluble vasoconstrictor agents more ready access to vascular smooth muscle. Thus, their effects would be potentiated.

Thus far, in vivo studies have not provided strong support for Henry's hypothesis. Rosendorff et al. [64] have shown that in awake dogs with hypercholesterolemia, subthreshold doses of norepinephrine cause coronary vasoconstriction. However, studies by Johannsen et al. [65] in anesthetized dogs with hypercholesterolemia have not shown any potentiation of coronary vasoconstriction to infusions of vasoactive agents, including norepinephrine. Recent studies in the coronary physiology laboratory at the University of Iowa suggest that, in vivo, atherosclerotic coronary vessels in cynomolgus monkeys are not particularly sensitive to the vasoconstrictor effects of either phenylephrine or ergonovine.

CLINICAL IMPORTANCE OF CORONARY SPASM

It is now certain that coronary spasm plays a significant role in the pathogenesis of ischemic heart disease. However, the extent to which coronary spasm participates in clinical syndromes other than variant angina remains to be defined. Recent data, however, suggest that coronary spasm could be important in unstable or rest angina [3–5], exercise-induced angina [43,44], acute myocardial infarction [3–5,9,10,17,24–26], and sudden cardiac death [3–5]. The concept that active coronary vasoconstriction plays a key role in the pathogenesis of ischemic heart disease is extremely attractive because pharmacologic therapeutic approaches hold great promise.

REFERENCES

1 Osler W: The Lumeleian lectures on angina pectoris. *Lancet* 1: 697, 1910.

2 Blumgart HL, Schlesinger MJ, Davis D: Studies on the relation of the clinical manifestations of angina pectoris, coronary thrombosis and myocardial infarction to the pathologic findings, with particular reference to the significance of the collateral circulation. *Am Heart J* 10: 567, 1935.

3 Prinzmetal M, Kemnamer R, Merliss R, Wade T, Born N: Angina pectoris. I. The variant form of angina pectoris. *Am J Med* 27: 375, 1959.

4 Maseri A: Variant angina and coronary vasospasm: Clues to a broader understanding of angina pectoris. *Cardiovasc Med* 4: 647, 1979.

5 Maseri A, Severi S, DeNes M, L'Abbate A, Chierchia S, Marzilli M, Ballestra AM, Parodi O, Biagini A, Distante A: "Variant" Angina: One aspect of a continuous spectrum of vasospastic myocardial ischemia. *Am J Cardiol* 42: 1019, 1978.

6 Hillis LD, Braunwald E: Coronary artery spasm. *N Engl J Med* 229: 695, 1978.

7 Helfant RH: Coronary arterial spasm and provocative testing in ischemic heart disease. *Am J Cardiol* 41: 787, 1978.

8 Heupler FA Jr: Provocative testing for coronary arterial spasm: Risk, method and rationale. *Am J Cardiol* 46: 335, 1980.

9 Conti CR: Coronary artery spasm. Cardiovasc Rev Rep 1: 17, 1980.

10 Braunwald E: Coronary artery spasm as a cause of myocardial ischemia. *J Lab Clin Med* 97: 299, 1981.

11 Roughgarden JW: Circulatory changes associated with spontaneous angina pectoris. *Am J Med* 41: 947, 1966.

11a Cannon DS, Harrison DC, Schroeder JS: Hemodynamic observations in patients with unstable angina pectoris. *Am J Cardiol* 33: 17, 1974.

11b Papapietro SE, Niess GS, Paine TD, Mantle JA, Rackley CE, Russell RO Jr, Rogers WJ: Transient electrocardiographic changes in patients with unstable angina: Relation to coronary arterial anatomy. *Am J Cardiol* 46: 28, 1980.

12 Gensini GG, Di Georgi S, Murad-Netto S, Black A: Arteriographic demonstration of coronary artery spasm and its release after the use of a vasodilator in a case of angina pectoris and in the experimental animal. *Angiology* 13: 550, 1962.

13 Dhurandar RW, Watt DL, Silver MD, Trimble AS, Adelman AG: Prinzmetal's variant form of angina with arteriographic evidence of coronary arterial spasm. *Am J Cardiol* 30: 902, 1972.

14 Oliva RB, Potts DE, Pluss RG: Coronary arterial spasm in Prinzmetal angina: Documentation by coronary arteriography. *N Engl J Med* 288: 745, 1973.

15 Schroeder J, Silverman JF, Harrison DC: Right coronary arterial spasm causing Prinzmetal's variant angina. *Chest* 65: 573, 1974.

16 Endo M, Kanda I, Hosada S, Hayashi H, Hirosawa K, Konno S: Prinzmetal's variant form of angina pectoris: Re-evaluation of mechanisms. *Circulation* 52: 33, 1975.

17 Maseri A, Mimmo R, Chierchia S, Marchesi C, Pesola A, L'Abbate A: Coronary spasm as a cause of acute myocardial ischemia in man. *Chest* 68: 625, 1975.

18 Higgins CB, Wexler L, Silverman J, Schroeder JS: Clinical and arteriographic features of Prinzmetal variant angina: Documentation of arterial spasm. *Am J Cardiol* 37: 831, 1976.

19 Maseri A, Parodi O, Severi S, Pesola A: Transient transmural reduction of myocardial blood flow, demonstrated by thallium-201 scintigraphy, as a cause of variant angina. *Circulation* 54: 280, 1976.

20 Selzer A, Langston M, Ruggeroli C, Cohn K: Clinical syndrome of variant angina with normal coronary arteriogram. *N Engl J Med* 295: 1344, 1976.

20a Bertrand ME, LaBlanche JM, Tilmant PY, Thieuleux FA, Delforge MR, Carre AG, Asseman P, Berzin B, Libersa C, Laurent JM: Frequency of provoked coronary arterial spasm in 1089 consecutive patients undergoing coronary arteriography. *Circulation* 65: 1299, 1982.

21 Perez-Gomez F, DeDios RM, Rey J, Aguado AG: Prinzmetal's angina: Reflex cardiovascular response during episode of pain. *Br Heart J* 42: 81, 1979.

22 Thames MD, Klopfenste NHS, Abboud FM, Mark AL, Walker JL: Preferential distribution of inhibitory cardiac receptors with vagal afferents to the inferoposterior wall of the left ventricle activated during coronary occlusion in the dog. *Circ Res* 43: 512, 1978.

23 Felder RB, Thames MD: Interaction between cardiac receptors and sinoartic baroreceptors in the control of efferent cardiac sympathetic nerve activity during myocardial ischemia in dogs. *Circ Res* 45: 728, 1979.

24 Hellstron HR: The injury-vasospasm hypothesis of ischemic heart disease, revisited. *Am Heart J* 94: 642, 1977.

25 Johnson AD, Detwiter JA: Coronary spasm, variant angina, and recurrent myocardial infarction. *Circulation* 55: 947, 1977.

26 Maseri A, L'Abbate A, Baroldi G, Chierchia S, Marzilli M, Ballestra AM, Severi S, Parodi O, Biagini A, Distante A, Pesola A: Coronary vasospasm as a possible cause of myocardial infarction. A conclusion derived from the study of "preinfarction" angina. *N Engl J Med* 299: 1271, 1978.

27 Ricci DR, Orlick AE, Doherty PW, Cipriano PR, Harrison DC: Reduction of coronary blood flow during coronary artery spasm occurring spontaneously and after provocation by ergonovine maleate. *Circulation* 57: 392, 1978.

28 Berman ND, McLaughlin P, Huckell V, Mahon W, Morch J, Adelman A: Prinzmetal's angina with coronary artery spasm: Angiographic, pharmacologic and radionuclide perfusion studies. *Am J Med* 60: 727, 1976.

29 Chierchia S, Brunelli C, Simonetti I, Lazzari M, Maseri A: Sequence of events in angina at rest: Primary reduction in coronary flow. *Circulation* 61: 759, 1980.

30 Curry RC Jr, Pepine CJ, Sabom MB, Feldman RL, Christie LG, Varnell JH, Conti CR: Hemodynamic and myocardial metabolic effects of ergonovine in patients with chest pain. *Circulation* 58: 648, 1978.

31 Conti RC, Levin DC, Grossman W: Coronary angiography, in *Cardiac Catheterization and Angiography*, 2d ed, W Grossman (ed). Philadelphia, Lea & Febiger, 1980, p. 167.

32 Chahine RA, Raizner AE, Ishimori T, Luchi RJ, McIntosh HD: The incidence and clinical implications of coronary artery spasm. *Circulation* 52: 972, 1975.

33 O'Reilly RJ, Spellberg RD, King TW: Recognition of proximal right coronary artery spasm during coronary arteriography. *Radiology* 95: 305, 1970.

34 Gensini GG: Coronary arteriography, in *Heart Disease: A Textbook of Cardiovascular Medicine*, Vol 1, E Braunwald (ed). Philadelphia, Saunders, 1980, chap 10, p 308.

35 Yasue H, Touyama M, Shimamoto M, Kato H, Tanaka S, Akiyama F: Role of autonomic nervous system in the pathogenesis of Prinzmetal's variant form of angina. *Circulation* 50: 534, 1974.

36 Yasue H, Touyama M, Kato H, Tanaka S, Akiyama F: Prinzmetal's variant form of angina as a manifestation of alpha-adrenergic receotormediated coronary artery spasm: Documentation by coronary arteriography. *Am Heart J* 91: 148, 1976.

37 Ricci DR, Orlick AE, Cipriano PR, Gunthaner DF, Harrison DC: Altered adrenergic activity in coronary arterial spasm: Insight into mechanism based on study of coronary hemodynamics and the electrocardiogram. *Am J Cardiol* 43: 1073, 1979.

38 Raizner AE, Chahine RA, Ishimori T, Verani MS, Zacca N, Jamal N, Miller RR, Luchi RJ: Provocation of coronary artery spasm by the cold pressor test: Hemodynamic, arteriographic and quantitative angiographic observations. *Circulation* 62: 925, 1980.

39 Mudge GH Jr, Grossman W, Mills RM Jr, Lesch M, Braunwald E: Reflex increase in coronary vascular resistance in patients with ischemic heart disease. *N Engl J Med* 295: 1333, 1976.

40 Endo M, Hirosawa K, Kancko N, Hase K, Inoue Y, Konno S: Prinzmetal's variant angina: Coronary arteriogram and left ventriculogram during angina attack induced by methacholine. *N Engl J Med* 294: 250, 1976.

41 Fernandez D, Rosenthal J, Cohen L, Hammond G, Wolfson S: Alcohol-induced Prinzmetal variant angina. *Am J Cardiol* 32: 238, 1973.

42 Yasue H, Nagao M, Omote S, Takizawa A, Miwa K, Tanaka S: Coronary arterial spasm and Prinzmetal's variant form of angina induced by hyperventilation and Tris-buffer infusion. *Circulation* 58: 56, 1978.

43 Specchia G, deServi S, Falcone C, Bramucci E, Angoli L, Mussini A, Marinoni P, Montemartini C, Bobba P: Coronary arterial spasm as a cause of exercise-induced ST segment elevation in patients with variant angina. *Circulation* 59: 948, 1979.

44 Yasue H, Omote S, Takizawa A, Nagao M, Miwa K, Tanaka S: Exertional angina pectoris caused by coronary arterial spasm: Effects of various drugs. *Am J Cardiol* 43: 647, 1979.

45 Buxton AE, Goldberg S, Harken A, Hirshfeld J Jr, Kastor JA: Coronary-artery spasm immediately after myocardial revascularization, recognition and management. *N Engl J Med* 304: 1249, 1981.

46 Oliva PB, Breckinridge JC: Arteriographic evidence of coronary arterial spasm in acute myocardial infarction. *Circulation* 56: 366, 1977.

47 Schroeder JS, Bolen JL, Quint RA, Clark DA, Hayden WG, Higgins CB, Wexler L: Provocation of coronary spasm with ergonovine maleate. New test with results in 57 patients undergoing coronary arteriography. *Am J Cardiol* 40: 487, 1977.

48 Heupler F, Proudfit W, Razavi M, Shirey E, Greenstreet R, Sheldon W: Ergonovine maleate provocative test for coronary arterial spasm. *Am J Cardiol* 41: 631, 1978.

49 Curry RC, Pepine CJ, Sabom MB, Feldman RL, Christie LG, Conti CR: Effects of ergonovine in patients with and without coronary artery disease. *Circulation* 56: 803, 1977.

50 Curry RC, Pepine, CJ, Sabom MB, Feldman FL, Christie LG, Varnell JA, Conti CR: Hemodynamic and myocardial metabolic effects of ergonovine in patients with chest pain. *Circulation* 58: 648, 1978.

51 Curry RC, Pepine CJ, Sabom MB, Conti CR: Similarities of ergonovine-induced and spontaneous attacks of variant angina. *Circulation* 59: 307, 1979.

52 Conti CR, Curry RC, Christie LG, Pepine CJ: Clinical use of provocative pharmacoangiography in patients with chest pain. *Adv Cardiol* 26: 44, 1979.

53 Innes IR: Identification of the smooth muscle excitory receptors for ergot alkaloids. *Br J Pharmacol* 19: 120, 1962.

53a Berde B: Pharmacology of ergot alkaloids in clinical use. *Med J* 2(suppl 3): 3, 1978.

53b Henry D, Yokoyama M: Supersensitivity of atherosclerotic rabbit aorta to ergonovine-mediation by a serotonergic mechanism. *J Clin Invest* 66: 306, 1980.

53c Yokoyama M, Akita H, Tetsuo M, et al: Hyperactivity of arterial smooth muscles exposed to hyperlipidemia in response to ergonovine mediated by serotonergic mechanism. *Circulation* 64(suppl 4): 122, 1981.

53d Yokoyama H, Akita H, Tetsuo M, et al: Serotonergic mechanism responsible for ergonovine-induced coronary contraction. *Circulation* 64(suppl 4): 121, 1981.

53e Stein I: Observations on the action of ergonovine on the coronary circulation and its use in the diagnosis of coronary artery insufficiency. *Am Heart J* 37: 36, 1949.

53f Meyers DG: Ergonovine provocation of coronary artery spasm. *Cardiovasc Rev Rep* 3: 855, 1982.

53g Buxton A, Goldberg S, Hirshfeld JW, et al: Refractory ergonovine-induced coronary vasospasm. *Am J Cardiol* 46: 329, 1980.

54 Antman E, Muller J, Goldberg S, MacAlpin R, Rubenfire M, Tabatznik B, Liang C, Heupler F, Achuff S, Reichek N, Geltman E, Kerin NZ, Neff RK, Braunwald E: Nifedipine therapy for coronary artery spasm: Experience in 127 patients. *N Engl J Med* 302: 1269, 1980.

55 Solberg L, Nissen R, Vlietstra R, Callahan J: Prinzmetal's variant angina—response to verapamil. *Mayo Clin Proc* 53: 256, 1978.

56 Rosenthal SJ, Ginsburg R, Lamb I, et al: Efficacy of diltiazem for control of symptoms of coronary arterial spasm. *Am J Cardiol* 46: 1027, 1980.

57 Mizgala HF, Crittin J, Water DD, et al: Results of immediate and long term treatment of variant angina with perhexiline maleate. *Circulation* 60: 181, 1979.

58 Endo M, Kanda I, Hosoda S, et al: Prinzmetal's variant form of angina pectoris. *Circulation* 52: 33, 1975.

59 Muller JE, Gunther SJ: Nifedipine therapy for Prinzmetal's angina. *Circulation* 57: 137, 1978.

60 Levi RI, Smith JB, Silver MS, et al: Detection of thromboxane B_2 in the peripheral blood of patients with Prinzmetal's angina. *Prostaglandins Med* 2: 243, 1979.

61 Folts JD, Crowell EB, Rowe GG: Platelet aggregation in partially obstructed vessels and its elimination with aspirin. *Circulation* 54: 365, 1976.

62 Yokoyama M, Henry PD: Sensitization of isolated canine coronary arteries to calcium ions after exposure to cholesterol. *Circ Res* 45: 479, 1979.

63 Yokoyama M, Goldman M, Henry PD: Supersensitivity of atherosclerotic arteries to ergonovine partially mediated by a serotonergic mechanism. *Circulation* 60: 100, 1979.

64 Rosendorff C, Hoffman JIE, Verrier ED, Rouleau J, Boerboom LE: Cholesterol potentiates the coronary artery response to norepinephrine in anesthetized and conscious dogs. *Circ Res* 48: 320, 1981.

65 Johannsen UJ, Mark AL, Marcus M, Armstrong ML: Effects of dietary hyperlipoproteinemia on coronary vascular responsiveness in vivo. *Circulation* 64: 267, 1980.

CHAPTER **13**

EFFECTS OF CARDIAC HYPERTROPHY ON THE CORONARY CIRCULATION

Clinicians have long suspected that hypertrophied hearts have an inadequate coronary circulation. This clinical suspicion was fostered by the observation that some patients with cardiac hypertrophy and anatomically normal epicardial coronary vessels complain of angina pectoris [1,2]. Also, electrocardiographic abnormalities suggestive of myocardial ischemia have been reported frequently in patients with cardiac hypertrophy in the absence of coronary obstructive disease [2,3].

Perfusion abnormalities in hypertrophied hearts may be caused by two mechanisms: (1) hemodynamic alterations related to the cause of the hypertrophy [4] and (2) architectural changes in the coronary vascular bed [5]. Hemodynamic alterations can produce abnormalities in both total coronary blood flow and the transmural distribution of myocardial perfusion (see Chapter 5). This chapter focuses on the physiological consequences of structural changes in the coronary vascular bed that occur in hypertrophied ventricles.

STRUCTURAL ALTERATIONS IN THE CORONARY CIRCULATION IN THE HYPERTROPHIED HEART

Cardiac hypertrophy is associated with vascular abnormalities at several levels in the coronary tree. The epicardial coronary vessels do not enlarge appropriately when ventricular hypertrophy occurs in response to a pressure load [6]. Because coronary blood flow via the conduit vessels is increased when the heart enlarges, it is likely that large vessel resistance is slightly increased in hypertrophied hearts. When hypertrophy occurs secondary to systemic hypertension, the wall/lumen ratio of coronary arterioles is increased because of hypertrophy of the vascular wall [7]. Hallback-Nordlander et al. [8] have shown that this type of structural change in coronary vessels limits coronary dilation and augments maximal coronary constriction. Capillary density in the myocardium is also altered in hypertrophied hearts. In both left and right ventricular hypertophy secondary to a pressure load, most laboratories have reported that capillary density decreased by 20 to 30 percent [9–11]. Pathologists have frequently observed that the subendocardium of hypertrophied ventricles is diffusely fibrotic [12]. This could result from myocardial ischemia secondary to inadequate coronary perfusion. Thus, there is anatomic evidence which supports the concept that the coronary circulation is inadequate in hypertophied hearts. However, in general, there is a paucity of precise quantitative information about the anatomic characteristics of the coronary circulation at multiple levels in the coronary bed in hypertrophied hearts.

EARLY PHYSIOLOGICAL STUDIES CONCERNING EFFECTS OF HYPERTROPHY ON THE CORONARY CIRCULATION

Several decades ago, investigators [13,14] measured flow per gram at rest in patients with hypertrophied ventricles and reported no abnormalities. In these studies, the transmural distribution of coronary flow was not assessed and measurements of flow during stress were not obtained.

CONCEPTUAL FRAMEWORK

In 1978 our group [15] published a conceptual diagram (Figure 13-1) concerning possible interactions between changes in cardiac mass and coronary vascular growth. This conceptual approach, with minor alterations, has served us very well. In this diagram, the size of the boxes represents cardiac mass and the circles depict the cross-sectional area of coronary resistance vessels. If cardiac enlargement were accompanied by excessive vascular growth (top right box in Figure 13-1), coronary resistance during maximal coronary dilation would decrease considerably. Such a result can be expected because the resistance across a parallel vascular bed decreases as the number of vascular channels and their cross-sectional area increase. If cardiac enlargement were accompanied by an appropriate degree of vascular growth (top left box in Figure 13-1), minimal vascular resistance per gram would remain unchanged and minimal vascular resistance in the entire hypertrophied

FIGURE 13-1
Conceptual diagram which relates ventricular mass to the cross-sectional area of the coronary resistance vessels. The center box reflects the normal situation; i.e., the ratio of ventricular mass (size of the box) to size of the vascular bed (total area of the circles within the box) is normal.

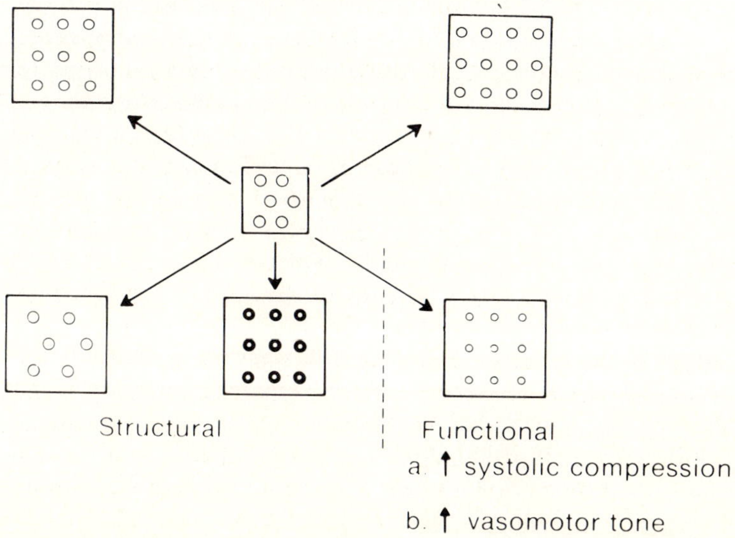

chamber would decrease in proportion to the increase in cardiac mass. Alternatively, if the change in the size of the cross-sectional area of the coronary vascular bed did not keep pace with the increase in cardiac mass, total vascular resistance would not decrease as the heart enlarged. At least three distinct mechanisms which are not mutually exclusive could limit the cross-sectional area of the coronary vascular bed (see bottom three boxes in Figure13-1). These mechanisms include decreased vascular growth (left bottom box), compromised cross-sectional area of resistance vessels secondary to vascular hypertrophy (center bottom box), and compression of coronary vascular channels by extravascular forces (right bottom box). Under various conditions, all three mechanisms contribute to impaired coronary vascular reserve in hypertrophied ventricles.

PHYSIOLOGICAL STUDIES IN ANIMALS

Since 1975, a large number of experiments in animals have examined the effects of various types of cardiac hypertrophy on coronary reserve. These studies have utilized sophisticated methodology and many different animal models of hypertrophy. Furthermore, many studies examined awake, chronically instrumented animals during a variety of perturbations which produce coronary vasodilation of variable intensity. Most studies focused on the effects of pressure-induced left ventricular hypertrophy on the coronary circulation.

EFFECTS OF PRESSURE-INDUCED LEFT VENTRICULAR HYPERTROPHY ON THE CORONARY CIRCULATION

Myocardial Perfusion at Rest

Almost all studies in animal models of left ventricular hypertrophy have shown that when the increase in muscle mass stabilizes following application of a stimulus which produces left ventricular hypertrophy, flow per gram in the enlarged left ventricle is normal (Figure 13-2) [15–27]. Sasayama et al. [28] demonstrated that left ventricular wall stress increased substantially immediately following the imposition of the pressure load. Over a period of weeks, increased ventricular wall thickness returned wall stress to control levels. Because the major determinants of myocardial oxygen consumption, wall stress, heart rate, and myocardial contractility are near normal in hypertrophied ventricles, it is not surprising that flow per gram is not altered. Even so, total flow to the enlarged ventricle should be increased. This can be demonstrated experimentally when hypertrophy is severe or differences in cardiac mass secondary to body mass or animal breed are minimized.

The transmural distribution of resting left ventricular perfusion is usually not altered unless hypertrophy is intense (greater than 75 percent increase in left ventricular mass). In dogs with severe left ventricular hypertrophy secondary to coarctation of the aorta, subendocardial flow is usually equal to or less than subepicardial flow and the greatest flow occurs in the midwall layers of the left

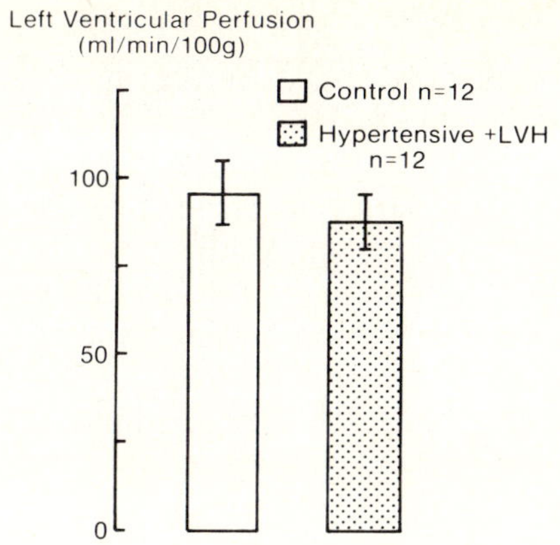

FIGURE 13-2
Left ventricular perfusion per gram of ventricle in normal and hypertrophied hearts. Stable pressure-induced left ventricular hypertrophy (hypertensive + LVH) does not increase flow per unit weigh in the left ventricle. *(Based on data originally presented by TM Mueller et al* [15].*)*

ventricle [16,17,19,24,25]. This unusual transmural distribution of coronary blood flow suggests that severe pressure-induced left ventricular hypertrophy may alter the transmural distribution of wall stress.

Effects of Tachycardia and Exercise

In normal hearts, when heart rate is doubled by pacing, coronary flow increases about twofold and the ratio of subendocardial to subepicardial flow usually decreases slightly [15,25]. In the pressure-hypertrophied left ventricle, flow invariably increases with pacing, but in some models the increase in subendocardial perfusion is limited [15,25].

The effects of exercise on myocardial perfusion in dogs with pressure-induced cardiac hypertrophy have been variable. If hypertrophy is mild and secondary to hypertension, moderate exercise does not elicit any abnormalities in myocardial perfusion [21,29]. In dogs [17] and miniswine [20] with severe hypertrophy secondary to coarctation of the aorta, strenuous exercise was associated with underperfusion of the subendocardium. It is not certain, however, that this underperfusion was associated with metabolic evidence of myocardial ischemia. In contrast to these studies, Bache et al. [24] noted only minimal perfusion abnormalities, which were limited to the posterior papillary muscle, during intense exercise in dogs with severe hypertrophy secondary to aortic coarctation. In Bache's study, during peak exercise coronary flow increased fivefold in the hypertrophied ventricle.

In summary, in dogs with pressure-induced left ventricular hypertrophy, pacing or exercise elicit mild abnormalities in the transmural distribution of myocardial perfusion. Furthermore, these abnormalities only occur when the stress imposed is near maximal. It should be noted that coronary vascular resistance during pacing or intense exercise is usually greater than the minimal coronary vascular resistance that can be achieved with pharmacologic coronary vasodilation [15,18,25,27].

Minimal Coronary Resistance

All studies that have assessed coronary vascular resistance during maximal coronary dilation have reported that minimal coronary vascular resistance is inappropriately high in animals with pressure-induced left ventricular hypertrophy [15,18,23,25,27] (Figures 13-3 and 13-4). Usually, coronary vascular resistance for the entire ventricle is similar in normal and enlarged hearts and minimal coronary vascular resistance per gram is increased (Figure 13-4). In light of the conceptual framework presented above, this implies that vascular growth has not kept pace with the increase in muscle mass. Although the finding of increased minimal coronary vascular resistance in pressure-induced left ventricluar hypertrophy has been consistent, the actual magnitude of the abnormality is quite small.

Effects of Vascular Hypertrophy Alone on Coronary Vascular Resistance

Wangler et al. [30] determined minimal coronary vascular resistance in the right ventricle of 15-month-old spontaneously hypertensive stroke-prone rats. In this model, hypertension is severe and long-standing, but the right ventricle is of normal size. Thus, the coronary vessels that perfuse the normal right ventricle are exposed to increased intravascular pressure which stimulates smooth muscle hypertrophy in coronary resistance vessels. In this model, minimal coronary vascular resistance in the right ventricle is increased twofold (Figure 13-5) [30]. Thus, coronary vascular hypertrophy, secondary to systemic hypertension, can decrease the cross-sectional area of coronary resistance vessels enough to significantly diminish maximal coronary vasodilator capacity. This same mechanism probably contributes to the decreased coronary vascular reserve in the left ventricle of patients and animals with systemic hypertension.

Effects of Duration of Cardiac Hypertrophy on Coronary Reserve

Because coronary vascular growth can continue throughout a significant portion of an animal's life span, it is possible that after a prolonged period of stable hypertrophy the coronary vasculature could increase sufficiently to return coronary vascular reserve to control levels. Wangler et al. [30] and Peters et al. [31] suggest that this can occur. In spontaneously hypertensive rats (SHR), left ventricular hypertrophy is maximal (30 percent increase in left ventricular mass) when the rats are 7 months old. Thereafter, left ventricular mass remains stable and hypertension persists. Coronary reserve is decreased when left ventricular hypertrophy in SHR is at its peak value (see Figure 13-6). However, after a period of stable left ventricular hypertrophy, coronary reserve returns to normal (Figure 13-6). If left ventricular hypertrophy is more intense (50 percent increase in left ventricular mass), as is the case in the stroke-prone SHR, the abnormality in coronary reserve persists throughout a long segment of the animal's life span (Figure 13-6). These studies indicate that if left ventricular hypertrophy is mild, a prolonged period of stable hypertrophy can modulate the interaction between changes in cardiac mass and coronary vascular growth [30,31]. Anatomic studies

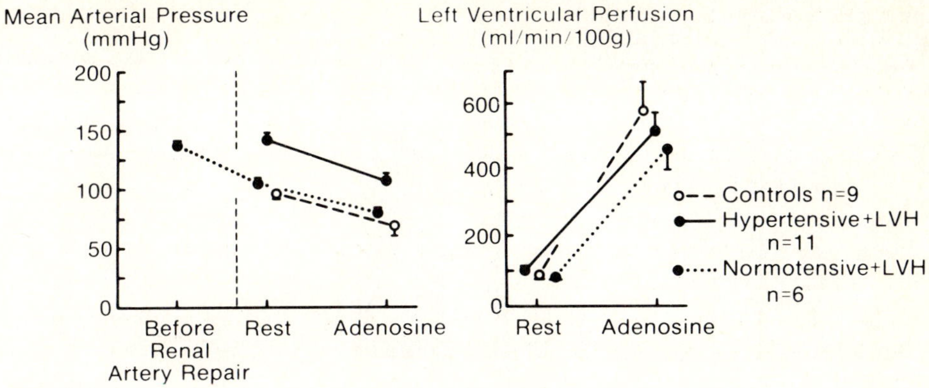

FIGURE 13-3
Effects of adenosine (4.7 μm/kg/min IV) on mean arterial pressure and left ventricular perfusion in three groups of awake dogs: control; renal hypertension + left ventricular hypertrophy (hypertensive + LVH); and left ventricular hypertrophy following relief of hypertension by renal artery repair (normotensive + LVH). Arterial pressure returned to control following renal artery repair. In all three groups adenosine markedly increased left ventricular perfusion. *(Redrawn from data originally presented by TM Mueller et al* [*15*].*)*

FIGURE 13-4
(Left) Minimal coronary vascular resistance expressed per gram or for *(right)* the total left ventricle in three groups of awake dogs: control; hypertension + left ventricular hypertrophy (hypertensive + LVH); and normotension + left ventricular hypertrophy (LVH). The graph shows derived values for coronary vascular resistance based on data presented in Figure 13-3. Minimal coronary vascular resistance was calculated during maximal coronary blood flow produced by IV infusion of adenosine (4.7 μm/kg/min). In the two groups of dogs with left ventricular hypertrophy, minimal coronary vascular resistance per gram was slightly increased *(left)*. Minimal coronary vascular resistance for the entire left ventricle was similar in all three groups of dogs (*right*). This indicates that cardiac hypertrophy was not accompanied by adequate growth of the coronary vasculature. If adequate growth of the coronary vessels had occurred in association with hypertrophy, minimal coronary vascular resistance per gram would be normal in the hypertrophied ventricles and total coronary vascular resistance per ventricle would be decreased in hypertrophied ventricles. *(Based on data presented by TM Mueller et al* [*15*].*)*

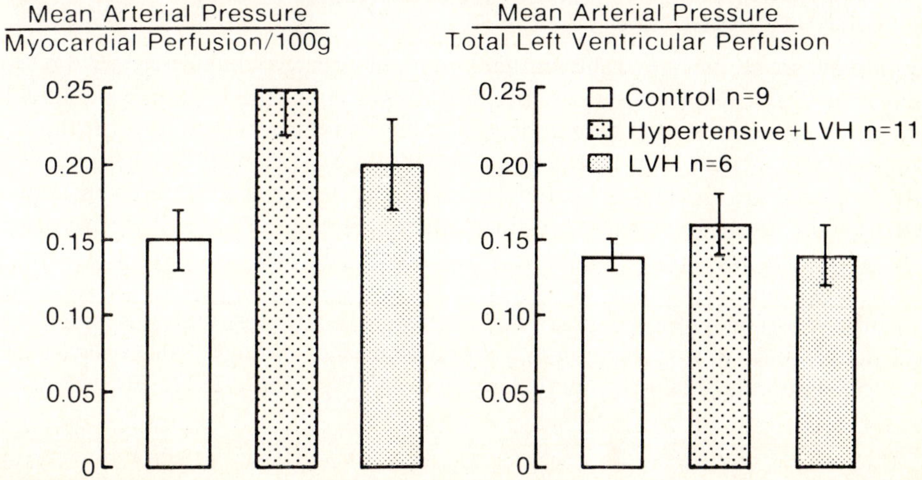

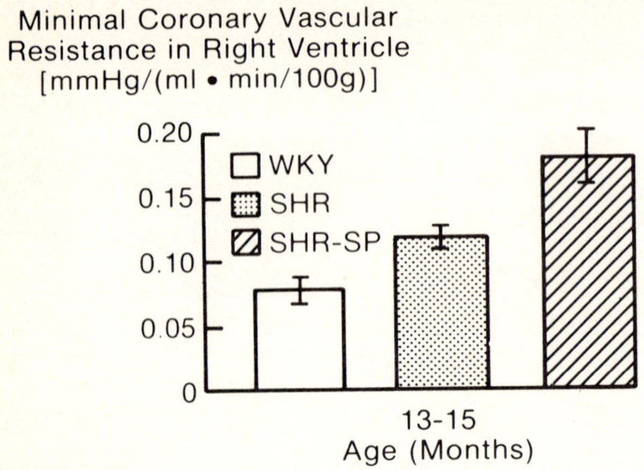

FIGURE 13-5
Effects of chronic hypertension on minimal coronary vascular resistance in the nonhypertrophied right ventricle of various genetic strains of rats. Minimal coronary vascular resistance was calculated from maximal right ventricular perfusion measured with microspheres and mean arterial pressure. Maximal coronary dilation was produced by infusion of dipyridamole. Three groups of chronically instrumented rats were studied: WKY = Wistar-Kyoto control; SHR = spontaneously hypertensive rats; and SHR-SP = stroke-prone SHR. The increase of minimal coronary vascular resistance in the SHR and SHR-SP strains reflects vascular hypertrophy in coronary resistance vessels secondary to chronic hypertension. (*Redrawn from a figure originally presented by RD Wangler et al* [30].)

of coronary vascular growth in SHR have shown that, when left ventricular hypertrophy stabilizes in this model, there is a significant acceleration in the growth rate of coronary capillaries [31a]. Thus, both physiological and anatomic studies support the notion that, given sufficient time, coronary vascular growth can keep pace with the development of moderate left ventricular hypertrophy.

Effects of Coronary Occlusion in Animals with Pressure-Induced Left Ventricular Hypertrophy

Epidemiologic studies have shown that when patients with hypertension and left ventricular hypertrophy sustain a myocardial infarction, the incidence of sudden cardiac death is increased threefold and other complications of myocardial infarction such as heart failure are more frequent than expected [32]. These adverse effects of coronary occlusion could be related to hypertension, left ventricular hypertrophy, or more extensive coronary disease in patients with these concomitant conditions. Koyanagi et al. [33,34] studied the effects of coronary occlusion in awake dogs with left ventricular hypertrophy secondary to renal hypertension. During the first 48 h following coronary occlusion, death presumably secondary to ventricular fibrillation occured much more frequently in dogs with hypertension and left ventricular hypertrophy than in controls (Figure 13-7) [33]. Furthermore,

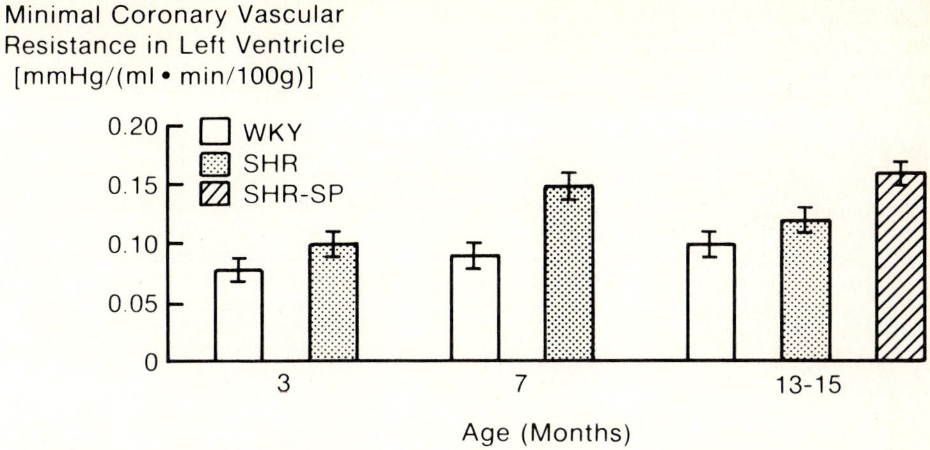

FIGURE 13-6
Interaction between age and coronary vascular growth in association with cardiac hypertrophy. In the rat species being examined (WKY and SHR), left ventricular hypertrophy is present at 3 months of age (SHR), maximal at 7 months of age, and stable thereafter. SHR-SP have more severe hypertension and hypertrophy than SHR. Minimal coronary vascular resistance was calculated from maximal coronary flow and mean arterial pressure in awake chronically instrumented rats. Maximal coronary flow was produced by IV infusion of dipyridamole. In the SHR, minimal coronary vascular resistance was abnormally increased when left ventricular hypertrophy was maximal (7 months of age); the abnormality was no longer present in SHR following a prolonged period of stable hypertrophy (13 to 15 months of age). SHR-SP demonstrated increased minimal coronary vascular resistance throughout a long segment of their life cycle. The data suggest that when left ventricular hypertrophy is not severe (SHR), given sufficient time, growth of coronary vasculature will keep pace with an increase in left ventricular mass. *(Redrawn from data originally presented by RD Wangler et al [30].)*

infarct size over a wide range of risk areas was increased in the dogs with left ventricular hypertrophy secondary to hypertension (Figure 13-8) [34]. Previous studies in this regard by Mueller et al. [35] were inconclusive because the methods employed were not sufficiently sensitive. Koyanagi's study provides the first experimental evidence that hypertrophy and hypertension alone adversely affect the response of myocardium to sudden coronary occlusion. These adverse affects could be related to electrophysiological abnormalities in hypertrophied cardiac muscle [36,37] or to abnormalities in coronary reserve or native collateral vessels in the hypertrophied ventricle.

EFFECTS OF VOLUME-INDUCED LEFT VENTRICULAR HYPERTROPHY ON THE CORONARY CIRCULATION

Two studies have evaluated coronary reserve in animals with volume-induced left ventricular hypertrophy [38,39]. In both, the degree of left ventricular hypertrophy produced was modest and no major abnormalities in coronary reserve were noted.

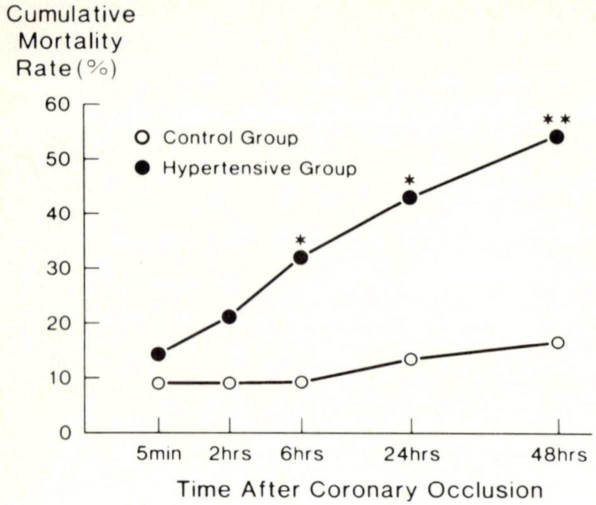

FIGURE 13-7
Effects of sudden coronary occlusion on mortality in control dogs (control group) and hypertensive dogs with left ventricular hypertrophy (hypertensive group). Mortality was much higher in the hypertensive group. The cause of death was primarily ventricular fibrillation. The data suggest that chronic hypertension and left ventricular hypertrophy adversely affect the consequences of sudden coronary occlusion in dogs.*$p <$ 0.05 vs. control; **$p<0.01$ vs. control. (*Data originally presented by S Koyanagi et al* [*33*].)

EFFECTS OF RIGHT VENTRICULAR HYPERTROPHY ON THE CORONARY CIRCULATION

Murray and Vatner [40,41a] produced severe right ventricular hypertrophy (70 to 110 percent increase in right ventricular mass) in dogs by creating severe supravalvular pulmonary stenosis. They noted that under resting condition right

FIGURE 13-8
Effects of chronic hypertension and left ventricular hypertrophy (HT-LVH) on the infarct-risk relationship. In this study, dogs were subjected to sudden coronary occlusion in the awake state. Forty-eight hours later, infarct size was determined by pathological techniques and the risk area was defined by postmortem coronary angiography. Over the entire range of risk areas examined, dogs with chronic hypertension and left ventricular hypertrophy had larger infarcts than controls. (*Data originally presented by S Koyanagi et al* [*34*].)

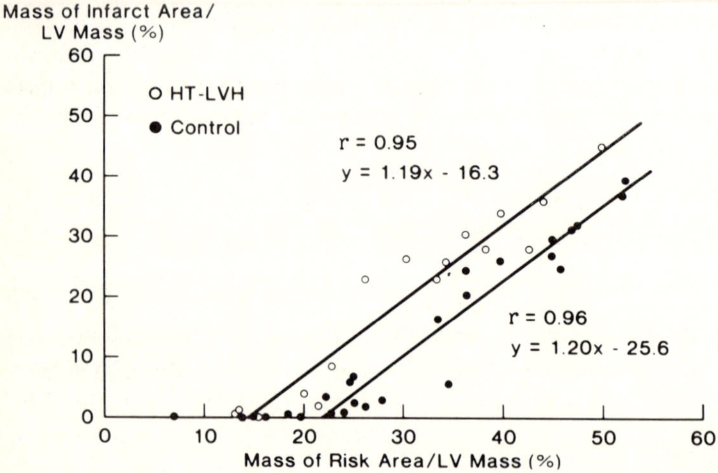

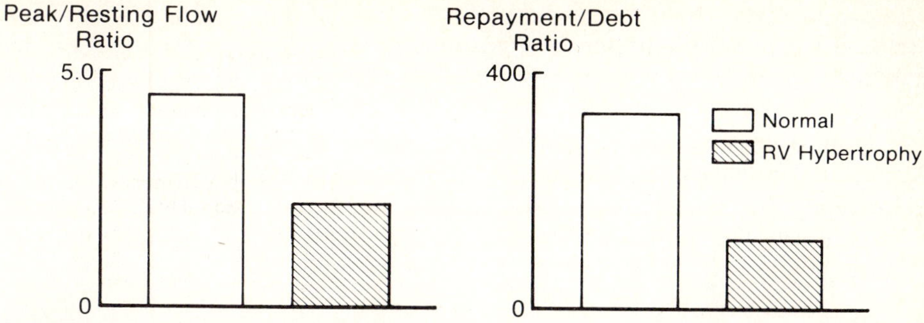

FIGURE 13-9
Characteristics of coronary reactive hyperemia in normal dogs and dogs with severe right ventricular hypertrophy (RV hypertrophy) secondary to supravalvular pulmonary obstruction. Coronary reactive hyperemic responses were examined in the right coronary artery. Following release of a 20-s coronary occlusion, peak-to-resting flow ratio and the repayment/debt ratio were markedly diminished in the dogs with right ventricular hypertrophy. (*Based on data originally presented by PA Murray and SF Vatner* [41].)

ventricular flow per gram doubled but that the transmural distribution of coronary flow was near normal. Responses to coronary dilator stimuli—infusion of adenosine, strenuous exercise, and transient coronary occlusion—indicated that in this model of cardiac hypertrophy right ventricular coronary reserve was profoundly impaired (Figure 13-9) [41,41a]. The magnitude of the coronary abnormalities in dogs with right ventricular hypertrophy noted by Murray and Vatner far exceeds that which has been observed in animal models of left ventricular hypertrophy.

EFFECTS OF PRESSURE-INDUCED RIGHT VENTRICULAR HYPERTROPHY IN NEONATAL ANIMALS

Several groups have produced right ventricular hypertrophy in lambs in utero or in lambs or calves immediately following birth [42–44]. In all studies, supravalvular pulmonary obstruction induced marked right ventricular hypertrophy. The remarkable observation in these studies was that right ventricular coronary reserve was normal or greater than expected. Thus, very early in the animal's development, right ventricular pressure overload produces an increase in muscle mass coupled with an appropriate augmentation in the coronary vasculature.

SUMMARY OF RESULTS OF PHYSIOLOGICAL STUDIES IN ANIMALS

It is now established that under most conditions, cardiac hypertrophy secondary to a pressure load is associated with normal myocardial perfusion at rest and a mild impairment in coronary vascular reserve. The limitation in coronary vascular capacity is engendered by inadequate growth of new vessels and vascular hypertrophy in coronary resistance vessels if systemic hypertension is present. The interaction between an increase in cardiac muscle mass and structural changes in the coronary vascular bed is mediated by (1) intensity of hypertrophy; (2) the ventricle involved (right versus left); (3) the type of stress employed (pressure versus volume); (4) the presence of systemic hypertension; (5) the duration that stable hypertrophy has been present; and (6) the time in the animal's life cycle when hypertrophy is produced.

The most dramatic abnormalities encountered thus far have been a marked decrease in coronary reserve in adult dogs with pressure-induced right ventricular hypertrophy [40–41] and a striking increase in the adverse affects of sudden coronary occlusion in dogs with left ventricular hypertrophy secondary to renal hypertension [33,34].

PHYSIOLOGICAL STUDIES IN HUMANS

There are three major reasons for studying the effects of cardiac hypertrophy on the coronary circulation in humans. First, the severity of cardiac hypertrophy in patients is much greater than that which can be produced in animals. Most animal models of hypertrophy have less than a twofold increase in ventricular mass. In contrast, patients with severe aortic stenosis occasionally have a two- to threefold increase in ventricular mass [45]. Second, the duration of cardiac hypertrophy in patients often extends over a period of many decades. Most animal studies employ preparations that have had cardiac hypertrophy over a small fraction of the animal's lifespan. Third, studies of coronary reserve in patients with cardiac hypertrophy are clinically relevant. Inferences from animal studies to the clinical arena must always be made with great caution.

EFFECTS OF PRESSURE-INDUCED LEFT VENTRICULAR HYPERTROPHY ON CORONARY RESERVE IN PATIENTS

Since 1979, my colleagues and I have obtained measurements of coronary reactive hyperemia in patients with cardiac hypertrophy at the time of cardiac surgery [46–53]. These studies were facilitated by the development of a Doppler probe which can be coupled to surface coronary vessels with suction [47] (see Chapter 2). With this device, phasic and mean coronary blood flow velocity can be measured and the quantitative characteristics of coronary reactive hyperemia can be assessed (Chapter 3). In all our studies the characteristics of coronary reactive hyperemia were measured prior to cardiopulmonary bypass. In humans, maximal coronary dilation follows release of a 20-s coronary occlusion [47] (see Figures 3-17 and 3-18).

In adult patients with normal coronary vessels and severe left ventricular hypertrophy secondary to valvular aortic stenosis we have found that the coronary reactive hyperemic response in the left anterior descending coronary artery was strikingly impaired (Figure 13-10) [48]. In contrast, the coronary reactive hyperemic response in vessels which perfuse the nonhypertrophied right ventricle are nearly normal (Figure 13-10). In most patients, coronary reserve is reduced to about one-third of normal (Figure 13-11) [48]. Similar results were obtained in children with supravalvular aortic stenosis [53]. Immediately following partial

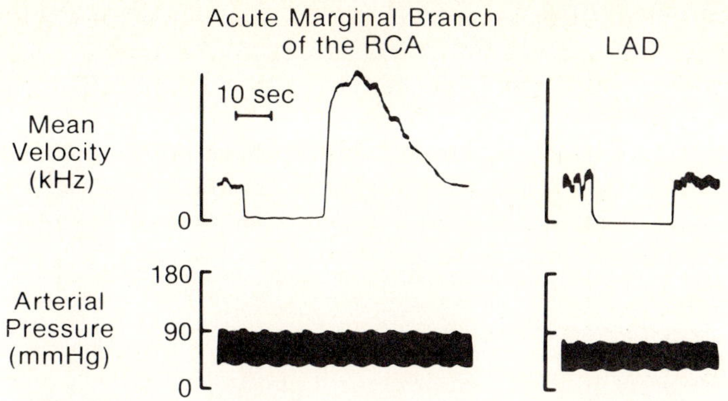

FIGURE 13-10
Coronary reactive hyperemic responses in a patient with severe aortic stenosis. These studies were obtained at the time of open heart surgery prior to cardiopulmonary bypass. The patient's right ventricle was of normal size; the left ventricle was severely hypertrophied; the coronary arteries were angiographically normal. The coronary reactive hyperemic response obtained from the acute marginal branch of the coronary artery (RCA) was normal; the coronary reactive hyperemic response obtained from the left anterior descending (LAD) coronary artery was strikingly attenuated. The data suggest that severe left ventricular hypertrophy in patients with aortic stenosis markedly limits coronary reserve. (*Based on data originally presented by ML Marcus et al* [*48*].)

relief of aortic valve obstruction, the coronary reactive hyperemic response in the left anterior descending coronary artery is not significantly improved [53]. This suggests that extravascular compressive forces are not responsible for the observed impairment in coronary reserve.

Strauer [54] and Tauchert et al. [55] have measured flow per gram with argon clearance in the left ventricle of patients with left ventricular hypertrophy secondary to aortic stenosis. Data were obtained at rest and during maximal coronary dilation produced by infusing a potent coronary dilator, dipyridamole. During maximal coronary dilation coronary reserve was substantially decreased. Patients with concomitant cardiac dilation and left ventricular failure demonstrated the greatest abnormalities in coronary reserve.

The studies demonstrated that coronary reserve in patients with severe left ventricular hypertrophy secondary to aortic stenosis is severely impaired in both adults and children. The magnitude of the abnormality in coronary reserve is sufficient to contribute significantly to the pathogenesis of angina in patients with aortic stenosis and normal coronary vessels. Furthermore, it is likely that intermittent episodes of subendocardial ischemia in these patients lead to subendocardial fibrosis, which in turn contributes to the genesis of congestive heart failure.

Strauer [2] has also examined coronary reserve in patients with various degrees

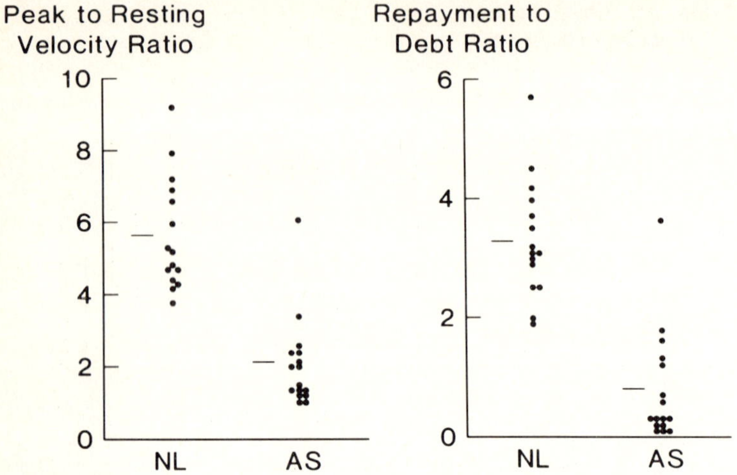

FIGURE 13-11
Characteristics of coronary reactive hyperemia in the left anterior descending coronary artery in patients with aortic stenosis (AS) and controls (NL). All studies were obtained at the time of open heart surgery prior to cardiopulmonary bypass. The left ventricles in the normal group were not enlarged and functioned normally; left ventricles in patients with aortic stenosis were markedly hypertrophied. All coronary vessels were angiographically normal. At the time the measurements were obtained, mean aortic pressure and heart rate were similar in both groups. Following release of a 20-s occlusion of the left anterior descending coronary artery, the peak-to-resting velocity ratios and the repayment/debt ratios were markedly decreased in patients with aortic stenosis. The horizontal bar to the left of each group of data points represents the mean value. These studies suggest that coronary reserve is markedly diminished in adult patients with severe aortic stenosis. (*Based on data originally presented by ML Marcus et al* [*48*].)

of systemic hypertension and left ventricular hypertrophy. These studies demonstrate that coronary reserve is frequently decreased in patients with cardiac hypertrophy secondary to hypertension even if the magnitude of the hypertrophy is relatively modest (30 percent increase in left ventricular mass) (Figure 13-12).

The results of these patient studies are in striking contrast to data reported from investigations in animals. Most animal studies of cardiac hypertrophy have detected a mild decrease in coronary reserves; patients with severe pressure-induced left ventricular hypertrophy have a profound decrease in coronary vasodilator reserve.

EFFECTS OF VOLUME-INDUCED LEFT VENTRICULAR HYPERTROPHY ON CORONARY RESERVE IN PATIENTS

Eastham et al. have examined the characteristics of coronary reactive hyperemia in patients with volume-induced cardiac hypertrophy secondary to severe mitral regurgitation (Figures 13-13 and 13-14) [51]. Coronary reserve was significantly diminished in vessels perfusing the hypertrophied left ventricle. Studies with the

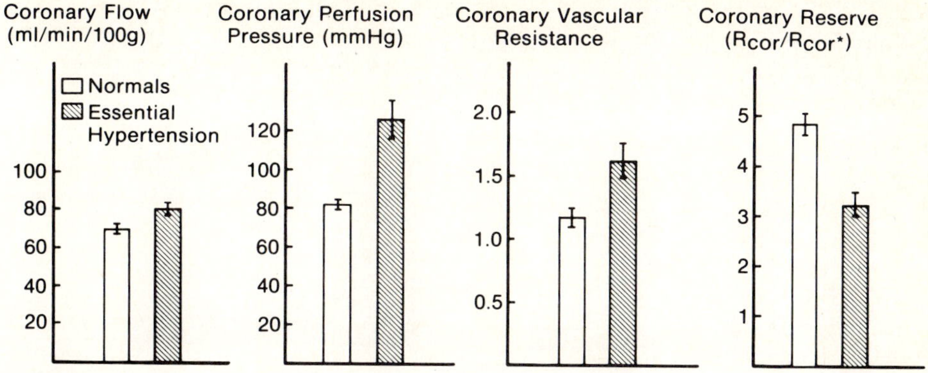

FIGURE 13-12
Characteristics of the coronary circulation in patients with essential hypertension and normals. Coronary flow was measured with the argon saturation technique. All patients included in the study had angiographically normal coronary vessels. Under control conditions flow per gram of left ventricle was not increased in patients with essential hypertension. However, coronary perfusion pressure and coronary vascular resistance were increased in patients with essential hypertension. The ratio of control coronary vascular resistance (R_{cor}) to minimal coronary vascular resistance (R_{cor*}) was decreased in patients with essential hypertension. This indicates that coronary reserve is less than normal in patients with essential hypertension. Maximal coronary dilation was produced by IV infusion of dipyridamole (0.5 mg/kg/min). (*Redrawn from data originally presented by BE Strauer* [54].)

argon clearance approach also indicate that coronary reserve is decreased in patients with volume-induced left ventricular hypertrophy secondary to mitral or aortic regurgitation [54,55]. Thus, left ventricular hypertrophy in patients secondary to volume overload is associated with impaired coronary reserve. Studies in animals have yielded the opposite result [38,39].

EFFECTS OF VOLUME-INDUCED RIGHT VENTRICULAR HYPERTROPHY ON CORONARY RESERVE IN PATIENTS

Patients with isolated large atrial septal defects and normal pulmonary artery pressure have marked right ventricular dilation and hypertrophy. Doty et al. have examined the characteristics of coronary reactive hyperemia in vessels perfusing the enlarged right ventricle of patients with atrial septal defects [49]. Two important abnormalities were observed: (1) the maximal dilator response was about one-half of that observed in control patients, and (2) the duration of the coronary reactive hyperemic response was markedly prolonged (Figures 13-15 and 13-16). The mechanism responsible for the prolongation of the reactive hyperemic response is uncertain.

EFFECTS OF PRESSURE-INDUCED RIGHT VENTRICULAR HYPERTROPHY ON CORONARY RESERVE IN PATIENTS

Pressure-induced right ventricular hypertrophy occurs in patients with various types of cyanotic congenital heart disease (e.g., tetrology of Fallot, transposition of

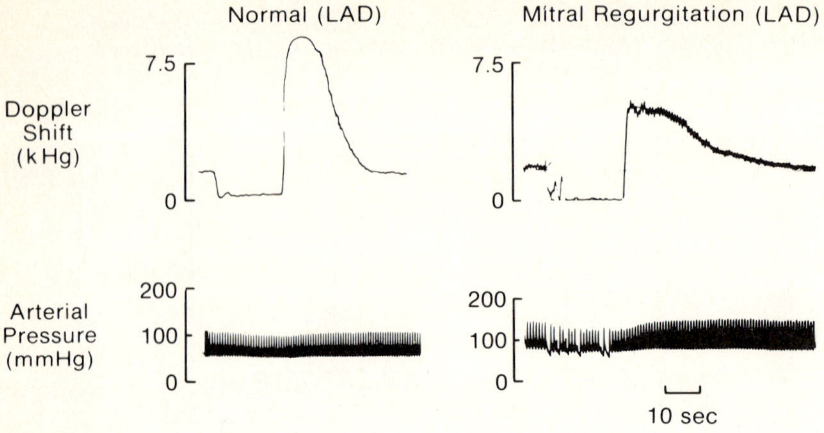

FIGURE 13-13
Coronary reactive hyperemic responses in a patient with a normal left ventricle (normal) and a patient with severe volume overload left ventricular hypertrophy secondary to mitral regurgitation. The coronary reactive hyperemic response following a 20-s occlusion was substantially diminished in the patient with mitral regurgitation. This suggests that coronary reserve is diminished in patients in a volume-induced left ventricular hypertrophy. In both patients, the left anterior descending (LAD) coronary artery was angiographically normal. (*Based on data reported originally by CL Eastham et al* [*51*].)

FIGURE 13-14
Quantitative characteristics of coronary reactive hyperemia in patients with normal or control left ventricles (cont), and patients with volume overload left ventricle hypertrophy (Vo-LHV) secondary to mitral regurgitation (MR). The coronary reactive hyperemic responses were assessed following release of the 20-s coronary occlusion of an angiographically normal left anterior descending coronary artery. The coronary reactive hyperemic responses were substantially reduced in patients with volume overload left ventricular hypertrophy secondary to mitral regurgitation. $p < 0.05$ vs. control. (*Based on data reported by CL Eastham et al* [*51*].)

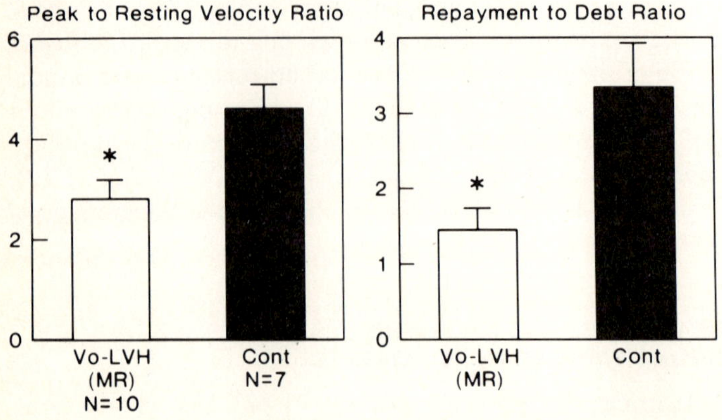

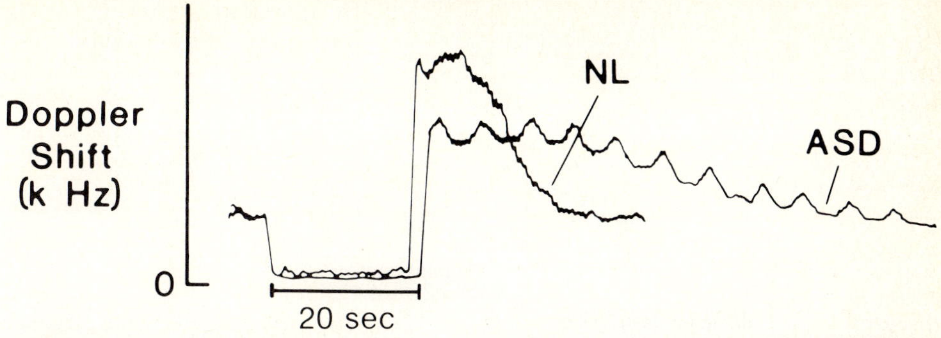

FIGURE 13-15
Coronary reactive hyperemic responses in a patient with a normal right ventricle (NL) and a patient with volume overload right ventricular hypertrophy secondary to a large atrial septal defect (ASD). The coronary reactive hyperemic responses were recorded in right ventricular branches of the right coronary artery following release of the 20-s coronary occlusion. The peak velocity was lower and the duration of the response was longer in the patient with the atrial septal defect. This suggests that volume overload right ventricular hypertrophy secondary to atrial septal defect decreases coronary reserve. In both patients, the right coronary arteries and their branches were angiographically normal. (*Based on data reported by D Doty et al* [*49*].)

FIGURE 13-16
Quantitative characteristics of coronary reactive hyperemia in patients with normal right ventricles (NL) and in patients with volume overload right ventricular hypertrophy secondary to an atrial septal defect (ASD). In all patients the right coronary arteries and their branches were normal. In patients with atrial septal defect, the duration of the reactive hyperemic response was longer and the peak velocity/resting velocity ratio was substantially reduced. (*Based on data reported by D Doty et al* [*49*].)

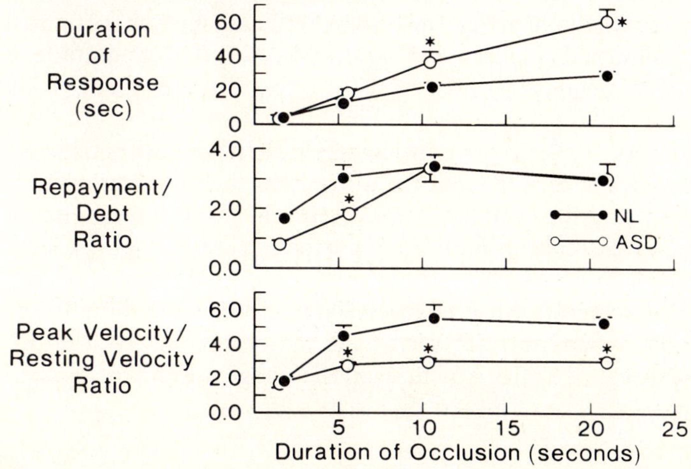

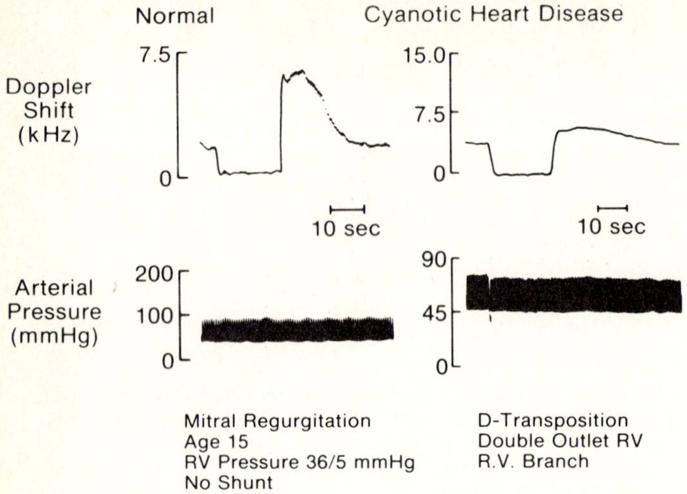

FIGURE 13-17
Coronary reactive hyperemic responses in a patient with a normal right ventricle (normal) and a patient with severe right ventricular hypertrophy associated with cyanotic congenital heart disease. Since both patients were less than 20 years old, it was assumed that the coronary vessels being studied were free of atherosclerosis. In both cases, coronary reactive hyperemic responses were recorded following release of a 20-s occlusion of a right ventricular branch of the right coronary artery. The coronary reactive hyperemic response was markedly diminished in the patient with right ventricular hypertrophy associated with a cyanotic congenital heart disease. This suggests that coronary reserve was reduced in the patient with cyanotic congenital heart disease. RV = right ventricle. No shunt = no intracardiac shunt. (*Based on data reported by ML Marcus et al* [52].)

the great vessels, etc.). My colleagues and I have noted that the coronary reactive hyperemic response in these patient groups in vessels perfusing the hypertrophied ventricle is markedly diminished (Figures 13-17 and 13-18) [52]. The magnitude of the abnormality observed is similar to the results of animal studies reported by Murray and Vatner [40–41].

Impaired coronary reserve in the right ventricle of children with cyanotic heart disease probably contributes to certain clinical features that such patients exhibit. For example, some patients with cyanotic heart disease have exertional angina which may result from impaired coronary dilator capacity. Also, such patients tolerate systemic hypotension poorly. This could result from inability of the coronary circulation to the hypertrophied ventricles to autoregulate. Finally, at postmortem examination, subendocardial necrosis is commonly observed in the hypertrophied right ventricle of patients with cyanotic congenital heart disease. Again, this may be a consequence of myocardial ischemia.

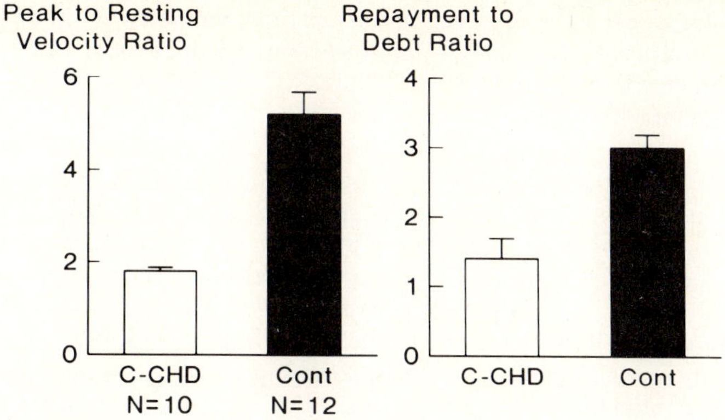

FIGURE 13-18
Quantitative characteristics of coronary reactive hyperemia in patients with normal or control right ventricles (cont) and patients with severe right ventricular hypertrophy associated with cyanotic congenital heart disease (C-CHD). The coronary reactive hyperemic responses were assessed following release of the 20-s coronary occlusion of a right ventricular branch of the right coronary artery. The coronary reactive hyperemic responses were substantially decreased in patients with cyanotic congenital heart disease. $p = <0.05$ vs. control. (*Based on data reported by ML Marcus et al* [52].)

SUMMARY OF RESULTS OF PHYSIOLOGICAL STUDIES IN HUMANS

In patients, coronary reserve is markedly decreased in volume- or pressure-induced hypertrophy of either the right or left ventricle. Studies in patients with mild to moderate hypertension associated with only a 30 percent increase in left ventricular mass indicate that even under these conditions there is a significant decrease in coronary reserve. It is likely that diminished coronary reserve in hypertrophied ventricles contributes significantly to the pathogenesis of angina and heart failure in patients with hypertrophied ventricles.

REFERENCES

1 Hurst JW, Logue RB, Schlant RB, Wenger NK: *The Heart, Arteries and Veins,* 4th ed. New York, McGraw-Hill, 1978, pp 1556–1590.
2 Strauer BE: *Hypertensive Heart Disease.* New York, Springer-Verlag, 1980.
3 Harris CN, Aronow WS, Parker DP, Kaplan MA: Treadmill stress in left ventricular hypertrophy. *Chest* 63: 353, 1973.
4 Buckberg GD, Fixler DE, Archie JP, Hoffman JIE: Experimental subendocardial ischemia in dogs with normal coronary arteries. *Circ Res* 30: 67, 1972.
5 Marcus ML, Mueller TM, Gascho JA, Kerber RE: Effects of cardiac hypertrophy secondary to hypertension on the coronary circulation. *Am J Cardio* 44: 1023, 1979.

6 Stack RS, Schirmer B, Greenfield JC Jr: Coronary artery luminal diameters in normal and hypertrophied canine ventricles (Abstr). *Circulation* 62(suppl III), October 1980.

7 Yamori Y, Mori C, Nishio T, Ooshima A, Horie R, Ohtaka M, Soeda T, Saito M, Abe K, Nara Y, Nakao Y, Kihara M: Cardiac hypertrophy in early hypertension. *Am J Cardiol* 44: 964, 1979.

8 Hallback-Nordlander M, Noresson E, Thoren P: Hemodynamic consequences of left ventricular hypertrophy in spontaneously hypertensive rats. *Am J Cardiol* 44: 986, 1979.

9 Rakusan K: Quantitative morphology of capillaries of the heart. Number of capillaries in animal and human hearts under normal and pathological conditions. *Methods Achiev Exp Pathol* 5: 272, 1971.

10 Wearn JT: The extent of the capillary bed of the heart. *J Exp Med* 47: 273, 1928.

11 Murray PA, Baig H, Fishbein MC, Vatner SF: Effects of experimental right ventricular hypertrophy on myocardial blood flow in conscious dogs. *J Clin Invest* 64: 421, 1979.

12 Buchner F: Qualitative morphology of heart failure. Light and electron microscopic characteristics of acute and chronic heart failure. *Methods Achiev Exp Pathol* 5: 60, 1971.

13 Bing RJ, Hammond MM, Handelsman JC, Powers SR, Spencer FC, Eckenhoff JE, Goodale WT, Hafkenschiel JF, Kety SS: The measurement of coronary blood flow, oxygen consumption, and efficiency of the left ventricle in man. *Am Heart J* 38: 1, 1949.

14 Rowe GG, Castillo CA, Maxwell GM, Crumpton CW: A hemodynamic study of hypertension including observations on coronary blood flow. *Ann Intern Med* 54: 405, 1961.

15 Mueller TM, Marcus ML, Kerber RE, Young JA, Barnes RW, Abboud FM: Effect of renal hypertension and left ventricular hypertrophy on the coronary circulation in dogs. *Circ Res* 42: 543, 1978.

16 Einzig S, Leonard JJ, Tripp MR, Lucas RV, Swayze CR, Fox IJ: Changes in regional myocardial blood flow and variable development of hypertrophy after aortic banding in puppies. *Cardiovasc Res* 15: 711, 1981.

17 Holtz J, Restorff WV, Bard P, Bassenge E: Transmural distribution of myocardial blood flow of coronary reserve in canine left ventricular hypertrophy. *Basic Res Cardiol* 72: 286, 1977.

18 O'Keefe DD, Hoffman JIE, Cheitlin R, O'Neill MJ, Allard JR, Shapkin E: Coronary blood flow in experimental canine left ventricular hypertrophy. *Circ Res* 43: 43, 1978.

19 Rembert JC, Kleinman LH, Fedor JM, Wechsler AS, Greenfield JC: Myocardial blood flow distribution in concentric left ventricular hypertrophy. *J Clin Invest* 62: 379, 1978.

20 White FC, Sanders M, Peterson T, Bloor CM: Ischemic myocardial injury after exercise stress in the pressure-overloaded heart. *Am J Pathol* 97: 473, 1979.

21 Bache RJ, Vrobel TR: Effects of exercise on blood flow in the hypertrophied heart. *Am J Cardiol* 44: 1029, 1979.

22 Breisch EA, Houser SR, Carey RA, Spann JF, Bove AA: Myocardial blood flow and capillary density in chronic pressure overload of the feline left ventricle. *Cardiovasc Res* 14: 469, 1980.

23 Mittmann U, Bruckner UB, Keller HE, Kohler U, Vetter H, Waag KL: Myocardial flow reserve in experimental cardiac hypertrophy. *Basic Res Cardiol* 75: 199, 1980.

24 Bache RJ, Vrobel TR, Ring WS, Emery RW, Andersen RW: Regional myocardial blood flow during exercise in dogs with chronic left ventricular hypertrophy. *Circ Res* 48: 76, 1981.

25 Bache RJ, Vrobel TR, Arentzen CE, Ring WS: Effect of maximal coronary vasodilation on transmural myocardial perfusion during tachycardia in dogs with left ventricular hypertrophy. *Circ Res* 49: 742, 1981.

26 Attarian DE, Jones RN, Currie WD, Hill RC, Sink JD, Olsen CO, Chitwood WR Jr, *Wechsler AS: Characteristics of chronic left ventricular hypertrophy induced by subcoronary valvular aortic stenosis. I. Myocardial blood flow and metabolism. J Thorac Cardiovasc Surg* 81: 382, 1981.

27 Marcus ML, Mueller TM, Eastham CL: Effects of short- and long-term left ventricular hypertrophy on coronary circulation. *Am J Physiol* 241: H358, 1981.

28 Sasayama S, Ross J, Franklin D, Bloor CM, Bishop S, Dilley RB: Adaptations of the left ventricle to chronic pressure overload. *Circ Res* 38: 172, 1976.

29 Mueller TM, Marcus ML, Eastham CL, Tipton CM: Effects of treadmill exercise in dogs with pressure induced left ventricular hypertrophy (abstr). *Fed Proc* 37: 647, 1979.

30 Wangler RD, Peters KG, Marcus ML, Tomanek RJ: Effects of duration and severity of arterial hypertension and cardiac hypertrophy on coronary vasodilator reserve. *Circ Res* 51: 10, 1982.

31 Peters KG, Wangler RD, Tomanek RJ, Marcus ML: Interaction of age and hypertrophy on coronary dilator capacity. *Fed Proc* 40: 546, 1981.

31a Tomanek RJ, Searls JC, Lachenbruch PA: Quantitative changes in the capillary bed during developing, peak and stabilized cardiac hypertrophy in the spontaneously hypertensive rat.

32 Kannel WB: Role of blood pressure in cardiovascular morbidity and mortality. *Prog Cardiovasc Dis* 17: 5, 1974.

33 Koyanagi S, Eastham C, Marcus ML: Effects of chronic hypertension and left ventricular hypertrophy on the incidence of sudden cardiac death following coronary occlusion in conscious dogs. *Circulation* 65: 1192, 1982.

34 Koyanagi S, Eastham CL, Harrison DG, Marcus ML: Increased size of myocardial infarction in dogs with chronic hypertension and left ventricular hypertrophy. *Circ Res* 50: 53, 1982.

35 Mueller TM, Tomanek RJ, Kerber RE, Marcus ML: Myocardial infarction in dogs with chronic hypertension and left ventricular hypertrophy. *Am J Physiol* 239(8): H731, 1980.

36 Aronson RS: Characteristics of action potentials of hypertrophied myocardium from rats with renal hypertension. *Circ Res* 47: 443, 1980.

37 Gelband H, Bassett A: Depressed transmembrane potentials during experimentally induced ventricular failure in cats. *Circ Res* 32: 625, 1973.

38 Gascho JA, Mueller TM, Eastham C, Marcus ML: Effect of volume-overload hypertrophy on the coronary circulation in awake dogs. *Cardiovasc Res* 16: 288–292, 1982.

39 Huntgren PB, Bove AA: Myocardial blood flow at rest and during exercise in dogs with volume overload induced left ventricular hypertrophy (abstr). *Fed Proc* 37: 647, 1978.

40 Murray PA, Vatner SF: Abnormal coronary vascular response to exercise in dogs with severe right ventricular hypertrophy. *J Clin Invest* 67: 1314, 1981.

41 Murray PA, Vatner SF: Reduction of maximal coronary vasodilator capacity in conscious dogs with severe right ventricular hypertrophy. *Circ Res* 48: 27, 1981.

42 Vlahakes GJ, Turley K, Verrier ED, Hoffman JIE: Greater maximal coronary flow in conscious lambs with experimental congenital right ventricular hypertrophy. *Circulation* 62(supp III), 1980.

43 Archie JP, Fixler DE, Ullyot DJ, Buckberg GD, Hoffman JIE: Regional myocardial blood flow in lambs with concentric right ventricular hypertrophy. *Circ Res* 34: 143, 1974.

44 Manohar M, Thurmon JC, Tranquilli WJ, Devous MD Sr, Theodorakis MC, Shawley RV, Feller DL, Benson JG: Regional myocardial blood flow and coronary vascular reserve in unanesthetized young calves with severe concentric right ventricular hypertrophy. *Circ Res* 48: 785, 1981.

45 Kennedy JW, Doces J, Stewart DK: Left ventricular function before and following aortic valve replacement. *Circulation* 56: 941, 1977.
46 Marcus ML, Wright C, Doty D, Eastham C, Fastenow C, Laughlin D, Krumm P: Characteristics of coronary reactive hyperemia in man. *Circulation* 59–60: 261, 1979.
47 Marcus ML, Wright C, Doty D, Eastham C, Laughlin D, Krumm P, Fastenow C, Brody M: Measurements of coronary velocity and reactive hyperemia in the coronary circulation of humans. *Circ Res* 49: 877, 1981.
48 Marcus ML, Doty DB, Hiratzka LF, Wright CB, Eastham CL: Decreased coronary reserve—A mechanism for angina pectoris in patients with aortic stenosis and normal coronary arteries. *N Engl J Med* 307: 1362–1367, 1982.
49 Doty D, Wright AC, Eastham C, Marcus ML: Coronary reserve in atrial septal defect. *Circulation* 62: III-115, 1980.
50 Eastham C, Doty D, Wright C, Marcus ML: Effects of age on coronary reserve in man. *Circulation* 62: III-64, 1980.
51 Eastham CL, Doty DB, Hiratzka LF, Wright CB, Marcus ML: Volume-overload left ventricular hypertrophy impairs coronary reserve in humans. *Circulation* 64(suppl IV), October 1981.
52 Marcus ML, Doty D, Hiratzka L, Wright C, Eastham C: Impaired coronary reserve in children with cyanotic congenital heart disease. *Circulation* 64: 127, 1981.
53 Doty D, Eastham C, Hiratzka L, Wright C, Marcus M: Determinants of coronary reserve in patients with supravalvular aortic stenosis. *Circulation* 64: 32, 1981.
54 Strauer BE: Ventricular function and coronary hemodynamics in hypertensive heart disease. *Am J Cardiol* 44: 999, 1979.
55 Tauchert M, Hilger HH: Application of the coronary reserve concept to the study of myocardial perfusion, in *The Patho-Physiology of Myocardial Perfusion*, W Schaper (ed). Amsterdam, Elsevier/North-Holland Biomedical Press, 1979, pp 141–167.

CHAPTER **14**

EFFECTS OF ANEMIA AND POLYCYTHEMIA ON THE CORONARY CIRCULATION

Oxygen delivery to the interstitial space in the myocardium is facilitated by hemoglobin. Because coronary vascular tone is closely coupled to oxygen demand (see Chapter 3), any factor that interferes with the efficient delivery of oxygen can potentially alter coronary vascular resistance. Thus, alterations in the concentration of hemoglobin or its functional characteristics may modify coronary vascular tone. Red cells also contribute significantly to the viscous properties of blood, a minor determinant of coronary vascular resistance. Thus, alterations in the hemoglobin concentration simultaneously affect the oxygen-carrying capacity and viscosity of blood.

Although the effect of anemia and polycythemia on the coronary circulation is usually modest, under some conditions alterations in the hemoglobin concentration in the blood can significantly influence the clinical manifestations of disease processes that affect the coronary circulation.

EFFECTS OF ANEMIA AND POLYCYTHEMIA ON SYSTEMIC HEMODYNAMICS

The effects of anemia on systemic hemodynamics depend on the cause of the anemia, rate of onset, severity, and the functional capacity of the cardiovascular system [1–8]. Severe anemia in a patient with mitral stenosis can produce life-threatening pulmonary edema. In contrast, in patients with a normal cardiovascular system, severe anemia which has developed very slowly may be well tolerated [2,3].

The effects of severe, chronic, anemia (hemoglobin = 4 to 6 g) on systemic hemodynamics in patients have been carefully examined [2]. Under such conditions, cardiac output was increased twofold, heart rate ranged from 65 to 120 beats per minute, and stroke volume was substantially elevated. Systolic arterial pressure was normal, but diastolic pressure was decreased. Hence, peripheral vascular resistance was substantially decreased. Pulmonary wedge pressure was normal. This combination of hemodynamic findings would probably modestly increase myocardial oxygen consumption.

Polycythemia is also associated with alterations in systemic hemodynamics. Usually, the effects on the systemic circulation are dominated by the cause of the polycythemia, i.e., severe pulmonary emphysema, etc. One clinical subgoup, patients with polycythemia vera, has a marked increase in their hemoglobin level without a superimposed condition that has major circulatory effects of its own, i.e., cyanotic congenital heart disease. In patients with polycythemia vera [9,10] blood volume is usually increased and resting cardiac output is modestly elevated. Heart rate is usually normal, and consequently stroke volume is elevated. Arterial pressure is modestly elevated but calculated peripheral vascular resistance is often near normal. The net effect of these hemodynamic alterations would probably result in a slight elevation in myocardial oxygen consumption.

In patients with either severe anemia or polycythemia exercise capacity is usually decreased [11].

Thus, both anemia and polycythemia have specific effects on systemic hemodynamics. However, in the usual clinical setting, the systemic hemodynamic abnormalities that accompany anemia and polycythemia are dominated by the disease process responsible for the changes in hemoglobin concentration.

SPECIFIC EFFECTS OF ANEMIA ON THE CORONARY CIRCULATION

Normovolemic anemia causes several important alterations in the coronary circulation [3,4,6–8,12–20a]. As the hemoglobin concentration decreases, coronary blood flow to all cardiac chambers rises substantially [17] and oxygen extraction across a coronary bed increases (Figure 14-1) [1,3,8,17]. The effects of anemia on coronary blood flow can be dramatic (Figure 14-2). For example, in chronically instrumented awake dogs, left ventricular blood flow was 43 ml/min/100 g at a hemoglobin of 15 g and 317 ml/min/100 g when the hemoglobin level was decreased to 4 g without a change in blood volume [17].

Usually, normovolemic anemia does not change myocardial oxygen consumption significantly [1,3]. However, in awake dogs acute hemodilution at a constant blood volume produces tachycardia and consequently a significant increase in myocardial oxygen consumption [17].

Anemia can also alter the transmural distribution of left ventricular perfusion [15,16,18]. In awake dogs, during severe anemia the transmural distribution of left

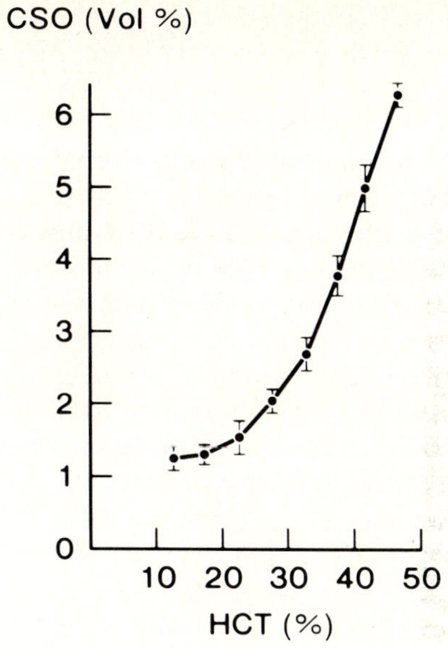

FIGURE 14-1
Relationship between coronary sinus oxygen saturation (CSO) expressed in volumes percent (Vol %) and hematocrit (HCT) in awake dogs with normovolemic anemia. The coronary circulation compensates in part for anemia by increasing oxygen extraction across the myocardium. Thus, in association with progressive anemia, coronary oxygen saturation decreases. *(Modified from an illustration originally presented by W von Restorff et al [17].)*

ventricular perfusion remains normal [18]. In anesthetized dogs, or dogs with superimposed hemodynamic abnormalities such as supravalvular aortic stenosis, anemia markedly decreases relative perfusion to the inner layers of the left ventricular myocardium [15,16]. Anemia shifts the relationship between the diastolic pressure time index/systolic pressure time index ratio and the subendocar-

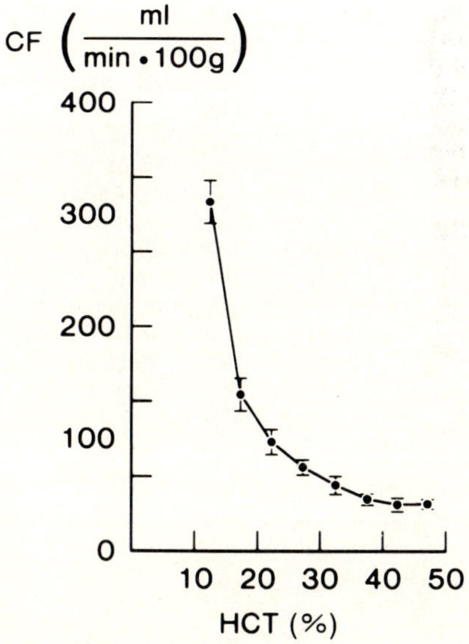

FIGURE 14-2
Relationship between left ventricular coronary flow (CF) and hematocrit (HCT) in awake dogs with normovolemic anemia. The coronary circulation compensates for anemia by significantly increasing coronary blood flow. *(Modified from an illustration originally presented by W von Restorff et al [17].)*

dial/subepicardial perfusion ratio to the left (see Figure 5-4). This occurs because the perfusion to the inner layers of the left ventricle is particularly sensitive to decreases in hemoglobin concentration.

In the presence of severe anemia (hemoglobin less than 5 g), coronary reserve is severely compromised (Figure 14-3). The coronary reactive hyperemic response appears blunted primarily because resting coronary flow is increased [8,12,17,18]. The limitation in coronary reserve is greatest in the inner layers of the left ventricle [18]. During severe anemia, autoregulation in the subendocardium is abolished [15–18]. Hence, modest decreases in perfusion pressure promptly lead to ischemia.

Marked anemia has one favorable effect on the coronary circulation. Because anemia increases the fluidity of the blood by decreasing its viscosity [17,18,21], minimal coronary vascular resistance actually decreases significantly [12,17,18]. Thus, in the presence of anemia, peak flow following release of a 12- to 20-s coronary occlusion is augmented in all layers of the left ventricular myocardium to a greater extent than what is observed when anemia is not present [12,17,18]. The decrease in minimal coronary vascular resistance is less than might be predicted from the decrease in viscosity that is associated with severe anemia because at high flow rates energy loss from nonviscous inertial factors presumably increases [18].

One study suggests that coronary blood flow to collateral-dependent zones increases modestly with severe anemia [21]. Chronic severe anemia stimulates the development of coronary collateral vessels [22,23].

Studies in patients also indicate that severe anemia is associated with a marked increase in coronary blood flow (Figure 14-4) [3,23a]. When the anemia is

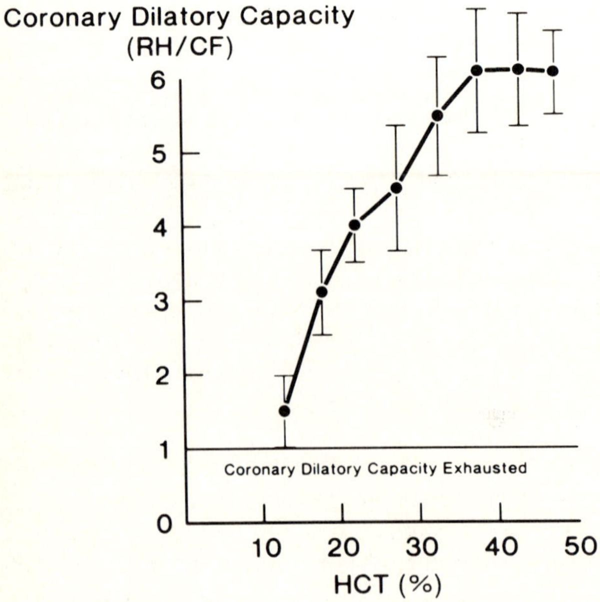

FIGURE 14-3
Effects of progressive normovolemic anemia in awake dogs in coronary reserve. Coronary reserve, or "dilatory capacity," was assessed by noting the ratio between peak flow following a 20-s occlusion (RH = reactive hyperemia) and control flow (CF). Coronary reserve declined strikingly with anemia. When the ratio of RH/CF equals unity, coronary dilatory capacity is exhausted. *(Modified from an illustration originally presented by W von Restorff et al [17].)*

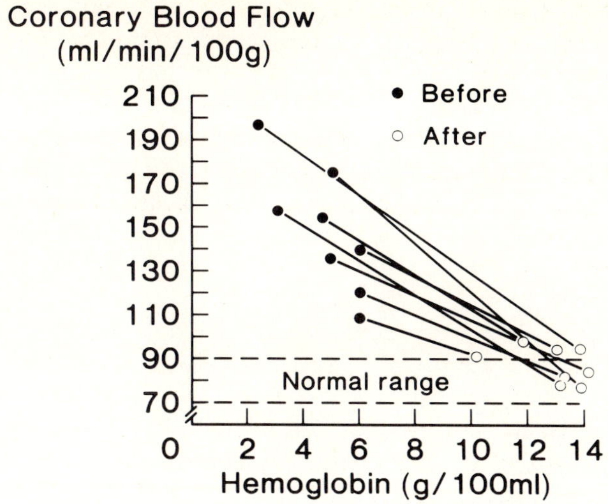

FIGURE 14-4
Effects of severe anemia on coronary blood flow. Coronary blood flow was measured before and after treatment of severe iron deficiency anemia. Each line connects before and after data in a single patient. These studies indicate that the coronary circulation in humans compensates for severe anemia by markedly increasing coronary blood flow. *(Redrawn from data originally presented by ML Bhatia et al* [23a].*)*

treated and hemoglobin levels are restored to normal, coronary blood flow returns to the normal range (Figure 14-4) [23a].

Thus, at rest, the normal coronary circulation compensates very well for the effects of severe anemia by decreasing vascular resistance and augmenting myocardial oxygen extraction. However, when superimposed abnormalities such as coronary stenosis, mild exercise, or aortic obstruction [1,15–17] are present, severe anemia will be associated with striking evidence of myocardial ischemia.

SPECIFIC EFFECTS OF POLYCYTHEMIA ON THE CORONARY CIRCULATION

The effects of normovolemic or hypervolemic polycythemia on the coronary concentration are just the opposite of what occurs with anemia. As the hemoglobin concentration rises beyond the normal range, coronary blood flow decreases and myocardial oxygen extraction remains constant or increases [1,20,24–26]. Polycythemia usually has little effect on myocardial oxygen consumption that cannot be attributed to changes in systemic hemodynamics [24,25]. Under control conditions, normovolemic polycythemia (hematocrit up to 74 percent) did not alter the transmural distribution of left ventricular perfusion [25]. Thus, when the oxygen-carrying capacity of the blood rises as a consequence of polycythemia, vasoconstriction occurs and coronary blood flow decreases.

When dogs with normovolemic polycythemia are subjected to coronary vasodilation (hypoxia, pacing, adenosine, coronary reactive hyperemia, decreased perfusion pressure, and supravalvular aortic stenosis), several abnormalities in the coronary circulation become manifest. Although vascular resistance decreased with these coronary dilator stimuli, minimal coronary vascular resistance was 50 percent higher at a hematocrit of 66 percent than at a hematocrit of 42 percent (see

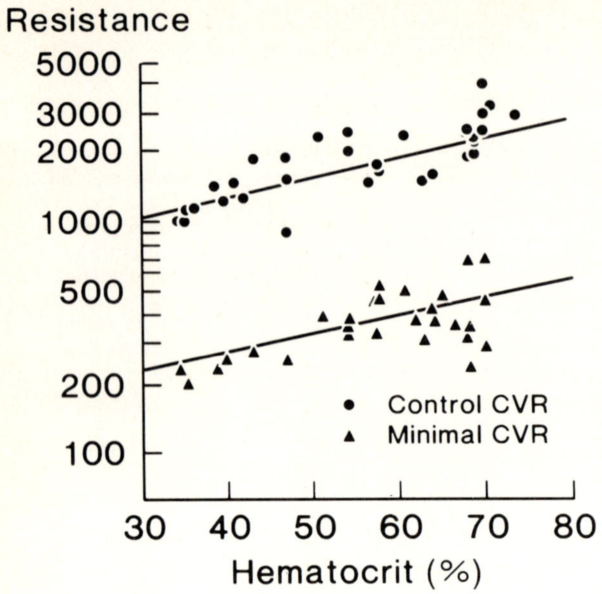

FIGURE 14-5
Effects of normovolemic polycythemia on control and minimal coronary vascular resistance (CVR) in anesthetized dogs. Note that resistance is plotted on a logarithmic scale. Control and minimal coronary vascular resistance increase progressively as hematocrit rises. *(Modified from an illustration originally presented by A Surjadhana et al* [25].*)*

FIGURE 14-6
Alteration in the inner and outer left ventricular (LV) flow ratio at various $DPTI_c$/SPTI ratios in normal and normovolemic polycythemia in anesthetized dogs. Polycythemia shifts the relationship between inner and outer flow and DPTI to the right. This indicates that the perfusion to the subendocardium of the left ventricle is adversely affected by normovolemic polycythemia. $DPTI_c$ = diastolic pressure time index; SPTI = systolic pressure time index. (*Modified from an illustration originally presented by A Surjadhana et al* [25].)

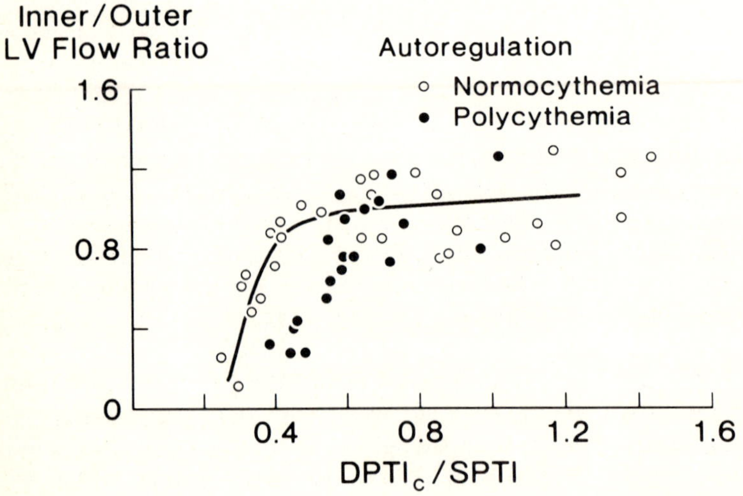

Figure 14-5) [25]. Furthermore, autoregulation in the inner layers of the left ventricle was compromised in the presence of normovolemic polycythemia (see Figure 14-6) [25].

The perfusion of collateral-dependent zones decreases with polycythemia [21].

Unfortunately, all experiments that relate to the effects of polycythemia on the coronary circulation have employed anesthetized dogs, and consequently extrapolation of the data to more physiological states must be guarded.

One clinical study measured coronary blood flow in patients living at high altitudes who had polycythemia as a consequence of chronic hypoxia. In these patients coronary vascular resistance was increased and resting coronary blood flow was decreased [26].

Thus, polycythemia has only modest adverse effects on the coronary circulation which become manifest only during intense coronary dilation. The abnormality in the coronary circulation is mainly due to an increase in blood viscosity that accompanies the polycythemia. It is conceivable that the adverse effects of severe polycythemia on the coronary circulation contribute to the pathogenesis of subendocardial infarction in children with cyanotic congenital heart disease [27].

SPECIFIC EFFECTS OF CHANGES IN BLOOD VISCOSITY

The original studies relating to the viscosity of blood simply related viscosity to hematocrit [28]. However, because blood is a non-Newtonian fluid, its effective viscosity is critically dependent on the shear rate (Figure 14-7). Classically, shear rate is calculated by the formula:

$$\text{Shear rate} = \frac{V}{\delta} \qquad \text{where } V = \text{blood velocity}$$

and δ = boundary layer thickness of the blood column

Thus, it follows that shear rates are relatively high in large arteries and very low in capillaries and venules [29–31]. Blood viscosity increases as a function of the hematocrit and decreases significantly as the shear rate increases (Figure 14-7) [29–31]. Therefore, at any one time, the effective viscosity of blood varies widely in different segments of the vasculature. Although shear rate and hematocrit are the dominant determinants of blood viscosity, several other factors (protein concentration, fibrogen level, and temperature) have minor effects on blood viscosity [30–32].

To assess the specific effects of blood viscosity on the coronary circulation, changes in the oxygen-carrying capacity of the blood which often accompany changes in viscosity must be minimized. A relatively uncommon disease, Waldenström's macroglobulinemia, provides a convenient experimental model [33].

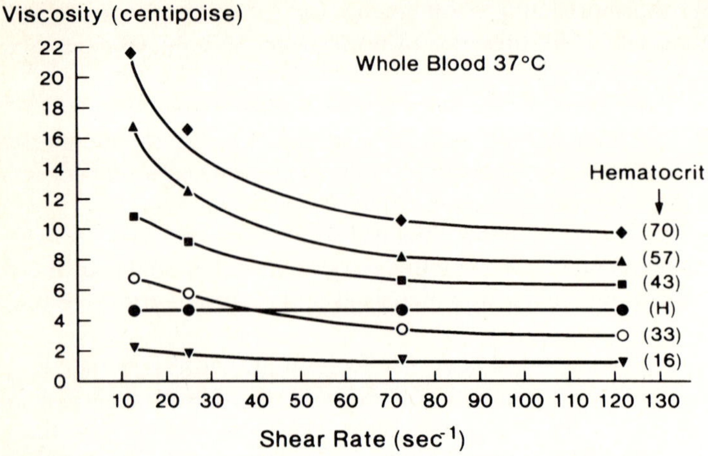

Figure 14-7
Effects of changes in hematocrit on the relationship between viscosity and shear rate. Because blood is a non-Newtonian fluid, effective viscosity increases as the shear rate decreases. With a Newtonian fluid (honey), changes in shear rate do not affect viscosity. (*Modified from an illustration originally presented by RE Wells and EW Merrill* [*29*].)

In this disease, abnormal proteins (macroglobulins) accumulate in the blood but red cell mass and oxygen-carrying capacity may remain in the normal range. The hyperproteinemia increases blood viscosity, and in some patients a "hyperviscosity syndrome" develops [34]. Strauer [35] has measured minimal coronary vascular resistance in a small group of patients with Waldenström's macroglobulinemia. His data indicate that minimal coronary vascular resistance is normal in these patients. The transmural distribution of coronary flow was not measured and, thus, a modest decrease in subendocardial perfusion cannot be excluded. Nonetheless, in humans, a modest increase in blood viscosity has very little effect on the regulation of the coronary circulation.

A second approach to this problem is to assess minimal coronary vascular resistance when the hemoglobin level is kept constant and the concentration of serum proteins is varied over a wide range. When this was done [32], major changes in the concentration of albumin (0.5 to 10 g) produced a small but detectable increase in minimal coronary vascular resistance [32].

Thus, these studies with macroglobulins and albumin support the notion that the plasma proteins have minimal effects on the regulation of the coronary circulation. This is so because these proteins are very minor determinants of blood viscosity.

The importance of red cell concentration on the regulation of the coronary circulation is dramatically demonstrated in the studies in which the effects of methemoglobinemia have been examined [24,36]. Methemoglobinemia can occur as a congenital abnormality [37]. It can also be acquired as a consequence of excessive oxidative stress imposed by exposure to certain chemical agents and drugs, including nitroprusside, a popular vasodilator [38]. Because methemoglobin cannot carry oxygen, methemoglobinemia decreases the oxygen-carrying capacity of blood without the concomitant decrease in viscosity that would occur if the oxygen-carrying capacity of the blood were decreased secondary to anemia. Two studies have measured blood flow when the oxygen-carrying capacity was decreased by producing severe methemoglobinemia [24,36]. Methemoglobinemia was associated with a limited increase in coronary blood flow, a substantial increase in myocardial oxygen extraction, and impaired coronary dilation in the subendocardium of the left ventricle in response to isoproterenol infusion. These studies suggest that the salutory effects of anemia on blood viscosity compensate in part for the loss of oxygen-carrying capacity of the blood.

SPECIFIC EFFECTS OF ALTERING THE OXYGEN-CARRYING CAPACITY OF HEMOGLOBIN

If the blood volume is unchanged, the functional capacity of hemoglobin to deliver oxygen to the tissues can be affected in several ways. First, the oxygen-hemoglobin dissociation curve can be shifted by changes in pH or temperature [39]. Second, structural alterations in the hemoglobin molecule can alter the affinity of hemoglobin for oxygen [40]. Third, the intracellular concentration of 2,3-DPG, which is known to vary in several disease states, can profoundly affect the binding of oxygen to hemoglobin [41,42]. In any of these situations, if the quantity of oxygen delivered to the myocardium is altered, compensatory alterations in coronary vascular resistance would almost certainly occur.

Four studies have examined the effects of a change in hemoglobin-oxygen affinity on either coronary flow [43–44a], the intensity of myocardial ischemia [45], or the extent of infarction following coronary occlusion [43,46]. The data indicate that a decrease in hemoglobin-oxygen affinity can increase coronary blood flow [44] and limit infarct size [43,46].

CLINICAL IMPLICATIONS

Whenever significant alterations occur in hemoglobin concentration, the functional characteristics of hemoglobin, or blood viscosity, the coronary circulation compensates by altering coronary vascular resistance and oxygen extraction across the coronary bed. Because coronary reserve is very great, the abnormalities noted above are of minor significance when they occur in otherwise healthy patients. However, when alterations in blood viscosity, hemoglobin concentration, or the functional capacity of hemoglobin occur in patients with limited coronary reserve, major clinical disturbances can occur.

The two most common clinical conditions which limit coronary reserve are obstructive coronary disease secondary to atherosclerosis (see Chapters 9 through 11) and severe cardiac hypertrophy from any cause (see Chapter 13). There are many reports of patients with coronary disease whose symptoms were exaggerated by anemia [47,48]. In this patient group anemia has two important adverse effects on the coronary circulation. Because the oxygen-carrying capacity of the blood is decreased, coronary flow increases; in effect, this decreases coronary reserve (Fig-

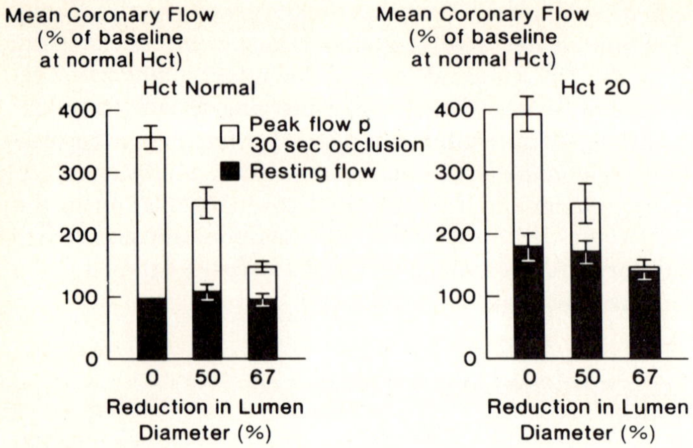

FIGURE 14-8
Effects of anemia on coronary reserve in the presence of experimentally induced coronary stenosis. Proximal coronary stenosis was produced in dogs by partial occlusion of a previously normal coronary artery. Luminal diameter was decreased by 50 and 67 percent of control. Coronary reserve was assessed by the peak-to-resting flow ratio following release of a complete coronary occlusion of the involved vessel. (*Left*) When hematocrit was normal, progressive coronary obstruction decreased coronary reserve but did not alter resting coronary blood flow. (*Right*) When the dogs were subjected to normovolemic anemia, resting coronary blood flow increased in the absence of coronary obstruction. With moderately severe obstruction (67 percent decrease luminal diameter) resting coronary blood flow decreased and coronary reserve was abolished. Thus, anemia adversely affected coronary reserve in the presence of experimentally induced coronary stenosis. Percent of baseline at normal Hct = percent of baseline mean coronary flow at a normal hematocrit; peak flow p 30 sec occlusion = peak flow following release of a 30-s coronary occlusion (*Redrawn from data originally presented by AS Geha et al* [49].)

ure 14-8) [49] and the pressure gradient across all coronary stenoses rises. In turn, perfusion pressure downstream is decreased. If the pressure drop is substantial, subendocardial ischemia will occur (see Chapters 4 and 11).

Whenever coronary reserve is limited by a disease process, superimposed abnormalities in blood viscosity, hemoglobin concentration, or the functional capacity of hemoglobin may produce clinical manifestations of myocardial ischemia. In such clinical situations, the hematologic disturbances should be corrected promptly.

REFERENCES

1 Case RB, Berglund E, Sarnoff SJ: Ventricular function: VII. Changes in coronary resistance and ventricular function resulting from acutely induced anemia and the effect thereon of coronary stenosis. *Am J Med* 18: 397, 1955.

2 Roy SB, Bhatia ML, Mathur VS, Virmani S: Hemodynamic effects of chronic severe anemia. *Circulation* 28: 346, 1963.
3 Regan TJ, Frank MJ, Lehan PH, Galante JG, Hellems HK: Myocardial blood flow and oxygen uptake during acute red cell volume increments. *Circ Res* 13: 172, 1963.
4 Race D, Dedichen H, Schenk WG Jr: Regional blood flow during dextran-induced normovolemic hemodilution in the dog. *J Thorac Cardiovasc Surg* 53: 578, 1967.
5 Neill WA, Oxendine JM, Moore SC: Acute and chronic cardiovascular adjustments to induced anemia in dogs. *Amer J Physiol* 217: 710, 1969.
6 Vatner SF, Higgins CB, Franklin D: Regional circulatory adjustments to moderate and severe chronic anemia in conscious dogs at rest and during exercise. *Circ Res* 30: 731, 1972.
7 von Restorff W, Höfling B, Holtz J, Bassenge E: Effect of increased blood fluidity through hemodilution on general circulation at rest and during exercise in dogs. *Pflügers Arch* 357: 25, 1975.
8 Geha AS: Coronary and cardiovascular dynamics and oxygen availability during acute normovolemic anemia. *Surgery* 80: 47, 1976.
9 Cobb LA, Kramer RJ, Finch CA: Circulatory effects of chronic hypervolemia in polycythemia vera. *J Clin Invest* 39: 1722, 1960.
10 Weber PM, Polycove M, Bacaner MB, Lawrence JH: Cardiac output in polycythemia vera. *J Lab Clin Med* 73: 753, 1969.
11 Rosenthall DS, Braunwald E: Hematologic-oncologic disorders and heart disease, in *Heart Disease: A Textbook of Cardiovascular Medicine*, E Braunwald (ed). Philadelphia, Saunders, 1980, vol 2, chap 48, p 1771.
12 Olsson RA, Gregg DE: Myocardial reactive hyperemia in the unanesthetized dog. *Am J Physiol* 208: 224, 1965.
13 Fowler NO, Holmes JC: Dextran-exchange anemia and reduction in blood viscosity in the heart lung preparation. *Am Heart J* 68: 204, 1964.
14 Murray JF, Rapaport E: Coronary blood flow and myocardial metabolism in acute experimental anaemia. *Cardiovasc Res* 6: 360, 1972.
15 Brazier J, Cooper N, Maloney JV, Buckberg G: The adequacy of myocardial oxygen delivery in acute normovolemic anemia. *Surgery* 75: 508, 1974.
16 Brazier J, Cooper H, Buckberg G: The adequacy of subendocardial oxygen content and myocardial oxygen need. *Circulation* 49: 968, 1974.
17 von Restorff W, Höfling B, Holtz J, Bassenge E: Effect of increased blood fluidity through hemodilution on coronary circulation at rest and during exercise in dogs. *Pflügers Arch* 357: 15, 1975.
18 Holtz J, Bassenge E, von Restorff W, Mayer E: Transmural differences in myocardial blood flow and in coronary dilatory capacity in hemodiluted conscious dogs. *Basic Res Cardiol* 71: 36, 1976.
19 Bing RJ, Hammond MM, Handelsman JC, Powers SR, Spencer FC, Eckenhoff JE, Goodale WT, Hafkenschiel JH, Kety SS: The measurement of coronary blood flow, oxygen consumption, and efficiency of the left ventricle in man. *Am Heart J* 38: 1, 1949.
20 Jan KM, Chien S: Effect of hematocrit variations on coronary hemodynamics and oxygen utilization. *Am J Physiol* 233: H106, 1977.
20a Fan F, Chen RYZ, Schuessler GB, Chien S: Effects of hematocrit variations on regional hemodynamics and oxygen transport in the dog. *Am J Physiol* 238: H545, 1980.
21 Johansson B, Linder E, Seeman T: Effects of hematocrit and blood viscosity on myocardial blood flow during temporary coronary occlusions in dogs. *Scand J Thor Cardiovasc Surg* 1: 165, 1967.

22 Scheel KW, Brody DA, Ingram LA, Keller F: Effects of chronic anemia on the coronary and coronary collateral vasculature in dogs. *Circ Res* 38: 553, 1976.

23 Eckstein RW: Development of interarterial coronary anastomoses by chronic anemia; disappearance following correction of anemia. *Circ Res* 3: 306, 1955.

23a Bhatia ML, Manchanda SC, Roy SB: Coronary haemodynamic studies in chronic severe anaemia. *Brit Heart J* 31: 365, 1969.

24 Regan TJ, Frank MJ, Lehan PH, Galante JG, Hellems HK: Myocardial blood flow and oxygen uptake during acute red cell volume increments. *Circ Res* 13: 172, 1963.

25 Surjadhana A, Rouleau J, Boerboom L, Hoffman JIE: Myocardial blood flow and its distribution in anesthetized polycythemic dogs. *Circ Res* 43: 619, 1978.

26 Moret P, Covarrubias E, Coudert J, Duchosal F: Cardiocirculatory adaptation to chronic hypoxia. Comparative study of coronary flow, myocardial oxygen consumption, and efficiency between sea level and high altitude residents. *Acta Cardiol* 27: 283, 1972.

27 Franciosi RA, Blanc WA: Myocardial infarcts in infants and children. I. A necropsy study in congenital heart disease *J Pediatrics* 73: 309, 1968.

28 Guyton AC: *Textbook of Medical Physiology*, 2d ed. Philadelphia, Saunders, 1961, p 345.

29 Wells RE Jr, Merrill EW: Influence of flow properties of blood upon viscosity-hematocrit relationships. *J Clin Med* 41: 1591, 1962.

30 Merrill EW: Rheology of blood. *Physiol Rev* 49: 863, 1969.

31 Benis AM, Usami S, Chien S: Effect of hematocrit and inertial losses on pressure-flow relations in the isolated hindpaw of the dog. *Circ Res* 27: 1047, 1970.

32 Avolio AP, Spaan JAE, Laird JD: Plasma protein concentration and control of coronary vascular resistance in isolated rat heart. *Am J Physiol* 238: H471, 1980.

33 Imhof JW, Baars H, Verloop MC: Clinical and hematological aspects of macroglobulinaemia of Waldenstrom. *Acta Med Scand* 163: 349, 1959.

34 Bloch KJ, Maki DG: Hyperviscosity syndromes associated with immunoglobulin abnormalities. *Semin Hematol* 10113, 1973.

35 Strauer B-E: Personal communication, Department of Medicine, University of Munich, August 1981.

36 Biro GP, Beresford-Kroeger D: Myocardial blood flow and O_2-supply following dextran-haemodilution and methaemoglobinaemia in the dog. *Cardiovasc Res* 13: 495, 1979.

37 Cartwright GE: Methemoglobinemia and sulfhemoglobinemia, in *Harrison's Principles of Internal Medicine*, MM Wintrobe, GW Thorn, RD Adams (eds). New York, McGraw-Hill, 1974, p 1644.

38 Bower PJ, Peterson JN: Methemoglobinemia after sodium nitroprusside therapy. *N Engl J Med* 293: 865, 1975.

39 Riggs A: Functional properties of hemoglobins. *Physiol Rev* 45: 619, 1965.

40 Wintrobe MM: *Clinical Hematology*. Philadelphia, Lea & Febiger, 1974.

41 Bunn HF, Jandl JH: Control of hemoglobin function within the red cell. *N Engl J Med* 282: 1414, 1970.

42 Grisolia S, et al: Binding of 2, 3-diphosphoglycerate (DPG) to oxhemoglobin; levels and effect of DPG on oxygen affinity of normal and abnormal blood, in *Red Cell Metabolism and Function*, G Brewer (ed). New York, Plenum Press, 1970, p 19.

43 Pantely GA, Oyama AA, Metcalfe J, Lawson MS, Welch JE: Improvement in the relationship between flow to ischemic myocardium and the extent of necrosis with glycolytic intermediates that decreases blood oxygen affinity in dogs. *Circ Res* 49: 395, 1981.

44 Mehmul HC, Duvelleroy MA, Laver MB: Response of coronary blood flow to pH-induced changes in hemoglobin-O_2 affinity. *J Appl Physiol* 35: 485, 1973.

44a Duvelleroy MA, Martin JL, Teisseire B, Gauduel Y, Duruble M: Abnormal hemoglobin oxygen affinity and the coronary circulation. *Biblthca Haemat* Basel, Karger, 46: 70, 1980.

45 Holsinger JW Jr, Salhany JM, Eliot RS: Evidence for a relationship between 2,3-diphosphoglycerate-depleted red blood cells, slow oxygen release and myocardial ischemia, in *Advances in Experimental Medicine and Biology*, HI Bicher, DF Bruley (eds). vol 37A, New York, Plenum Press 1973, p 187.

46 Rude RE, Kloner RA, Tumas J, DeBoer LWV, Gunst M, Laver M, Moroko PR: Reduction of experimental myocardial infarction size by ortho-idio sodium benzoate. *Am J Cardiol* 45: 485, 1980.

47 Ellis LB, Faulkner JM: The heart in anemia. *N Engl J Med* 220: 943, 1939.

48 Elliot AH: Anemia as the cause of angina pectoris in the presence of healthy coronary arteries and aorta: Report of case. *Am J Med Sci* 181: 135, 1934.

49 Geha AS, Baue AE: Graded coronary stenosis and coronary flow during acute normovolemic anemia. *World J Surg* 2: 645, 1978.

CHAPTER **15**

RARE DISEASES OF THE CORONARY VASCULATURE WHICH CAN IMPAIR MYOCARDIAL PERFUSION

CONGENITAL ABNORMALITIES
ARTERITIS
SMALL VESSEL CORONARY ARTERY DISEASE SECONDARY TO SYSTEMIC HYPERTENSION
CORONARY MURAL THICKENING
CORONARY EMBOLI
DISSECTION AND TRAUMA
ANEURYSM
MYOCARDIAL BRIDGES
OTHER SOURCES OF EXTERNAL COMPRESSION OF CORONARY VESSELS
SYNDROME X

Coronary vessels are susceptible to disease processes that affect other vascular beds. These include congenital abnormalities, trauma, infection, dissection, embolism, aneurysm, vasculitis, and external compression. These disease processes are usually not considered in the initial evaluation of patients with myocardial ischemia because their combined prevalence is probably less than 5 percent of that associated with atherosclerotic coronary vascular disease.

CONGENITAL ABNORMALITIES

In the absence of other congenital heart defects, anomalous origin of a coronary artery occurs in 1.2 percent of patients [1–3]. The incidence of such abnormalities is presumably higher in patients with coexistent congenital heart defects [4,5]. Most of the abnormalities concerning the origin of major coronary vessels are of no physiological significance [1–3]. For example, the most common major abnormality—origin of the circumflex coronary artery from the proximal right coronary artery or the right sinus of Valsalva—has no adverse effects on myocardial perfusion.

Three congenital abnormalities of the coronary vessels can adversely affect the myocardial perfusion: origin of one or both coronary vessels from the pulmonary artery, origin of the right and left coronary arteries from one sinus of Valsalva, and coronary arteriovenous fistulas.

When one or more coronary vessels arise from the pulmonary artery, coronary driving pressure is low and the blood perfusing the anomalous coronary vessel(s) is moderately desaturated [2,6–11]. If the right coronary artery arises from the pulmonary artery the abnormality in myocardial perfusion is of little consequence. This anomaly can be tolerated for decades [2].

If both coronary arteries arise from the pulmonary artery, death ensues soon after birth [2,6]. On rare occasions patients with anomalous origin of both coronary arteries from the pulmonary artery are protected by a coexistent high pressure–high flow shunt [12]. Under these conditions, because pulmonary artery pressure and the oxygen saturation of pulmonary arterial blood are high, coronary perfusion is adequate. Failure to recognize this coronary abnormality prior to surgical correction of the defect responsible for the shunt would have devastating effects.

When the left coronary artery arises from the pulmonary artery, about 85 percent of patients do not survive until adulthood [7–11]. In most patients, massive anterolateral myocardial infarction occurs in infancy and is frequently accompanied by left ventricular failure and mitral regurgitation [7–11]. Patients tolerate this abnormality only if adequate collaterals between the right and left coronary arteries develop (Figure 15-1) [13]. Under these conditions, a type of "coronary

FIGURE 15-1
Composite drawing of anomalous left coronary artery which filled retrogradely from the right coronary, causing contrast medium to spill into the pulmonary artery. PA = pulmonary artery. (*From M Verani et al* [*13*].)

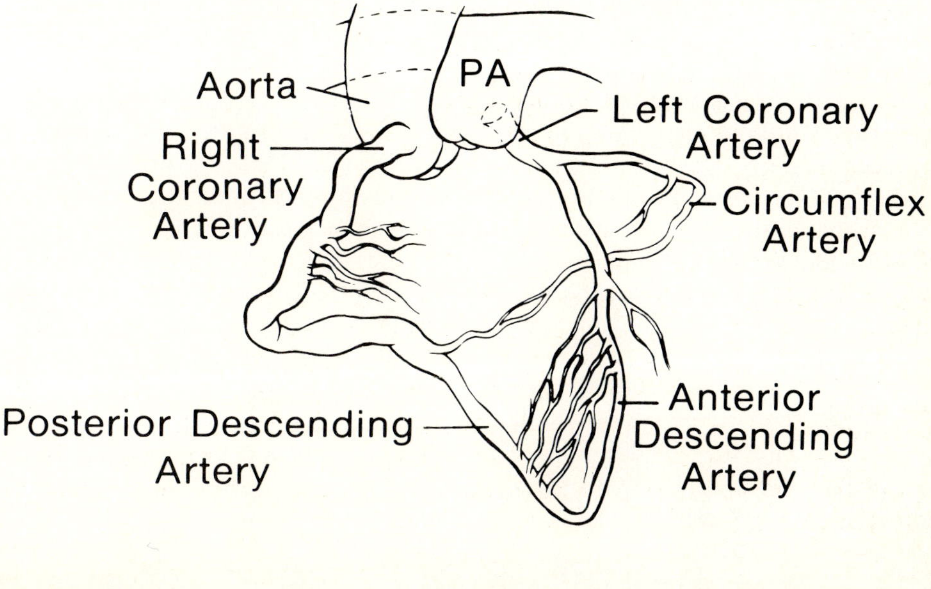

steal" occurs. Blood from the right coronary artery under high pressure perfuses the left coronary system and some of the blood reaches the pulmonary artery. Consequently, a small left-to-right shunt develops.

Multiple major coronary arteries occasionally arise from one sinus of Valsalva (right coronary artery from the left sinus of Valsalva; left anterior descending, circumflex, or main left coronary artery from the right sinus of Valsalva) [2,3,14–15]. These abnormalities are of particular importance if the left main coronary artery arises from the right sinus of Valsalva because of the acute angle the vessel takes as it passes leftward behind the pulmonary artery.

It has been postulated that during exercise the great vessels dilate and compression of the coronary vessel passing between the great vessels can impair perfusion in the distribution of the anomalous vessel. Exertional angina, acute myocardial infarction, and sudden cardiac death have been noted in patients in whom the main left coronary artery arises from the right sinus of Valsalva [14].

Although congenital coronary abnormalities that are of physiological significance are very infrequent; they can be responsible for major abnormalities in myocardial perfusion.

The older literature suggests that when the right coronary artery arises from the left sinus of Valsalva, no abnormalities in myocardial perfusion occur [15]. A recent report by Roberts et al. (15a) challenges this notion. Roberts noted that 12 of 41 cases of this anomaly studied during life had manifestations of myocardial ischemia (two acute myocardial infarction; five angina pectoris; eight either syncope, nonfatal ventricular fibrillation or sudden death). We have recently studied a patient with this anomaly in the operating room with a Doppler probe. Because the patient had suffered a subendocardial infarction and ventricular fibrillation presumably related to the anomalous right coronary artery, the vessel was bypassed. When the downstream branches of the anomalous right coronary artery were perfused by the graft, the reactive hyperemia response (20-s coronary occlusion) was 50 percent greater than when the vessels were perfused by the anomalous vessel. This data suggests that the anomalous right coronary artery was partially obstructed.

Coronary fistulae may link the right and left coronary vessels, or the coronary vessels may drain directly into the coronary sinus or one of the cardiac chambers. In recent reviews, Upshaw [16] and Rittenhouse et al. [16a] noted that the great majority of such fistulas drain to chambers on the right side of the heart. Coronary fistulas that drain to the right sided cardiac chambers result in left to right shunts which are usually very small [16,16a]. Electrocardiographic manifestations of myocardial ischemia and angina pectoris [17–17b] have occasionally been attributed to coronary fistulas.

ARTERITIS

Generalized vascular inflammatory diseases (see Table 15-1) may occasionally involve coronary vessels [18]. In this regard, two specific diseases warrant particular mention: luetic arteritis and systemic lupus erythematosus.

TABLE 15-1
TYPES OF CORONARY ARTERITIS

Luetic
Granulomatous (Takayasu disease)
Infectious
Polyarteritis nodosa
Rheumatoid arthritis
Rheumatic fever
Ankylosing spondylitis
Systemic lupus erythematosus

Obliterative endarteritis involving the coronary ostia occurs in 26 percent of patients with luetic cardiovascular involvement [19]. Most patients with luetic involvement of the coronary arteries also have other manifestations of cardiovascular syphilis, such as aortic regurgitation or aortic aneurysm. The coronary ostial lesions characteristic of syphilis can produce severe coronary obstruction and all its attendant complications, including angina pectoris, acute myocardial infarction, and sudden cardiac death.

Lupus erythematosus is a collagen vascular disease that occasionally involves coronary vessels [18,20–22]. Although initially the coronary involvement characteristic of lupus erythematosus was thought to be limited to small intramural coronary arteries [20], the arteritis can occasionally involve major coronary vessels and precipitate acute myocardial infarction [21,22]. Strauer [23] has measured coronary reserve in a small group of patients with systemic lupus erythematosus who had normal coronary angiograms. In this patient group, coronary dilator capacity assessed by measuring maximal coronary blood flow during infusion of dipyridamole was moderately decreased. When these patients were treated with steroids for several months, symptoms of myocardial ischemia were ameliorated and coronary reserve returned toward normal. This study by Strauer provides the best evidence to date that a collagen-vascular disease, by virtue of isolated small coronary involvement, can have functionally important effects on the coronary circulation.

SMALL VESSEL CORONARY ARTERY DISEASE SECONDARY TO SYSTEMIC HYPERTENSION

Increased intraluminal pressure in coronary vessels stimulates the growth of smooth muscle in the vascular wall [24]. As a consequence, the wall-to-lumen ratio of coronary resistance vessels decreases and coronary reserve is impaired (see Chapter 13). This process occurs in patients with moderate hypertension and can cause all the classic manifestations of myocardial ischemia [25]. Unfortunately, this abnormality usually escapes recognition because (1) patients with systemic hypertension have concomitant atherosclerotic disease of the large coronary ves-

TABLE 15-2
CAUSES OF CORONARY MURAL THICKENING

Mucopolysaccharidosis (Hurler disease)
Homocystinuria
Fabry's disease
Amyloidosis
Juvenile intimal sclerosis (idiopathic arterial calcification of infancy)
Intima hyperplasia associated with contraceptive steroids or with the postpartum period
Pseudoxanthoma elasticum
Coronary fibrosis caused by radiation therapy

sels and (2) coronary reserve is rarely assessed in hypertensive patients with angiographically normal coronary vessels and a clinical syndrome suggesting myocardial ischemia. Strauer [25], has characterized this clinical entity in a very thorough manner. Clinical cardiologists should be encouraged to consider this diagnosis in the evaluation of hypertensive patients with angina pectoris and normal coronary arteriograms.

CORONARY MURAL THICKENING

Cheitlin et al. [18] have reviewed a number of clinical syndromes and metabolic diseases that occasionally cause mural thickening of coronary vessels (see Table 15-2). In most of these conditions, the pathology has been described from postmortem material, but the functional significance of the pathological lesions has not been assessed in a subgroup of patients affected with the disease entity. For the most part, the coronary involvement in these conditions contributes in a minor way to the patient's clinical profile.

CORONARY EMBOLI

Because the coronary vessels are the first branches of the aorta, the source of coronary embolic material must reside in the heart or the coronary vessels [18,26]. This anatomic arrangement coupled with the small percentage of cardiac output that perfuses the heart limits the susceptibility of coronary vessels to emboli. Consequently, coronary emboli are less common than embolic occlusions involving other major vascular beds [26].

Bacterial emboli incorporated in vegetations from infected cardiac valves on the left side of the heart are the predominant source of coronary embolism [26].

Less common sources of coronary emboli include: intracardiac thrombi, intracardiac tumors, atherosclerotic or syphilitic plaques, fat, and fibrin or thrombotic material that accumulates on left-sided prosthetic valves [26]. There are two iatrogenic sources of coronary emboli. Rarely, a clot or air bubble in a coronary catheter is flushed into a coronary vessel. Also, during cardiopulmonary bypass with or without coronary cannulation and perfusion, clots, air bubbles, or other debris from diseased or prosthetic valves can embolize the coronary vessels.

Whenever coronary embolism occurs, the consequences depend on the size and composition of the embolus and the vessel involved. The complications of emboli vary from no detectable abnormality (small air bubble injected into the right coronary artery) to sudden death (large thrombotic embolus in the main left coronary artery). The manifestations of embolic coronary occlusion are similar to other types of coronary occlusion (see Chapter 9).

DISSECTION AND TRAUMA

Dissection of a coronary vessel, when it occurs spontaneously, is usually associated with concomitant dissection of the aortic root [27,28]. This clinical catastrophe usually results in myocardial infarction and death [27,28]. Rarely, spontaneous coronary dissection is confined to a single coronary artery [29–31]. Cystic medial degeneration in the involved vessel associated with Marfan's syndrome or polyarteritis nodosa are the most frequent predisposing conditions [29,30]. For unexplained reasons, isolated coronary dissection occurs more frequently than expected in young women in the peripartum period [31].

Coronary dissection can be iatrogenic. This complication can occur during coronary angiography [32], coronary angioplasty [33], or as a result of coronary cannulation associated with cardiac surgery [34]. Myocardial infarction often ensues following iatrogenic coronary dissections [32–34].

Coronary vessels are occasionally injured as a result of trauma [35–37]. Lacerations of the coronary vessel usually produce pericardial tampanode. The patient succumbs from cardiac compression before other manifestations of the coronary injury become evident [35,36]. Myocardial contusion, secondary to blunt-chest trauma, usually produces microvascular injury and myocardial infarction. Although previous studies suggested that myocardial contusion provoked coronary spasm, it is now clear that the perfusion abnormalities associated with myocardial contusion are unrelated to involvement of the epicardial coronary vessels [37]. In general, even when blunt-chest trauma damages the myocardium, the coronary arterial system is spared.

Although dissection and trauma to coronary vessels occur, these problems are rare and frequently unrecognized unless they are iatrogenically induced.

ANEURYSM

Coronary artery aneurysms do not in themselves alter myocardial perfusion. However, superimposed complications, including thrombosis, rupture, or embolism from the aneurysmal sac, can produce myocardial ischemia or infarction [38]. The most common cause of coronary aneurysm is atherosclerosis [38]. Recent studies have called attention to the frequency with which coronary aneurysms develop in children afflicted with mucocutaneous lymph node syndrome (Kawasaki's disease) [38a].

MYOCARDIAL BRIDGES

The major coronary arteries usually lie on the surface of the heart. Occasionally, a segment of a major coronary artery may penetrate the cardiac surface and follow an intramural course for a short distance. Thus, a short segment of the vessel is covered by a "myocardial bridge." Pathological studies indicate that this anomaly occurs in 23 percent of patients [39]. Angiographic studies suggest that during systole, the subepicardial segment is compressed to a variable degree [40]. Angiographic evidence of such compression is noted in 0.5 percent of angiograms performed in patients with chest pain syndromes [40a].

The functional consequences of myocardial bridges has been controversial. On theoretical grounds, one would predict that systolic compression of a coronary vessel would not significantly alter myocardial perfusion. Normally, less than 20 percent of coronary flow recorded in an epicardial vessel perfusing the left ventricle occurs in systole (see Chapter 4). Furthermore, some of this "systolic flow" reflects the capacitive function of epicardial vessels rather than anterograde tissue perfusion in systole (see Chapter 4). In the dog, the interventricular septum is perfused by a large septal artery which is intramyocardial throughout most of its course. In essence, this vessel is totally "surrounded" by a myocardial bridge. Yet, the septum in dogs is well perfused during intense exercise [41]. Furthermore, minimal vascular resistance in the septum is similar to that of the left ventricular free wall [42]. My colleagues and I have recently studied a patient who had a prominent myocardial bridge. We measured phasic coronary blood flow velocity and the coronary reactive hyperemic response in the affected vessel with our Doppler probe. In this vessel, coronary reserve was nearly normal (Figure 15-2) and diastolic inflow to the vessel was not delayed (Figure 15-3). Taken together these theoretical and physiological considerations suggest that myocardial bridges should not significantly alter myocardial perfusion.

Data from the clinical literature suggests the opposite conclusion. Clinicians have noted that "myocardial bridges" are occasionally associated with angina pectoris, electrocardiographic abnormalities suggestive of myocardial ischemia, perfusion defects, decreases in coronary flow, and metabolic evidence of myocardial ischemia [43–46]. Also, following surgical division of cardiac muscle compressing a subepicardial major coronary vessel, clinical evidence of myocardial ischemia that was present preoperatively may no longer be detectable [45–47].

There is no way to reconcile all the data. Krawczyk et al. [48] and Mays et al. [49] suggested that "delayed opening" of a coronary vessel following systolic occlusion by a myocardial bridge could contribute importantly to the genesis of myocardial ischemia in patients with prominent myocardial bridges. In an animal model,

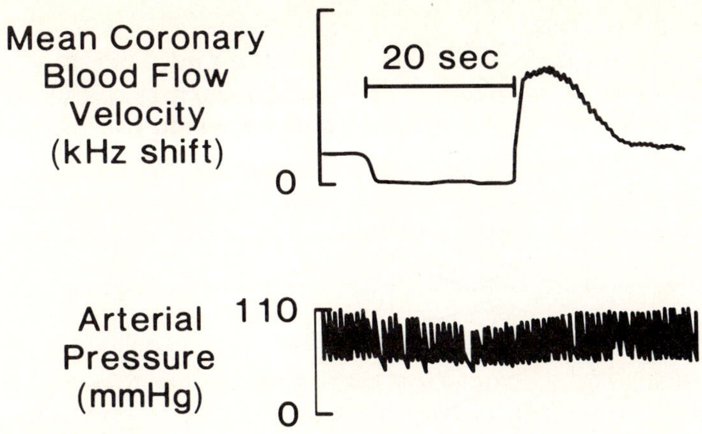

FIGURE 15-2
Coronary reactive hyperemic response in a vessel with a prominent myocardial bridge. This recording was obtained at the University of Iowa by L Hiratzka (Division of Thoracic and Cardiovascular Surgery, Department of Surgery) and CL Eastham (Cardiovascular Research Center) at the time of cardiac surgery. Coronary blood flow velocity was measured with a Doppler probe (see Chapter 2) prior to cardiopulmonary bypass. Following release of a 20-s coronary occlusion, coronary blood flow velocity increased substantially. The peak-to-resting velocity ratio was 3.2:1, which is slightly below the normal range in our laboratory (see Chapter 3). Thus, the myocardial bridge in this patient only moderately decreased coronary reserve.

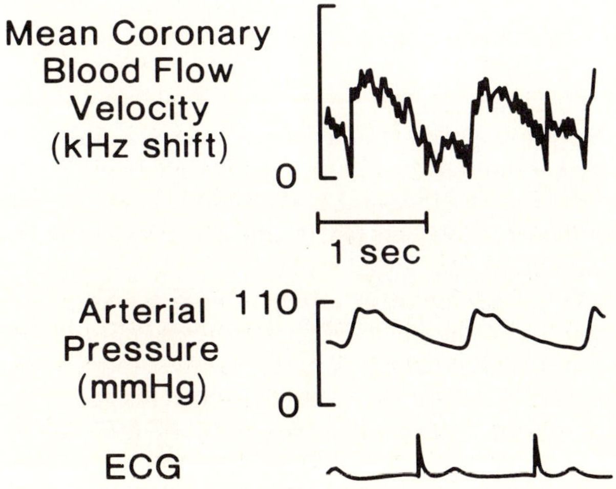

FIGURE 15–3
Phasic coronary blood flow velocity in a vessel with a prominent myocardial bridge. This recording was obtained at the University of Iowa by L Hiratzka (Division of Thoracic and Cardiovascular Surgery, Department of Surgery) and CL Eastham (Cardiovascular Research Center) at the time of cardiac surgery. Coronary blood flow velocity was measured with a Doppler probe (see Chapter 2) prior to cardiopulmonary bypass. The rapid upstroke in diastolic coronary blood flow velocity indicates that there was no delay in coronary inflow. Thus, in this instance, delayed opening of the vascular segment as a result of the myocardial bridge was probably not present.

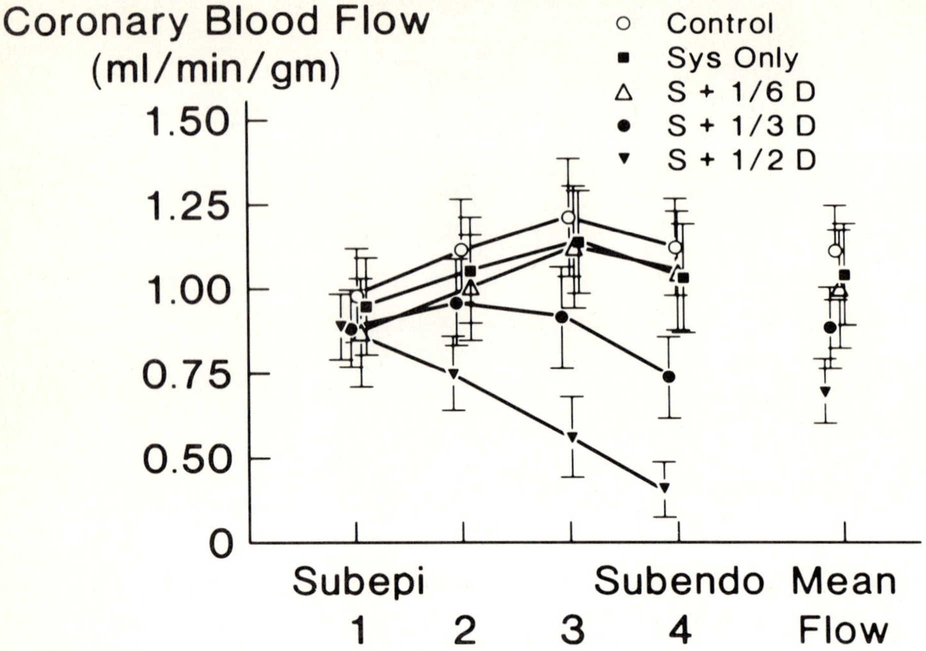

FIGURE 15-4
Effects of a simulated myocardial bridge on regional left ventricular coronary blood flow measured with microspheres. In this study, a myocardial bridge was simulated in an awake dog by transiently occluding a major coronary artery with a balloon occluder in systole (S) or systole plus a fraction of diastole (D). Left ventricular coronary blood flow was not altered until coronary occlusion involved all of systole and at least one-third of diastole. Subepi = subepicardium; Subendo = subendocardium; integers at the bottom of figure represent the number of layers of left ventricular myocardium. (*From AE Mays Jr, PA McHale, and JC Greenfield Jr* [*49*].)

however, the simulated delay in diastolic opening of a coronary vessel required to produce significant ischemia was substantial—¼ to ½ of the diastolic interval at a heart rate of 60 to 120 beats/min (Figures 15-4 and 15-5) [48,49]. These experimental studies indicate that insufficient inflow time [48,49] and decreased coronary perfusion pressure distal to the simulated myocardial bridge [49] contributed to the perfusion abnormalities noted. One case report in a patient with a myocardial bridge suggested complete reopening of the involved coronary segment did not occur until 50 percent of the diastolic interval had elapsed [50]. At surgery, measurements of phasic coronary blood flow in this patient indicated that diastolic flow was delayed. After the myocardial bridge was divided, the coronary inflow delay resolved.

Clinical studies concerning the potential significance of myocardial bridges have many deficiencies, including the following.

1 The criteria for identifying a myocardial bridge angiographically are not quantitative. Ideally, a significant myocardial bridge should produce a given de-

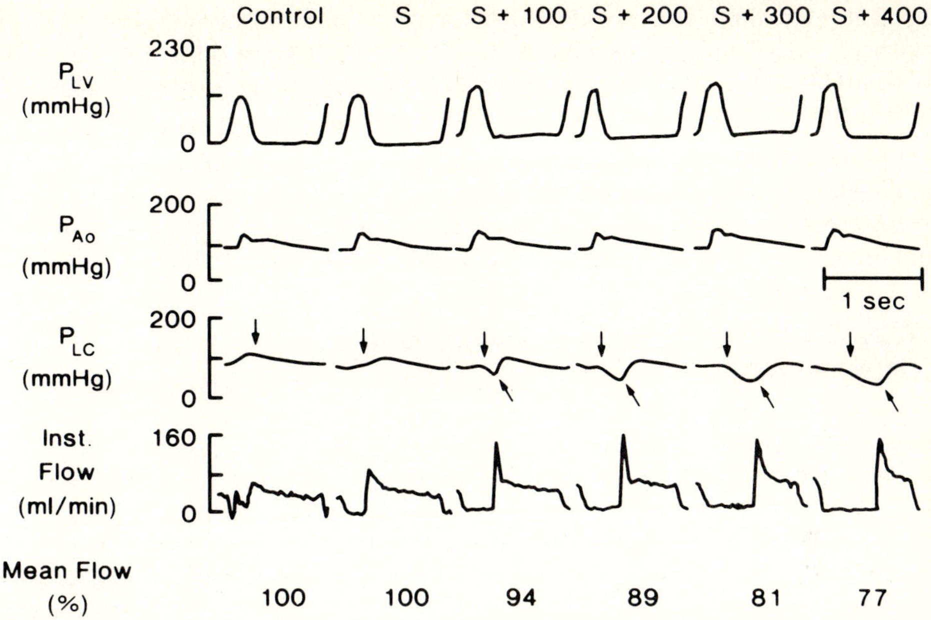

FIGURE 15-5
Effects of a simulated myocardial bridge on systemic and coronary hemodynamics in an anesthetized dog. P_{LV} = left ventricular pressure; P_{AO} = aortic pressure; P_{LC} = left circumflex coronary pressure distal to the coronary occluder; inst. flow = instantaneous coronary blood flow in circumflex coronary artery; Mean Flow = % mean flow in the circumflex coronary artery as a percent of control; S = systolic coronary occlusion; S + = systolic coronary occlusion plus number of milliseconds of diastolic coronary occlusion. In this study, coronary occlusion was accomplished by inflating a balloon occluder around the circumflex artery for specific time intervals. Transient coronary occlusion had no effect on left ventricular or aortic pressure. Systolic coronary occlusion alone did not affect circumflex coronary artery pressure or coronary flow. By progressively increasing the duration of transient occlusion to include progressively longer segments of diastole, the transient occlusions did decrease distal pressure and coronary flow in the left circumflex coronary artery. These data indicate that transient coronary occlusion does not significantly affect coronary hemodynamics unless the occlusion includes systole and a significant percentage of diastole. (*Modified from an illustration originally presented by JA Krawczyk et al* [*48*].)

crease in the *luminal area* of the involved vessel. The effect of changes in myocardial contractility on the magnitude of systolic compression should be considered. Also, delayed reopening of the involved vascular segment should be sought.

2 It is possible that some patients reported to have a hemodynamically significant myocardial bridge had undetected obstructive coronary lesions or fixed obstructions whose significance was underestimated (see Chapter 11).

3 Many noninvasive procedures for detecting myocardial ischemia, such as the exercise electrocardiogram and thallium 201 perfusion scintigrams, have relatively high false-positive rates [51,52]. Hence, in selected cases, the chance occurrence of a false-positive noninvasive test which suggests myocardial ischemia and a myocardial bridge could lead to clinical misinterpretation. This fortuitous combination can be excluded only by examining a large group of consecutive patients with myocardial bridges and an appropriate control population. Such data have not been reported.

My view is that myocardial bridges are of minimal functional importance in the vast majority of patients with this anomaly. However, rarely such myocardial bridges may be of physiological significance, particularly when they are prominent and occur in patients with coexistent ventricular hypertrophy [43].

OTHER SOURCES OF EXTERNAL COMPRESSION OF CORONARY VESSELS

One study has suggested that constrictive pericarditis, or sudden cardiac dilation, could alter coronary hemodynamics. Studies by Allard et al. suggest that severe, acute cardiac dilation can increase wall tension sufficiently to impair coronary flow [54]. In the experiments of Allard et al., fulminant heart failure associated with acute cardiac dilation was produced in anesthetized dogs by infusing phenformin intravenously. When the pericardium was left open, marked subendocardial perfusion of the left ventricle developed. This effect did not occur if the pericardium was closed. These data suggest that gross, acute, left ventricular distention may adversely alter myocardial perfusion.

SYNDROME X

Recently, in a group of patients with exertional angina and normal coronary arteries, it has been found that the coronary vessels cannot dilate appropriately in response to pacing or an infusion of dipyridamole [55,56]. A few such patients developed metabolic evidence of myocardial ischemia during pacing [55]. This clinical entity has been called syndrome X. The mechanism of impaired coronary reserve in these patients remains unexplained.

REFERENCES

1 Edwards JE: Anomalous coronary arteries with special reference to arteriovenous-like communications (editorial). *Circulation* 17: 1001, 1958.

2 Blake HA, Manion WC, Mattingly TW, Baroldi G: Coronary artery anomalies. *Circulation* 30: 927, 1964.

3 Engel HJ, Torres C, Page HL: Major variations in anatomical origin of the coronary arteries: Angiographic observations in 4,250 patients without associated congenital heart disease. *Cath Cardiovasc Diag* 1: 157, 1975.

4 Elliot LP, Amplatz K, Edwards JE: Coronary artery patterns in transposition complexes: Anatomic and angiographic studies. *Am J Cardiol* 17: 362, 1966.

5 White RJ: The nature and significance of anomalous coronary arteries in tetrology of Fallot. *Am J Roent* 114: 350, 1972.

6 Tedeschi CG, Helpern MM: Heterotopic origin of both coronary arteries from the

pulmonary artery: Review of literature and report of a case not complicated by associated defects. *Pediatrics* 14: 53, 1954.

7 Wesselhoeft H. Fawcett JS, Johnson AL: Anomalous origin of the left coronary artery from the pulmonary trunk: Its clinical spectrum, pathology, and pathophysiology based on a review of 140 cases with 7 further cases. *Circulation* 38: 403, 1968.

8 Askenazi J, Nadas AS: Anomalous left coronary artery originating from the pulmonary artery. *Circulation* 51: 976, 1975.

9 Edwards JE: The direction of blood flow in coronary arteries arising from the pulmonary trunk. *Circulation* 29: 163, 1964.

10 Bland EF, White PD, Garland J: Congenital anomalies of the coronary arteries: Report of an unusual case associated with cardiac hypertrophy. *Am Heart J* 8: 787, 1933.

11 Keith JD: Anomalous origin of left coronary artery from pulmonary artery. *Brit Heart J* 21: 149, 1959.

12 Tow A: Cor biloculare with truncus arteriosus and endocarditis. *Am J Dis Child* 42: 1413, 1939.

13 Verani M, Marcus M, Ehrhardt J, Doty D: Demonstration of improved myocardial perfusion following aortic implantation of anomalous left coronary artery. *J Nucl Med* 19: 1032, 1978.

14 Cheitlin MD, DeCastro CM, McAllister HA: Sudden death as a complication of anomalous left coronary origin from the anterior sinus of Valsalva. A not-so-minor congenital anomaly. *Circulation* 50: 780, 1974.

15 Thompson SI, Vieweg WVR, Alpert JS, Hagan AD: Anomalous origin of the right coronary artery from the left sinus of Valsalva with associated chest pain: Report of two cases. *Cath Cardiovasc Diag* 2: 397, 1976.

15a Roberts WC, Siegel RJ, Zipes DP: Origin of the right coronary artery from the left sinus of valsalva and its functional consequences: Analysis of 10 necropsy patients. *Am J Cardiol* 49: 863, 1982.

16 Upshaw CB Jr: Congenital coronary arteriovenous fistula. Report of a case with an analysis of 73 reported cases. *Am Heart J* 63: 399, 1962.

16a Rittenhouse EA, Doty DB, Ehrenhaft JL: Congenital coronary artery—cardiac chamber fistula. Review of operative management. *Ann Thorac Surg* 20: 468, 1975.

17 Sakakibara S, Yokoyama M, Takao A, Nogi M Gomi H: Coronary arteriovenous fistula: Nine operated cases. *Am Heart J* 72: 307, 1966.

17a Ghosh MB, Chia BL, Tan NC: Coronary artery fistula. *Aust NZ J Med* 1: 233, 1971.

17b Oldham HN, Ebert PA, Young WG, Sabiston DC: Surgical management of congenital coronary artery fistula. *Ann Thorac Surg* 12: 503, 1971.

18 Cheitlin MD, McAllister HA, deCastro CM: Myocardial infarction without atherosclerosis. *JAMA* 231: 951, 1975.

19 Heggtveit HA: Syphilitic aortitis: A clinicopathologic autopsy study of 100 cases. 1950 to 1960. *Circulation* 29: 346, 1964.

20 Klemperer P, Pollack A, Baehr G: Pathology of disseminated lupus erythematosus. *Arch Pathol* 32: 569, 1941.

21 Bonfiglio TA, Botti RE, Hagstrom JW: Coronary arteritis, occlusion and myocardial infarction due to lupus erythematosus. *Am Heart J* 83: 153, 1972.

22 Benisch BM, Pervez H: Coronary artery vasculitis and myocardial infarction with systemic lupus erythematosus. *NY State J Med* 74: 873, 1974.

23 Strauer BE: Department of Medicine, University of Munich, Personal communication. July 1981.

24 Folkow B, Hallback M, Lundgren Y, Sivertsson R, Weiss L: Importance of adaptive changes in vascular design for establishment of primary hypertension, studied in man and in spontaneously hypertensive rats. *Circ Res* 32/33: 2, 1973.

25 Strauer BE: *Hypertensive Heart Disease*, Berlin, Springer-Verlag, 1980.

26 Wenger NK, Bauer S: Coronary embolism: Review of the literature and presentation of fifteen cases. *Am J Med* 25: 549, 1958.

27 Hirst AE Jr, Johns VJ Jr, Kime SW Jr: Dissecting aneurysm of the aorta: Review of 505 cases. *Medicine* 37: 217, 1958.

28 Wheat MW Jr, Palmer RF: Dissecting aneurysms of the aorta. *Curr Probl Surg* July: 2, 1971.

29 Smith JC: Dissecting aneurysms of coronary arteries. *Arch Pathol* 99: 117, 1975.

30 Benson PA: Dissecting aneurysms of right and left coronary arteries. *J Forensic Sci* 15: 65, 1970.

31 Claudon DG, Claudon DB, Edwards JE: Primary dissecting aneurysm of coronary artery. A cause of acute myocardial ischemia. *Circulation* 45: 259, 1972.

32 Kitamura K, Gobel FL, Wang Y: Dissection of the left coronary artery complicating retrograde left heart catheterization. *Chest* 57: 587, 1970.

33 Gruentzig AR, Senning A, Siegenthaler WE: Nonoperative dilation of coronary-artery stenosis. *N Eng J Med* 301: 61, 1979.

34 Fishman NG, Youker JE, Roe BB: Mechanical injury to the coronary arteries during operative cannulation. *Am Heart J* 75: 26, 1968.

35 Parmley LF, Manion WC, Mattingly TW: Nonpenetrating traumatic injury of the heart. *Circulation* 18: 371, 1958.

36 Liedtke AJ, DeMuth WE: Nonpenetrating cardiac injuries: A collective review. *Am Heart J* 86: 687, 1973.

37 Liedtke AJ, Allen RP, Nellis SH: Effects of blunt cardiac trauma on coronary vasomotion, perfusion, myocardial mechanics and metabolism. *J Trauma* 20: 777, 1980.

38 Daoud AS, Pankin D, Tulgan H, Florentin RA: Aneurysms of the coronary artery: Report of ten cases and review of the literature. *Am J Cardiol* 11: 228, 1963.

38a Chung J, Brandt L, Fulton DR, Kreidberg MB: Cardiac and coronary arterial involvement in infants and children from New England with mucocutaneous lymph node syndrome (Kawasaki disease). *Am J Cardiol* 50: 136, 1982.

39 Geiringer E: The mural coronary. *Am Heart J* 41: 359, 1951

40 Amplatz K, Anderson R: Angiographic appearance of myocardial bridging of the coronary artery. *Invest Radiol* 3: 213, 1968.

40a Noble J, Bourassa MG, Petitclerc R, Dyrda I: Myocardial bridging and milking effect of the left anterior descending coronary artery: Normal variant or obstruction. *Am J Cardiol* 37: 993, 1976.

41 Ball RM, Bache RJ,Cobb FR, Greenfield JC Jr: Regional myocardial blood flow during graded treadmill exercise in the dog. *J Clin Invest* 75: 43, 1975.

42 Mueller TM, Marcus ML, Kerber RE, Young JA, Barnes RW, Abboud FM: Effect of renal hypertension and left ventricular hypertrophy on the coronary circulation in dogs. *Circ Res* 42: 543, 1978.

43 Noble J, Bourassa MG, Petitclerc R, Dyrda I: Myocardial bridging and milking effect of the left anterior descending coronary artery: Normal variant or obstruction? *Am J Cardiol* 37: 993, 1976.

44 Morales AR, Romanelli R, Boucek RJ: The mural left anterior descending coronary artery, strenuous exercise and sudden death. *Circulation* 62: 230, 1980.

45 Faruqui AMA, Maloy WC, Felner JM, Schlant RC, Logan WD, Symbas P: Symptomatic myocardial bridging of coronary artery. *Am J Cardiol* 41: 1305, 1978.

45a Pichard AD, Casanegra P, Marchant E, Rodriguez JA: Abnormal regional myocardial flow in myocardial bridging of the left anterior descending coronary artery. *Am J Cardiol* 47: 978, 1981.

46 Raizner AS, Ishimori T, Verani MS, Spencer WH, Guinn G, Chahine RA, Howell JF, Miller RR: Surgical relief of myocardial ischemia due to myocardial bridges. *Am J Cardiol* 45: 417, 1980.

47 Grondin P, Bourassa MG, Moble J, Petitclerc R, Dydra I: Successful course after supra arterial myotomy for myocardial bridging and milking effect of the left anterior descending artery. *Ann Thorac Surg* 24: 422, 1977.

48 Krawczyk JA, Dashkoff N, Mays A, Klocke FJ: Reduced coronary flow in a canine model of "muscle bridge" with inflow occlusion extending into diastole; possible role of downstream vascular closure. *Transac Assoc Am Physicians* 93: 100, 1980.

49 Mays AE, Jr, McHale PA, Greenfield JC Jr: Transmural myocardial blood flow in a canine model of coronary artery bridging. *Circ Res* 49: 726, 1981.

50 Hill RC, Chitwood WR, Bashore TM, Sink JD, Cox JL, Wechsler AS: Coronary flow and regional function before and after supraarterial myotomy for myocardial bridging. *Ann Thorac Surg* 31: 176, 1981.

51 Weiner DA, Ryan TJ, McCabe CH, Kennedy JW, Schloss M, Tristani F, Chaitman BR, Fisher LD: Correlations among history of angina, ST-segment response and prevalence of coronary-artery disease in the coronary artery surgery study (CASS). *N Engl J Med* 301: 230, 1979.

52 Pohost GM, Alpert NM, Ingwall JS, Strauss HW: Thallium redistribution: Mechanism and clinical utility. *Sem Nucl Med* 10: 70, 1980.

53 Goldberg E, Stein J, Berger M, Berdoff RL: Diastolic segmental coronary artery obliteration in constrictive pericarditis. *Cath Cardiovasc Diag* 2: 397, 1976.

54 Allard JR, Gertz EW, Bristow JD, Hoffman JIE: Beneficial effect of the pericardium in acute heart failure. *Clin Res* 26: 481A, 1978.

55 Greenberg MA, Neuburger N, Grose R, Kramer K, Yipintsoi T: Decreased coronary reserve in syndrome X. *Circulation* 64(supp IV): 305, 1981.

56 Tillmans H: Personal communication. London, June 1982.

PART **FIVE**

DIFFERENCES IN THE CORONARY CIRCULATION OF THE RIGHT AND LEFT VENTRICLES

CHAPTER **16**

DIFFERENCES IN THE REGULATION OF CORONARY PERFUSION TO THE RIGHT AND LEFT VENTRICLES

Throughout this volume, I have briefly noted differences in the regulation of myocardial perfusion to the right and left ventricles. The purpose of this chapter is to focus on these differences and to emphasize those which may be clinically relevant.

ANATOMY

The perfusion field of the right coronary artery is much smaller than that of the left (left anterior descending plus circumflex) in all species. This difference is particularly prominent in the dog. In this species, 37 percent of the free wall of the right ventricle and the entire left ventricle, including the interventricular septum, are supplied by branches of the left coronary artery [1]. In the pig, the perfusion field of the right coronary artery includes a significant portion of the right ventricular free wall as well as the inferior wall of the left ventricle and the posterior third of the interventricular septum (see Chapter 1). In humans, when the posterior descending coronary artery arises from the right coronary artery, the free wall of the right ventricle, the inferior wall of the left ventricle, and the posterior third of the interventricular septum are supplied by the right coronary artery. In some patients, a significant portion of the lateral and posterior walls of the left ventricle are also supplied by branches of the right coronary artery (see Chapter 1) [2,3].

Vascular density in general [4] and capillary density in particular [5–7] are similar in the right and left ventricles. In addition, minimal coronary vascular resistance is similar in these two cardiac chambers [4,8–10].

METABOLIC REGULATION

Metabolic regulation of coronary blood flow is similar in the right and left ventricles [11–13c]. Oxygen extraction [14,15] and the quantitative characteristics of coronary reactive hyperemia [16] are similar in the right and left ventricles (see Chapter 3). Under normal conditions, however, flow per gram in the right ventricle is about two-thirds of that in the left ventricle [8,9,13b,13c]. This presumably reflects differences in wall stress in these two chambers.

PHASIC FLOW, AUTOREGULATION, AND TRANSMURAL BLOOD FLOW

Extravascular compressive forces are markedly different in the right and left ventricles under normal conditions. As a consequence, systolic flow expressed as a fraction of diastolic flow is much greater in vessels that perfuse the right ventricle than the left ventricle [16–18] (see Chapter 4). If right ventricular systolic pressure exceeds aortic systolic pressure, retrograde systolic flow occurs in epicardial coronary vessels that perfuse the right ventricle [19,20].

Under normal conditions in awake and anesthetized animals, the subendocardial/subepicardial flow ratio in the right ventricular free wall and left ventricle are similar [1,5,9,10,13,13b,21,22]. During systole, in the left ventricle there is a steep gradient of transmural perfusion which favors the subepicardium [23–25]. In the normal right ventricle, however, systolic coronary perfusion is uniformly distributed across the wall of the right ventricle [26].

Critical closing pressure during maximum coronary dilation ranges from 11 to 37 mmHg in vessels which perfuse the right ventricle [27] and 12 to 18 mmHg in vessels which perfuse the left ventricle [28,29].

In the left ventricle, changes in coronary perfusion pressure within the range of 60 to 130 mmHg are not associated with major changes in mean left ventricular perfusion because autoregulation is very effective [30–35]. Although the relationship between changes in coronary driving pressure and right ventricular pressure have not been extensively investigated, a recent study by Murray and Vatner [36] reported that a moderate increase in aortic pressure (91 vs. 122 mmHg) was accompanied by a 55 percent increase in right ventricular perfusion. In this study, the autonomic nervous system was blocked with hexamethonium and right ventricular hemodynamics and heart rate were stable during the rise in aortic pressure. Therefore, the response observed was not related to reflex changes or alterations in right ventricular metabolism. Nonethelsss, an increase in coronary driving pressure was associated with a decrease in right ventricular coronary resistance. The data suggest that the effectiveness of autoregulation in vessels that perfuse the right and left ventricles is strikingly different.

In the left ventricle, changes in perfusion pressure have selective effects on coronary flow to various layers of the left ventricular myocardium. As perfusion pressure is decreased from 100 to 30 mmHg, flow to the subepicardium is better preserved than flow to the subendocardium [37]. Thus, autoregulation is more effective in the subepicardium than in the subendocardium of the left ventricle [37]. The effects of alterations in perfusion pressure over a broad range on flow to various layers in the right ventricular myocardium have not been studied.

Acute increases in ventricular pressure also have different effects on right and left ventricular perfusion. When the left ventricle is subjected to a sudden increase in aortic pressure, flow to the subendocardium is much lower than that to the subepicardium [38] and electrocardiographic changes suggestive of ischemia develop [39]. However, in less than 30 s, the subendocardial flow increases and the transmural distribution flow across the left ventricle returns to normal [38].

When right ventricular pressure is suddenly increased to extreme levels (right ventricular systolic pressure 60 to 100 mmHg), persistent right ventricular dysfunction occurs [13a,40]. It has been shown that this occurs in part because of inadequate perfusion of the right ventricular free wall [13a,40]. In the right ventricle, the inadequate perfusion that accompanies a sudden increase in right ventricular pressure is not transient. It persists and can be accompanied by metabolic evidence of right ventricular ischemia [40,41]. Brooks et al. [13a] and Gold et al. [40] have shown that this can be reversed by increasing coronary driving pressure. Unfortunately, when sudden right ventricular hypertension occurs in a clinical setting (massive pulmonary embolism), it is often accompanied by systemic hypotension.

Sudden increases in right ventricular pressure are accompanied by an enormous increase in circulating catecholamines and probably a major augmentation of sympathetic outflow [42]. Thus, one might postulate that when right ventricular pressure is suddenly increased, the inadequate perfusion that occurs is in part a response to alpha-adenergic coronary vasoconstriction. This neurally mediated coronary vasoconstriction may contribute importantly to the pathogenesis of right ventricular ischemia that accompanies sudden increases in right ventricular pressure.

Patients who experience massive pulmonary emboli occasionally develop increased right ventricular pressure, acute right ventricular failure, and systemic hypotension [43–45]. This clinical syndrome, which is often associated with decreased cardiac output and decreased left ventricular filling pressure, may occur as a consequence of right ventricular ischemia.

In summary, phasic coronary blood flow, autoregulation, and the effects of sudden increases in ventricular pressure on transmural perfusion are very different in vessels that perfuse the right and left ventricles. These basic differences in the regulation of perfusion to the right and left ventricles will affect the responses of their respective vascular beds to a variety of physiological and pathological stimuli.

NEURAL CONTROL

The integrated response of the coronary circulation to neural stimuli reflects a balance between direct vasomotor effects and indirect metabolic consequences of neural activation. In the left ventricle, the metabolic effects usually dominate the integrated response to neural activation. In the right ventricle, metabolic responses are blunted because changes in aortic pressure do not directly alter right ventricular metabolism. Thus, one might hypothesize that the direct vasomotor effects of neural activation may be more important in the right ventricle. One recent study concerning modulation of right ventricular coronary vascular resistance by the baroreceptor reflex supports this hypothesis [36]. In the left coronary circulation, baroreflex activation results in transient coronary vasoconstriction followed by prolonged coronary vasodilation (Figure 16-1) [46,47]. In the right coronary circulation, baroreflex activation produced by bilateral carotid occlusion was accompanied by persistent coronary vasoconstriction (Figure 16-1) [36].

FIGURE 16-1
Schematic diagram which illustrates the effects of activation of the baroreceptor reflex (bilateral carotid artery occlusion) on aortic pressure, right and left ventricular coronary flow, and resistance. Activation of the baroreceptor reflex produces a persistent elevation in right coronary artery (RCA) resistance and a biphasic alteration in left coronary artery (LCA) resistance. (*Based on data presented in Refs. 36,46,47.*)

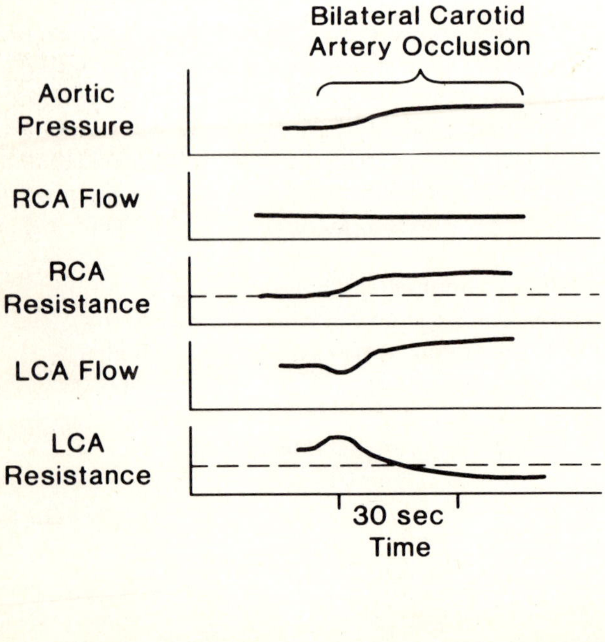

HUMORAL AND PHARMACOLOGIC REGULATION

The effects of the humoral and pharmacologic agents on the coronary circulation are determined by a balance between the direct vasomotor and indirect metabolic effects of these agents on coronary vessels. As noted above, vasomotor effects will usually dominate the response of coronary vessels which perfuse the right ventricle, whereas metabolic effects will predominate in the left ventricle. Coronary responses to angiotensin II infusion are an example of this differential response [48]. Angiotensin II markedly increases aortic pressure but only slightly increases pulmonary artery pressure. Thus angiotensin II increases left ventricular metabolism more than right ventricular metabolism. This may partially explain why increases in coronary vascular resistance in response to angiotensin II infusion are greater in vessels which perfuse the right ventricle than those which supply the left ventricle (Figure 16-2) [48].

Very few studies have sought differences in the response of the right and left coronary vascular beds to humoral or pharmacologic stimuli.

CORONARY OCCLUSION, CORONARY SPASM, AND THE CORONARY COLLATERAL CIRCULATION

Occlusion of the right coronary atery in patients as a result of thrombotic obstruction or spasm is frequently associated with bradyarrhythmias, atrioventricular block, and inappropriately low systemic vascular resistance [49,50]. Atrioventricular block occurs in this setting because the arterial supply of the atrioventricular node usually arises from the right coronary artery [2,3]. Bradycardia and decreases in systemic vascular resistance occur because ischemia of the inferior-

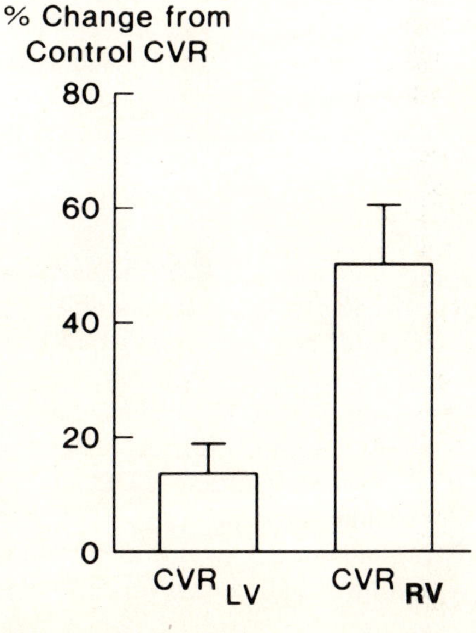

FIGURE 16-2
Effects of angiotensin (0.2 μg/kg/min IV) on coronary vascular resistance (CVR) in the left ventricle (LV) and the right ventricle (RV). The coronary vasoconstrictor effects of angiotensin are more prominent in the right ventricle than in the left ventricle. *(Based on data presented by S Gunther and PJ Cannon [48].)*

posterior wall of the left ventricle activates stretch receptors which restrain sympathetic outflow [51,52]. Occlusion of the left anterior descending coronary artery by spasm or thrombus often produces tachycardia [49,50]. In the anterior wall, left ventricular stretch receptors are presumably less abundant and exert a lesser effect on sympathetic outflow [51,52].

Because the right coronary artery in humans usually supplies a small perfusion field, right coronary artery occlusion does not often result in the devastating hemodynamic consequences that often occur with proximal occlusion of major coronary vessels which perfuse the left ventricle [53–55]. Although right ventricular infarction accompanies infarction of the inferior wall of the left ventricle in as many as one-third of patients who suffer a proximal occlusion of the right coronary artery, usually the right ventricular infarction plays a minimal role in the patient's clinical course [54]. Massive right ventricular infarction, however, can produce right ventricular failure and systemic hypotension [53,55].

In the dog, although occlusion of the proximal right coronary artery produces right ventricular infarction, this response is very inconsistent. Furthermore, if right ventricular pressure is normal in the dog, right coronary occlusion has only modest effects on right ventricular function [13a]. Even if severe right ventricular destruction is produced, right ventricular dysfunction is often not very striking [57]. Proximal occlusion of a large coronary artery perfusing the left ventricle in the dog almost always results in some area of myocardial infarction [58].

The resistance of native collateral vessels to and from the perfusion field of the right coronary artery in the dog is greater than that of the resistance of native collaterals between major branches of the left coronary artery [59,60]. The resistance of stimulated coronary collaterals from the perfusion field of the right coronary artery in dogs has not been reported. It is known, however, that when dogs are subjected to progressive simultaneous coronary occlusion of the circumflex and right coronary arteries, infarction usually does not occur. Furthermore, when the coronary collaterals are fully developed, perfusion of both the right and left ventricles is normal at rest and during moderate exercise [61]. In pigs with right ventricular hypertrophy, the development of collaterals to the right ventricle following gradual occlusion of the right coronary artery appears to be impaired [62].

CARDIAC HYPERTROPHY

Moderate or severe right ventricular hypertrophy increases right ventricular flow per gram substantially [8,9]. However, the ratio of subendocardial to subepicardial flow in the hypertrophied right ventricular free wall remains normal [8,9]. In contrast, with moderate to severe left ventricular hypertrophy, flow per gram is unchanged in the enlarged left ventricle [4,10,63–66]. Severe left ventricular hypertrophy secondary to supravalvular aortic obstruction, however, decreases the subendocardial to subepicardial perfusion ratio in the left ventricle [63,65,66].

There is no explanation for why right ventricular flow per gram increases substantially in right ventricular hypertrophy and left ventricular flow per gram is unchanged in left ventricular hypertrophy. It is known that when left ventricular pressure is increased chronically, left ventricular wall thickness increases sufficiently to normalize wall stress [67]. If chronic right ventricular hypertension was associated with an inadequate increase in right ventricular wall thickness, right ventricular wall stress would remain elevated and, hence, flow per gram would not return to normal.

In dogs, severe pressure overload right ventricular hypertrophy markedly decreases coronary reserve [8]; moderate and severe left ventricular hypertrophy secondary to pressure overload only slightly decreases coronary reserve [4,10, 63–66]. In patients, right or left ventricular hypertrophy secondary to pressure overload profoundly diminishes coronary vascular reserve [68–72].

Experimental studies in fetal lambs, newborn lambs, or calves [73–75] suggest that when right ventricular hypertrophy is produced early in life, coronary growth keeps pace with or exceeds hypertrophy of the right ventricular muscle. Hence, coronary reserve is well preserved. These animal studies suggest that infants with congenital heart defects may have normal coronary reserve because their cardiac hypertrophy developed early in life. Unfortunately, studies of coronary reserve in infants with cardiac enlargement secondary to congenital heart defects have demonstrated that coronary reserve is severely impaired [70].

In summary, many differences exist between the regulation of perfusion to the right and left ventricles. All to often, these differences are ignored by investigators and clinicians. Discrepancies in the regulation of perfusion to the right and left ventricles deserve much more attention than they have been given in the past.

REFERENCES

1 Murray PA, Vatner SF: Fractional contributions of the right and left coronary arteries to perfusion of normal and hypertrophied right ventricles of conscious dogs. *Circ Res* 47: 190, 1980.

2 Baroldi G, Scomazzoni G: *Coronary Circulation in the Normal and the Pathologic Heart.* Washington, Office of the Surgeon General, 1967.

3 James TH: *Anatomy of the Coronary Arteries.* New York, Harper & Row, 1961.

4 O'Keefe DD, Hoffman JIE, Cheitlin R, O'Neill MJ, Allard JR, Shapkin E: Coronary blood flow in experimental canine left ventricular hypertrophy. *Circ Res* 43: 43, 1978.

5 Murray PA, Baig H, Fishvein MC, Vatner SF: Effects of experimental right ventricular hypertrophy on myocardial blood flow in conscious dogs. *J Clin Invest* 64: 421, 1979.

6 Rakusan K: Quantitative morphology of capillaries of the heart. Number of capillaries in animal and human hearts under normal and pathological conditions. *Methods Achiev Exp Pathol* 5: 272, 1971.

7 Rembert JC, Kleinman LH, Fedor JM, Wechsler AS, Greenfield JC: Myocardial blood flow distribution in concentric left ventricular hypertrophy. *J Clin Invest* 62: 379, 1978.

8 Murray PA, Vatner SF: Reduction of maximal coronary vasodilator capacity in conscious dogs with severe right ventricular hypertrophy. *Circ Res* 48: 27, 1981.

9 Manohar M, Thurmon JC, Tranquilli WJ, Devous MD Sr, Theodorakis MC, Shawley RV, Feller DL, Benson JG: Regional myocardial blood flow and coronary vascular

reserve in unanesthetized young calves with severe concentric right ventricular hypertrophy. *Circ Res* 48: 785, 1981.

10 Mueller TM, Marcus ML, Kerber RE, Young JA, Barnes RW, Abboud FM: Effect of renal hypertension and left ventricular hypertrophy on the coronary circulation in dogs. *Circ Res* 42: 543, 1978.

11 Eckenhoff JE, Hafkenschiel JH, Lanmesser CM, Harmel M: Cardiac oxygen metabolism and control of the coronary circulation. *Am J Physiol* 149: 634, 1947.

12 Berne RM, Rubio R: Coronary circulation, in *Handbook of Physiology*, vol 1, sect 2, The cardiovascular system, RM Berne (ed). Bethesda, Maryland, American Physiological Society, 1979, p 873.

13 Fixler DE, Archie JP, Ullyot DJ, Buckberg GD, Hoffman JIE: Effect of acute right ventricular systolic hypertension on regional myocardial blood flow in anesthetized dogs. *Am Heart J* 85: 491, 1973.

13a Brooks H, Kirk ES, Vokonas PS, Urschel CW, Sonnenblick EH: Performance of the right ventricle under stress: Relation to right coronary flow. *J Clin Invest* 50: 2176, 1971.

13b Manohar M, Bisgard GE, Bullard V, Will JA, Anderson D, Rankin JHG: Myocardial perfusion and function during acute right ventricular systolic hypertension. *Am J Physiol* 235: H628, 1978.

13c Domenech RJ, Ayuy AH: Total and regional coronary blood flow during acute right ventricular pressure overload. *Cardiovasc Res* 8: 611, 1974.

14 Weiss HR, Sinha AK: Regional oxygen saturation of small arteries and veins in the canine myocardium. *Circ Res* 42: 119, 1978.

15 Vinten-Johansen J, Weiss HR: Oxygen consumption in subepicardial and subendocardial regions of the canine left ventricle: The effect of experimental acute valvular aortic stenosis *Circ Res* 46: 139, 1980.

16 Marcus M, Wright C, Doty D, Eastham C, Laughlin D, Krumm P, Fastenow C, Brody M: Measurements of coronary velocity and reactive hyperemia in the coronary circulation of humans. *Circ Res* 49: 877, 1981.

17 Gregg DE: *The Coronary Circulation in Health and Disease.* Philadelphia, Lea & Febiger, 1950.

18 Khouri EM, Gregg DE, Rayford CR: Effect of exercise on cardiac output, left coronary flow and myocardial metabolism in the unanesthetized dog. *Circ Res* 17: 427, 1965.

19 Bellamy RF, Lowensohn HS: Effect of systole on coronary pressure-flow relations in the right ventricle of the dog. *Am J Physiol* 238: H481, 1980.

20 Lowensohn HS, Khouri EM, Gregg DE, Pyle RL, Patterson RE: Phasic right coronary artery blood flow in conscious dogs with normal and elevated right ventricular pressures. *Circ Res* 39: 760, 1976.

21 Manohar M, Bisgard GE, Bullard V, Will JA, Anderson D, Rankin JHG: Regional myocardial blood flow and myocardial function during acute right ventricular pressure overload in calves. *Circ Res* 44: 531, 1979.

22 Cobb RF, Bache RJ, Greenfield JC Jr: Regional myocardial blood flow in awake dogs. *J Clin Invest* 53: 1618, 1974.

23 Downey JM, Kirk ES: Distribution of the coronary blood flow across the canine heart wall during systole. *Circ Res* 35: 251, 1974.

24 Hess DS, Bache RJ: Transmural distribution of myocardial blood flow during systole in the awake dog. *Circ Res* 38: 5, 1976.

25 Rembert JC, Greenfield JC Jr, Alexander JA, Cobb FR: Transmural distribution of systolic myocardial blood flow in the awake dog, in *Cardiovascular System Dynamics*,

J Baan, A Noodergraaf, J Raines (eds). London, MIT Press, p 40, 1978.
26 Hess DS, Bache RJ: Transmural right ventricular myocardial blood flow during systole in the awake dog. *Circ Res* 45: 88, 1979.
27 Bellamy RF: Calculation of coronary vascular resistance. *Cardiovasc Res* 5: 261, 1980.
28 Klocke FJ, Weinstein IR, Klocke JF, Ellis AK, Kraus DR, Mates RE, Canty JM, Anbar RD, Romanowski RR, Wallmeyer KW, Echt MP: Zero-flow pressures and pressure-flow relationships during single long diastoles in the canine coronary bed before and during maximum vasodilation; Limited influence of capacitive effects. *J Clin Invest* 68: 970, 1981.
29 Eng C, Jentzer JH, Kirk ES: The effects of coronary capacitance on the interpretation of diastolic pressure-flow relationships. *Circ Res* 50: 334, 1982.
30 Rouleau J, Boerboom LE, Surjadhana A, Hoffman JIE: The role of autoregulation and tissue diastolic pressures in the transmural distribution of left ventricular blood flow in anesthetized dogs. *Circ Res* 45: 804, 1979.
31 Scott JB, Hardin RA, Haddy FJ: Pressure-flow relationships in the coronary vascular bed of the dog. *Am J Physiol* 199: 765, 1960.
32 Cross CE, Rieben PA, Salisbury PF: Coronary driving pressure and vasomotor tonus as determinants of coronary blood flow. *Circ Res* 9: 589, 1961.
33 Mosher P, Ross J Jr, McFate PA, Shaw RF: Control of coronary blood flow by an autoregulatory mechanism. *Circ Res* 14: 250, 1964.
34 Driscol TE, Moir TW, Eckstein RW: Autoregulation of coronary blood flow: Effect of interarterial pressure gradients. *Circ Res* 15: 103, 1964.
35 Dole WP, Montville WJ, Bishop VS: Dependency of myocardial reactive hyperemia on coronary artery pressure in the dog. *Am J Physiol* 240: H709, 1981.
36 Murray PA, Vatner SF: Carotid sinus baroreceptor control of right coronary circulation in normal, hypertrophied, and failing right ventricles of conscious dogs. *Circ Res* 49: 1339, 1981.
37 Guyton RA, McClenathan JH, Newman GE, Michaelis LL: Significance of subendocardial S-T segment elevation caused by coronary stenosis in the dog. *Am J Cardiol* 40: 373, 1977.
38 Walston A, Rembert JC, Tedor JM, Greenfield JC: Regional myocardial blood flow after sudden aortic constriction in awake dogs. *Circ Res* 42: 419, 1978.
39 Monroe RG, Gamble WJ, LaFarge CG, Kumar AE, Stark J, Sanders GL, Phornphutkul C, Davis M: The Anrep effect reconsidered. *J Clin Invest* 51: 2573, 1972.
40 Gold FL, Bache RJ: Transmural right ventricular blood flow during acute pulmonary artery hypertension in the awake dog: Evidence for subendocardial ischemia during right ventricular failure despite residual vasodilator reserve. *Circ Res* 51: 196, 1982.
41 Vlahakes GJ, Turley K, Hoffman JIE: The pathophysiology of failure in acute right ventricular hypertension. Hemodynamic correlations. *Circulation* 63: 87, 1981.
42 Gold FL, Horwitz LD, Bache RJ: Anatagonism of the coronary vasodilator effect of adenosine during acute right ventricular systolic hypertension in the awake dog: Evidence for adrenergic coronary vasoconstriction (in press).
43 McIntyre KM, Sasahara AA: Hemodynamic and ventricular responses to pulmonary embolism. *Prog Cardiovasc Dis* 17: 175, 1974.
44 Stein PD, Alshabkhoun S, Hatem C, Pur-Shahriari AA, Haynes F, Harken DE, Dexter L: Coronary artery blood flow in acute pulmonary embolism. *Am J Cardiol* 21: 32, 1968.
45 Sasahara AA: Current problems in pulmonary embolism. *Prog Cardiovasc Dis* 17: 161, 1974.
46 Feigl EO: Carotid sinus reflex control of coronary blood flow. *Circ Res* 23: 223, 1968.

47 Powell JR, Feigl EO: Carotid sinus reflex coronary vasoconstriction during controlled myocardial oxygen metabolism in the dog. *Circ Res* 44: 44, 1979.

48 Gunther S, Cannon PJ: Modulation of angiotensin II coronary vasoconstriction by cardiac prostaglandin systhesis. *Am J Physiol* 238: H895, 1980.

49 Perez-Gomez F, DeDios RJ, Rey J, Aguado AG: Prinzmetal's angina: Reflex cardiovascular response during episode of pain. *Br Heart J* 42: 81, 1979.

50 Pantridge JF, Adgey AAJ, Geddes JS, Webb SW: *The Acute Coronary Attack*. New York, Grune & Stratton, 1975.

51 Felder RB, Thames MD: Interaction between cardiac receptors and sinoaortic baroreceptors in the control of efferent cardiac sympathetic nerve activity during myocardial ischemia in dogs. *Circ Res* 45: 728, 1979.

52 Thames MD, Klopfenstein HS, Abboud FM, Mark AL, Walker JL: Preferential distribution of inhibitory cardiac receptors with vagal afferents to the inferoposterior wall of the left ventricle activated during coronary occlusion in the dog. *Circ Res* 43: 512, 1978.

53 Cohn JN, Guiha NH, Broder MI, Limas CJ: Right ventricular infarction: Clinical and hemodynamic features. *Am J Cardiol* 33: 209, 1974.

54 Sharpe DN, Botvinick EH, Shames DM, Schiller NB, Massie BM, Chatterjee K, Parmley WW: The noninvasive diagnosis of right ventricular infarction. *Circulation* 57: 483, 1978.

55 Cohn JN: Right ventricular infarction revisited. *Am J Cardiol* 43: 556, 1979.

56 Schaper W, Sass S: Right ventricular infarct size and collateral blood flow following occlusion of the right coronary artery in the dog. *Circulation* 64: 118, 1981.

57 Guiha NH, Limas CJ, Cohn JN: Predominant right ventricular dysfunction after right ventricular destruction in the dog. *Am J Cardiol* 33: 254, 1974.

58 Koyanagi S, Eastham CL, Harrison DG, Marcus ML: Transmural variation in the relationship between myocardial infarct size and risk area. *Am J Physiol* 242: H867, 1982.

59 Scheel KW, Ingram LA, Wilson JL: Effects of exercise on the coronary and collateral vasculature of beagles with and without coronary occlusion. *Circ Res* 48: 523, 1981.

60 Scheel KW, Rodriguez RJ, Ingram LA: Directional coronary collateral growth with chronic circumflex occlusion in the dog. *Circ Res* 40: 384, 1977.

61 Schaper W: Influence of physical exercise on coronary collateral blood flow in chronic experimental two vessel occlusion. *Circulation* 65: 905, 1982.

62 Peter RH, Ramo BW, Ratliff N, Morris JJ Jr: Collateral vessel development after right ventricular infarction in the pig. *Am J Cardiol* 29: 58, 1972.

63 Rembert JC, Kleinman LC, Fedor JM, Wechsler AS, Greenfield JC Jr: Myocardial blood flow distribution in concentric left ventricular hypertrophy *J Clin Invest* 62: 379, 1978.

64 Bache RJ, Vrobel TR: Effects of exercise on blood flow in the hypertrophied heart. *Am J Cardiol* 44: 1029, 1979.

65 Holtz J, von Restorff W, Bard P, Bassenge E: Transmural distribution of myocardial blood flow and of coronary reserve in canine left ventricular hypertrophy. *Basic Res Cardiol* 72: 286, 1977.

66 Einzig S, Leonard JJ, Tripp MR, Lucas RV, Swayze CR, Fox IJ: Changes in regional myocardial blood flow and variable development of hypertrophy after aortic banding in puppies. *Cardiovasc Res* 15: 711, 1981.

67 Sasayama S, Ross J, Franklin D, Bloor CM, Bishop S, Dilley RB: Adaptations of the left ventricle to chronic pressure overload. *Circ Res* 38: 172, 1976.

68 Marcus ML, Doty DB, Hiratzka LF, Wright CB, Eastham CL: Decreased coronary reserve–A mechanism for angina pectoris in patients with aortic stenosis and normal coronary arteries. *N Eng J Med* 307: 1362–1367, 1982.

69 Doty D, Eastham C, Hiratzka L, Wright C, Marcus M: Determinants of coronary reserve in patients with supravalvular aortic stenosis. *Circulation* 64(suppl IV): 32, 1981.

70 Marcus ML, Doty D, Hiratzka L, Wright C, Eastham C: Impaired coronary reserve in children with cyanotic congenital heart disease. *Circulation* 64(suppl IV): 127, 1981.

71 Eastham CL, Doty DB, Hiratzka LF, Wright CB, Marcus ML: Volume-overload left ventricular hypertrophy impairs coronary reserve in humans. *Circulation* 64: 26, 1981.

72 Doty D, Wright C, Eastham C, Marcus ML: Coronary reserve in atrial septal defect. *Circulation* 62: 115, 1980.

73 Archie JP, Fixler DE, Ullyot DJ, Buckberg GD, Hoffman JIE: Regional myocardial blood flow in lambs with concentric right ventricular hypertrophy. *Circ Res* 34: 143, 1974.

74 Manohar M, Thurmon JC, Tranquilli WJ, Devous MD Sr, Theodorakis MC, Shawley RV, Feller DL, Benson JG: Regional myocardial blood flow and coronary vascular reserve in unanesthetized young calves with severe concentric right ventricular hypertrophy. *Circ Res* 48: 785, 1981.

75 Vlahakes GJ, Turley K, Verrier ED, Hoffman JIE: Greater maximal coronary flow in conscious lambs with experimental congenital right ventricular hypertrophy. *Circulation* 62(suppl III), 1980.

PART **SIX**

MEDICAL AND SURGICAL INTERVENTIONS THAT MODIFY THE CORONARY CIRCULATION

CHAPTER **17**

CORONARY BYPASS GRAFTS

In 1969, Johnson, Flemma, Lepley, and Ellison [1] reported that they had successfully placed saphenous vein grafts in the distal segments of coronary vessels in a large series of patients with proximal coronary obstructive disease. In this initial clinical report, 91 percent of 105 grafts studied postoperatively were patent. This was the first large patient series that demonstrated the feasibility of coronary bypass surgery [2]. Coronary bypass surgery has revolutionized the treatment of patients with coronary obstructive disease. The operation involves interposing a conduit vessel, usually a saphenous vein, between the ascending thoracic aorta and the coronary arterial segment distal to an obstructive lesion. The procedure requires microvascular surgical techniques because the usual diameter of the coronary segment receiving the graft is 1 to 3 mm. Since 1969, many variations of this basic operative procedure have been described [3,4]. At present, about 200,000 patients a year have coronary bypass surgery in the United States. Although the effects of this operative procedure on survival in various patient subgroups continues to be a subject surrounded by controversy [3–5], there is indisputable evidence that this procedure improves myocardial perfusion and the symptomatic status of the patient [3–5].

INTRAOPERATIVE EVALUATION OF CORONARY BYPASS GRAFTS (GENERAL CONSIDERATIONS)

Intraoperative evaluation of coronary bypass grafts has long been of interest to cardiac surgeons [3,4]. Although many approaches have been applied, none is completely satisfactory. I will briefly discuss the reasons why the results of intraoperative studies to evaluate the functional capacity of coronary grafts are difficult to interpret.

Graft/Coronary Diameter Ratio

Animal studies [6,7] and data gleaned from models [6–8] indicate that the fraction of distal flow in a grafted vessel which comes from the graft is dependent upon the graft/artery cross-sectional area ratio (Figure 17-1); the larger the ratio, the more the flow supplied by the graft. In patients who receive saphenous vein bypass grafts, the diameter of the graft is usually much larger than the recipient coronary vessel.

Severity of Proximal Obstruction in the Recipient Vessel

If the graft/coronary diameter ratio is 1, the fraction of distal coronary flow that originates from the graft will vary with the extent of proximal stenosis in the recipient vessel (Figure 17-2) [6–9]. The converse is also true; i.e., stenosis of the graft at the proximal or distal anastomosis will have a similar effect. Because the extent of stenosis differs from vessel to vessel, one might expect highly variable graft flow rates on this basis alone.

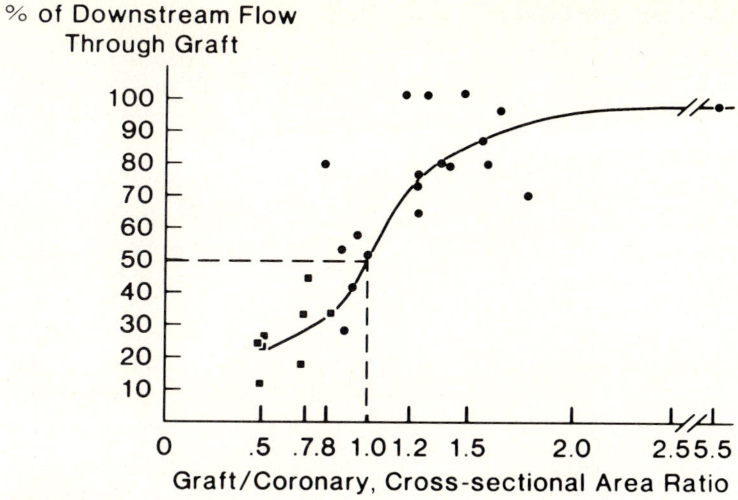

FIGURE 17-1
Effects of graft/coronary cross-sectional area ratio on the percent of downstream flow which originates from the bypass graft. Flow measurements were made 1 h after graft insertion when the heart was working and mean arterial pressure was 70 to 80 mmHg. When the graft/coronary cross-sectional area ratio is 1, 50 percent of downstream flow originates from the bypass graft, and 50 percent originates from the proximal artery. When this ratio is 2, almost all of the downstream flow originates from the graft. Most saphenous vein bypass grafts placed in patients with coronary disease have a cross-sectional area which is two times larger than that of the recipient coronary vessel. Therefore, in most grafted vessels, the majority of downstream flow originates from the bypass graft. (*From JB Overton et al* [7].)

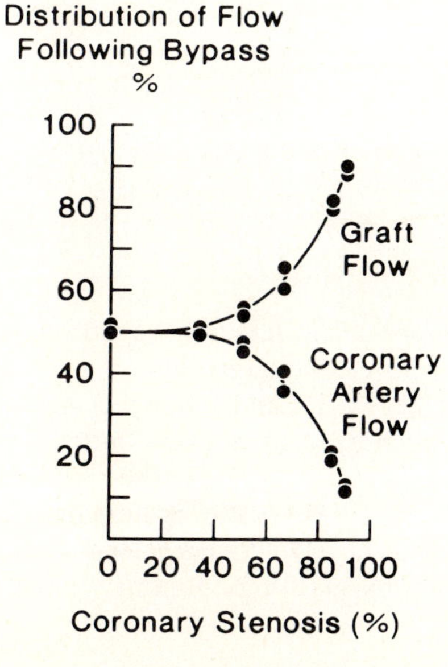

FIGURE 17-2
Effects of proximal coronary stenosis on the distribution of flow to the downstream vessel following placement of a coronary bypass graft assuming that the graft/coronary cross-sectional area ratio is unity. Measurements were obtained in a hydraulic model simulating the cardiovascular system. Proximal coronary stenosis has a profound effect on the distribution of flow following placement of a coronary bypass graft. (*From PD Stein, HN Sabbah, and M Marzilli* [8].)

Perfusion Field of the Recipient Vessel

The area of the myocardium perfused by a single graft is dependent on the number of distal anastomoses and the extent to which the graft may perfuse adjacent vascular beds via collaterals. Studies which have employed intragraft installation of radiolabeled particles [10,11] have demonstrated that the perfusion field of individual grafts is quite variable. The largest graft flow rates have been measured in "circular grafts" [12,13], which have side to side anastomosis with several major arteries and their branches. Thus, the variable size of the perfusion field of any given graft contributes to the diversity of the measurements of blood flow in bypass grafts.

Operative Conditions

Graft flow is dependent on the resistance of the distal vascular bed. Consequently, all the determinants which alter coronary vascular resistance (metabolic, autoregulatory, neural, and humoral factors) will affect graft flow. Furthermore, because graft flow rates are usually measured minutes after termination of cardiopulmonary bypass, body temperature, hematocrit, and anesthetic drug effects must also be considered [14,15]. Studies by Greenfield et al. [14] indicate that graft flow declined significantly during the first 20 to 30 min following cessation of cardiopulmonary bypass. Hiratzka et al. [16] have shown that, following cardiopulmonary bypass, resting coronary blood flow is probably increased and the coronary reactive hyperemic response is attenuated in normal coronary vessels. Also, intraoperative studies in patients are by necessity performed expeditiously, and sometimes this promotes technical errors.

In view of the problems listed above, intraoperative measurements of blood flow in bypass grafts should be interpreted with considerable caution.

INTRAOPERATIVE EVALUATION OF CORONARY BYPASS GRAFTS (SPECIFIC METHODS)

The specific methods which are currently used in the operating theater to assess bypass graft function are described below.

Studies with Electromagnetic Flow Meters

Most of our knowledge concerning the intraoperative function of coronary bypass grafts is based upon studies performed with electromagnetic flow meters. This approach was initially employed by Johnson et al. [17] and Mitchel et al. [18] in 1970 to measure graft flow and has subsequently been used by numerous investigators. Studies with electromagnetic flow meters have had three general purposes: (1) to examine the characteristics of phasic coronary flow in humans, (2) to relate intraoperative graft flow rates to long-term graft patency, and (3) to analyze graft flow responses to physiological and pharmacologic stimuli.

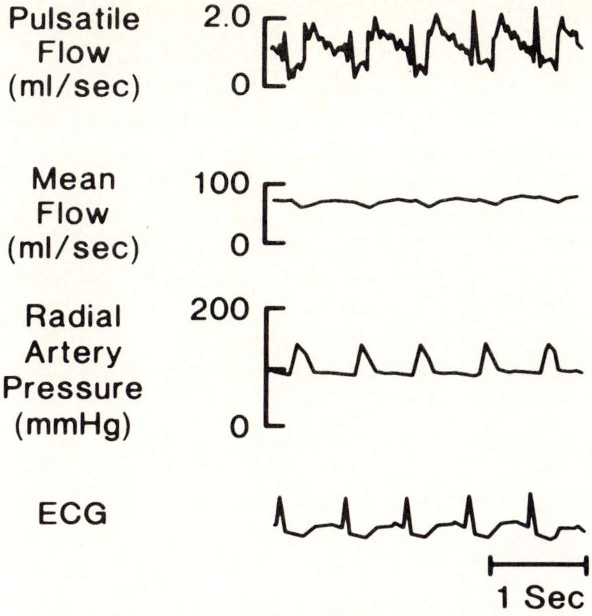

FIGURE 17-3
Phasic blood flow (pulsatile flow) measured with an electromagnetic flow probe placed on a saphenous vein bypass graft to a coronary vessel perfusing the left ventricle. These recordings were made in the operating room 30 to 40 min following cardiopulmonary bypass. The phasic character of flow in the bypass graft is similar to that observed in a native coronary vessel perfusing the left ventricle. (*From JC Greenfield Jr et al* [*14*].)

Phasic Coronary Blood Flow in Bypass Grafts The phasic character of flow in a bypass graft to an artery perfusing the left ventricle is similar [14,19,20] to the pattern of flow reported in native coronary vessels of dogs and humans (Figure 17-3) [21,22]. Greenfield et al. [14] reported that the ratio of systolic to total flow in such grafts ranged from 19 to 34 percent. If the bypass graft perfuses a vessel primarily serving the right ventricle [19,20] or an area of scar [19], the percent of total flow occurring in systole is substantially increased. Folts et al. [20] have reported that low systolic/diastolic flow ratios in grafts that perfused the circumflex or left anterior descending vessels indicated that long-term graft patency was unlikely.

Intraoperative Graft Flow Rates and Graft Patency Reported blood flow measurements in vein bypass grafts have varied from less than 20 ml/min [23–25] to more than 300 ml/min [12,13]. Most investigators, however, have noted that in the great majority of bypass grafts, flow varies from 30 to 100 ml/min [14,15,17–20,23–29]. Although many factors contribute to the variability of these flow measurements (see above), Kreulen et al. [26] have emphasized the importance of the pressure gradient between the aorta and the coronary segment receiving the graft in this regard (Figure 17-4). The size of this pressure gradient reflects the severity of the proximal obstruction in the recipient vessel. Several groups have found a significant relationship between intraoperative measurements of graft flow and the likelihood of early or late graft closure (Figure 17-5)

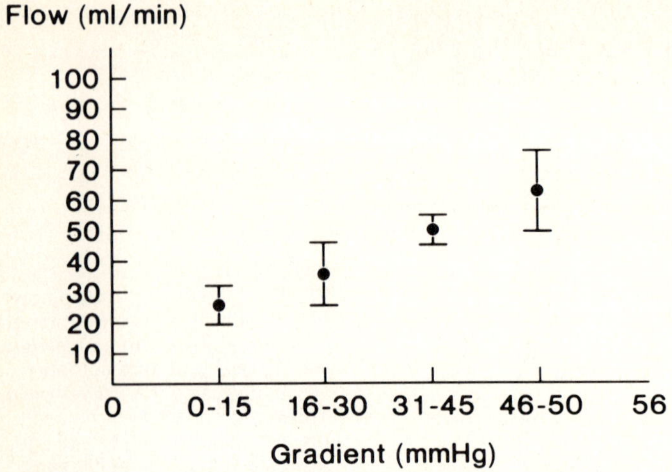

FIGURE 17-4
Relationship between the gradient between aortic pressure and coronary pressure distal to the point of graft insertion and graft flow in patients. Graft flow was measured after cardiopulmonary bypass in the operating theater. Graft flow increased significantly as the magnitude of the gradient increased. The magnitude of the gradient reflects the severity of proximal coronary stenosis. These clinical data are compatible with the experimental data presented in Figure 17-2. (*Modified from an illustration originally presented by TH Kreulen et al* [*26*].)

FIGURE 17-5
Relationship between intraoperative measurements of graft flow rates with an electromagnetic flow meter and the incidence of graft occlusion 1 week or 1 week to 1 year postoperatively as assessed by coronary angiography. Flows are given in units of ml/min. Low graft flows were associated with high rates of early and late graft closure. (*Based on data originally presented by CM Grondin et al* [*13*].)

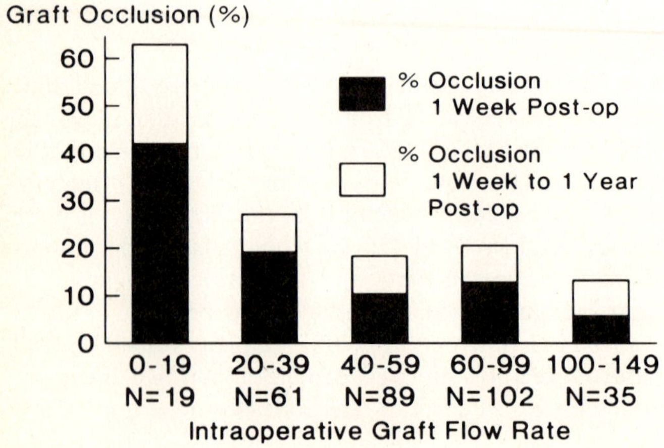

[13,24,25]. Other studies [20,27,29], however, have not observed this. In view of the numerous determinants of intraoperative graft flow rates (see above), diversity in the reported flow measurements and their predictive value is not unexpected.

Alterations in Graft Flow in Response to Physiological and Pharmacologic Stimuli Many studies have described the effects of transient graft occlusion on graft blood flow [14,19,20,25,29–36], and a few have noted a significant relationship between the magnitude of the reactive hyperemic response and long-term graft patency [20,25].

The coronary reactive hyperemic responses measured in bypass grafts are peculiar in several respects. First, the responses are remarkably feeble compared to the coronary reactive hyperemic responses of normal coronary vessels [21,22]. Following release of a 10- or 20-s coronary occlusion, peak flow in a bypass graft usually increases less than twofold above baseline. In a normal coronary vessel, flow increases five- or sixfold following release of a 20-s coronary occlusion [21,22]. Second, in a significant percentage of bypass grafts (10 to 40 percent) no coronary reactive hyperemic response can be elicited by graft closure alone. Third, although increasing the duration of graft occlusion from 5 to 15 s augments the coronary reactive hyperemic response [27], 30- and 60-s graft occlusions yield coronary reactive hyperemic responses which are substantially less than the response following a 10-s occlusion of the bypass graft [14]. Fourth, maximal reactive hyperemic responses yield peak flows which are substantially less than those which occur in response to pharmacologic stimuli [33–35].

Why do coronary reactive hyperemic responses measured in bypass grafts have such unusual characteristics? First, the distal vascular bed of the recipient vessel is often abnormal because of diffuse atherosclerosis [37]. Second, the coronary vasculature is usually dilated in the early period following cardiopulmonary bypass when measurements of graft flow are usually performed [14–16]. Third, graft occlusion alone does not produce myocardial ischemia unless the proximal stenosis in the recipient vessel is severe [27,29–31,33]. Hence, in the absence of severe proximal stenosis in the vessel receiving the bypass graft, coronary reactive hyperemia following graft occlusion will be attenuated or absent (Figure 17-6). Fourth, preexisting collateral channels or adjacent patent bypass grafts may prevent myocardial ischemia from occurring during graft occlusion.

In my view, the data obtained from coronary reactive hyperemic responses following occlusion of vein bypass grafts are of little value in the intraoperative assessment of the functional capacity of coronary bypass grafts. If coronary reactive hyperemic responses are to be of value in this regard, three conditions must be met: (1) both the bypass graft and the recipient vessel must be occluded simultaneously, (2) evidence of myocardial ischemia during the occlusion in the perfusion field of the involved vessels must be documented, and (3) the vasomotor state of the vasculature prior to occlusion should be quantified. Until these three conditions can be satisfied, intraoperative measurements of coronary reactive hyperemia and vein bypass should be abandoned.

Responses of graft flow to intravenous or intragraft injections of drugs and

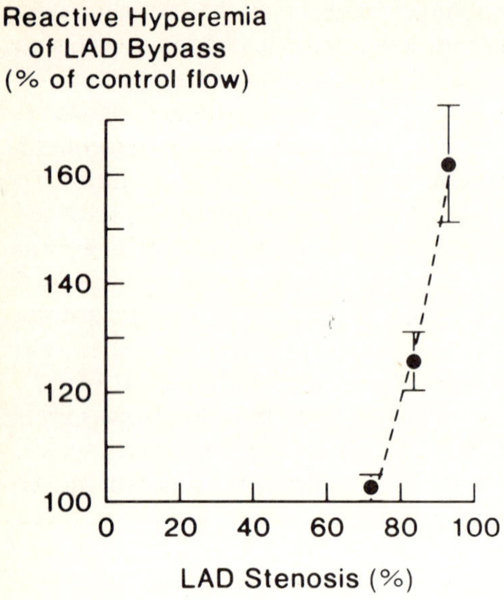

FIGURE 17-6
Effects of the severity of proximal left anterior descending coronary artery stenosis (LAD stenosis) on the reactive hyperemic response in a left anterior descending coronary bypass graft. Reactive hyperemia was assessed by occluding the graft only for 20 s. Percent of control flow = peak reactive hyperemia. Flow expressed as a percent of the control flow. No reactive hyperemic response occurred unless the severity of proximal stenosis in the left anterior descending coronary artery was at least 70 percent. Even when the percent stenosis in the left anterior descending coronary artery was greater than 90 percent, the magnitude of the reactive hyperemic response in the bypass graft was less than 200 percent of control. This reactive hyperemic response is much less than observed in normal native coronary arteries in patients prior to or following cardiopulmonary bypass. (*Modified from an illustration originally presented by F Schwarz et al* [*30*].)

humoral substances have been the subject of numerous investigations. The pharmacologic agents examined have included isoproterenol [14,38], norepinephrine [14,38], epinephrine [38], phenylephrine [14,38], metaraminol [27], propranolol [15], nitroglycerine [14], nitroprusside [37,40], diazepam [40], papaverine [13,24,35,39], and dipyridamole [33]. The responses reported are qualitatively similar to what has been noted when these agents were administered into native coronary vessels (Chapters 7 and 21). The most important contribution of these pharmacologic studies is that they demonstrate that blood flow in bypass grafts is responsive to a wide variety of pharmacologic stimuli.

Frequently, intragraft administration of vasodilators such as papaverine [13,24,35,39] or dipyridamole [33] has been utilized to assess the vasodilator reserve of the bypass graft and the distal vascular bed. Two problems beset the interpretation of such studies: (1) the dose of the drug administered and (2) the vasomotor state of the coronary circulation. It is difficult to assess the effects of any pharmacologic agent without a dose-response relationship. It is always possible that a blunted dilator response occurred simply because the concentration of the drug administered was inadequate to produce maximal dilation. When a drug is administered into a bypass graft, the effective concentration of the drug delivered to the coronary resistance vessels is dependent upon two factors: (1) the amount of drug administered and (2) the ratio of the flow in the graft to flow delivered to the coronary resistance vessel by the native coronary artery and coronary collateral channels. The latter is important because the perfusion to the vascular bed that does not originate in the graft will dilute the concentration of the drug in the blood delivered to the myocardium served by the graft. Because flow from the native vessel, collateral channels, and the graft is extremely variable (see above), it is an absolute necessity to perform dose-response curves when one attempts to produce maximal coronary dilation by pharmacologic means. Unfortunately, dose-response curves have rarely been reported by investigators who have examined the pharmacologic regulation of blood flow in vein bypass grafts.

The vasodilator state of the coronary bed will also affect the magnitude of the dilator response that occurs following administration of a vasoactive substance. If the coronary vessels are already markedly dilated, responses to any additional dilator stimulus will be blunted. This is an important consideration because the vasodilator state of the coronary bed is quite variable (see above) under the conditions which prevail when intraoperative graft flow studies are performed.

Although studies of flow in bypass grafts with electromagnetic flow meters have been used extensively to assess the functional capacity of coronary bypass grafts, the interpretation of the data should be guarded. In most instances, one can be certain only that blood was flowing through the graft at a particular rate provided that the flow meter was properly calibrated and the probe was applied correctly.

Studies with Doppler Flow Probes

The use of Doppler probes for intraoperative assessment of bypass grafts has several advantages (see Chapter 2). The zero flow is stable and the flow signal is not so critically dependent on contact between the ultrasonic crystal and the vessel. If the probe is coupled to the coronary vessel with suction, blood flow velocity can be measured in the native coronary vessel beyond the point of graft insertion. This is a major advantage because zero flow in the downstream vessels can be verified following simultaneous occlusion of the graft and the recipient vessel. This provides some assurance that vascular occlusion is producing myocardial ischemia. Hence, one might expect that coronary dilation would follow release of the occlusion. Hiratzka et al. [16] have shown that by measuring blood flow velocity in coronary vessels downstream from the point of graft insertion, the independent contribution of the native vessel and the graft to resting flow and coronary reactive hyperemic response can be assessed (Figure 17-7). By using a protocol similar to that illustrated in Figure 17-7, a good deal of information about graft function can be obtained. *In my view, the Doppler approach yields more useful information than simply measuring flow in the graft with an electromagnetic flow meter.*

Although the Doppler studies offer some advantages, several problems still remain. First, until a gated Doppler system is available which can permit measurements of integrated blood flow velocity across the vessel as well as vessel diameter and thereby permit calculations of blood flow, it will be possible to measure only changes in coronary blood flow velocity. As a consequence, the vasomotor state of the vascular bed under control conditions cannot be quantified. This is a major concern (see above). Even if one records zero flow in a native

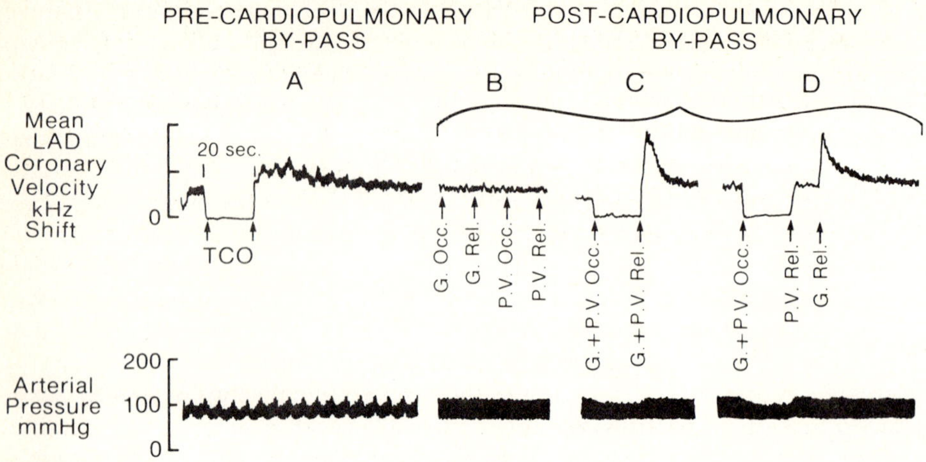

FIGURE 17-7
Recordings of coronary blood flow velocity in the left anterior descending coronary artery (LAD) and arterial pressure before (precardiopulmonary bypass) and after (postcardiopulmonary bypass) placement of a saphenous vein bypass graft in the left anterior descending coronary artery beyond the point of a severe proximal obstruction. These studies were performed by Dr. Loren Hiratzka (Department of Cardiovascular-Thoracic Surgery) and Charles Eastham (Cardiovascular Research Center), at the University of Iowa. The studies were done in a patient during the course of a coronary bypass surgical operation. TCO = transient coronary occlusion; G.Occ. = graft occlusion; G. Rel. = graft release; P.V. Occ. = proximal left anterior descending coronary artery occlusion; P.V. Rel = proximal left anterior descending coronary artery release. (*a*) The reactive hyperemic response following a 20-s coronary occlusion of the left anterior descending coronary artery was markedly attenuated. This indicates that the proximal obstruction of the left anterior descending coronary artery was hemodynamically significant. (*b*) Occlusion of the graft or the proximal left anterior descending coronary artery alone did not alter downstream coronary blood flow velocity. Thus, both the graft and the left anterior descending coronary artery could deliver adequate flow to maintain the control level of coronary blood flow velocity in the left anterior descending coronary artery. Therefore, occlusion of either vessel alone did not alter downstream coronary blood flow velocity. (*c*) Simultaneous occlusion of the graft and the proximal left anterior descending coronary artery decreased downstream blood flow velocity to 0. Following release of a 20-s occlusion of both the graft and the proximal left anterior descending coronary artery there was a substantial reactive hyperemic response. The improved reactive hyperemic response in (*c*) compared to the preoperative study in (*a*) indicates that placement of the coronary bypass graft distal to the obstruction in the left anterior descending artery improved the coronary vasodilator reserve of the downstream vascular bed. (*d*) Simultaneous occlusion of the graft and the proximal left anterior descending coronary artery decreased downstream coronary blood flow velocity to 0. Following a 20-s occlusion, release of the proximal left anterior descending coronary artery alone while graft occlusion was maintained resulted in a markedly blunted reactive hyperemic response. Subsequent release of the graft occlusion a few seconds later permitted a significant vasodilator response of the downstream vascular bed to become manifest.

coronary vessel distal to the point of graft insertion during occlusion of the graft and a proximal segment of the recipient vessel, collateral flow could still prevent myocardial ischemia from developing in the perfusion field being examined. Such collateral flow can be excluded only by demonstrating functional evidence of ischemia, i.e., segmental dyskinesis, during the time that zero flow is measured. Although studies with the Doppler are encouraging, much remains to be done before this technique will be of significant value in the intraoperative assessment of the functional capacity of vein bypass grafts.

Measurements of Segmental Wall Motion

Segmental left ventricular wall motion can be determined intraoperatively with echocardiographic techniques [41] or implanted sonomicrometers [42]. These studies have shown that in patients regional myocardial ischemia or infarction is associated with localized mechanical dysfunction. Although such measurements of segmental wall motion can be used to assess the contractile state of cardiac muscle, it is almost impossible to assess the functional capacity of bypass grafts with this approach because ventricular function is similar if coronary flow is normal or six times normal. Even if segmental function improves following placement of a bypass graft, the change could reflect enhanced perfusion or some alteration in the loading condition of the ventricle.

Other Intraoperative Approaches to Studying Coronary Bypass Grafts

In the early 1970s, several approaches to assessing graft function were introduced. These included intragraft infusions of xenon 133 (^{133}Xe) [26,33,43,44] or hydrogen [45] to measure myocardial perfusion, mass spectrometry to determine intramyocardial gas tensions [46], thermocouples to estimate graft flow [47], and intraoperative coronary angiography [48,49] to assess graft anatomy. These methods of evaluating bypass grafts intraoperatively were either impractical or not quantitative. Hence, they are not widely employed at present. In 1977, Oldham et al. [50] utilized intragraft injection of labeled albumin macroaggregates coupled with electromagnetic flow measurements to assess both the volume and distribution of graft flow. This innovative approach may be particulary helpful in studying collateral flow in humans.

In summary, at present all approaches to the intraoperative evaluation of coronary bypass grafts have significant limitations. Studies with the Doppler probe represent the most promising technique available. It is likely that sophisticated intraoperative studies of the functional capacity of vein bypass grafts would lead to improvements in operative techniques and perhaps to better patient selection. Therefore, efforts to improve the intraoperative assessment of bypass grafts should be encouraged.

POSTOPERATIVE EVALUATION OF CORONARY BYPASS GRAFTS

Since 1969, many approaches to the postoperative evaluation of coronary bypass grafts have been introduced. Although none of these techniques is ideal, each of them can be of value in studying the functional capacity of coronary bypass grafts.

Coronary Angiography

Postoperative coronary angiography is the most widely used technique for evaluating coronary bypass grafts and the only method that is used to make definitive decisions about patient care [1,3–5,10,11,13,17,18,20,25,27,48,49]. In essence, the angiograms define the anatomic state of the grafts and the native coronary vessels. Postoperative angiograms provide the following specific data:

1 Native coronary vessels Location of obstructive lesions; assess progression of disease from the time of previous catheterization in vascular segments proximal and distal to the point of graft insertion.

2 Bypass grafts Determine graft patency, geometry of the proximal and distal anastomosis, appropriateness of the distal anastomosis site selected, and the size of the bed perfused by the graft.

Postoperative angiographic studies indicate that 75 to 87 percent of bypass grafts are patent 1 year following the operative procedure [51–56]. Studies from Montreal [54,56] have shown that 50 percent of grafts that close in 6 to 12 months following surgery do so in the first 2 to 4 weeks in the postoperative period. Although 10 to 25 percent of grafts close in the first year, for the subsequent 6 to 8 years the vein graft occlusion rate is only 2 percent per year [54–56]. Although coronary angiography can define the anatomic state of bypass grafts, the functional capacity of the grafts cannot be determined quantitatively with angiography alone.

Perfusion Field of Coronary Bypass Grafts

By injecting albumin microspheres labeled with gamma-emitting isotopes into bypass grafts at the time of cardiac catheterization, the perfusion field of the graft can be ascertained [10,11]. Unfortunately, the resolution of the currently available gamma cameras for detecting the distribution of these radioactive particles is far from ideal. Although these microsphere studies provide a better definition of the perfusion field of the vein bypass graft than does coronary angiography [10,11], such measurements do not permit one to measure the flow rate or the transmural distribution of flow.

Postoperative Measurements of Flow in Bypass Grafts

Four techniques are currently used to measure the flow in bypass grafts in the postoperative period: videodensitometry, ^{133}Xe clearance, hydrogen clearance, and measurements of blood flow velocity with various types of Doppler probes.

Videodensitometry Rutishauser et al. [57] pioneered the use of videodensitometry for measurements of blood flow (see Chapter 2). Over the years, this approach has been utilized occasionally to measure flow in coronary vessels and bypass grafts [58–62]. When this technique is used in association with coronary angiography, a major artifact is introduced: The contrast media required to produce the angiograms from which videodensitometry measurements are made, significantly alter blood flow in the bypass graft [61–63]. Studies which have employed videodensitometry indicate that flow rates in saphenous vein bypass grafts under resting conditions average 68 ml/min [61,62].

Computed transmission tomography tremendously enhances the potential value of measurements of bypass graft flow with videodensitometry (see Chapter 2). With computed transmission tomography, only a small amount of contrast material that can be injected intravenously is needed [64–66]. Thus, at once the two drawbacks of conventional videodensitometry are eliminated: coronary angiography is no longer required and flow rates are not artificially distorted by the injection of large volumes of contrast media directly into the graft. Initial experience with this approach is extremely encouraging [64–66].

^{133}Xe Clearance At the time of coronary angiography, myocardial perfusion can be measured if ^{133}Xe is injected intracoronary or intragraft and the clearance of the isotope is quantified with the gamma detector (Chapter 2). The limitations of this technique have been reviewed in Chapter 2 of this monograph. When ^{133}Xe is employed to assess the functional capacity of coronary bypass grafts [44,67–70], the flows measured reflect total perfusion from all sources (graft, proximal vessel, and collaterals) to the myocardial region being examined. Thus, with the ^{133}Xe clearance technique, it is not possible to determine the component of perfusion to a specific region that traverses the bypass graft.

Studies that have employed the ^{133}Xe clearance method indicate that myocardial perfusion averages 40 to 100 ml/min/100 g in zones which are within the perfusion field of bypass grafts. In addition, ^{133}Xe clearance studies have suggested that exercise [33] and isoproterenol infusion [69] can substantially increase flow to areas served by patent bypass grafts.

Hydrogen Clearance Hydrogen clearance was utilized to assess flow in coronary bypass grafts by Green et al. [45] in 1972. The limitations of this technique have been described in Chapter 2. Like ^{133}Xe, hydrogen clearance measures total tissue perfusion. Consequently, the component of tissue flow which traverses the bypass graft cannot be measured.

Doppler Probes Catheter-mounted [71,72] and transcutaneous [73–75] Doppler probes have been used to study blood flow velocity in bypass grafts. With this method, phasic blood flow velocity can be recorded and responses to vasoactive stimuli easily determined [72]. The reported studies have not employed sophisticated Doppler instruments which can assess the velocity profile and vessel diameter [76]. Without this information flow cannot be computed. The best results to date with this technique have been reported by Diebold et al. [75]. In a series of 163 vein grafts examined, 127 patent and 14 occluded grafts were correctly identified, 11 patent grafts could not be recorded, and 11 occluded grafts were falsely diagnosed as patent. Sensitivity and specificity of the method were 92 percent and 56 percent, respectively. It is likely that technological advances in Doppler instrumentation in the near future will greatly improve the value of this approach to studying the functional capacity of vein bypass grafts postoperatively.

Presently available methods for measuring blood flow in vein bypass grafts in the postoperative period have many deficiencies. The most promising approaches at this time are videodensitometry coupled with computed transmission tomography and transcutaneous Doppler measurements with sophisticated instrumentation.

INDIRECT METHODS OF EVALUATING THE POSTOPERATIVE FUNCTION OF CORONARY BYPASS GRAFTS

All the clinical procedures that have been applied to diagnose coronary disease preoperatively have also been utilized to assess the functional status of coronary bypass grafts. Most patients who undergo bypass surgery have multivessel coronary disease and require multiple coronary bypasses. Hence, the most frequent clinical concern is: how many and which of the bypass grafts are open? Unfortunately, the standard noninvasive tests for evaluating patients with coronary disease share a common deficiency: they cannot accurately determine the extent of coronary disease. This limitation is an enormous handicap when these diagnostic procedures are used in the postoperative evaluation of coronary bypass grafts. Nonetheless, clinical symptoms, electrocardiographic monitoring during treadmill exercise tests, thallium 201 perfusion scintigrams, and rest and exercise ventricular function studies are widely used to evaluate the functional status of coronary bypass grafts.

Clinical Symptoms

Preoperatively, most patients who are going to have coronary bypass surgery have symptoms that may be related to myocardial ischemia. The most prevalent symptoms are angina pectoris and previous myocardial infarction. If, following coronary bypass surgery, the symptoms are no longer present, the coronary bypass grafts are probably open. Clinical studies have shown that symptomatic relief is correlated with the completeness of the revascularization procedure [77–79]. Assad-Morell and coworkers [77] reported that 80 percent of completely revascularized patients became asymptomatic in the postoperative period. If one or two diseased vessels remained ungrafted, the percentage of asymptomatic patients decreased to 60 percent and 16 percent, respectively. Although these clinical correlates are helpful in predicting the clinical course of groups of patients, they are of little assistance in the evaluation of a single patient. The absence of symptoms following coronary bypass surgery could occur because (1) the angina producing myocardial segment infarcted during the operative procedure and the grafts are closed, (2) the patient severely limits exercise activities, (3) the original cause of the angina pectoris was muscular skeletal pain which has since been relieved with aspirin, (4) the psychological effects of the operation, and (5) the grafts are open and functioning well.

The relief of symptoms of myocardial ischemia following coronary bypass surgery suggests that the bypass grafts probably are open. Conversely, persistent symptoms in the postoperative course imply that one or more of the ischemic zones present preoperatively are not being adequately perfused. These clinical impressions can be used to estimate roughly the outcome of the operative procedure; however, as noted above, clinical evaluation of such patients is often inaccurate.

Graded Exercise Treadmill Tests with Electrocardiographic Monitoring

In general, one cannot accurately determine the patency of coronary bypass grafts from the results of graded exercise tolerance tests with electrocardiographic monitoring. However, the frequency of negative treadmill exercise tolerance tests increases with the completeness of the revascularization procedure]77–78]. Ninety-one percent of completely revascularized patients have negative graded exercise tolerance tests [77]. If one diseased vessel is ungrafted, 30 percent of patients have a negative graded treadmill exercise tolerance test [77]. Four percent of patients with two ungrafted diseased vessels have negative exercise tests [77]. Unfortunately, an abnormal test is not specific; it could be due to a long list of factors [80] which are associated with false-positive exercise electrocardiographic responses. Alternatively, an abnormal test could reflect inadequate perfusion of the myocardium served by an occluded or obstructed coronary bypass graft.

Thallium 201 Perfusion Scintigrams

Thallium 201 perfusion scintigrams are widely used to assess the relative distribution of myocardial perfusion [81]. In theory, a preoperative scintigram which showed diminished uptake of thallium 201 in a region perfused by an obstructed vessel preoperatively would demonstrate a normal thallium 201 distribution postoperatively if the graft to the obstructed vessel was patent [82–85]. Although clinical studies have shown that most patients with multivessel coronary disease have positive thallium 201 scintigrams, the defect in the perfusion scintigrams is often confined to one area. Hence, when large groups of patients have conventional thallium 201 scintigrams prior to coronary bypass surgery, normal thallium 201 uptake is noted in most areas served by obstructed coronary vessels. If the zone of myocardium served by a severely obstructed coronary vessel had normal thallium 201 uptake on both the pre- and postoperative scintigrams, the status of the bypass graft would be unpredictable (Figure 17-8) [83]. Also, if the segment of myocardium contains a substantial amount of fibrous tissue as a result of previous myocardial infarction, a thallium 201 defect may persist postoperatively even if the region is perfused by an open bypass graft [81,83].

In my view, thallium 201 scintigrams performed in the conventional manner (planar scintigrams without quantitative analysis) are of little value in the postoperative evaluation of coronary bypass grafts.

A few recent studies which have analyzed thallium 201 scintigrams with quantitative technique indicate that these improved scintigraphic procedures may be of value in assessing the functional capacity of coronary bypass grafts in the postoperative period [86–88].

Rest and Exercise Left Ventriculargrams

When rest and exercise studies of ventricular wall motion are used to assess the functional capacity of coronary bypass grafts, the problems encountered are similar to those noted for thallium 201 scintigrams. Many areas served by ob-

FIGURE 17-8
Relationship between postoperative thallium 201 (TL^{201}) perfusion scintigrams and coronary bypass graft patency. In this study, 15 patients had pre- and postoperative thallium 201 scintigrams during exercise. Perfusion was graded in five ventricular segments in each patient ($5 \times 15 = 75$). Bypass graft patency was determined by coronary angiography. Most myocardial segments showed no change in thallium 201 uptake (TL^{201} unchanged) when the pre- and postoperative scintigrams were compared; in this group, 8 of 46 bypass grafts were occluded. In the eight myocardial segments which showed a worsened thallium 201 uptake postoperatively, only five were served by occluded grafts. In the 21 segments which showed improved thallium 201 uptake, one was served by an occluded graft. These studies demonstrate that worsened, unchanged, or improved thallium 201 uptake postoperatively can be associated with either patent or occluded bypass grafts. Hence, postoperative thallium 201 perfusion images are not a particularly effective way to determine coronary bypass graft patency. (*Based on data originally presented by JA Sbarbaro et al* [*83*].)

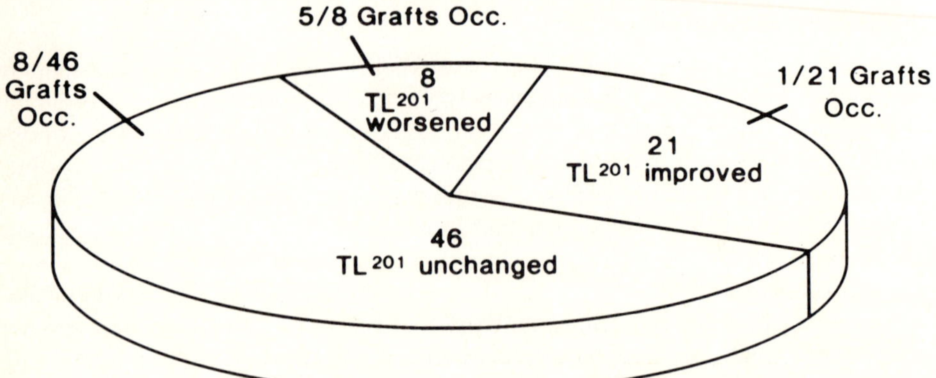

structed vessels do not demonstrate ventricular wall motion abnormalities during exercise [89,90]. Hence, normal segmental wall motion during rest or exercise can occur in segments perfused by occluded or open coronary bypass grafts. Furthermore, areas of previous infarction usually do not improve their segmental wall function following surgery even if the bypass graft perfusing the segment is open and functioning well [91].

Under specific circumstances, exercise ventricular function can be helpful in assessing the functional capacity of coronary bypass grafts. In a patient with normal ventricular function preoperatively and single vessel disease, if exercise produces preoperatively a segmental wall motion abnormality which disappears postoperatively at the same exercise stress, it is likely that the bypass graft perfusing the region is open (Figure 17-9) [92].

The standard noninvasive tests for evaluating the functional capacity of coronary bypass grafts are not precise. Hence, clinicians should be hesitant to make definitive therapeutic decisions on the basis of the results of these procedures alone.

FIGURE 17-9
Effects of coronary artery bypass grafts on global left ventricular function at rest and during exercise. In this study, all patients had normal left ventricular function preoperatively (left ventricular [LV] ejection fraction greater than 50 percent). Preoperatively, with intense exercise, myocardial ischemia was provoked and global left ventricular function decreased. Postoperatively, at the same level of exercise, no myocardial ischemia occurred and global left ventricular function actually improved slightly. All patients had patent coronary bypass grafts determined by angiography. Left ventricular ejection fraction was determined by radionuclide ventriculography. (*Based on data originally presented by KM Kent et al* [92].)

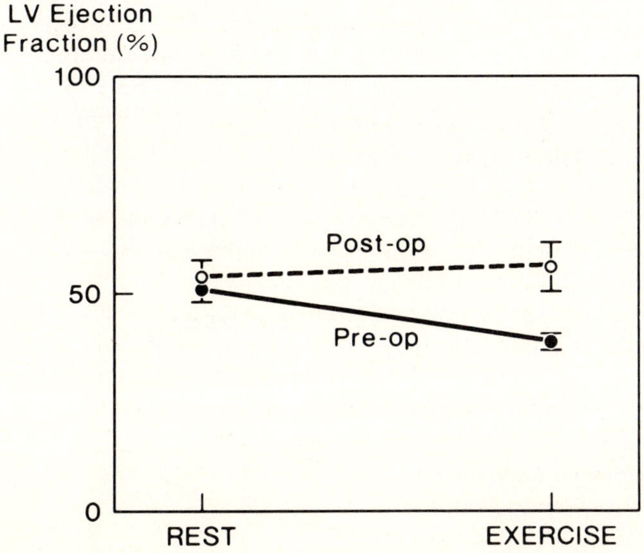

POTENTIAL DELETERIOUS EFFECTS OF CORONARY BYPASS GRAFTS ON THE CORONARY CIRCULATION

Coronary bypass grafts can adversely affect the coronary circulation if complications associated with the operative procedure develop. These include aortic dissection, stenosis at the anastomosis sites, improper placement of the bypass graft, myocardial infarction, coronary dissection, and coronary ligation. In addition, even in the best medical centers, coronary bypass graft surgery is associated with a mortality rate of 0.5 to 1 percent in good surgical candidates [5]. Even if the grafts are properly placed, open, and functioning well, bypass grafts potentially can have two adverse effects on the coronary circulation: (1) functioning grafts can promote closure of previously existing mature coronary collateral vessels and (2) the graft may hasten the progression of atherosclerosis in native coronary vessels proximal and distal to the site of anastomosis.

Effects on the Coronary Collateral Circulation

The function of coronary collateral vessels depends on the existence of a pressure gradient between the collateral channel and the recipient coronary bed. If a bypass graft is placed distal to a severe obstruction, pressure in the distal vascular segment will increase and the pressure gradient from the coronary collateral channel to the distal vascular segment will decrease commensurately. A similar phenomenon occurs following successful balloon angioplasty (Chapter 19). When the pressure gradient between the obstructed vessel and the coronary collateral channel no longer exists, coronary collateral vessels are not detectable by coronary angiography. One study suggests that coronary collaterals begin to close within minutes following placement of an effective bypass graft [14].

Postoperative coronary arteriograms have defined several courses that coronary collateral channels follow after coronary bypass surgery [93–97]. If the severely diseased coronary vessel that had previously received adequate collaterals is effectively bypassed, the collaterals will no longer be visible at the time of postoperative angiography [93–97]. This change has been documented to occur within 2 weeks following coronary bypass surgery [97] but probably takes place immediately following graft insertion. If, following this sequence, the graft becomes occluded, the coronary collaterals will usually reappear [93,94,97]. Animal studies by Khouri [98], performed in the prebypass era, suggested that "dormant coronary collaterals" could reappear if coronary occlusion reoccurred (see Chapter 10). If graft occlusion, progressive atherosclerotic occlusion of native vessels, or both occur in a vascular bed that did not appear to receive collateral flow on a preoperative coronary arteriogram, the postoperative arteriogram will often demonstrate that newly developed coronary collateral channels delivered blood to the diseased vessel [93,97]. *These angiographic studies demonstrate that the coronary collateral circulation in humans is dynamic and can respond quickly to alterations in the functional state of native coronary vessels.*

Effects on the Progression of Coronary Atherosclerosis

Two to four years following placement of a coronary bypass graft distal to a coronary obstruction, follow-up coronary arteriograms demonstrate progression of disease in 47 percent of vascular segments proximal and 4 percent of vascular segments distal to the site of graft insertion [99,100]. Progression of a proximal stenosis to total occlusion occurs almost exclusively in proximal segments that had at least 75 percent stenosis noted on the preoperative coronary angiogram [99,100]. Some investigators have suggested that the progression of atherosclerotic disease, particularly in the proximal segment, may be hastened by the presence of a patent coronary bypass [101]. The graft decreases flow in the proximal segment by competing with the parent vessel. This decrease in flow could promote occlusion of the diseased vascular segment. Also, blood entering the coronary vessel from the bypass graft causes moderate alterations in the blood velocity profile within the vessel, and this could also promote atherosclerosis.

Unfortunately, the available data related to this question are difficult to interpret [99–107]. The problems with previous clinical studies in this area are as follows:

1 Progression of coronary disease is almost always defined by measurements of percent diameter stenosis from coronary arteriograms obtained prior to and following bypass surgery. Percent diameter stenosis correlates poorly with the functional severity of coronary obstructive lesions [108,109]. When the severity of a coronary obstruction is defined by percent stenosis, one assumes that the coronary lesion is symmetrical and that the segments proximal and/or distal to the obstructive lesion are uninvolved by atherosclerosis. Furthermore, percent stenosis measurements between the pre- and postoperative coronary arteriograms assume that the condition of the vascular segments proximal and distal to the obstruction did not change. All these assumptions are erroneous (see Chapter 11).

2 There are major problems with the quality of postoperative angiograms because the vascular segment proximal to the graft is often perfused anterograde from the aorta and retrograde from the graft. Because the arteriograms are performed by selective injection of contrast into either the graft or the native coronary vessel, the proximal segment often receives both opacified and nonopacified blood. Under such conditions, identification of the borders of the proximal vessel can be exceedingly difficult.

3 In the reported clinical studies, no attempt has been made to match the pre- and postoperative arteriograms with respect to major determinants of coronary diameter, which include distending pressure, coronary vascular tone, and nitroglycerine administration during and prior to the angiographic procedure.

4 It is tacitly assumed that coronary lesions of differing severity progress toward occlusion at a similar rate. In fact, mild lesions progress slowly, and severe obstructions progress rapidly toward total occlusion. The mass of atheroma needed to increase the percent diameter stenosis of a vessel 3 mm in diameter from 15 to 25 percent is two times greater than the mass of atheroma needed to increase percent diameter stenosis from 70 to 100 percent.

5 In any given patient, the rate of progression of atherosclerosis will depend on the presence of various factors which tend to promote atherosclerosis, such as smoking, hypertension, and hypercholesterolemia. Thus, to determine if a patent bypass graft hastened the progression of atherosclerosis, one would have to identify patients with two coronary vessels that had a similar degree of obstruction in each vessel and bypass only one vessel. Thereafter, one could determine the rate of progression in the vessel that was bypassed and its control. Such data are obviously not available.

6 Finally, unless pre- and postoperative coronary arteriograms are analyzed quantitatively (see Chapter 11), *errors* related to intra- and interobserver variability in the interpretation of the arteriograms would almost certainly obscure any real differences in the rate of progression of atherosclerosis that could be induced by placement of a patent bypass graft.

In my view, there is no convincing data to either confirm or deny the notion that coronary bypass grafts alter the rate at which atherosclerotic coronary obstructions progress toward total occlusion.

Although coronary bypass grafts can potentially have deleterious effects on the coronary circulation, in the vast majority of patients the operative procedure alleviates the symptoms of myocardial ischemia and improves myocardial perfusion. In selected patient subgroups, coronary bypass surgery may also prevent myocardial infarction and prolong life.

REFERENCES

1 Johnson WD, Flemma RJ, Lepley D, Ellison EH: Extended treatment of severe coronary artery disease: A total surgical approach. *Ann Surg* 170: 460, 1969.

2 Miller DW Jr: A short history of myocardial revascularization, in *The Practice of Coronary Artery Bypass Surgery.* New York, Plenum Medical, 1977, chap 1, p 1.

3 Norman JC (ed): *Coronary Artery Medicine and Surgery: Concepts and Controversies.* New York, Appleton-Century-Crofts, 1975.

4 Yu PN, Goodwin JF (eds): *Progress in Cardiology*, vol 6. Philadelphia, Lea & Febiger, 1977.

5 Rahimatoola SH: Coronary bypass surgery for chronic angina—1981—a perspective. *Circulation* 65: 225, 1982.

6 Furuse A, Klopp EH, Brawley RK, Gott VL: Hemodynamics of aorta-to-coronary artery bypass, experimental and analytical studies. *Ann Thorac Surg* 14: 282, 1972.

7 Overton JB, Smith JC, Robel SB, Spencer MP, Mansfield PB, Sauvage LR: Origin of downstream flow in nonobstructed coronary arteries. *Arch Surg* 107: 764, 1973.

8 Stein PD, Sabbah HN, Marzilli M: Reduction of coronary flow in the circulation after bypass. Observations in a hydraulic model of the cardiovascular system. *J Thorac Cardiovasc Surg* 78: 772, 1979.

9 Kakos GS, Oldham HN Jr, Dixon SH Jr, Davis RW, Hagan P-O, Sabiston DC Jr: Coronary artery hemodynamics after aorto-coronary artery vein bypass. *J Thorac Cardiovasc Surg* 63: 849, 1972

10 Hamilton GW, Murray JA, Lapin E, Allen D, Hämmermeister KE, Ritchie JL: Evaluation of myocardial perfusion by direct injection of radioactive particles following coronary bypass surgery, in *Coronary Artery Medicine and Surgery: Concepts and Controversies*, JC Norman (ed). New York, Appleton-Century-Crofts, 1975, p 860.

11 Kolibash AJ, Lewis RP, Goodenow JS, Bush CA, Tetalman MR: Extensive myocardial blood flow distribution through individual coronary artery bypass grafts. *Chest* 77:17, 1980.

12 Bartley TD, Bigelow JC, Page US: Aortocoronary bypass grafting with multiple sequential anastomoses to a single vein. *Arch Surg* 105: 915, 1972.

13 Grondin CM, Vouhé P, Bourassa MG, Lespérance J, Bouvier M, Campeau L: Optimal patency rates obtained in coronary artery grafting with circular vein grafts. *J Thorac Cardiovasc Surg* 75: 161, 1978.

14 Greenfield JC Jr, Rembert JC, Young WG Jr, Oldham HN Jr, Alexander JA, Sabiston DC Jr: Studies of blood flow in aorta-to-coronary venous bypass grafts in man. *J Clin Invest* 51: 2724, 1972.

15 Tyers GF, O'Neil MJ, Messner JT, Waldhausen JA: Nonmechanical factors affecting aortocoronary vein graft flow. *Circulation* 51 & 52: 178, 1975.

16 Hiratzka L, Eastham C, Carter J, Moyers J, Elliot D, Wright C, Doty D, Marcus M: Coronary dilation after cardiopulmonary bypass. *Am J Cardiol* 49: 969, 1982.

17 Johnson WD, Flemma RJ, Lepley D Jr: Determinants of blood flow in aortic-coronary saphenous vein bypass grafts. *Arch Surg* 101: 806, 1970.

18 Mitchel BF, Adam M, Lambert CJ, Sungu U, Shiekh S: Ascending aorta-to-coronary artery saphenous vein bypass grafts. *J Thorac Cardiovasc Surg* 60: 457, 1970.

19 Olinger GN, Mulder DG, Maloney JV, Buckberg GD: Phasic coronary flow: Intraoperative evaluation of flow distribution, myocardial function, and reactive hyperemic response. *Ann Thorac Surg* 21: 397, 1976.

20 Folts JD, Kahn DR, Bittar N, Rowe GG: Effects of partial obstruction of phasic flow in aortocoronary grafts. *Circulation* 52(suppl 1): 148, 1975.

21 Olsson RA, Gregg DE: Myocardial reactive hyperemia in the unanesthetized dog. *Am J Physiol* 208: 224, 1965.

22 Marcus M, Wright C, Doty D, Eastham C, Laughlin D, Krumm P, Fastenow C, Brody M: Measurements of coronary velocity and reactive hyperemia in the coronary circulation of humans. *Circ Res* 49: 877, 1981.

23 Grondin CM, Castonguay YR, Lespérance J, Bourassa MG, Campeau L, Grondin P: Attrition rate of aorta-to-coronary artery saphenous vein grafts after one year. *Ann Thorac Surg* 14: 223, 1972.

24 Nitter-Hauge S, Hall KV, Troysaker T: Aorto-coronary saphenous vein bypass graft. *Scan J Thor Cardiovasc Surg* 12: 235, 1978.

25 Marco JD, Barner HB, Kaiser GC, Codd JE, Mudd JG, Willman V: Operative flow measurements and coronary bypass graft patency. *J Thorac Cardiovasc Surg* 71: 545, 1976.

26 Kreulen TH, Kirk ES, Gorlin R, Cohn LH, Collins JJ: Coronary artery bypass surgery: Assessment of revascularization by determination of blood flow and myocardial mass. *Am J Cardiol* 34: 129, 1974.

27 Stinson EB, Olinger GN, Glancy DL: Anatomical and physiological determinants of blood flow through aortocoronary vein bypass grafts. *Surgery* 74: 390, 1973.

28 Walter P, Schwarz F, Flameng W, Hehrlein F: Determinants of restricted aorta-coronary bypass graft flow. *Thorac Cardiovasc Surg* 27: 5, 1979.

29 Roth JA, Cukingnan RA, Brown BG, Gocka E, Carey JS: Factors influencing patency of saphenous vein grafts. *Ann Thorac Surg* 28: 176, 1979.

30 Schwarz AF, Flameng W, Thiedemann K-U, Schaper W, Schlepper M: Effect of coronary stenosis on myocardial function, ultrastructure and aortocoronary bypass graft hemodynamics. *Am J Cardiol* 42: 193, 1978.

31 Bittar H, Kroncke GM, Dacumos GC Jr, Rowe GG, Young WP, Chopra PS, Folts JD, Kahn DR: Vein graft flow and reactive hyperemia in the human heart. *J Thorac Cardiovasc Surg* 64: 855, 1972.

32 Brower RW, Serruys PW, Bos E, Nauta J: Regional myocardial shortening in relation to graft-reactive hyperemia and flow after coronary bypass surgery. *J Thorac Cardiovasc Surg* 77: 92, 1979.

33 Flameng W, Schwarz F, Hehrlein FW: Intraoperative evaluation of the functional significance of coronary collateral vessels in patients with coronary artery disease. *Am J Cardiol* 42: 187, 1978.

34 McKelvie RS, Kline RL, Black LL, McKenzie FN, Heimbecker RO: Influence of alternate sources of blood flow on the reactive hyperemia response in aorta-coronary saphenous vein bypass grafts in man. *J Thorac Cardiovasc Surg* 78: 62, 1979.

35 Barner HB, Kaiser GC, Codd JE, Willman VL: Coronary graft flow and glucose tolerance: Evidence against the existence of myocardial microvascular disease. *Vasc Surg* 9: 220, 1975.

36 Skotnicki S, Vonk J, Sleegers TH, Dercksen S, Linssen LL, Kuijpers P: Aortocoronary graft flow and reactive hyperaemia in relation to postoperative myocardial infarction. *Thorax* 31: 172, 1976.

37 Arnett EN, Isner JM, Redwood DR, Kent KM, Baker WP, Ackerstein H, Roberts WC: Coronary artery narrowing in coronary heart disease: Comparison of cineangiographic and necropsy findings. *Ann Int Med* 91: 350, 1979.

38 McCormick JR, Kaneko M, Baue AE, Geha AS: Blood flow and vasoactive drug effects in internal mammary and venous bypass grafts. *Circulation* 52(suppl 1): 72, 1975.

39 Larsen PB, Yeh BK, Gentsch TO, Traad EA, Faraldo AR, Gosselin AJ, Swaye PS: Sodium nitroprusside as a coronary vasodilator in man: A comparison of the effects of sodium nitroprusside and papaverine hydrochloride on aortocoronary saphenous vein graft flow. *Ann Thorac Surg* 21: 16, 1976.

40 Stoelting RK, King RD: Aortocoronary vein graft flow in response to peripheral venous administration of sodium nitroprusside or diazepam. *Ann Thorac Surg* 24: 59, 1977.

41 Likoff M, Reichek N, Macoviak J, Harken A, Sutton MST, Muhammed A, Plappert T, Kastor JA: High frequency epicardial echo mapping of segmental myocardial performance at multiple sites on right and left ventricles. *Am J Cardiol* 47: 403, 1981.

42 Kleinman LH, Hill RC, Chitwood WR Jr, Hammon JW Jr, Jones KW, Wechsler AS: Regional myocardial dimensions following coronary artery bypass grafting in patients. Relationship of functional deterioration to graft occlusion. *J Thorac Cardiovasc Surg* 77: 13, 1979.

43 Smith SC Jr, Gorlin R, Herman MV, Taylor WJ, Collins JJ Jr: Myocardial blood flow in man: Effects of coronary collateral circulation and coronary artery bypass surgery. *J Clin Invest* 51: 2556, 1972.

44 Korbuly DE, Formanek A, Gypser G, Moore R, Ovitt TW, Tuna N, Amplatz K: Regional myocardial blood flow measurements before and after coronary bypass surgery. *Circulation* 52: 38, 1975.

45 Green DG, Klocke FJ, Schimert GL, Bunnell IL, Wittenberg SM, Lajos T: Evaluation of venous bypass grafts from aorta to coronary artery by inert gas desaturation and direct flowmeter techniques. *J Clin Invest* 51: 191, 1972.

46 Gardner TJ, Brantigan JW, Perna AM, Bender HW, Brawley RK, Gott VL: Intramyocardial gas tensions in the human heart during coronary artery-saphenous vein bypass. *J Thorac Cardiovasc Surg* 62: 844, 1971.

47 Tanimoto Y, Watanabe T, Endo M, Hayashi H: Noninvasive assessment of aorta-coronary saphenous vein bypass graft patency using thermocouple. *Jpn Heart J* 19: 252, 1978.

48 Diethrich EB, et al: Intraoperative coronary arteriography. *Am J Surg* 124: 815, 1972.

49 Kaplitt MJ, Frantz SL, Tortolani AJ, Newman FA, Stein HL, Gulotta SJ: Review of intraoperative coronary antiography in aortocoronary bypass surgery, in *Coronary Artery Medicine and Surgery: Concepts and Controversies.* New York, Appleton-Century-Crofts, 1975.

50 Oldham HN, Jr, Jones RH, Harris CC, Howe WR, Goodrich JK, Sabiston DC Jr: Intraoperative relationships between regional myocardial distribution of bypass graft flow and the coronary collateral circulation. *J Thorac Cardiovasc Surg* 77: 32, 1979.

51 Fitzgibbon GM, Burton JR, Leach AJ: Coronary bypass graft fate: Angiographic grading of 1400 consecutive grafts early after operation and of 1132 after one year. *Circulation* 57: 1070, 1978.

52 Lawrie GM, Morris GC Jr, Chapman DW, Winters WL, Lie JT: Patterns of patency of 596 vein grafts up to 7 years after aorta-coronary bypass. *J Thorac Cardiovasc Surg* 73: 433, 1977.

53 Kouchoukos NT, Karp RB, Oberman A, Russell RO, Jr, Alison HW, Holt JH Jr: Long-term patency of saphenous veins for coronary bypass grafting. *Circulation* 58: 96, 1978.

54 Campeau L, Lespérance J, Corbara F, Hermann J, Grondin C, Bourassa MG: Aorto-coronary saphenous vein bypass graft changes 5–7 years after surgery. *Circulation* 59: 117, 1978.

55 Rimm AH, Blumlein S, Barboriak JJ, Anderson AJ, Walker JA, Johnson WD: The probability of closure in aortocoronary vein bypass grafts. *JAMA* 236: 2637, 1976.

56 Bourassa MG, Campeau L, Lespérance J: Effects of bypass surgery on the coronary circulation: Incidence and effects of vein graft occlusion, in *Coronary Bypass Surgery*, SH Rahimtoola (ed). Philadelphia, Davis, 1977, p 107.

57 Rutishauser W, Simon H, Stucky JP, Schad N, Nosida G, Wellauer J: Evaluation of roentgen cinedensitometry for flow measurement in models and in the intact circulation. *Circulation* 36: 951, 1967.

58 Smith HC, Frye RL, Davis GD, Pluth JR, Sturm RE, Wood EH: Simultaneous indicator dilution curves at selected sites in the coronary circulation and determination of blood flow in coronary artery-saphenous vein grafts by roentgen videodensitometry, in *Roentgen-, Cine- and Videodensitometry: Fundamentals and Applications for Blood Flow and Heart Volume Determination*, PH Heintzen (ed). Stuttgart, Georg Thieme, 1971, p 152.

59 Smith HC, Sturm RE, Wood EH: Videodensitometric system for measurement of vessel blood flow, particularly in the coronary arteries, in man. *Am J Cardiol* 32: 144, 1973.

60 Hamby RI, Aintablian A, Wisoff BG, Hartstein ML: Comparative study of the post-operative flow in the saphenous vein and internal mammary artery bypass grafts. *Am Heart J* 93: 306, 1977.

61 Schmiel FK, Hackbarth W, Korfer R, Politz B, Spiller P, Bircks W: Flow measurements and simultaneously performed angiography of aorto-coronary bypass grafts during bypass surgery. *Thorac Cardiovasc Surg* 27: 386, 1979.

62 Chesebro JH, Ritman EL, Frye RL, Smith HC, Connolly DC, Rutherford BD, Davis

GD, Danielson GK, Pluth JR, Barnhorst DA, Wallace RB: Videometric analysis of regional left ventricular function before and after aortocoronary artery bypass surgery: Correlation of peak rate of myocardial wall thickening with late postoperative graft flows. *J Clin Invest* 158: 1339, 1976.

63 Bussman WD, Rutishauser W, Noseda G, Preter B, Meier W: Influence of a new contrast medium (Metrizoate) on coronary blood flow. in *Roentgen-, Cine- and Videodensitometery*, PH Heintzen (ed). Stuttgart, Georg Thieme, 1971, p 133.

64 Brundage BH, Lipton MJ, Herfrens RJ, Berninger WH, Redington RW, Chatterjee K, Carlsson E: Detection of patent coronary bypass grafts by computed tomography. A Preliminary Report. *Circulation* 61: 826, 1980.

65 Boyd DP, Gould RG, Quinn JR, Sparks R, Stanley RH, Herrmannsfeldt WG: A proposed dynamic cardiac 3-D densitometer for easy detection and evaluation of heart disease. *IEEE Trans Sci NS*-26: 2724, 1979.

66 Goldberg AD, Crawley JCW, Raftery EB, Yacoub MH: Myocardial blood flow following saphenous vein bypass surgery. *Circulation* 51 & 52: 215, 1975.

67 Cannon PJ: Measurement of coronary blood flow and evaluation of regional myocardial perfusion by intracoronary injection techniques, in *Cardiovascular Nuclear Medicine, Prog Nucl Med* 6: 85, Basel, Karger, 1980.

68 Lichtlen P, Moccetti T, Halter J, Schonbeck M, Senning A: Postoperative evaluation of myocardial blood flow in aorta-to-coronary artery vein bypass grafts using the senon-residue detection technic. *Circulation* 46: 445, 1972.

69 Schmidt DH, Blau F, Hellman C, Grzelak L, Johnson WD: Isoproterenol-induced flow responses in mammary and vein bypass grafts. *J Thorac Cardiovasc Surg* 80: 319, 1980.

70 Cannon PJ: Measurement of coronary blood flow and evaluation of regional myocardial perfusion by intracoronary injection techniques, in *Cardiovascular Nuclear Medicine*, Prog nucl med 6, Basel, Karger, 1980, p 85.

71 Benchimol A, Desser KB, Raizada V: Effects of amyl nitrite on phasic aortocoronary bypass graft blood velocity in man. *Am Heart J* 93: 592, 1977.

72 Benchimol A, Desser KB: Measurement of phasic aortocoronary bypass graft blood flow velocity in conscious man. *Am J Cardiol* 32: 895, 1973.

73 Gould KL, Mozersky DJ, Hokanson DE, Baker DW, Kennedy JW, Summer DS, Strandness ED Jr: A noninvasive technic for determining patency of saphenous vein coronary bypass grafts. *Circulation* 46: 595, 1972.

74 Pisko-Dubienski Z, Baird RJ, Wilson DR: Noninvasive assessment of aorta-coronary saphenous vein bypass graft patency using directional Doppler. *Circulation* 52(2 suppl 1): 188, 1975.

75 Diebold B, Theroux P, Bourassa MG, Peronneau P, Guermonprez JL: Noninvasive assessment of aortocoronary bypass graft patency using pulsed Doppler echocardiography. *Am J Cardiol* 43: 10, 1979.

76 Peronneau PA, Bournat JP, Bugnon A, Barbet A, Xhaard M: Theoretical and practical aspects of pulsed Doppler flowmetry: Real-time application to the measure of instantaneous velocity profiles in vitro and in vivo, in *Cardiovascular Applications of Ultrasound*, RS Reneman (ed). New York, Elsevier, 1974, chap 6, p 66.

77 Assad-Morell JL, Frye RL, Connolly DC, Davis GD, Pluth JR, Wallace RB, Barnhorst DA, Elveback LR, Danielson GK: Aorta-coronary artery saphenous vein bypass surgery. Clinical and angiographic results. *Mayo Clin Proc* 50: 379, 1975.

78 Peduzzi P, Hultgren HN: Effect of medical vs. surgical treatment on symptoms in stable angina pectoris. The Veterans Administration Cooperative Study of Surgery for Coronary Arterial Occlusive Disease. *Circulation* 60: 888, 1979.

79 Assad-Morell JL, Frye RL, Connolly DC, Gau GT, Pluth JR, Barnhorst DA, Wallace RB, Davis GD, Elveback LR, Danielson GK: Relation of intraoperative or early postoperative transmural myocardial infarction to patency of aortocoronary bypass grafts and to diseased ungrafted coronary arteries. *Am J Cardiol* 35: 767, 1975.

80 Weiner DA, Ryan TJ, McCabe CH, Kennedy JW, Schloss M, Tristani F, Chaitman BR, Fisher LD: Correlations among history of angina, ST-segment response and prevalence of coronary-artery disease in the coronary artery surgery study (CASS). *N Engl J Med* 301: 230, 1979.

81 Pohost GM, Alpert NM, Ingwall JS, Strauss HW: Thallium redistribution: Mechanism and clinical utility. *Sem Nucl Med* 10: 70, 1979.

82 Verani MS, Marcus ML, Spoto G, Rossi NP, Ehrhardt JC, Razzak MA: Thallium-201 myocardial perfusion scintigrams in the evaluation of aorto-coronary saphenous bypass surgery. *J Nucl Med* 19: 765, 1978.

83 Sbarbaro JA, Harischandra K, Cantez S, Harper PV, Resnekov L: Thallium-201 imaging in assessment of aortocoronary artery bypass graft patency. *Br Heart J* 42: 553, 1979.

84 Ritchie JL, Narahara KA, Trobaugh G, Williams DL, Hamilton GW: Thallium 201 myocardial imaging before and after coronary revascularization: Assessment of myocardial blood flow and graft patency. *Circulation* 56: 830, 1977.

85 Ritchie JL, Hamilton GW, Wachers FJT: *Thallium-201 Myocardial Imaging*. New York, Raven Press, 1978.

86 Francisco DA, Collins SM, Go RT, Ehrhardt JC, Van Kirk OC, Marcus ML: Tomographic thallium-201 myocardial perfusion scintigrams following maximal coronary artery vasodilation with intravenous dipyridamole. A comparison of qualitative and quantitative approaches. *Circulation* 66: 370, 1982.

87 Garcia E, Maddahi J, Berman D, Waxman A: Space/Time quantitation of thallium-201 myocardial scintigraphy. *J Nucl Med* 22: 309, 1981.

88 Watson DD, Campbell NP, Read EK, Gibson RS, Teates CD, Beller GA: Spatial and temporal quantitation of plane thallium myocardial images. *J Nucl Med* 22: 577, 1981.

89 Sharma B, Goodwin JF, Raphael MJ, Steiner RE, Rainbow RG, Taylor SH: Left ventricular function in ischemic disease. *Br Heart J* 38: 59, 1976.

90 Borer J, Bacharach SL, Green MV, Kent KM, Epstein SE, Johnston GS: Real-time radionuclide cineangiography in the noninvasive evaluation of global and regional left ventricular function at rest and during exercise in patients with coronary artery disease. *N Engl J Med* 296: 839, 1977.

91 Ehsani A, Rahimtoola SH, Sinno MZ, Loeb HS, Rosen KM, Gunnar RM: Left ventricular performance after acute myocardial infarction: Spectrum of functional abnormalities and significance of wall motion disturbances. *Arch Intern Med* 135: 1539, 1975.

92 Kent KM, Borer JS, Green MV, Bacharach SL, McIntosh CL, Conkle DM, Epstein SE: Effects of coronary artery bypass on global and regional left ventricular function during exercise. *N Engl J Med* 298: 1434, 1978.

93 McLaughlin PR, Berman ND, Morton BC, McLoughlin MJ, Aldridge HE, Adelman AG, Goldman BS, Trimble AS, Morch JE: Saphenous vein bypass grafting. Changes in native circulation and collaterals. *Circulation* 52: 66, 1975.

94 Valle M, Wiljasalo M, Frick MH, Korhola O, Souranta H, Tallroth K: Collateral circulation before and after coronary artery reconstruction. *Ann Clin Res* 7(4): 251, 1975.

95 Di Luzio V, Roy PR, Sowton E, Dow J: Fate of coronary collateral circulation after aorto-coronary saphenous vein bypass grafts. *Br Heart J* 37: 397, 1975.

96 Glassman E, Krauss KR, Weisinger B, Spencer FC: The effect of bypass grafting on the coronary circulation. *Circulation* 4: 53, 1973.

97 Bourassa MG, et al: Regression and appearance of coronary collaterals in humans during life. *Circulation* 49,50: 127, 1974.

98 Khouri EM, Gregg DE, McGranahan GM Jr: Regression and reappearance of coronary collaterals. *Am J Physiol* 220: 655, 1971.

99 Bourassa MG, Goulet C, Lespérance J: Progression of coronary arterial disease after aortocoronary bypass grafts. *Circulation* 48: 127, 1973.

100 Bourassa MG, Lespérance J, Saltiel J, Corbara F, Campeau L: Progression of obstructive coronary disease 5–7 years after aortocoronary bypass surgery. *Circulation* 58: 100, 1978.

101 Aldridge HE, Trimble AS: Progression of proximal artery lesions to total occlusion after aorta-coronary saphenous vein bypass grafting. *J Thorac Cardiovasc Surg* 62: 7, 1971.

102 Itscoitz SB, Redwood DR, Stinson EB, Reis RL, Epstein SE: Saphenous vein bypass grafts: Long-term patency and effect on the native coronary circulation. *Am J Cardiol* 36: 739, 1975.

103 Griffith LSC, Achuff SC, Conti CR, Humphries JO, Brawley RK, Gott VL, Ross KS: Changes in intrinsic coronary circulation and segmental ventricular motion after saphenous vein coronary bypass graft surgery. *N Engl J Med* 288: 589, 1973.

104 Gensini GG, Esente P, Kelly, A: Natural history of coronary disease in patients with and without bypass surgery. *Circulation* 50: 98, 1974.

105 BenZvi, J, Hildner FJ, Javier RP, Fester A, Samet P: Progression of coronary artery disease. Cine-arteriographic and clinical observations in medically and surgically treated patients. *Am J Cardiol* 34: 295, 1974.

106 Nitter-Hauge S, Levorstad K: Does aortocoronary saphenous vein bypass surgery change the native coronary arteries? *Acta Med Scand* 207: 189, 1980.

107 Palac RT, Hwang MH, Meadows WR, Croke RP, Pifarre R, Loeb HS, Gunnar RM: Progression of coronary artery disease in medically and surgically treated patients 5 years after randomization. *Circulation* 64, 1981.

108 Wright C, White C, Fruda J, Doty D, Eastham C, Laughlin D, Marcus M: Can the coronary arteriogram predict the functional significance of a coronary stenosis? *Circulation* 62: 214, 1980.

109 Harrison DG, White CW, Hiratzka LF, Wright CB, Doty DB, Miller MR, Eastham CL, Marcus ML: Can the significance of a coronary stenosis be predicted by quantitative coronary angiography? *Circulation* 64: 160, 1981.

CHAPTER **18**

CARDIOPULMONARY BYPASS WITH COLD CHEMICAL CARDIOPLEGIA

Clinical open heart surgery, which began in the early 1950s [1–5], was tremendously aided by the development of effective cardiopulmonary bypass [6,7]. Once the problem of maintaining the circulation to the brain had been solved, interest focused on myocardial protection during open heart surgical procedures. This issue has always reflected a conflict between satisfying the needs of the cardiac surgeon and those of the myocardium. The cardiac surgeon would prefer to operate on a flaccid heart, without time constraints, in a still, bloodless field. Ideal cardiac protection would occur if the beating heart were continuously perfused with oxygenated blood delivered to all areas of the myocardium at normal perfusion pressure. Because these two utopian situations are incompatible, for almost three decades investigators in this field have been seeking an acceptable compromise.

During the past 29 years, four primary approaches to myocardial preservation have been discarded: hyperthermia alone, continuous coronary perfusion, intermittent coronary perfusion, and ischemic cardiac arrest. The reasons why these techniques for myocardial protection are no longer widely employed have recently been reviewed by Hearse et al. [8,9]. At present, most surgical centers utilize cold chemical cardioplegia administered intermittently during open heart procedures. This approach to cardiac protection provides the surgeon with a still, bloodless operative field, a flaccid heart, and several hours of operating time. Simultaneously, in most situations, the myocardial protection afforded by cold chemical cardioplegia is sufficient to prevent clinically important cardiac damage.

Before the discussion of specific aspects of cold chemical cardioplegia, three closely related topics are reviewed briefly below: (1) effects of asystole and ventricular fibrillation on myocardial oxygen consumption and coronary blood flow, (2) effects of hypothermia on the myocardium, and (3) noncoronary collateral blood flow.

EFFECTS OF ASYSTOLE AND VENTRICULAR FIBRILLATION ON CORONARY BLOOD FLOW AND MYOCARDIAL OXYGEN CONSUMPTION

Cardiac asystole can be broadly classified as *systolic* or *diastolic* cardiac arrest. Systolic cardiac arrest occurs when cold chemical cardioplegia is inadequate or when prolonged ischemia associated with severe depletion of high-energy phosphates in the myocardium [10] produces cardiac contracture [10–12a] (Figures 18-1 and 18-2). In its most severe form, cardiac contracture, or the "stone heart syndrome," results in the death of the patient because of irreversible cardiac rigor.

Diastolic cardiac arrest has three desirable characteristics: (1) It eliminates extravascular compressive forces and, hence, decreases coronary vascular resistance (see Chapter 4); (2) it decreases myocardial oxygen consumption by about 75 to 80 percent (see Figure 18-3) [13,14]; and (3) it facilitates complex intracardiac surgical procedures by keeping the heart flaccid.

Myocardial oxygen consumption in a spontaneously fibrillating left ventricle is

FIGURE 18-1
The onset and progression of ischemic contraction in an isolated, beating rat heart. Following the onset of ischemia produced by eliminating coronary flow, effective contraction ceases in a few minutes. Contracture, assessed by measuring an increase in diastolic ventricular pressure, begins about 15 min following the onset of ischemia and is maximal 15 min later. (*From DJ Hearse, PB Garlick, and SM Humphrey* [10].)

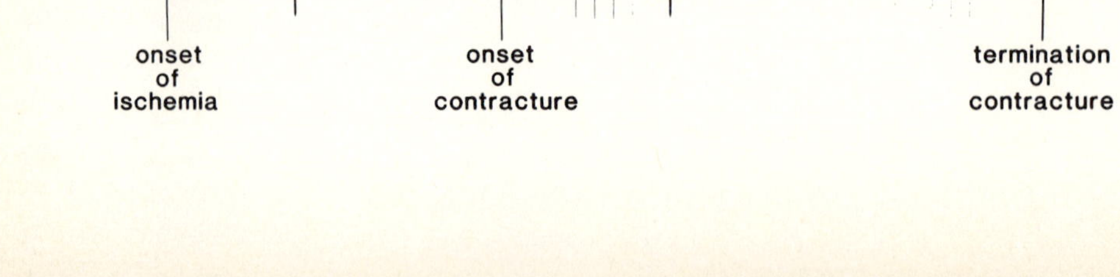

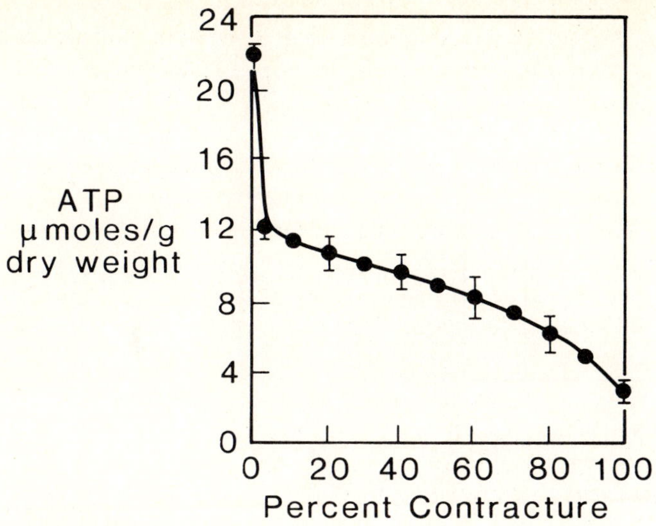

FIGURE 18-2
Relationship between the course of contracture and ATP content in totally ischemic rat hearts. Contracture does not begin until ATP content is reduced by almost 50 percent. When contracture is maximal, ATP content is less than 20 percent of the control level. (*From DJ Hearse, PB Garlick, and SM Humphrey* [*10*].)

FIGURE 18-3
Effects of various conditions on myocardial oxygen consumption. Vagal or potassium (K^+) arrest decreased myocardial oxygen consumption to almost 25 percent of that noted in a working heart (Cont = control). During vagal arrest, changes in intraventricular volume had no effect on myocardial oxygen consumption. During ventricular fibrillation (Vent. Fib.) myocardial oxygen consumption was much greater than that observed in the arrested heart. (*Based on data presented by WP McKeever et al* [*14*].)

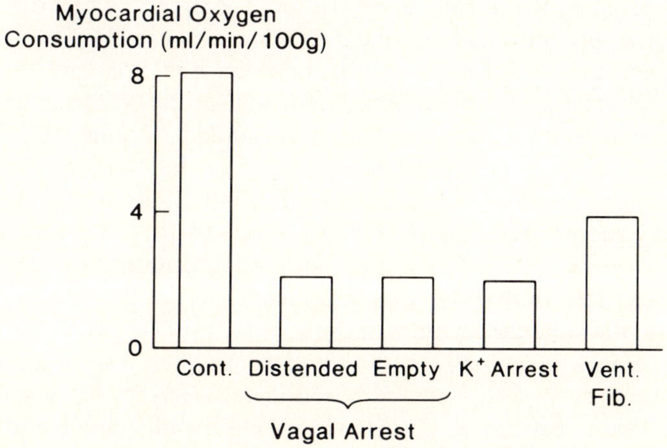

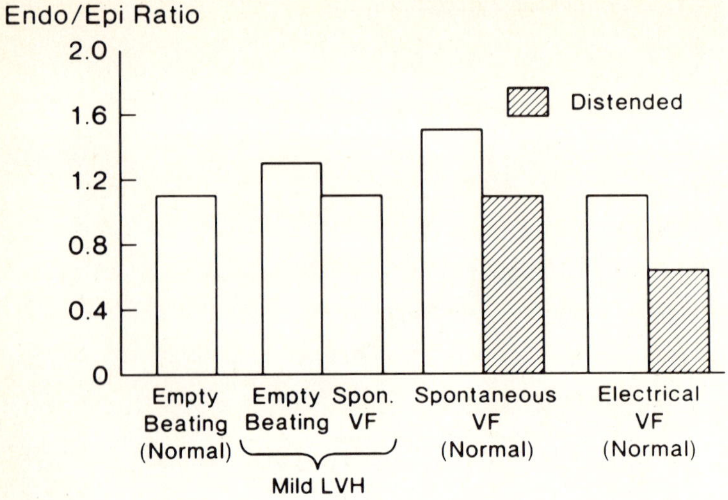

FIGURE 18-4
Effects of various conditions on the transmural distribution (Endo/Epi Ratio-subendocardial/subepicardial ratio) of left ventricular perfusion. In hearts with mild pressure-induced left ventricular hypertrophy (mild LVH) the endo/epi ratio did not increase during spontaneous ventricular fibrillation (VF). In contrast, in normal hearts (Normal) the endo/epi ratio increased during spontaneous ventricular fibrillation. The endo/epi ratio also did not increase during electrically induced ventricular fibrillation. In normal hearts, during either spontaneous or electrically induced ventricular fibrillation, ventricular distenion had an adverse effect on the transmural distribution of left ventricular perfusion. Empty Beating = empty beating heart. (*Based on data presented by CE Hottenrott et al [15–17a]*.)

50 to 70 percent greater than that in an empty beating left ventricle [14–18] (Figure 18-3). Even so, because adverse alterations in the transmural distribution of left ventricular perfusion are not associated with spontaneous ventricular fibrillation (Figure 18-4), it is well tolerated by the normal myocardium if oxygenated blood is provided at normal perfusion pressure and cardiac distention is avoided [15–18]. During spontaneous ventricular fibrillation, severe myocardial ischemia can develop if any of three conditions is present: left ventricular distention, left ventricular hypertrophy, or coronary perfusion pressure less than 50 mmHg. (Figure 18-5) [15–18]. In the latter three conditions, left ventricular subendocardial perfusion is inadequate in the presence of spontaneous ventricular fibrillation (Figure 18-4) and metabolic evidence of ischemia develops (Figure 18-5) [15–18].

When ventricular fibrillation is sustained by application of alternating current (60 cps) to the left ventricle, left ventricular ischemia occurs promptly because blood is diverted away from the subendocardium of the left ventricle (Figures 18-4 and 18-5) [15–18]. Thus, during electrically maintained ventricular fibrillation, myocardial ischemia develops even if oxygenated blood is delivered to the coronary vessels at normal perfusion pressures and the left ventricle is undistended and normal in size.

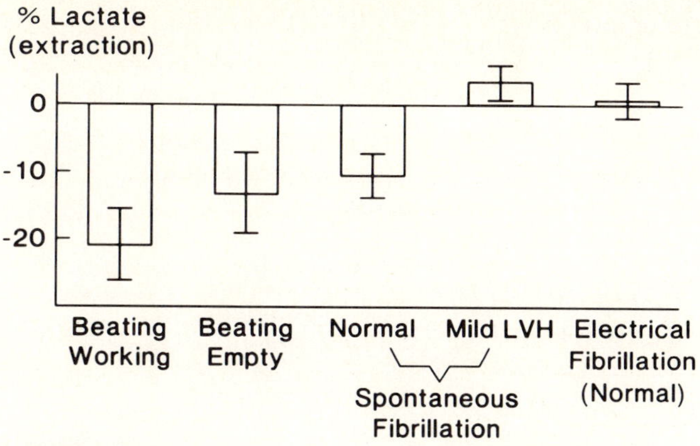

FIGURE 18-5
Effects of various conditions on left ventricular metabolism. Working (beating working), empty (beating empty), and normal hearts (normal), with spontaneous ventricular fibrillation (spontaneous fibrillation) continue to extract lactate normally. Hearts with mild pressure-induced left ventricular hypertrophy (Mild LVH) that developed spontaneous ventricular fibrillation produced lactate. Normal hearts with electrically maintained ventricular fibrillation also produced lactate. Thus, these latter two conditions are associated with metabolic evidence of myocardial ischemia. (*Based on studies presented by CE Hottenrott et al* [*15–17a*].)

Why does ventricular fibrillation impair perfusion to the left ventricular subendocardium? Cardiac relaxation facilitates perfusion of the subendocardium. During ventricular fibrillation, cardiac relaxation is adversely affected because the relaxation phase of the cardiac cycle is uncoordinated.

In addition to promoting myocardial damage, sustained ventricular fibrillation can interfere with the conduct of the surgical procedure. Although the fibrillating ventricles are relatively still, the heart muscle is difficult to manipulate. Hence, complex intracardiac operative procedures are difficult to perform.

In summary, during open heart surgical procedures, ventricular fibrillation has adverse effects on the myocardium and operative conditions. At present ventricular fibrillation is avoided whenever possible during cardiac surgery.

EFFECTS OF HYPOTHERMIA ON THE MYOCARDIUM AND THE CORONARY CIRCULATION

As temperatures decrease, all metabolic processes in the myocardium are depressed, albeit in a heterogenous fashion [19,20]. The marked slowing of phase four of the action potential that occurs with hypothermia causes heart rate to decrease significantly [19–22]. The less impressive decrease in phase two of the cardiac action potential that is associated with decreases in temperature permits additional calcium to enter the myocardial cells [19,20]. As a result, myocardial contractility increases progressively as temperature decreases [19–22]. Because

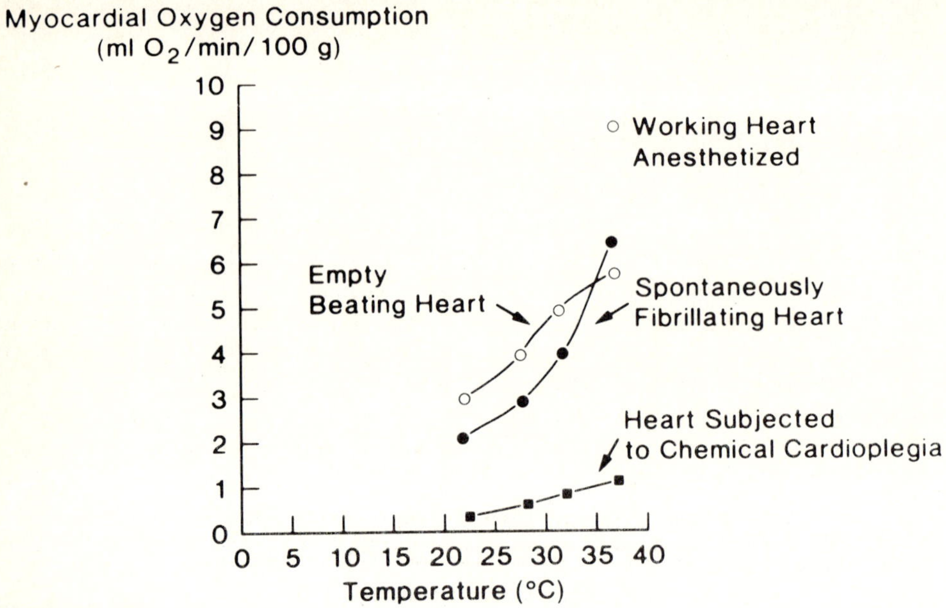

FIGURE 18-6
Effects of hypothermia on myocardial oxygen consumption in various experimental preparations. In all preparations, hypothermia reduced myocardial oxygen consumption considerably. In hearts subjected to cold chemical cardioplegia, at a temperature of 20°C myocardial oxygen consumption is less than 5 percent of control. (*Based on data originally presented by GD Buckberg et al* [23].)

declines in heart rate outstrip increases in myocardial contractility during hypothermia, myocardial oxygen consumption and coronary blood flow decrease significantly as temperature is lowered [21–25] (see Figure 18-6). Hypothermia also significantly decreases myocardial oxygen consumption in the presence of cold chemical cardioplegia [23–25] (Figure 18-6). Hypothermia does not adversely affect the transmural distribution of left ventricular perfusion [23,25].

Hypothermia tends to increase arterial pH [25a]. Although several lines of investigation suggest that increases in pH during hypothermia may have salutary effects on coronary flow and myocardial metabolism [25b], much work remains to be done in this area.

Hypothermia has many other effects on the myocardium, including: decreases in the fluidity of membrane lipids, impaired ionic homeostasis, alterations in the physical properties of water, alterations in the cellular response to drugs and hormones, and alterations in the oxygen affinity of hemoglobin in blood and adverse alterations in clotting mechanisms [19–26a].

Progressively lower temperatures conserve cellular energy. However, with extremely low cardiac temperatures, cellular homeostasis is impaired as a result of ionic redistribution, cellular swelling, and cold-induced injury [19]. Although the myocardial temperature that maximizes the salutary effects of hypothermia and minimizes the adverse effects remains controversial, most available data suggest that myocardial temperatures between 10 and 20°C are probably ideal for myocardial protection during cardiac surgery.

NONCORONARY COLLATERAL BLOOD FLOW

The existence of noncoronary sources of myocardial perfusion has been acknowledged for many decades [27,28]. Noncoronary flow emanates from mediastinal vessels which connect with atrial myocardium at the pericardial reflection. Extracardiac anastomoses to coronary arteries were described in 1932 by Hudson et al. [27]. In 1966 Björk observed that noncoronary vessels could deliver x-ray contrast media to the coronary vasculature [28]. The advent of cardiac surgery permitted certain clinical observations which strongly support the existence of noncoronary collateral channels in patients. When the aorta is cross-clamped and the coronary sinus and left ventricle adequately vented, occasionally arterial blood is observed emanating from the coronary ostia when the aorta is opened to facilitate aortic valve replacement. Furthermore, when single-dose cold chemical cardioplegia is employed, ventricular fibrillation often recurs and myocardial temperature rises with time [30].

In 1975, Brazier et al. [29] quantified the extent of noncoronary collateral flow in dogs and emphasized the importance of such perfusion with regard to myocardial preservation during open heart surgery [29,31,32]. Noncoronary collateral flow contributes to washout of cardioplegic solutions and increases in myocardial temperature. Consequently, when cold chemical cardioplegia is employed during long operative procedures for myocardial preservation, the solution must be administered either continuously or intermittently. Studies with microspheres in dogs indicate that during cardiopulmonary bypass (mean arterial pressure 100 mmHg) with the aorta cross-clamped and the heart arrested in diastole, the left ventricle received between 0.4 and 16 ml/min/100 g of blood via these noncoronary collateral channels [29]. Noncoronary collateral flow was delivered to the atria, right and left ventricles. However, the proportion of total flow delivered to the atria and right ventricle was greater than that observed when coronary flow is delivered via normal channels [29]. Within the left ventricle, the transmural and apex-to-base distribution of noncoronary collateral flow was similar to that observed during normal perfusion [29]. Noncoronary collateral flow was diminished in the beating, working heart (left ventricular perfusion = 0.25 ml/min/100 g) and was nearly zero when perfusion pressure was lowered to 50 mmHg [29]. The highest noncoronary collateral flows (left ventricular perfusion = 12 to 16 ml/min/100 g) were observed in hypertrophied left ventricles during diastolic arrest with an aortic perfusion pressure of 100 mmHg [29]. One clinical study measured noncoronary collateral flow in the contracting left ventricle with aortic pressure 70 to 90 mmHg. Under these conditions with the aorta cross-clamped, coronary sinus effluent varied from 0 to 14.7 ml/min and averaged 2.4 ml/min, or 6 percent of normal left ventricular flow [33].

Although noncoronary collateral flow is of minimal importance to the heart under normal conditions, during cardiopulmonary bypass with cold chemical cardioplegia, the oxygen delivered to the myocardium via these collateral channels could amount to 0.3 ml/min/100 g [34]. This is close to the oxygen requirements of the left ventricle during effective chemical cardioplegia if the myocardial temperature is kept at 20°C [34].

COLD CHEMICAL CARDIOPLEGIA

The standard technique for myocardial preservation employed today during open heart surgery is cold chemical cardioplegia. With this method, myocardial oxygen consumption can be reduced to less than 5 percent of that observed in a normal working heart (see Figure 18-6). In addition, the myocardium is still and flaccid and the operative field is bloodless. Although this general technique of myocardial preservation has gained worldwide acceptance, many specific aspects of the method remain controversial. Improved cardiac preservation will probably not translate to better surgical results in ideal patient subgroups, i.e., adult patients with nonhypertrophied hearts and normal coronary vessels who require relatively short (less than 90 min) cardiac operations. On the other hand, when the patient's condition may compromise the ability of the surgical team to achieve ideal myocardial protection (e.g., infants with complex congenital heart defects; patients with severe cardiac hypertrophy; patients with severe coronary obstructive disease; or long operative procedures, i.e., greater than 2.5 h), improved methods of myocardial protection may substantially improve the long-term results of the operative intervention.

VARIATIONS IN THE MANNER IN WHICH COLD CHEMICAL CARDIOPLEGIA IS EMPLOYED

This section addresses specific aspects of myocardial protection with cold chemical cardioplegia which are currently under intensive investigation.

Components of Cardioplegic Solutions

In 1955, Melrose et al. in England [35] and Lamb et al. in the United States [36] suggested that cold chemical cardioplegia may be of value in cardiac preservation during open heart surgery. Since then, dozens of cardioplegic solutions have been proposed [34].

Cardioplegic solutions are designed to produce rapid, reversible diastolic cardiac arrest and protect the myocardium from ischemic damage during the operative period. Some components of the cardioplegic solutions contribute to both of these goals (i.e., low Ca^{2+}, increased Mg^{2+} and procaine). Other components either promote rapid reversible arrest (i.e., high K^{+}) or limit ischemic damage (pH control, intracellular buffering, high-energy phosphates) [34]. Although there is no consensus on the ideal formulation of cardioplegic solutions, present evidence favors the use of isotonic solutions which contain high K^+ (10 to 40 mm/liter), low or normal Ca^{2+}, and slightly reduced Na^+ concentrations. Inclusion of other components (increased Mg^{2+}, beta blockers, Ca^{2+} blockers, procaine, various substrates, hormones, and osmotic agents) remains controversial [34].

Methods of Administering Cardioplegic Solutions

Cardioplegic solutions can be administered continuously or intermittently by two routes: infusion into the ascending aorta below the aortic cross-clamp or via intracoronary cannulas. In addition, the components of the cardioplegic solution can be added to blood or delivered in an oxygenated asanguinous solution with or without fluorocarbons. If the operative procedure necessitates opening the proximal ascending aorta, i.e., aortic valve replacement, cardioplegia must be achieved by intracoronary administration of the solution.

At present, most surgical centers employ intermittent administration of cardioplegic solutions delivered in an oxygenated asanguinous solution [37].

In patients with severe coronary obstructive disease, the effectiveness of cold chemical cardioplegia may be limited because delivery of the solution to the myocardium is impaired. One possible way of resolving this problem is to administer cardioplegic solutions both anterograde via the ascending aorta and retrograde via the coronary sinus. This approach deserves investigation.

Methods of Achieving Cardiac Hypothermia

The temperature of the myocardium can be reduced in four ways during open heart surgery: cooling the cardioplegic solution prior to infusion; topical hypothermia (i.e., ice slush surrounding the heart); intracavitary administration of cold solutions; and systemic hypothermia achieved by cooling the blood delivered to the systemic circulation through the cardiopulmonary bypass machine. Although intracavitary administration of cold solutions has been discarded, the remaining three approaches are often used simultaneously to achieve and maintain adequate cardiac hypothermia during open heart surgical procedures.

EFFECTS OF COLD CHEMICAL CARDIOPLEGIA ON THE MYOCARDIUM AND THE CORONARY CIRCULATION

To accomplish ideal myocardial protection, diastolic cardiac arrest and cardiac hypothermia should be achieved promptly (less than 1 min) following administration of the cold cardioplegic solution. Hypothermic diastolic arrest should be completely maintained in all areas of the myocardium throughout the operative procedure and quickly reversed (less than 1 min) following restoration of coronary perfusion. Delayed induction, inadequate maintenance, or lengthy reversal of cold chemical cardioplegia will consume myocardial energy stores and lead to myocardial damage.

Following the reversal of cardioplegia, the status of the myocardium depends upon the preoperative condition of the heart, the positive or negative consequences of the operative procedure (aortic valve replacement, intraoperative myocardial infarction), and the effectiveness of myocardial protection during the operation. At present, severe cardiac damage rarely occurs as a result of totally inadequate myocardial protection during a cardiac surgical procedure. However, some adverse effects on the myocardium which can be detected by sophisticated diagnostic procedures still occur in many patients who undergo open heart surgery [38].

Several investigators have suggested that some of the cardiac damage that occurs as a consequence of inadequate cardiac protection may be attributed to reperfusion injury [34]. They suspect that abrupt reperfusion of the heart with systemic blood following a sustained period of cold chemical cardioplegia may injure the myocardium. One suggested mechanism for this effect is the phenomenon of calcium paradox [34]. In vitro studies have shown that if hearts are perfused with a calcium-free crystaloid solution, reperfusion with a calcium-containing medium can result in the sudden induction of massive tissue injury characterized by contracture, severe ultrastructural damage, cell swelling, and enzyme leakage (calcium paradox). Calcium paradox occurs only if the cardioplegic solution is absolutely calcium-free. Although some cardioplegic solutions contain very low concentrations of calcium, very few in current use are truly calcium-free. The possibility of calcium paradox can be minimized by employing adequate hypothermia, avoiding alkalosis and ischemia, and having appropriate concentrations of sodium and magnesium in the cardioplegic solutions. In addition, some surgeons perfuse the ascending aorta with a specially modified blood solution to reverse the effects of cardioplegic solutions before perfusion the circulation with blood.

Reperfusion injury is most effectively prevented by adequate myocardial protection during the period of cardioplegia with a solution which is not totally free of calcium.

Little information is available on the effects of cardioplegia on the coronary circulation. Studies by Hiratzka et al. [39] indicate that when normal dogs are subjected to 1 h of cold chemical cardioplegia in the immediate postperfusion period the coronary vessels are slightly dilated but myocardial oxygen consumption, the transmural distribution of left ventricular perfusion, and minimal coronary vascular resistance are near normal. Coronary reactive hyperemic responses are decreased in the immediate postoperative period because resting coronary flow is modestly elevated and arterial pressure is lower than that prior to cardiopulmonary bypass.

In summary, cardiopulmonary bypass coupled with cold chemical cardioplegia has many effects on the myocardium and the coronary vasculature. These effects have a major influence on the outcome of the surgical procedure and on the results of the studies of the myocardium and coronary vasculature in the immediate postoperative period.

REFERENCES

1 Lewis FJ, Taufic M: Closure of atrial septal defects with the aid of hypothermia: Experimental accomplishments and the report of one successful case. *Surgery* 33: 52, 1953.

2 Lillehei CW, Cohen M, Warden HE, Varco RL: The direct-vision intracardiac correction of congenital anomalies by controlled cross-circulation. *Surgery* 38: 11, 1955.

3 Kirklin JW, DuShane JW, Patrick RT, Donald DE, Hetzel PS, Harshbarger HG, Wood EH: Intercardiac surgery with the aid of a mechanical pump oxygenator system (Gibbon-type). Report of 8 cases. *Proc Mayo Clin* 30: 201, 1955.

4 Kirklin JW, Donald DE, Harshbarger HG, Hetzel PS, Patrick RT, Swan HJC, Wood EH: Studies in extracorporeal circulation. 1. Applicability of Gibbon-type oxygenator to human intracardiac surgery: 40 cases. *Ann Surg* 144: 2, 1956.

5 Cooley DA, Belmonte BA, DeBakey ME, Latson JR: Temporary extracorporeal circulation in the surgical treatment of cardiac and aortic disease: Report of 98 cases. *Ann Surg* 145: 898, 1957.

6 Gibbon JH Jr: Application of mechanical heart and lung apparatus to cardiac surgery. *Minn Med* 37: 171, 1954.

7 Kirklin JW, Conti VR, Blackstone EH: Prevention of myocardial damage during cardiac operations. *N Engl J Med* 301: 135, 1979.

8 Hearse DJ, Braimbridge MV, Jynge P: Historical review, in *Protection of the Ischemic Myocardium: Cardioplegia.* New York, Raven Press, 1981, chap 1, p 3.

9 Hearse DJ, Braimbridge MV, Jynge P: Comparison of methods, in *Protection of the Ischemic Myocardium: Cardioplegia.* New York, Raven Press, 1981, chap 4, p 95.

10 Hearse DJ, Garlick PB, Humphrey SM: Ischemic contracture of the myocardium: Mechanisms and prevention. *Am J Cardiol* 39: 986, 1977.

11 Cooley DA, Reul GJ, Wukasch DC: Ischemic contracture of the heart: "Stone heart." *Am J Cardiol* 29: 575, 1972.

12 Katz AM, Tada M: The "stone heart": A challenge to the biochemist. *Am J Cardiol* 29: 578, 1972.

12a Katz AM, Tada M: The "stone heart" and other challenges to the biochemist. *Am J Cardiol* 39: 1073, 1977.

13 Sabiston DC, Gregg DE: Coronary arterial inflow, coronary sinus drainage and myocardial oxygen consumption in asystole and ventricular fibrillation. *Fed Proc* 14: 127, 1955.

14 McKeever WP, Gregg DE, Canney PC: Oxygen uptake of the non-working left ventricle. *Circ Res* 6: 612, 1958.

15 Hottenrott CE, Maloney JV, Buckberg G: Studies of the effects of ventricular fibrillation on the adequacy of regional myocardial flow. I. Electrical vs. spontaneous fibrillation. *J Thorac Cardiovasc Surg* 68: 615, 1974.

16 Hottenrott C, Buckberg G: Studies on the effects of ventricular fibrillation on the adequacy of regional myocardial flow. II. Effects of ventricular distention. *J Thorac Cardiovasc Surg* 68: 626, 1974.

17 Hottenrott C, Maloney JV, Buckberg G: Studies of effects of ventricular fibrillation on the adequacy of regional myocardial flow. III. Mechanisms of ischemia. *J Thorac Cardiovasc Surg* 68: 634, 1974.

17a Hottenrott CE, Towers B, Kurkji HJ, Maloney JV, Buckberg G: The hazard of ventricular fibrillation in hypertrophied ventricles during cardiopulmonary bypass. *J Thorac Cardiovasc Surg* 66: 742, 1973.

18 Buckberg GD, Hottenrott CE: Ventricular fibrillation: Its effect on myocardial flow, distribution and performance. *Ann Thorac Surg* 20: 76, 1975.

19 Hearse DJ, Braimbridge MV: *Protection of the Ischemic Myocardium: Cardioplegia.* New York, Raven Press, 1981, p 167.

20 Coraboeuf E, Weidmann S: Temperature effects on the electrical activity of Purkinje fibres. *Helv Physiol Acta* 12: 32, 1954.

21 Archie JP, Kirklin JW: Effect of hypothermic perfusion on myocardial oxygen consumption and coronary resistance. *Surg Forum* 24: 186.

22 Monroe RG, Strang RH, La Farge CG, Levy J: Ventricular performance, pressure-volume relationships, and O_2-consumption during hypothermia. *Am J Physiol* 206: 67, 1964.

23 Buckberg GD, Brazier JR, Nelson RH, Goldstein SM, McConnell DH, Cooper N: Studies on the effects of hypothermia on regional myocardial blood flow and metabolism during cardiopulmonary bypass. I. The adequately perfused beating, fibrillating, and arrested heart. *J Thorac Cardiovasc Surg* 73: 87, 1977.

24 Greenberg JJ, Edmunds H Jr, Brown RB: Myocardial metabolism and postarrest function in the cold and chemically arrested heart *Surgery* 48: 31, 1960.

25 Chitwood WR, Sink JD, Hill RC, Wechsler AS, Sabiston DC: The effects of hypothermia on myocardial oxygen consumption and transmural coronary blood flow in the potassium-arrested heart. *Ann Surg* 190: 106, 1979.

25a White FN: A comparative physiological approach to hypothermia. *Thorac Cardiovasc Surg* 82: 821, 1981.

25b MConnell DH, White FN, Nelson RL, Goldstein SM, Mahoney JV, DeLand EC, Buckberg GD: Importance of "alkalosis" in maintenance of ideal blood pH during hypothermia. *Surg Forum* 26: 263, 1975.

26 Swan H: Clinical hypothermia: A lady with a past and some promise for the future. *Surgery* 73: 736, 1973.

26a Swan H: *Thermoregulation and Bioenergetics.* New York, American Elsevier, 1974.

27 Hudson CL, Moritz AR, Wearn JR: The extracardiac anastomoses of the coronary arteries. *Soc Exp Med* 56: 919, 1932.

28 Björk L: Angiographic demonstration of extracardial anastomoses to the coronary arteries. *Radiology* 87: 274, 1966.

29 Brazier JR, Hottenrott C, Buckberg GD: Non-coronary collateral myocardial blood flow. *Ann Thorac Surg* 19: 426, 1975.

30 Schaper W, Schaper J, Palmowski J, et al: Ischemia tolerance following cardioplegic arrest in human patients and in experimental animals. *J Cardiovasc Surg* (Torino) 16: 268, 1975.

31 Buckberg GD: Left ventricular subendocardial necrosis. *Ann Thorac Surg* 24: 379, 1977.

32 Buckberg GD: A proposed "solution" to the cardioplegic controversy. *J Thorac Cardiovasc Surg* 77: 803, 1979.

33 Hetzer R, Warnecke H, Wittrock H, Engel HJ, Borst HG: Extracoronary collateral myocardial blood flow during cardioplegic arrest. *Thorac Cardiovasc Surg* 28: 191, 1980.

34 Hearse DJ, Braimbridge MV, Jynge P: Components of cardioplegic solutions, in *Protection of the Ischemic Myocardium: Cardioplegia.* New York, Raven Press, 1981, p 209.

35 Melrose DG, Dreyer B, Bentall HH, Baker JBE: Elective cardiac arrest. *Lancet* 2: 21, 1955.

36 Lamb CR, Geoghegan T, Lepore A: Induced cardiac arrest for intracardiac surgical procedures. *J Thorac Surg* 30: 620, 1955.
37 Hearse DJ, Braimbridge MV, Jynge P: Principles of formulation and administration, in *Protection of the Ischemic Myocardium: Cardioplegia.* New York, Raven Press, 1981, p 300.
38 Hearse DJ, Braimbridge MV, Jynge P: Methods of assessment and results of cardiac surgery using cardioplegia, in *Protection of the Ischemic Myocardium: Cardioplegia.* New York, Raven Press, 1981, p 375.
39 Hiratzka L, Eastham C, Carter J, Moyers J, Elliot D, Wright C, Doty D, Marcus M: Coronary dilation after cardiopulmonary bypass. *Am J Cardiol* 49: 969, 1982.

CHAPTER **19**

INTRAAORTIC BALLOON COUNTERPULSATION

One approach to increasing coronary perfusion in a failing, ischemic heart is to augment selectively arterial diastolic pressure with an external force. This idea was originally put forth by Kantrowitz and Kantrowitz in 1953 [1]. Subsequently, Clauss et al. [2] in 1962 suggested that in addition to diastolic augmentation of arterial pressure, reducing systolic pressure might further improve the status of ischemic myocardium. In the following year, Moulopoulos et al. [3] demonstrated that cyclical reductions in systolic arterial pressure and augmentation of diastolic pressure could be produced with ECG synchronized inflation and deflation of an intraaortic balloon with carbon dioxide. Such a device was first utilized in patients by Kantrowitz et al. [4] in 1967. In 1969, Kantrowitz et al. reported that intraaortic balloon pumping favorably affected the course of 27 patients in cardiogenic shock. Since then, thousands of patients have been treated with intraaortic balloon counterpulsation. Although some of the recently proposed indications for balloon counterpulsation remain controversial (limitation of infarct size [6], unstable or preinfarction angina [7–10], poor left ventricular function [11], and various prophylactic applications [12,13]), several indications for this form of therapy are well established (major complications of acute myocardial infarction such as cardiogenic shock, acute ventricular septal defect, and acute mitral regurgitation [13–17], or inability to come off cardiopulmonary bypass [18,19]). The salutary effects of balloon counterpulsation occur because this intervention improves both systemic and coronary hemodynamics [19a].

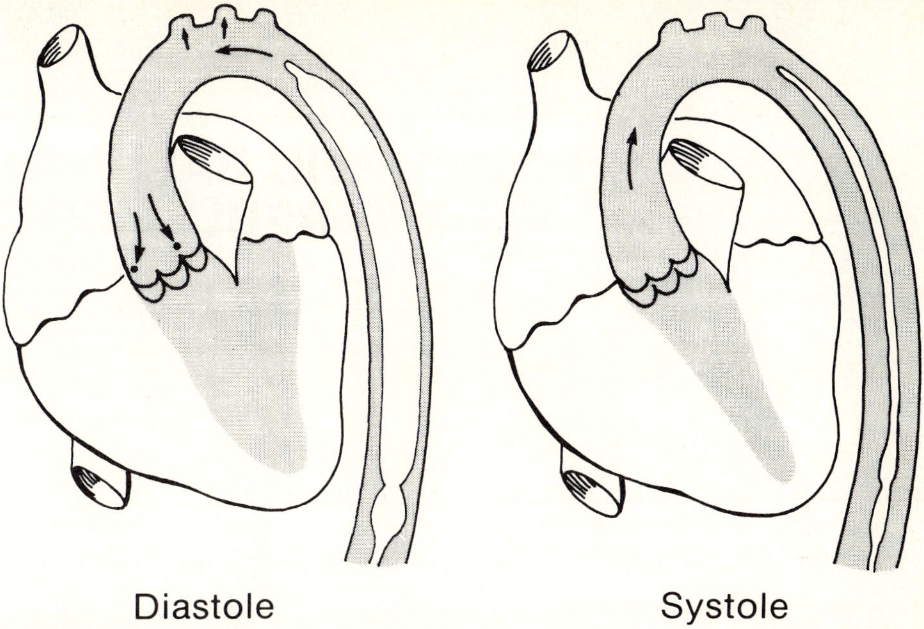

FIGURE 19-1
(*Left*) Diagrammatic illustration of aortic balloon counterpulsation. During diastole, the intraaortic balloon is expanded to increase diastolic pressure. (*Right*) During systole, the intraaortic balloon is collapsed to decrease aortic systolic pressure.

EFFECTS OF INTRAAORTIC BALLOON COUNTERPULSATION ON SYSTEMIC HEMODYNAMICS

Counterpulsation is accomplished by expanding a balloon placed in the descending aorta during systole and rapidly collapsing it during diastole (see Figure 19-1). The hemodynamic effects of this mechanical procedure depend on several physical characteristics of the device: size, shape, and position of the balloon in the aorta; the percent aortic occlusion achieved during balloon inflation; and the rapidity of inflation and deflation [20,20a]. In addition, several important biological variables modulate the effects of balloon counterpulsation. These biological variables include: heart rate, cardiac rhythm, and the pressure-volume relationship in the aorta [20,20a]. Finally, certain pathological conditions (e.g., acute mitral regurgitation or an acute ventricular septal defect) are more responsive to intraaortic balloon counterpulsation than are others (e.g., severe pump failure unrelated to myocardial ischemia) [13]. Because many factors influence the hemodynamic effects that can be achieved with balloon counterpulsation, the clinical response to this procedure is quite variable.

The largest group of patients that have been treated with balloon counterpulsation are those with cardiogenic shock (systolic pressure less than 80 mmHg; peripheral signs of intense vasoconstriction) secondary to acute myocardial infarction. In this patient group, balloon counterpulsation decreases systolic pressure about 20 percent and increases diastolic arterial pressure about 30 percent (Figure

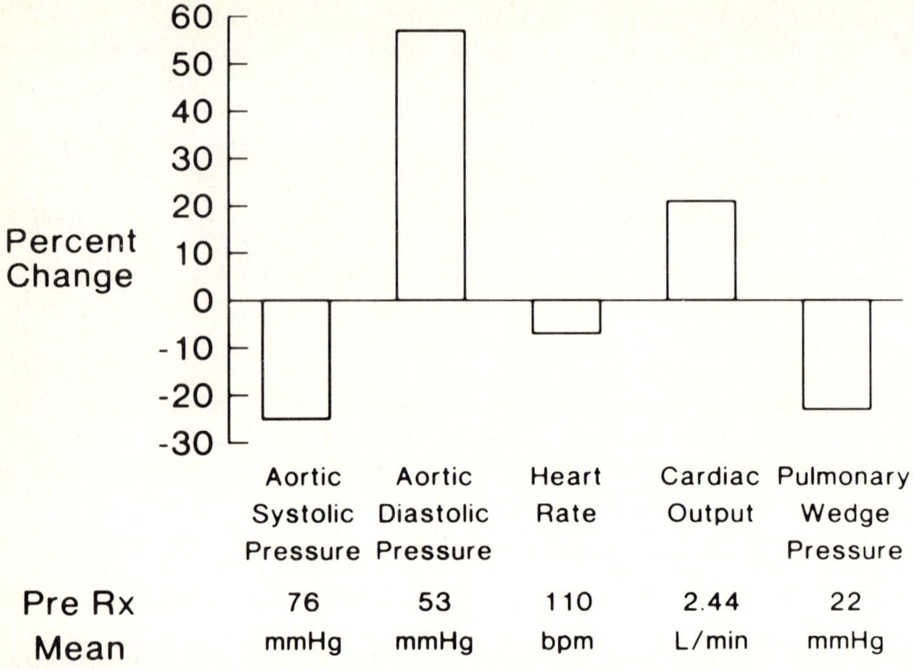

FIGURE 19-2
Effects of aortic balloon counterpulsation on systemic hemodynamics in patients with cardiogenic shock. Instituting aortic balloon counterpulsation in this patient group produced a modest decrease in aortic systolic pressure, a marked increase in aortic diastolic pressure, a minimal change in heart rate, a modest increase in cardiac output, and a modest decrease in pulmonary wedge pressure. Thus, aortic balloon counterpulsation in this patient group clearly caused a net substantial improvement in systemic hemodynamics. PreRx = value for each parameter prior to starting aortic balloon counterpulsation. (*Based on data reported by S Scheidt et al* [*16*].)

19-2) [16]. Heart rate decreases by less than 10 percent [16], cardiac output increases by 21 percent [16], and mean pulmonary capillary wedge pressure decreases by 23 percent [14] (Figure 19-2). In association with these improved hemodynamics, perfusion to the periphery improves and urine output increases significantly. Thus, balloon counterpulsation improves systemic hemodynamics in patients with cardiogenic shock secondary to acute myocardial infarction. Furthermore, the net effects of these hemodynamic alterations would tend to decrease myocardial oxygen consumption.

EFFECTS OF INTRAAORTIC BALLOON COUNTERPULSATION ON MYOCARDIAL PERFUSION

Animal Studies

Most information concerning the effects of balloon counterpulsation on myocardial perfusion is based on animal studies. Unfortunately, none of the animal studies reported has used an appropriate model, i.e., an awake preparation with acute myocardial infarction, cardiogenic shock, multivessel coronary obstructions, and variable coronary collateral channels. The animal studies reported have been performed in anesthetized preparations following occlusion of one coronary vessel perfusing a relatively small area of myocardium. The unoccluded coronary vessels were free of disease. Furthermore, in these experimental studies coronary occlusion was not associated with the development of cardiogenic shock or severe left ventricular failure. In view of the major differences between these animal preparations and patients treated with intraaortic balloon counterpulsation, one must be very cautious about extending the results of these animal studies to clinically relevant situations.

Most animal studies have reported that intraaortic balloon counterpulsation has little effect on perfusion to myocardial segments served by occluded or severely obstructed coronary vessels (Figure 19-3) [21–25]. In the few studies that have reported that intraaortic balloon counterpulsation increased perfusion to ischemic myocardium [26,27] the magnitude of the increase in flow was probably of minimal functional significance. For example, in the study reported by Gill et al. [27] intraaortic balloon counterpulsation increased perfusion to the ischemic zone from 11 to 16 ml/min/100 g. Both of these flows were less than 20 percent of the perfusion to adjacent normal myocardium (Figure 19-3) [27]. Why did intraaortic balloon counterpulsation have such a feeble effect on the perfusion of the ischemic myocardium in these experimental studies? First, resistance through native collateral vessels in the dog is extremely high (see Chapter 10). Second, the

FIGURE 19-3
Effects of aortic balloon counterpulsation on myocardial perfusion in open chest dogs subjected to acute coronary occlusion. In this animal model, aortic balloon counterpulsation had a minimal effect on flow to normally perfused or severely ischemic areas of the myocardium. (*Based on data reported by CC Gill et al* [27].)

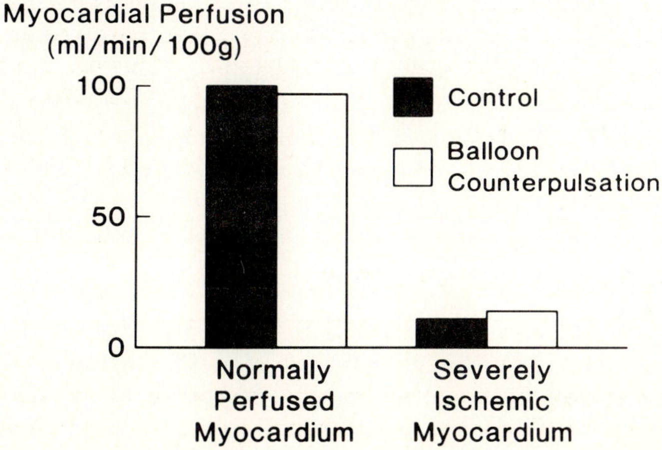

increase in coronary driving pressure achieved in these experimental studies was usually small (less than 10 mmHg) compared to what has been reported in clinical studies (Figure 19-2).

Animal studies have also reported that intraaortic balloon counterpulsation has very little effect on perfusion to normal myocardium (Figure 19-3) [21,27]. Typically, during intraaortic balloon counterpulsation perfusion to normal myocardium was unchanged or decreased by less than 10 percent [21,27]. This occurs because in the absence of cardiogenic shock or severe left ventricular failure intraaortic balloon counterpulsation has minimal effects on the major determinants of myocardial oxygen consumption, left ventricular wall stress, myocardial contractility, and heart rate. If intraaortic balloon counterpulsation does not alter myocardial oxygen consumption, one would not expect coronary blood flow to change significantly (Chapter 3). Even if balloon counterpulsation increased diastolic perfusion pressure substantially, this would not increase coronary flow because autoregulation is very effective in a normal coronary bed (Chapter 4). Increases in diastolic perfusion pressure secondary to intraaortic balloon counterpulsation could affect coronary vascular resistance by passively distending coronary vessels. Recent studies by Schwartz et al. [27a] suggest that this effect produces a minimal decrease in coronary vascular resistance.

Although these experimental studies indicate that intraaortic balloon counterpulsation has minimal effects on the perfusion of ischemic or normal myocardium, because the experimental preparations employed do not simulate the clinical situation (see above) the relevance of these observations to patient care is severely limited.

Patient Studies

Four groups of investigators have assessed the effects of intraaortic balloon counterpulsation on some aspect of coronary flow or myocardial metabolism. Mueller et al. [28] demonstrated that, following institution of intraaortic balloon counterpulsation in patients with cardiogenic shock secondary to acute myocardial infarction, mean arterial pressure and coronary sinus flow increased significantly (Figure 19-4). The increase in coronary flow was associated with a decrease in oxygen extraction by the myocardium (Figure 19-5). In addition, measurements of coronary sinus and arterial lactate levels indicated that prior to the onset of intraaortic balloon counterpulsation the myocardium produced lactate; following intraaortic balloon counterpulsation the myocardium extracted lactate (Figure 19-5). Scheidt et al. [16] noted that coronary sinus lactate in patients with cardiogenic shock secondary to acute myocardial infarction decreased substantially during intraaortic balloon counterpulsation. Calculated lactate extraction improved in 18 of 19 patients. Bregman et al. [29] noted that during intraaortic balloon counterpulsation blood flow in a vein bypass graft at cardiac surgery increased substantially (Figure 19-6). Recently, Whittle et al. [30] reported that during intraaortic balloon counterpulsation coronary blood flow (coronary sinus thermal dilution technique) in the ischemic zone increased from 50 to 61 ml/min, whereas flow in the nonischemic region was unchanged (96 vs. 92 ml/min).

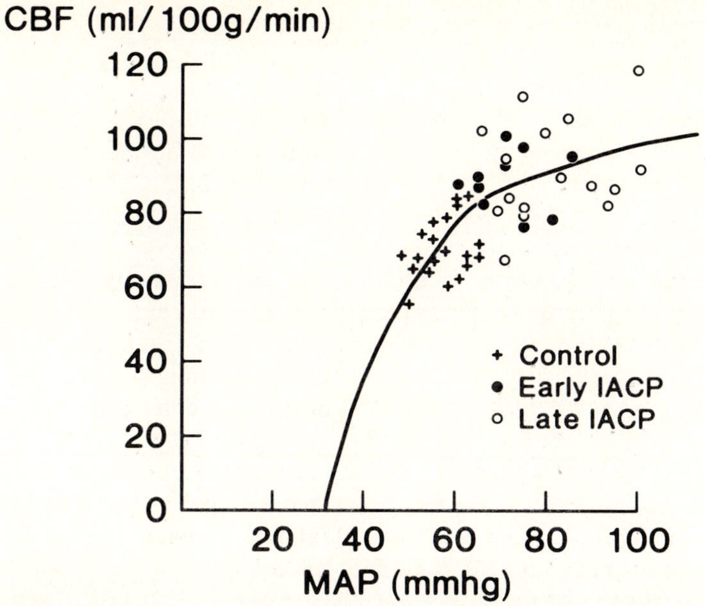

FIGURE 19-4
Effects of intraaortic balloon counterpulsation (IACP) on coronary blood flow (CBF) and mean arterial pressure (MAP) in patients with cardiogenic shock secondary to acute myocardial infarction. Following institution of intraaortic balloon counterpulsation, mean aortic pressure and coronary blood flow increased substantially. Each symbol represents data obtained from one patient in the designated subgroup. Control = data obtained prior to intraaortic counterpulsation. Early IACP = data obtained 4 to 6 h following institution of intraaortic balloon counterpulsation. Late IACP = data obtained 12 to 72 h following institution of intraaortic balloon counterpulsation. (*Modified from an illustration originally presented by H Mueller et al* [28].)

Although these clinical studies have significant technical limitations (Chapter 2) and may not be quantitatively precise, *it is reasonable to conclude that in patients with cardiogenic shock secondary to acute myocardial infarction intraaortic balloon counterpulsation improves coronary perfusion and metabolism in ischemic myocardium.*

EFFECTS OF INTRAAORTIC BALLOON COUNTERPULSATION ON VARIOUS MANIFESTATIONS OF MYOCARDIAL ISCHEMIA

Animal Studies

The effects of intraaortic balloon counterpulsation on regional wall motion and the extent of this ST segment elevation in ischemic regions have been reported. When regional wall motion was assessed with either an echocardiographic technique [21] or with sonomicrometers [31] intraaortic balloon counterpulsation did not favorably alter the contractile function of acutely ischemic myocardium.

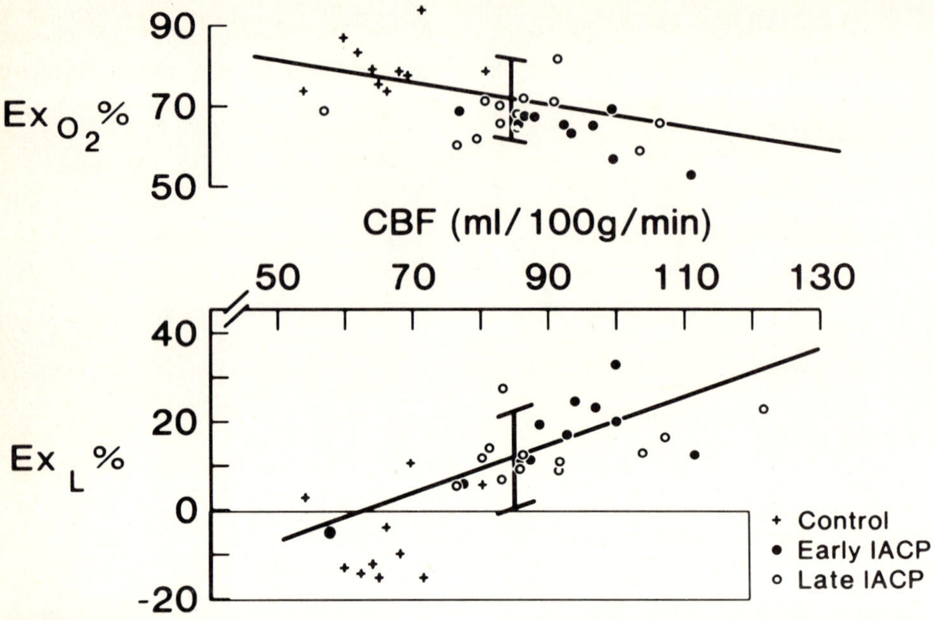

FIGURE 19-5
Effects of intraaortic balloon counterpulsation (IACP) on oxygen extraction across the coronary bed (Ex_{O_2}, lactate extraction by the myocardium (Ex_L), and coronary blood flow (CBF) in patients with cardiac shock secondary to acute myocardial infarction. Following institution of intraaortic balloon counterpulsation, oxygen extraction decreased and lactate metabolism changed from production (negative lactate extraction) to lactate uptake by the myocardium (positive lactate extraction). Thus, intraaortic counterpulsation in this patient subgroup improved myocardial metabolism. Control = data obtained prior to institution of intraaortic balloon counterpulsation. Early IACP = data obtained 4 to 6 h following institution of intraaortic balloon counterpulsation. Late IACP = data obtained 12 to 72 h following institution of intraaortic balloon counterpulsation. (*Modified from an illustration originally presented by H Mueller et al* [28].)

One study, which assessed wall motion abnormalities with contrast ventriculography, reported that intraaortic balloon counterpulsation significantly improved wall motion in the ischemic zone [30]. Several investigators have reported that intraaortic balloon counterpulsation decreased the extent of epicardial ST segment elevation in an ischemic area of the myocardium [32]. One study indicates that intraaortic balloon counterpulsation may decrease infarct size [32].

Although these experimental studies suggest that intraaortic balloon counterpulsation decreases ST segment elevation, limits infarct size, and occasionally improves segmental ventricular function in ischemic myocardium, studies in more clinically relevant animal preparations are obviously needed.

Patient Studies

The effects of intraaortic balloon counterpulsation on ST segment abnormalities have been assessed in patients with acute infarction or preinfarction angina [6,7].

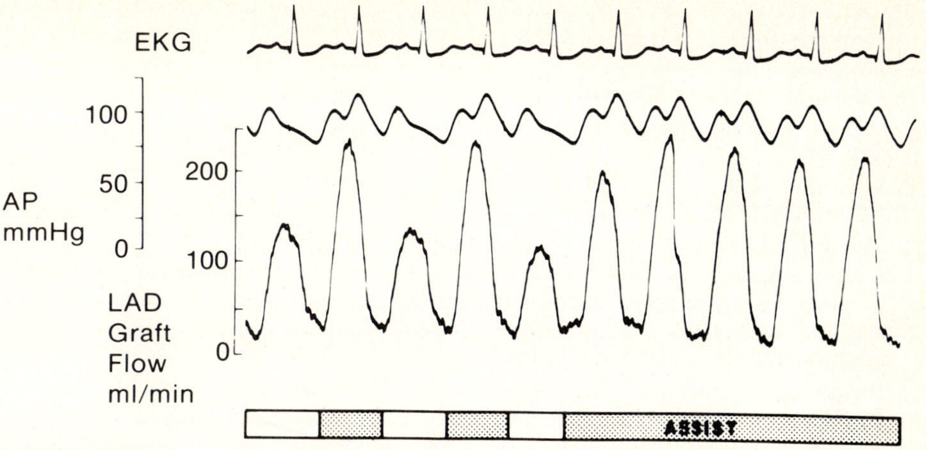

FIGURE 19-6
Effects of intraaortic balloon counterpulsation (ASSIST) on arterial pressure (AP) and graft flow in a saphenous vein bypass graft in the left anterior descending coronary artery (LAD). These studies were obtained in the operating room following cardiopulmonary bypass and placement of the bypass graft. Intraaortic balloon counterpulsation (ASSIST) increased diastolic arterial pressure and strikingly increased graft flow. (*Modified from an illustration originally presented by D Bregman et al* [29].)

Usually, ST segment abnormalities improve or disappear when intraaortic balloon counterpulsation is instituted in patients with severe myocardial ischemia or acute myocardial infarction. One study involving 11 patients suggested that intraaortic balloon counterpulsation decreased infarct size if the coronary vessel supplying the ischemic region was not totally occluded [6]. This provocative observation warrants further investigation.

In summary, although intraaortic balloon counterpulsation can significantly alter myocardial perfusion and metabolism, the efficacy of this intervention is very dependent on many factors (presence of severe heart failure, cardiogenic shock, coronary occlusion, etc.) which vary considerably from patient to patient.

REFERENCES

1 Kantrowitz A, Kantrowitz A: Experimental augmentation of coronary flow by retardation of arterial pressure pulse. *Surgery* 34: 678, 1953.

2 Clauss RH, Birtwell WC, Albertal G, Lunzer S, Taylor WJ, Fosberg AM, Harken DE: Assisted circulation. I. The arterial counterpulsator. *J Thorac Cardiovasc Surg* 41: 447, 1961.

3 Moulopoulos SD, Topaz S, Kolff WJ: Diastolic balloon pumping (with carbon dioxide) in the aorta—a mechanical assistance to the failing circulation. *Am Heart J* 63: 669, 1962.

4 Kantrowitz A, Tjønneland S, Freed PS, Phillips SJ, Butner AN, Sherman JL Jr: Initial clinical experience with intraaortic balloon pumping in cardiogenic shock. *JAMA* 203: 135, 1968.

5 Kantrowitz A, Krakauer JS, Rosenbaum A, et al: Phase-shift balloon pumping in medically refractory cardiogenic shock. Results in 27 patients. *Arch Surg* 99: 739, 1969.

6 Leinback RC, Gold HK, Harper RW, Buckley MJ, Austen WG: Early intraaortic balloon pumping for anterior myocardial infarction without shock. *Circulation* 58: 204, 1978.

7 Weintraub RM, Voukydis PC, Aroesty JM, Cohen SI, Ford P, Kurland GS, LaRaia PJ, Morkin E, Paulin S: Treatment of preinfarction angina with intraaortic balloon counterpulsation and surgery. *Am J Cardiol* 34: 809, 1974.

8 Langou RA, Geha AS, Hammond GL, Cohen LS: Surgical approach for patients with unstable angina pectoris: Role of the response to initial medical therapy and intraaortic balloon pumping in perioperative complications after aortocoronary bypass grafting. *Am J Cardiol* 42: 629, 1978.

9 Weintraub RM, Aroesty JM, Paulin S, Levine FH, Markis JE, LaRaia PJ, Cohen SI, Kurland GF: Medically refractory unstable angina pectoris. I. Long-term follow-up of patients undergoing intraaortic balloon counterpulsation and operation. *Am J Cardiol* 43: 877, 1979.

10 Aroesty JM, Weintraub RM, Paulin S, O'Grady GP: Medically refractory unstable angina pectoris. II. Hemodynamic and angiographic effects of intraaortic balloon counterpulsation. *Am J Cardiol* 43: 883, 1979.

11 Feola M, Wiener L, Walinsky P, Kasparian H, Duca P, Gottlieb R, Brest A, Templeton J: Improved survival after coronary bypass surgery in patients with poor left ventricular function: Role of intraaortic balloon counterpulsation. *Am J Cardiol* 39: 1021, 1977.

12 Rajai HR, Hartman CW, Innes BJ, Bartel AG, Brickman RD, Crisler C, Grinnan GLB: Prophylactic use of intra-aortic balloon pump in aortocoronary bypass for patients with left main coronary artery disease. *Ann Surg* 187: 118, 1978.

13 McEnany MT, Kay HR, Buckley MJ, Daggett WM, Erdmann AJ, Mundth ED, Rao RS, deToeuf J, Austen WG: Clinical experience with intraaortic balloon pump support in 728 patients. *Circulation* 58: 124, 1978.

14 Dunkman WB, Leinbach RC, Buckley MJ, Mundth ED, Kantrowitz AR, Austen WG, Sanders CA: Clinical and hemodynamic results of intraaortic balloon pumping and surgery for cardiogenic shock. *Circulation* 46: 465, 1972.

15 Gold HK, Leinbach RC, Sanders CA, Buckley MJ, Mundth ED, Austen WG: Intraaortic balloon pumping for ventricular septal defect or mitral regurgitation complicating acute myocardial infarction. *Circulation* 47: 1191, 1973.

16 Scheidt S, Wilner G, Mueller H, Summers D, Lesch M, Wolff G, Krakauer J, Rubenfire M, Fleming P, Noon G, Oldham N, Killip T, Kantrowitz A: Intra-aortic balloon counterpulsation in cardiogenic shock. *N Engl J Med* 288: 979, 1973.

17 Willerson JT, Curry GC, Watson JT, Leshin SJ, Ecker RR, Mullins CB, Platt MR, Sugg WL: Intraaortic balloon counterpulsation in patients in cardiogenic shock, medically refractory left ventricular failure and/or recurrent ventricular tachycardia. *Am J Med* 58: 183, 1975.

18 Buckley MJ, Craver JM, Gold HK, Mundth ED, Daggett WM, Austen WG: Intraaortic balloon pump assist for cardiogenic shock after cardiopulmonary bypass. *Circulation* 47 & 48: 90, 1973.

19 Scanlon PJ, O'Connell J, Johnson SA, Moran JM, Gunnar R, Pifarre R: Balloon counterpulsation following surgery for ischemic heart disease. *Circulation* 54: 90, 1976.

19a Scheidt S, Collins M, Goldstein J, Fisher J: Mechanical circulatory assistance with the intraaortic balloon pump and other counterpulsation-devices. *Prog Cardiovasc Dis* 25: 55, 1982.

20 Weber KT, Janicki JS: Intraaortic balloon counterpulsation. *Ann Thorac Surg* 17: 602, 1974.

20a Bolooki H (ed): Clinical Application of Intra-aortic Balloon Pump, Mount Kisco, New York, Futura, 1977.

21 Kerber RE, Marcus ML, Ehrhardt J, Abboud FM: Effect of intra-aortic balloon counterpulsation on the motion and perfusion of acutely ischemic myocardium. *Circulation* 53: 853, 1976.

22 Reneman RS, Jageneau AHM, Schaper WKA, Brouwer FAS, Gervan WV: Influence of counterpulsation on collateral circulation after acute occlusion of the left anterior descending coronary artery in dogs. *Cardiovasc Res* 6: 45, 1972.

23 Saini VK, Hood WB Jr, Hechtman HB, Berger RL: Nutrient myocardial ischemia: effects of intraaortic balloon counterpulsation and coronary reperfusion. *Circulation* 52: 1086, 1975.

24 Watson JT, Willerson JT, Fixler DE, Sugg WL: Temporal changes in collateral coronary blood flow in ischemic myocardium during intra-aortic balloon pumping. *Circulation* 50: 249, 1974.

25 Shaw J, Taylor DR, Pitt B: Effects of intra-aortic balloon counterpulsation on regional coronary blood flow in experimental myocardial infarction. *Am J Cardiol* 34: 552, 1974.

26 Gundel WD, Brown BG, Gott VL: Coronary collateral flow studies during variable aortic root pressure waveforms. *J Appl Physiol* 29: 579, 1970.

27 Gill CC, Wechsler AS, Newman GE, Oldham HN Jr: Augmentation and redistribution of myocardial blood flow during acute ischemia by intraaortic balloon pumping. *Ann Thorac Surg* 16: 445, 1973.

27a Schwartz GG, McHale PA, Greenfield JC: Coronary vasodilation after a single ventricular extra-activation in the conscious dog. *Circ Res* 50: 38, 1982.

28 Mueller H, Ayres SM, Conklin EF, Giannelli S Jr, Mazzara JT, Grace WT, Nealon TF Jr: The effects of intra-aortic counterpulsation on cardiac performance and metabolism in shock associated with acute myocardial infarction. *J Clin Invest* 50: 1885, 1971.

29 Bregman D, Parodi EN, Reemtsma K, Malm JR: Advances in clinical intraaortic balloon pumping, in *Coronary Artery Medicine and Surgery: Concepts and Controversies*, JC Norman, EP Lawrence, T Cooper (eds). New York, Appleton-Century-Crofts, 1975, p 413.

30 Whittle JL, Feldman RL, Pepine CJ, Nichols WW, Selby J, Kelly T, Conti CR: Effects of intra-aortic balloon pumping on regional and total coronary flow in patients with coronary disease. *Am J Cardiol* 45: 395, 1980.

31 Sasayama S, Osakada G, Takahashi M, Hamashima H, Nishimura E, Kawai C: Effects of intraaortic balloon counterpulsation on regional myocardial function during acute coronary occlusion in the dog. *Am J Cardiol* 43: 59, 1979.

32 Roberts AJ, Alonso DR, Combes JR, Jacobstein JG, Post MR, Cahill PT, Ho ST, Abel RM, Subramanian VA, Gay WA Jr: Role of delayed intraaortic balloon pumping in the treatment of experimental myocardial infarction. *Am J Cardiol* 41: 1202, 1978.

CHAPTER **20**

CORONARY ANGIOPLASTY

In 1978, Andreas Grüntzig, working in Zurich, Switzerland, performed the first successful dilation of an obstructed coronary artery with a specially designed balloon catheter [1]. Although similar catheter dilations have been performed in peripheral vessels since 1964 [2], extending this approach to the coronary circulation represents a major clinical advance. Since 1978, over 1500 percutaneous transluminal coronary angioplasty procedures have been performed in various medical centers [3]. A review of this initial experience indicates the following findings:

1 About 5 to 10 percent of patients with operable coronary obstructive disease may be suitable candidates for percutaneous transluminal coronary angioplasty [4,5]. (As indications for the procedure are liberalized, this percentage will undoubtedly increase.)

2 In medical centers with the largest experience, clinically significant dilation can be accomplished in two-thirds of patients in whom the angioplasty procedure is attempted [6–11]. (With improved catheters and more experience, the success rate of this procedure will probably increase.)

3 A small percentage of patients have one or more major complications as a result of the procedure [3]. These complications include acute myocardial infarction (5 percent), important peripheral vascular problems (1 percent), death (1 percent), and need for emergency coronary bypass surgery (7 percent). The clinical importance of the latter complication is minimized if the patients selected for angioplasty would otherwise have required coronary bypass surgery.

SALUTARY EFFECTS OF PERCUTANEOUS TRANSLUMINAL CORONARY ANGIOPLASTY

Patients subjected to percutaneous transluminal coronary angioplasty have been evaluated following the procedure with a wide variety of diagnostic techniques aimed at determining the effects of this therapeutic modality on coronary anatomy and myocardial perfusion.

Lumen Size

Coronary angiograms performed immediately following angioplasty indicate that in up to two-thirds of patients lumen size increases in the diseased vascular segment subjected to balloon dilation (see Figures 20-1 and 20-2) [6–11]. These studies based their assessment of lumen size on measurement of percent diameter stenosis. Although this index is a very crude method of estimating luminal area in coronary vessels with eccentric obstructive lesions (see Chapter 11), a decrease in percent stenosis observed in two angiographic projections indicates that luminal area of the segment increased following the dilation. Coronary angiograms obtained 2 to 9 months following successful percutaneous transluminal coronary angioplasty indicate that in 80 percent of patients the caliber of the dilated segment remains unchanged or actually increases (see Figure 20-1) [6,7].

Recent unpublished studies by Gail Brayden at the University of Iowa, which have employed quantitative coronary angiography (see Chapter 11), have shown that the luminal area of an obstructed coronary segment more than doubled following balloon angioplasty. Also, six months following the procedure the luminal area enlarges by an additional 35 percent. The final luminal area achieved, however, is only about one-half of the luminal area of the dilating balloon.

Stenosis Pressure Gradient

After the balloon angioplasty catheter is properly positioned, pressure distal to the obstructive lesion can be measured prior to dilation. In the experience of Grüntzig et al. [6], the pressure gradient between the aorta and the vascular segment distal to the obstruction averaged 60 mmHg. Following successful dilation, the gradient decreased significantly (see Figures 20-2 and 20-3).

Although the decrease in the pressure gradient following angioplasty implies that the obstruction has been partially relieved, the quantitative interpretation of such data must be cautious. The pressure gradient across an obstruction is criti-

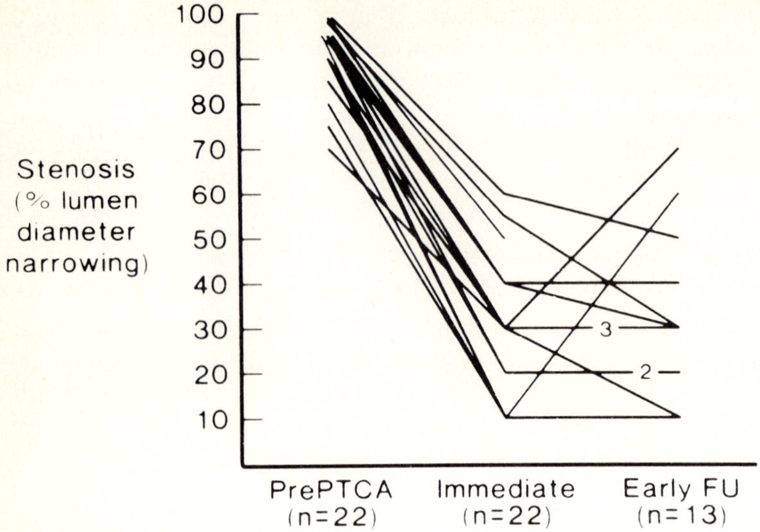

FIGURE 20-1
Effects of percutaneous transluminal coronary angioplasty (PTCA) on a percent coronary stenosis expressed as percent lumen diameter narrowing. Immediately following percutaneous transluminal coronary angioplasty (Immediate) in all patients in whom the procedure was successful, the severity of coronary stenosis decreased. Repeat cardiac catheterization in an early follow-up period (Early FU) showed that in most patients the decrease in lumen diameter narrowing immediately following percutaneous transluminal coronary angioplasty was either maintained or the vascular segment dilated further. Early follow-up catheterizations were performed within 2 months following the angioplasty procedure. The integers in lines connecting immediate and early followup data indicate that several patients had identical responses. (*From RE Vlietstra et al* [7].)

cally dependent on blood flow velocity. Also, the catheter which traverses the lesion contributes to the obstruction. The magnitude of this contribution increases significantly as the ratio between the cross-sectional area of the vascular lumen and the cross-sectional area of the catheter decreases.

Tissue Perfusion

When thallium 201 is injected during exercise, the distribution of the isotope reflects the distribution of myocardial perfusion [12]. In greater than 90 percent of patients in whom percutaneous transluminal coronary angioplasty is successful, abnormal thallium 201 images revert to normal [6,8,13–15].

Studies which have employed the xenon 133 technique have indicated that the flow in the perfusion field of a severely obstructed vessel increases following successful angioplasty [15].

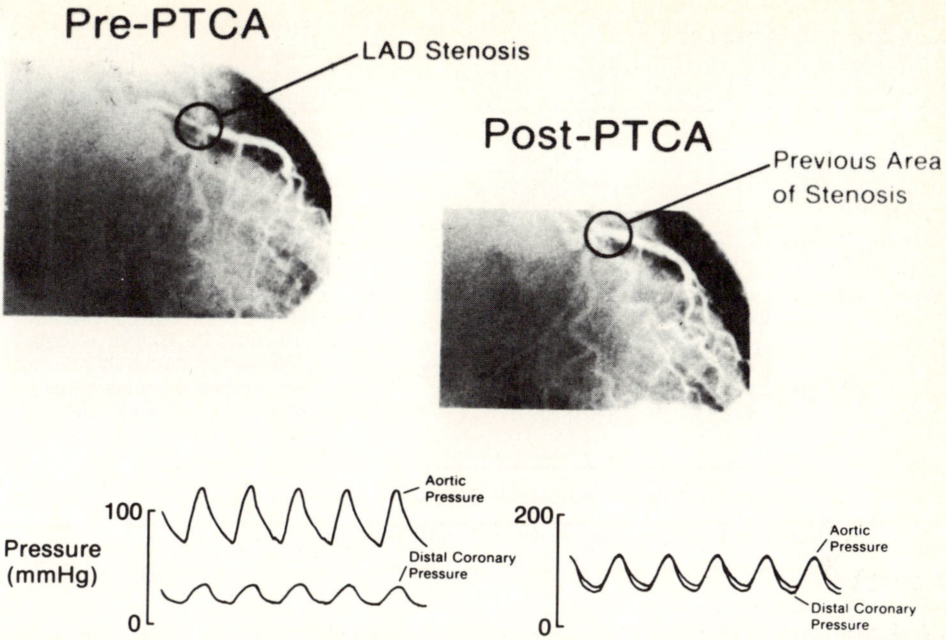

FIGURE 20-2
(*Left*) Effects of percutaneous transluminal coronary angioplasty (PTCA) on angiographic coronary anatomy and (*right*) the transstenosis pressure gradient prior to (pre-PTCA) and following (post-PTCA) coronary angioplasty. Prior to PTCA there was a severe narrowing in the proximal left anterior descending coronary artery (*left*) and an 81-mm pressure gradient between the aorta and the left anterior descending coronary artery distal to the coronary obstruction (*right*). Immediately following PTCA the narrowed segment of the left anterior descending coronary artery was restored toward normal (*left*) and the transstenosis pressure gradient decreased to 4 mmHg. In this patient, PTCA obviously improved coronary hemodynamics. (*Courtesy of C White, Associate Professor of Medicine, University of Iowa, and D Ferguson, Instructor in Medicine, University of Iowa.*)

Ventricular Function

When patients with severe isolated coronary stenosis are subjected to exercise, the myocardium served by the obstructed vessel contracts abnormally [16,17]. Such exercise-induced wall motion abnormalities are eliminated in most patients following successful angioplasty (Figure 20-4) [9,18].

Left ventricular diastolic filling, which is usually diminished in patients with coronary obstructive disease, returns to normal if significant coronary dilation in the diseased vascular segment is achieved with the coronary angioplasty (Figure 20-4) [18].

Exercise Tolerance and Angina

Following successful balloon dilation of a diseased coronary vascular segment, the clinical manifestations of ischemic heart disease are markedly ameliorated [3–11].

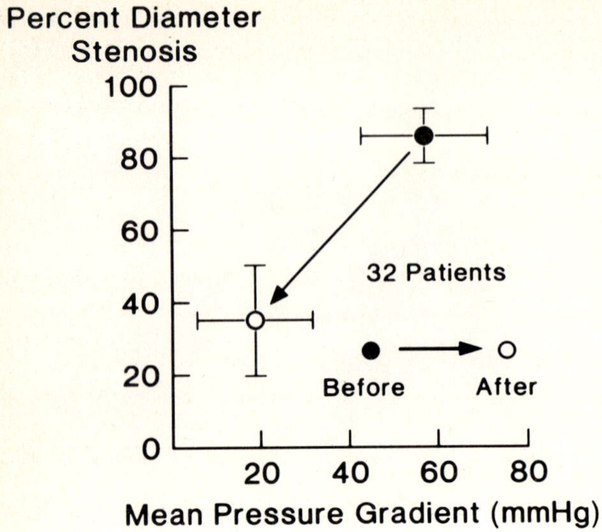

FIGURE 20-3
Effects of percutaneous transluminal coronary angioplasty on the mean pressure gradient across the coronary vascular segment being dilated and percent diameter stenosis of the obstructed vascular segment. After successful percutaneous transluminal coronary angioplasty percent diameter stenosis and mean pressure gradient decreased substantially. Before = data obtained immediately prior to percutaneous transluminal coronary angioplasty. (*From AR Grüntzig, A Senning, and WE Siegenthaler* [6].)

FIGURE 20-4
Effects of percutaneous transluminal coronary angioplasty on left ventricular (LV) ejection fraction during exercise and left ventricular diastolic filling rate at rest. Both left ventricular ejection fraction during exercise and left ventricular diastolic filling rate increased following successful percutaneous transluminal coronary angioplasty. End-diastolic vol/sec = End-diastolic volumes per second. Pre = data obtained several days following the angioplasty procedure. (*Based on data originally presented by KM Kent et al* [9].)

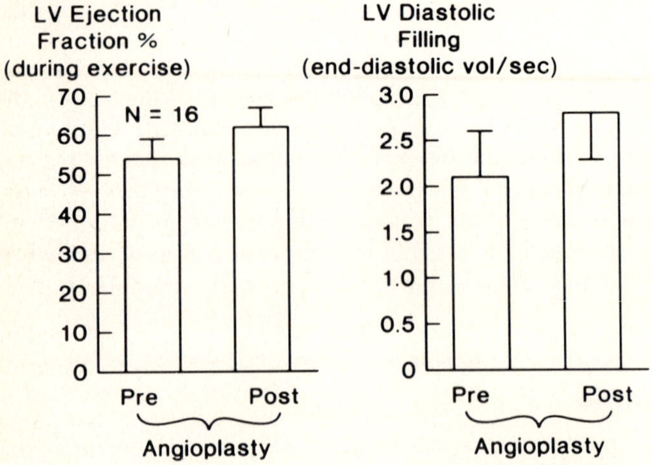

Angina pectoris occurs much less often or not at all, exercise tolerance improves substantially, and electrocardiographic manifestations of myocardial ischemia during exercise are usually no longer detectable [6–11].

MECHANISMS RESPONSIBLE FOR LUMINAL DILATION FOLLOWING CORONARY ANGIOPLASTY

Grüntzig originally hypothesized that percutaneous luminal coronary angioplasty enlarged the vascular lumen of the diseased artery by compressing the atherosclerotic plaque [19]. Studies in an animal model [20,21], human cadaver hearts [22–24], and limited autopsy specimens from patients who died soon after coronary angioplasty [24] indicate that plaque compression is not the mechanism whereby balloon angioplasty dilates coronary vessels. These studies indicate that two mechanisms are responsible: superficial plaque disruption and intimal splitting. Focal intimal splitting occurs as the inelastic plaque is overstretched by the inflated balloon. The plaque ruptures or splits at its weakest point leaving the more elastic media intact but slightly stretched. The split in the atherosclerotic plaque is usually confined to the area of the angioplasty and does not propagate. Following this "controlled vascular injury," reparative processes are activated which in effect maintain the caliber or further dilate the involved vascular segment.

EFFECTS OF CORONARY ANGIOPLASTY ON CORONARY COLLATERAL CIRCULATION

Immediately following successful balloon dilation, coronary collateral vessels which could be seen angiographically prior to the procedure are no longer apparent on a follow-up coronary arteriogram [25]. Flow through coronary collateral vessels depends on the presence of a pressure gradient between the normal and obstructed coronary vessels (see Chapter 10). If the pressure gradient is eliminated by relief of the obstruction, the coronary collateral channels are no longer functional. A similar phenomenon occurs following successful coronary bypass surgery [26–28]. Experimental studies in dogs indicate that these "dormant collateral channels" can be quickly restored to their previous functional state if obstruction recurs in the involved vessel [29]. The potential function of such dormant coronary collateral vessels in humans has not been extensively studied.

CLINICAL SIGNIFICANCE

There is indisputable evidence that successful percutaneous transluminal coronary angioplasty dilates obstructive coronary segments and improves myocardial perfusion. Although the long-term effects of this therapeutic modality remain to be defined, it is likely that this approach will be widely applied in the treatment in patients with coronary obstructive disease.

REFERENCES

1 Grüntzig AR: Transluminal dilation of coronary-artery stenosis. *Lancet* 1: 263, 1978.

2 Dotter CT, Judkins MP: Transluminal treatment of arteriosclerotic obstruction: Description of a new technic and a preliminary report of its application. *Circulation* 30: 654, 1964.

3 Levy RI, Mock MB, Willman VL, Passamani ER, Frommer PL: Editorial: Percutaneous transluminal coronary angioplasty–A status report. *N Engl J Med* 305: 399, 1981.

4 Gosselin AJ, Fisher L, Judkins MP, Ryan TJ, Vlietstra RE, Kemp HC, Gillespie MJ, Mock MB: Percutaneous transluminal angioplasty: An estimate of the number of possible candidates for the CASS registry, in proceedings of the Workshop on Percutaneous Transluminal Coronary Angioplasty, Washington, DC, June 1979, NIH Publication 80-2030, 1980, p 89.

5 Hamby RI, Katz S: Percutaneous transluminal coronary angioplasty: Its potential impact on surgery for coronary artery disease. *Am J Cardiol* 45: 1161, 1980.

6 Grüntzig AR, Senning A, Siegenthaler WE: Nonoperative dilation of coronary-artery stenosis. Percutaneous transluminal coronary angioplasty. *N Engl J Med* 301: 61, 1969.

7 Vlietstra RE, Holmes DR, Smith HC, Hartzler GO, Orszulak TA, Orszulak TA: Percutaneous transluminal coronary angioplasty. Initial Mayo Clinic experience. *Mayo Clin Proc* 56: 287, 1981.

8 Block PC: Percutaneous transluminal coronary angioplasty. *Prim Cardiol Clin* 2: 13, 1976.

9 Kent KM, Bonow RO, Rosing DR, Ewels CJ, Lipson LC, McIntosh CL, Bacharach S, Green M, Epstein SE: Improved myocardial function during exercise after successful percutaneous transluminal coronary angioplasty. *N Engl J Med* 306: 441, 1982.

10 Stertzer SH, Myler RH, Bruno MS, Wallsh E: Transluminal coronary artery dilation. *Prac Cardiol* 5: 25, 1979.

11 Kent D, Banka V, Bentivoglio L, Block P, Cowley M, Diamond G, Dorros G, Ellestad M, Faxon D, Fiedotin A, Goldberg S, Grüntzig A, Hamby R, Hirshfeld J, Kaltenbach M, Kober G, Lach R, Leatherman L, Lee G, Meyer J, Myler R, Ockene I, Robert E, Rosing D, Simpson J, Sosa J, Spring D, Stertzer S, Vlietstra R, Walton J, Williams D, Fisher L, Gillespie M, Mullin S, Mock M: Percutaneous transluminal coronary angioplasty (PTCA): Update from the NHLBI registry. *Circulation* 62: 160, 1980.

12 Pohost GM, Alpert NM, Ingwall JS, Strauss HW: Thallium redistribution:Mechanisms and clinical utility. *Sem Nucl Med* 10: 70, 1980.

13 Hirzel HO, Grüntzig A, Neusch K, Krayenbuehl HP, Horst W: Thallium-201 imaging for the evaluation of myocardial perfusion after percutaneous transluminal angioplasty of coronary artery stenosis. *Circulation* 58: 180, 1978.

14 National Heart, Lung and Blood Institute: Workshop on percutaneous transluminal coronary angioplasty. Bethesda, Maryland, June 15–16, 1979.

15 Schmidt DH, Dymond DS, Ray G: Qualitative and quantitative assessment of myocardial perfusion following coronary angioplasty. *Clin Res* 29: 753, 1981.

16 Borer JS, Bacharach SL, Green MV, Kent KM, Epstein SE, Johnston GS: Real-time radionuclide cineangiography in the noninvasive evaluation of global and regional left ventricular function at rest and during exercise in patients with coronary artery disease. *N Engl J Med* 296: 839, 1977.

17 Rerych SK, Scholz PM, Newman GE, Sabiston DC, Jones RH: Cardiac function at rest and exercise in normals and patients with coronary disease: Evaluation by radionuclide angiocardiography. *Ann Surg* 187: 449, 1978.

18 Bonow RO, Kent KM, Rosing DR, Lipson LC, Bacharach SL, Green MV, Epstein SE: Improved left ventricular diastolic filling in patients with coronary artery disease following coronary angioplasty. *Circulation* 64: 79, 1981.

19 Grüntzig A: *Die perkutane transluminale Rekanalisation chronischer Arterienverschlusse mit einer neuen Dilationstechnik.* Baden-Baden, West Germany, Witszstrock, 1977–1980.

20 Block PC, Baughman KL, Pasternak RC, Fallon JT: Transluminal angioplasty: Correlation of morphologic and angiographic findings in an experimental model. *Circulation* 61: 778, 1980.

21 Block PC, Fallon JT, Elmer D: Experimental angioplasty: Lessons from the laboratory. *Am J Radiol* 135: 907, 1980.

22 Lee G, Ikeda RM, Joye JA, Bogren HG, DeMaria AN, Mason DT: Evaluation of transluminal angioplasty of chronic coronary artery stenosis: Value and limitations assessed in fresh human cadaver hearts. *Circulation* 61: 77, 1980.

23 Castaneda-Zuniga WR, Formanek A, Tadavarthy M, Vlodaver Z, Edwards JE, Zollikofer C, Amplatz K: The mechanism of balloon angioplasty. *Radiology* 135: 565, 1980.

24 Block PC, Myler RK, Stertzer S, Fallon JT: Morphology after transluminal angioplasty in human beings. *N Engl J Med* 305: 382, 1981.

25 Grüntzig A, Pyle R, Goebel N, Schlumpf M: The fate of collaterals after percutaneous transluminal coronary angioplasty (PTCA). *Circulation* 62: 161, 1980.

26 Bourassa MG, Solignac A, Goulet C, Lespérance J: Regression and appearance of coronary collaterals in humans during life. *Circulation* 50: 127, 1974.

27 Valle M, Wiljasalo M, Frick MH, Korhola O, Souranta H, Tallroth K: Collateral circulation before and after coronary artery reconstruction. *Ann Clin Res* 7: 251, 1975.

28 DiLuzio V, Roy PR, Sowton E, Dow J: Fate of coronary collateral circulation after aorto-coronary saphenous vein bypass grafts. *Br Heart J* 37: 397, 1975.

29 Khouri EM, Gregg DE, McGranahan GM, Jr: Regression and reappearance of coronary collaterals. *Am J Physiol* 220: 655, 1971.

CHAPTER **21**

INTRACORONARY THROMBOLYSIS

Fletcher et al., in 1959, suggested that thrombolytic therapy may be useful in the treatment of patients with acute myocardial infarction [1]. For more than two decades, however, physicians have hesitated to employ this therapeutic modality. Two problems have limited the widespread use of thrombolytic treatment for myocardial infarction. First, there has been continued controversy concerning the role of coronary thrombosis in the pathogenesis of acute myocardial infarction [2]. Second, clinical trials which have assessed the efficacy of intravenously administered thrombolytic agents on mortality from acute myocardial infarction have produced results which were often equivocal or negative [3–6]. Recent clinical studies have resolved these problems to some extent and thereby have ushered in a bold new therapeutic approach to myocardial infarction—intracoronary thrombolysis.

IS ACUTE MYOCARDIAL INFARCTION SECONDARY TO CORONARY THROMBOSIS?

Pathologists have vacillated in their response to this question for decades. In the 1940s, pathological studies by Master et al. [7] and Blumgart et al. [8,9] supported the view that coronary thrombosis played a causal role in the pathogenesis of many cases of acute myocardial infarction. In the 1950s, pathological studies began to question the concept that thrombosis was the cause of acute myocardial infarction [10,11]. Some pathologists even championed the view that myocardial infarction, by producing low cardiac output and shock, actually caused thrombosis rather than vice versa [11]. Pathological studies in the late 1960s and early 1970s concluded that coronary thrombosis was present in about 86 to 97 percent of patients who sustained an acute, large, or transmural myocardial infarction [12–15]. One influential pathologist, William Roberts, from the National Institute of Health, has maintained that coronary thrombosis is found in only 54 percent of patients with acute transmural myocardial infarction. Roberts noted that a thrombus was particularly unlikely to be found in patients who died suddenly of myocardial infarction but would often be present in those who died of cardiogenic shock secondary to acute myocardial infarction. On the basis of these observations, Roberts concluded that "coronary thrombi are consequences rather than causes of acute myocardial infarction" [16].

Pathological studies concerning the relationships between coronary thrombosis and acute myocardial infarction have several inherent deficiencies. The patients who die of infarction may not be representative of those who survive. Most pathological studies are based on examinations of patients with histological evidence of infarction. Because light microscopy does not detect necrosis unless the infarction is at least 6 h old, patients with very recent infarctions are often excluded from pathological series. Also, many pathological studies have included many patients who died days or weeks following acute myocardial infarction. In these cases, a thrombus which caused the infarct could have spontaneously lysed between the time of the acute myocardial infarction and the postmortem examination. Finally, most studies do not separate their patients into subgroups with subendocardial or small infarctions vs. transmural or large infarctions. This distinction is of importance because it has been shown that coronary thrombosis is primarily associated with transmural infarctions [15–17]. These limitations of pathological studies have contributed to the controversy concerning the relationship between coronary thrombosis and acute myocardial infarction.

Results of Angiographic and Surgical Studies

In 1979, two groups of investigators [18–19] studied the frequency of complete coronary occlusion assessed by coronary angiography in patients with acute transmural myocardial infarction. In patients studied within 4 h for the onset of symptoms of myocardial infarction, 87 percent had complete occlusion of the coronary vessel serving the infarcted zone (Figure 21-1) [18a]. As the time between the onset of symptoms and the time of cardiac catheterization lengthened, the incidence of complete coronary occlusion detected by coronary angiography decreased. Twelve to twenty-four hours following acute myocardial infarction only 65 percent of patients had complete coronary occlusion (Figure 21-1) [18a]. Many of the patients included in the angiographic studies were treated acutely with coronary bypass surgery. Hence, at surgery, the presence of the coronary thrombosis could be ascertained by opening the occluded vessel and extracting the clot. These intraoperative evaluations demonstrated that thrombus was present in 88 percent of patients in whom coronary angiography showed complete occlusion in

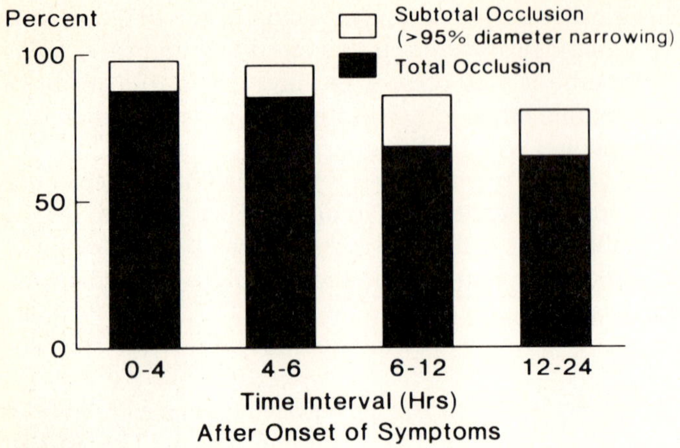

FIGURE 21-1
Incidence of total and subtotal coronary occlusion in patients with acute myocardial infarctions studied at various time intervals after the onset of symptoms. In patients studied within 4 h of the onset of symptoms, coronary angiography demonstrated that 87 percent had total occlusion of the vessel serving the infarct zone. (*Based on data originally presented by MA DeWood et al* [*18a*].)

a vessel serving the infarcted zone and definite angiographic features of thrombus [18a]. Since 1979, many groups of investigators [20–25a] have confirmed the notion that intracoronary thrombus is the predominant cause of transmural acute myocardial infarction in patients.

Thus, it is now certain that acute transmural myocardial infarction in humans is almost always caused by coronary thrombosis which is superimposed on an atherosclerotic coronary obstruction of variable severity.

APPROACHES TO RECANALIZING ACUTELY OCCLUDED CORONARY VESSELS

Four approaches to opening acutely occluded coronary vessels have been introduced. As noted above, coronary bypass surgery with extraction of the intracoronary thrombus can be accomplished [19,26]. Although this procedure is relatively safe [19], at most medical centers it cannot be performed with sufficient dispatch to salvage much of the myocardium at risk from infarction. It is likely, therefore, that this therapeutic option will have limited use. Intracoronary thrombi can be dislodged by passing a wire through the thrombus at the time of coronary angiography [27,28]. Also, if coronary occlusion is due to spasm, this can be alleviated with intracoronary nitroglycerin or administration of a calcium blocking agent [28,29]. Recent studies, however, indicate that the most successful way to recanalize an occluded artery is intracoronary infusion of streptokinase (Figure 21-2) [20–25a,28].

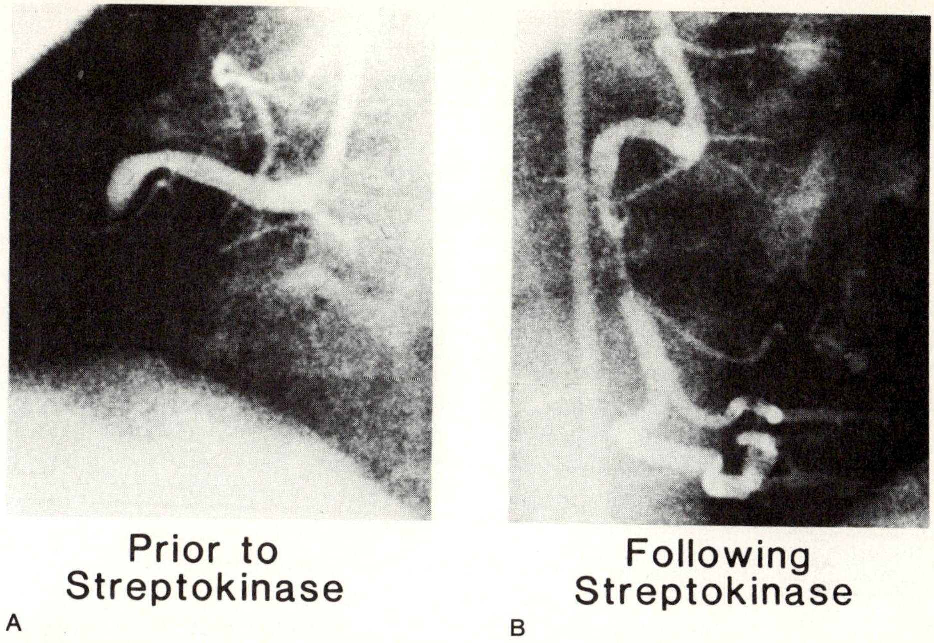

FIGURE 21-2
(*a*) Coronary arteriogram prior to infusion of streptokinase demonstrating complete occlusion of the right coronary artery. (*b*) Coronary arteriogram demonstrating reperfusion of the occluded right coronary artery 30 min following intracoronary infusion of streptokinase. (*Courtesy of C White, Associate Professor of Medicine, University of Iowa.*)

Intracoronary Thrombolysis

Recanalization of coronary thrombi is currently being achieved by infusion of intracoronary streptokinase or a mixture of streptokinase and plasminogen [20–25a,28]. Streptokinase is a single-chain protein of molecular weight 45,000 which is a catabolic by-product of β-hemolytic streptococcus [30–32]. This enzyme activates plasminogen indirectly by way of a proactivator-activator system. Streptokinase binds with plasminogen and produces a conformational change in plasminogen. Once the streptokinase-plasminogen complex has been formed, activation of other plasminogen molecules proceeds by the cleavage of a single arginyl-valine bond. The streptokinase-plasminogen complex is gradually converted to streptokinase-plasmin, which can also activate plasminogen. In the presence of a thrombus, plasmin digests fibrin and thereby dissolves the thrombus.

When intracoronary streptokinase is administered to patients with acute myocardial infarction, within 6 h of the onset of symptoms, between 75 and 95 percent of occluded coronary arteries can be recanalized [20–22,24–25a]. In the majority of patients, the occluded vessel opens in less than 30 min from the onset of streptokinase infusion [20,22–25a]. In 90 percent of patients, the occluded vessel remains open for at least several weeks following the streptokinase infusion [21]. During this interim period, the patients are treated with anticoagulants, nitrates, and calcium blocking drugs. The mortality associated with intracoronary streptokinase treatment is less than 5 percent, and major morbidity is infrequent [20–25a].

Salutary Effects of Intracoronary Thrombolysis

Although measurements of regional myocardial perfusion following successful recanalization of an occluded coronary vessel have not been reported, clinical observations suggest myocardial perfusion in the involved zone does improve following this therapeutic procedure. In most patients, chest pain disappears immediately following reperfusion of the occluded vessel with streptokinase [21]. Electrocardiographic evidence of ischemia disappears or improves almost immediately following recanalization [20–22]. In several reported patients with severe systemic hypotension, arterial pressure increased dramatically as soon as the occluded vessel was opened and perfusion of the involved zone was restored [21,22]. Markis et al. [23] and Schwarz et al. [25a] have reported that thallium 201 uptake in the perfusion field of the occluded vessel improved significantly following reperfusion of the occluded vessel. This implies that thallium 201 was being delivered to the involved zone and that viable cells were able to accumulate the cation. Mathey et al. [22], Reduto et al. [24], and Rentrop et al. [25] have reported that global and segmental left ventricular function improve in patients in whom intracoronary streptokinase successfully recanalized the occluded vessel (Figure 21-3).

Even if intracoronary streptokinase does successfully recanalize an occluded vessel, most patients demonstrate electrocardiographic, enzymatic, and ventriculographic evidence of infarction [20–25a]. It is not known if the infarction which occurs following recanalization is smaller than it might have been in the absence of coronary reperfusion.

POTENTIAL COMPLICATIONS OF CORONARY REPERFUSION

Studies in dogs have shown that coronary reperfusion can be associated with a high incidence of lethal ventricular arrhythmias (see Chapter 9). Such arrhythmias seldom occur in patients in whom an occluded vessel has been reopened with streptokinase [20–25a]. This discrepancy between the results of animal studies and clinical experience is best explained by differences in the underlying state of the coronary vessels (with or without superimposed stenosis), the state of alertness (awake vs. anesthetized), and the duration of the occlusion.

Reperfusion can occasionally produce hemorrhagic infarction (see Chapter 9). Although some have suggested such hemorrhage could extend the size of an infarct, in my view this is unlikely. Hemorrhage into an acute myocardial infarction occurs as a late manifestation of the no-reflow phenomenon and is confined to zones of myocardium which are completely necrotic. There is no convincing evidence that such hemorrhage actually extends the size of an existing infarct.

Recanalization of an acutely occluded vessel often eliminates angiographically apparent coronary collaterals which delivered flow to the jeopardized region. This

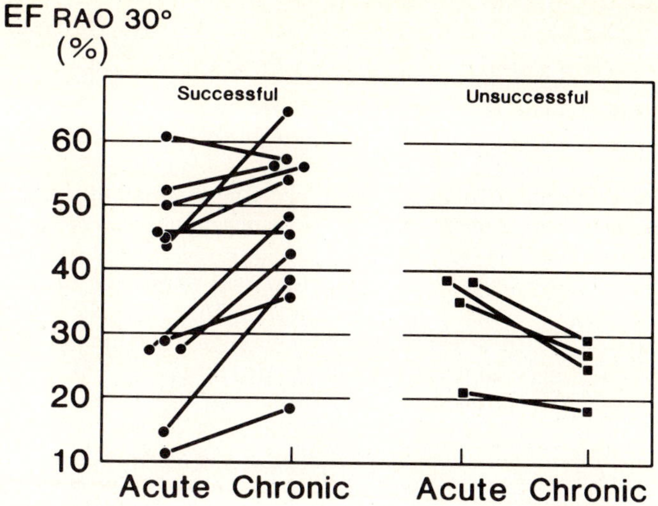

FIGURE 21-3
Effects of successful and unsuccessful coronary thrombolysis on global left ventricular function. All patients included in this study had acute myocardial infarction presumably secondary to thrombotic occlusion of a major coronary artery. Left ventricular function was assessed by measuring left ventricular ejection fraction (EF) from a 30° right anterior oblique (RAO) contrast ventriculargram. The acute study was performed prior to thrombolysis. The chronic study was done 7 to 21 days following thrombolysis. Patients who had successful thrombolysis had an improvement in global left ventricular function. (*Modified from an illustration originally presented by Mathey et al* [22].)

is reminiscent of the effects of coronary bypass surgery on angiographically apparent coronary vessels (see Chapter 16). The long-term effects of coronary thrombolysis on coronary collateral circulation remain to be ascertained.

If recanalization of an acutely occluded coronary vessel leads to the salvage of the myocardium, the patient's clinical course will depend in part on the characteristics of the "salvaged myocardium" (see Chapter 10). Salvaged myocardium could have positive effects (increased global left ventricular function) or negative effects (promote the genesis of lethal arrhythmias).

In summary, intracoronary thrombolysis is an exciting approach to the treatment of acute myocardial infarction. Critically important questions in this area to be answered include (1) What is the available time in which treatment may be effective? and (2) Can other adjunctive treatments (infusion of a substrate; percutaneous transluminal angioplasty of the stenosis in the involved vessel) improve on the results of streptokinase alone? and (3) Can an effective thrombolytic agent be developed which can be administered intravenously? The value of thrombolytic therapy must be determined by carefully controlled, randomized studies which employ techniques that allow investigators to determine if infarct size expressed as a percent of the risk area (see Chapter 10) is favorably altered by this method of treatment.

REFERENCES

1 Fletcher AP, Sherry S, Alkjaersig N, Smyrniotis FE, Jick S: The maintenance of a sustained thrombolytic state in man. II. Clinical observations on patients with myocardial infarction and other thrombo-embolic disorders. *J Clin Invest* 38: 1111, 1959.

2 Chandler AB, Chapman I, Erhardt LR, Roberts WC, Schwartz CJ, Sinapius D, Spain DM, Sherry S, Ness PM, Simon TL: Coronary thrombosis in myocardial infarction: Report of a workshop on the role of coronary thrombosis in the pathogenesis of acute myocardial infarction. *Am J Cardiol* 34: 823, 1974.

3 Duckert F: Thrombolytic therapy in myocardial infarction. *Prog Cardiovasc Dis* 21: 342, 1979.

4 Aber CP, Bass NM, Berry LL, et al: Streptokinase in acute myocardial infarction: A controlled multicentre study in the United Kingdom. *Br Med J* 2: 1100, 1976.

5 European collaborative study: A controlled trial of urokinase in myocardial infarction. *Lancet* 2: 624, 1975.

6 European cooperative study group for streptokinase treatment in acute myocardial infarction: Streptokinase in acute myocardial infarction. *N Engl J Med* 301: 979, 1979.

7 Master AM, Gubner R, Dack S, Jaffe HL: Differentiation of acute coronary insufficiency with myocardial infarction from coronary occlusion. *Arch Int Med* 67: 647, 1941.

8 Blumgart HL, Schlesinger MJ, Davis D: Studies on the relation of the clinical manifestations of angina pectoris, coronary thrombosis, and myocardial infarction to the pathologic findings. *Am Heart J* 19: 1, 1940.

9 Blumgart HL, Schlesinger MJ, Zoll PM: Angina pectoris, coronary failure and acute myocardial infarction. *JAMA* 116: 91, 1941.

10 Miller RD, Burchell HB, Edwards JE: Myocardial infarction with and without acute coronary occlusion. *Arch Intern Med* 88: 597, 1951.

11 Branwood AW, Montgomery GL: Observations on the morbid anatomy of coronary artery disease. *Scot Med J* 1: 367, 1956.

12 Chapman I: Relationships of recent coronary artery occlusion and acute myocardial infarction. *J Mt Sinai Hosp* 35: 149, 1968.

13 Schwartz CJ, Walsh WJ: The pathologic basis of sudden death. *Prog Cardiovasc Dis* 13: 465, 1971.

14 Sinapius D: Beziehungen zwischen Koronarthrombosen und Myokardinfarkten. *Dtsch Med Wochenschr* 97: 443, 1972.

15 Spain DM: The pathologic spectrum of myocardial infarction, in *Atherosclerosis and Coronary Heart Disease,* W Likoff et al. (eds). New York, Grune & Stratton, 1972, p. 133.

16 Roberts WC, Buja LM: The frequency and significance of coronary arterial thrombi and other observations in fatal acute myocardial infarction. A study of 107 necropsy patients. *Am J Med* 52: 425, 1972.

17 Friedberg CK, Horn H: Acute myocardial infarction not due to coronary artery occlusion. *JAMA* 112: 1675, 1939.

18 DeWood MA, Spores J, Notske RN, Mouser LT, Burroughs R, Mohiuddin S: Incidence of total coronary occlusion and thrombosis in the early phase of acute transmural myocardial infarction. *Clin Res* 27: 162, 1979.

18a DeWood MA, Spores J, Notske R, Mouser LT, Burroughs R, Golden MS, Lang HT: Prevalence of total coronary occlusion during the early hours of transmural myocardial infarction. *N Eng J Med* 303: 897, 1980.

19 Phillips SJ, Kongtahworn C, Zeff RH, Benson M, Iannone L, Brown T, Gordon DF: Emergency coronary artery revascularization: A possible therapy for acute myocardial infarction. *Circulation* 60: 241, 1979.

20 Ganz W, Buchbinder N, Marcus H, Mondkar A, Maddahi J, Charuzi Y, O'Connor L, Shell W, Fishbein MC, Kass R, Miyamoto A, Swan HJC: Intracoronary thrombolysis in evolving myocardial infarction. *Am Heart J* 101: 4, 1981.

21 Rentrop P, Blanke H, Karsch KR, Kaiser H, Kostering H, Leitz K: Selective intracoronary thrombolysis in acute myocardial infarction and unstable angina pectoris. *Circulation* 63: 307, 1981.

22 Mathey DG, Kuck K-H, Tilsner V, Krebber H-J, Bleifeld W: Nonsurgical coronary artery recanalization in acute transmural myocardial infarction. *Circulation* 63: 489, 1981.

23 Markis JE, Malagold M, Parker JA, Silverman KJ, Barry WH, Als AV, Paulin S, Grossman W, Braunwald E: Myocardial salvage after intracoronary thrombolysis with streptokinase in acute myocardial infarction. Assessment by intracoronary thallium-201. *N Engl J Med* 305: 777, 1981.

24 Reduto LA, Smalling RW, Freund GC, Gould KL: Intracoronary infusion of streptokinase in patients with acute myocardial infarction: Effects of reperfusion on left ventricular performance. *Am J Cardiol* 48: 403, 1981.

25 Rentrop KP, Blanke H, Karsch KR: Effects of nonsurgical coronary reperfusion on the left ventricle in human subjects compared with conventional treatment. Study of 18 patients with acute myocardial infarction treated with intracoronary infusion of streptokinase. *Am J Cardiol* 49: 1, 1982.

25a Schwarz F, Schuller G, Katus H, Hemel HC, von Olshausen K, Hofmann M, Herrmann H-J, Kubler W: Intracoronary thrombolysis in acute myocardial infarction: Correlations among serum enzyme, scintigraphic and hemodynamic findings. *Am J Cardiol* 50: 32, 1982.

26 DeWood MA, Spores J, Notske RN, et al: Medical and surgical management of acute myocardial infarction. *Am J Cardiol* 44: 1356, 1979.

27 Rentrop P, DeVivie ER, Karsch KR, Kreuzer H: Acute coronary occlusion with impending infarction as angiographic complication relieved by a guide-wire recanalization. *Clin Cardiol* 1: 101, 1978.

28 Rentrop KP, Blanke H, Karsch KR, Wiegand V, Kostering H, Oster H, Leitz K: Acute myocardial infarction: Intracoronary application of nitroglycerin and streptokinase. *Clin Cardiol* 2: 354, 1979.

29 Maseri A, L'Abbate A, Baroldi G, Chierchia S, Marzilli M, Ballestra AM, Severi S, Parodi O, Biagini A, Distante A, Pesola A: Coronary vasospasm as a possible cause of myocardial infarction. *N Engl J Med* 299: 1271, 1978.

30 Castellino FJ, Violand BJ: The fibrinolytic system—Basic considerations. *Prog Cardiovasc Dis* 21: 241, 1979.

31 Barlow GH: Pharmacology of fibrinolytic agents. *Prog Cardiovasc Dis* 21: 315, 1979.

32 Bell WR, Meek AG: Guidelines for the use of thrombolytic agents. *N Engl J Med* 301: 1266, 1979.

CHAPTER **22**

PHARMACOLOGIC AGENTS

Modulating the coronary circulation by pharmacologic means has been actively pursued for more than 100 years [1]. Hundreds of drugs have been shown to affect myocardial perfusion. In general, pharmacologic agents can alter coronary flow in two ways: (1) indirectly, by affecting the primary factors that control coronary vascular resistance (see Chapters 3 through 8) or (2) directly, by acting on the smooth muscle in coronary vessels. Furthermore, pharmacologic agents can selectively affect a specific segment of the coronary vascular bed [2–4].

This chapter will focus on major classes of pharmacologic agents that have significant effects on the coronary circulation. No attempt will be made to catalog all the drugs that have been demonstrated to affect coronary vascular resistance.

INOTROPIC DRUGS

In this section, four classes of inotropic drugs will be discussed: cardiac glycosides, methylxanthines, dobutamine, and the endogenous catecholamines. These agents include all the important inotropic drugs in current clinical use.

Cardiac Glycosides

Although cardiac glycosides have been used for the treatment of heart failure since 1775 [4a], their effects on the coronary circulation have been under investigation only since 1932 [5].

The interactions between the cardiac glycosides and the coronary circulation are complex because these agents alter coronary resistance by affecting four basic mechanisms that modulate coronary flow: cardiac metabolism, neurocontrol, extravascular compressive forces, and direct effects on smooth muscle in coronary vessels.

Cardiac metabolism is influenced by the glycosides because the drugs can change the fundamental determinants of myocardial oxygen consumption, that is, myocardial contractility, heart rate, wall stress, and shortening (see Figure 3-5). Although, the major effect of these compounds is to enhance contractility [6], they can have marked effects on heart rate, wall stress, and shortening, particularly when administered to patients with heart failure and atrial fibrillation associated with a rapid ventricular response [7].

Neuroexcitation is a very important effect of digitalis [8]. The neural effects of digitalis include direct vagal stimulation, augmentation of the gain of the baroreceptor reflex, excitation of autonomic ganglia, and centrally mediated enhancement of peripheral sympathetic activity [8]. Because coronary vasomotor tone is modulated in part by neural mechanisms (see Chapter 5), the neuroexcitatory effects of digitalis influence the coronary circulation.

The cardiac glycosides influence extravascular compressive forces by altering systolic wall stress, ventricular end-diastolic pressure, heart rate, and myocardial contractility (see Chapter 4). These effects are of minimal importance when coronary tone is normal. However, when normal coronary vessels are markedly dilated or the myocardium is perfused via collateral channels, extravascular compressive forces contribute importantly to vascular conductance (see Chapter 4).

Many studies have shown that digitalis produces constriction in the peripheral [9,10], mesenteric [11,12] and coronary vascular beds (Figure 22-1) [13–17]. In vitro, isolated coronary vessels contract in response to the cardiac glycosides [18,19]. Furthermore, intracoronary injection of digitalis preparations produces prompt coronary vasoconstriction [14]. Following intravenous injection of digitalis preparations, the coronary constriction that occurs is mediated by four mechanisms: direct stimulatory effect on coronary smooth muscle [14,18,19], centrally mediated sympathetic activation of alpha receptors [15–17] (Figure 22-2), decreased metabolism related to slight bradycardia that occurs in response to the drug [13], and autoregulatory coronary vasoconstriction that occurs in response to

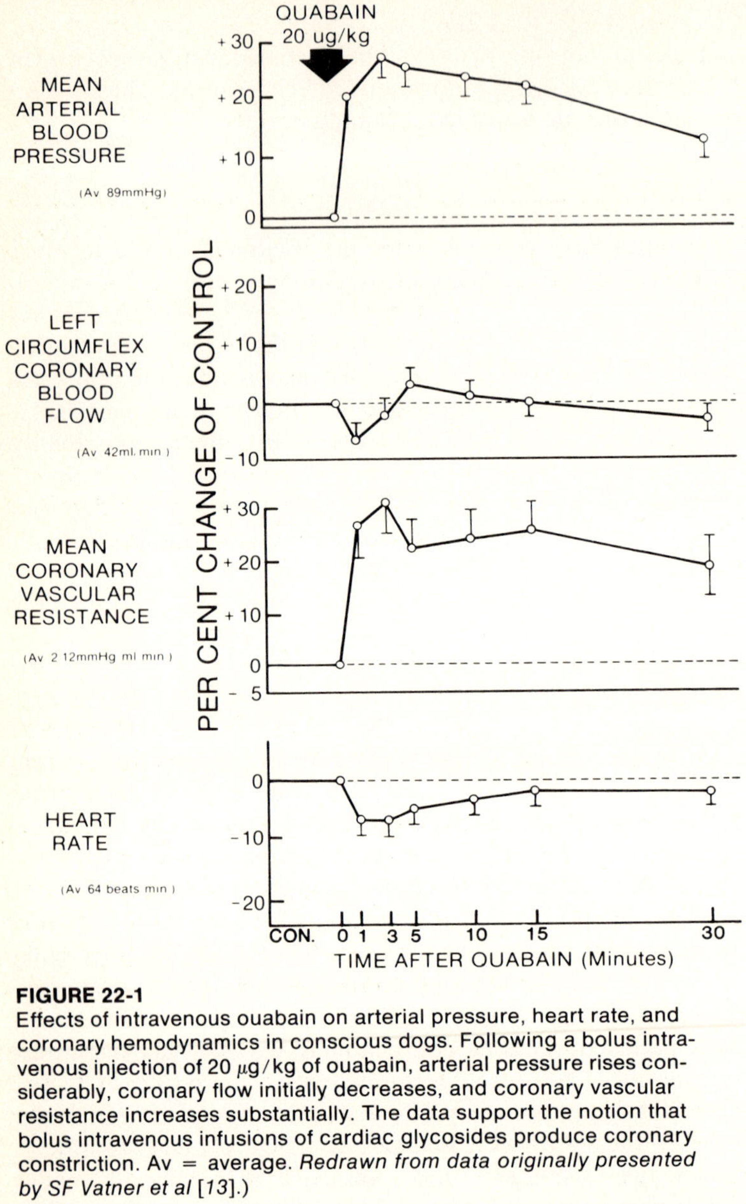

FIGURE 22-1
Effects of intravenous ouabain on arterial pressure, heart rate, and coronary hemodynamics in conscious dogs. Following a bolus intravenous injection of 20 μg/kg of ouabain, arterial pressure rises considerably, coronary flow initially decreases, and coronary vascular resistance increases substantially. The data support the notion that bolus intravenous infusions of cardiac glycosides produce coronary constriction. Av = average. *Redrawn from data originally presented by SF Vatner et al* [*13*].)

effects of the cardiac glycosides on systemic pressure [13]. The segment(s) in the coronary vascular tree where the constriction occurs (large vessels, small resistance vessels, collateral channels) has not been determined.

Although coronary vasoconstriction in response to administration of cardiac glycosides is well documented, in my view this response has minimal clinical significance. This view is based upon the following observations. First, the coronary vasocon-

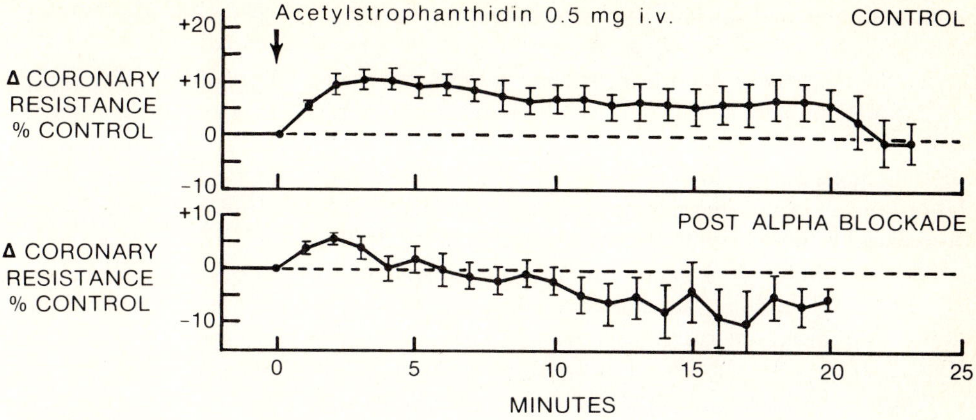

FIGURE 22-2
Effects of intravenous acetylstrophanthidin on coronary vascular resistance in anesthetized dogs. The increase in coronary vascular resistance that occurs following intravenous acetylstrophanthidin, a cardiac glycoside, is mediated by alpha-adrenergic coronary constriction. Δ = change; post alpha blockade = following alpha-adrenergic blockade with phentolamine. (*Modified from data originally presented by NP Hamlin et al* [*16*].)

striction that occurs in response to bolus intravenous injection of a cardiac glycoside is usually mild (about a 20 percent increase in coronary vascular resistance) and dissipates within 15 to 45 min [13–17,20,21]. Second, the vasoconstrictor response to digitalis preparations is minimal if the drug is administered slowly over a 10- to 20-min period [22,23]. This is best explained by studies that demonstrate that the inotropic effects of the digitalis compounds have a slow onset which is dependent on contraction frequency [24], whereas the vascular effects of the cardiac glycosides are maximal immediately after injection [13–17,20,21]. The temporal disparity in these effects is important because they have opposite actions on coronary vascular resistance. Increasing myocardial contractility augments myocardial oxygen consumption and indirectly decreases coronary vascular resistance; the direct effects of the cardiac glycosides on coronary smooth muscle increase coronary resistance. Third, when large doses of cardiac glycosides are infused intracoronary over a 30- to 60-min period, responses to a metabolic stress such as transient coronary occlusion are not attenuated [22]. Fourth, in awake dogs, the cardiac glycosides increase perfusion to acutely ischemic myocardium [20,21]. Finally, despite some scattered clinical reports [25–28] there is no convincing evidence that administration of cardiac glycosides in clinically relevant doses actually produces myocardial ischemia secondary to direct coronary constriction.

Studies in animals indicate that, in the normal coronary circulation of a nonfailing heart, administration of digitalis has minimal effects on coronary flow and does not alter the transmural distribution of myocardial perfusion [20,21]. If myocardial contractility increases substantially, a modest increase in coronary flow will occur.

Clinical studies indicate that, in patients with a normal coronary circulation and a nonfailing heart, cardiac glycosides have only modest effects on coronary blood flow [23].

In the presence of conditions such as heart failure, acute myocardial infarction, or cardiogenic shock, the net effect of the digitalis glycosides on the coronary circulation will depend upon the overall effects of the drug on cardiac function. If digitalis is employed in the treatment of heart failure associated with atrial fibrillation and a rapid ventricular response, the drug will decrease heart rate, wall stress, and reflex peripheral sympathetic vasoconstriction and will increase myocardial contractility [7]. As a consequence, coronary flow will probably decrease. Alternatively, in the presence of cardiogenic shock and normal sinus rhythm, digitalis preparations often have no major effects on overall hemodynamics and, consequently, coronary blood flow would probably be unchanged.

Experimental studies [20,21] indicate that the cardiac glycosides increase perfusion to ischemic myocardium and redistribute left ventricular perfusion toward the subendocardium [20,21]. The effects of cardiac glycosides on stimulated or mature coronary collaterals have not been reported. In addition, studies that relate to the effects of the cardiac glycosides on large coronary vessels have not been reported.

Clinicians have often noted that digitalis decreases the severity of angina in patients with coexistent heart failure and has no effect on or occasionally increases angina in patients with coronary heart disease and normal left ventricular function [29]. No data are available concerning the effects of digitalis preparations on the perfusion of ischemic myocardium in patients in the presence or absence of congestive heart failure.

Methylxanthines

The methylxanthines (caffeine, theophylline, and theobromine) are related alkaloids that have effects on many physiologic functions [30]. Aminophylline is the most commonly used methylxanthine in the treatment of patients with cardiovascular disease. It is a combination of theophylline and ethylenediamine. Ethylenediamine is biologically inert but serves to increase the solubility of theophylline. The actions of the methylxanthines include central nervous system stimulation, smooth muscle relaxation, stimulation of secretion from several endocrine and exocrine tissues, and promotion of water and electrolyte excretion by the kidney [30].

The actions of the methylxanthines on the cardiovascular system are modulated by direct and indirect effects of these compounds. By promoting the release of catecholamines and thereby activating $alpha_1$, $beta_1$, and $beta_2$ receptors, the methylxanthines indirectly alter many functional characteristics of the cardiovascular system [31–33]. By directly increasing myocardial contractility and relaxing vascular smooth muscle, the methylxanthines exert significant influences on cardiovascular function [30,32,33].

Since 1929, the effects of aminophylline on the coronary circulation have been studied in animals [33–40] and humans [41]. Although it has been generally

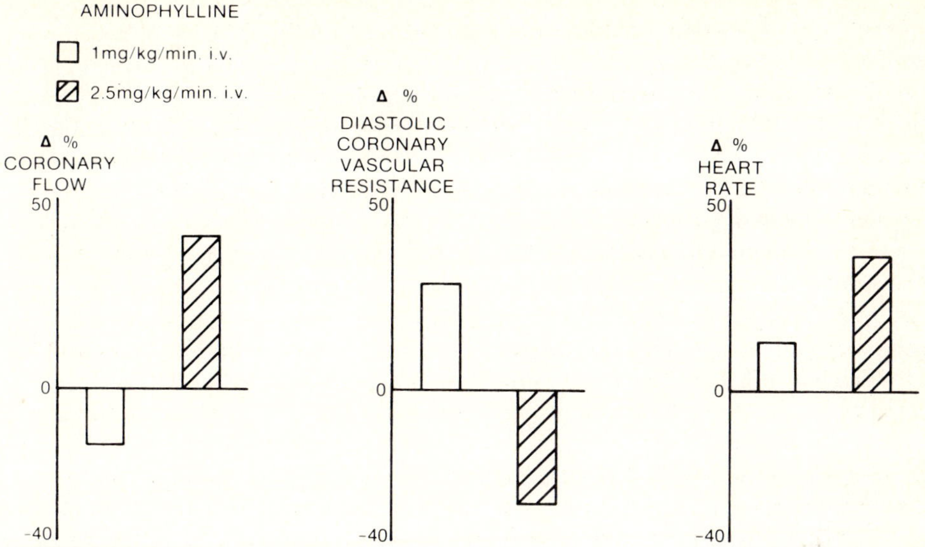

FIGURE 22-3
Effects of low-dose (1 mg/kg/min IV) and high-dose (2.5 mg/kg/min IV) aminophylline on coronary hemodynamics and heart rate in conscious dogs. Low doses of aminophylline produce small increases in heart rate and coronary constriction; high doses are associated with substantial tachycardia and coronary dilation. Δ % = percent change. (*Based on data originally presented by JD Rutherford et al* [33].)

concluded that the net effect of aminophylline is to cause coronary dilation [34–40], it is now clear that the directional effects of aminophylline on coronary vascular resistance are dose-dependent [33] (Figure 22-3). At relatively low doses of aminophylline that produce little or no tachycardia the drug increases coronary vascular resistance [33,41]. This occurs because in this dose range the dominant factor influencing the action of aminophylline on coronary vascular resistance is an increase in alpha-adrenergic stimulation [33]. Doses of aminophylline that are sufficient to produce substantial tachycardia are invariably associated with increases in coronary blood flow and decreases in coronary vascular resistance [33–40]. The coronary dilation occurs as a consequence of several actions. Activation of $beta_1$ receptors (see Chapter 5) [33] and augmentation of myocardial contractility by direct means [32,33] both lead to an increase in myocardial oxygen consumption [35], and this indirectly produces coronary dilation (see Chapter 3). By stimulating the release of epinephrine, aminophylline stimulates $beta_2$ receptors in coronary vessels and, thereby, relaxation of coronary smooth muscle. This response promotes coronary vasodilation. These combined dilator influences overshadow the two coronary vasoconstrictor actions that occur concomitantly, that is, increased alpha-adrenergic tone [33] and increased extravascular compressive forces (see Chapter 4). The coronary dilation that occurs with moderate doses of aminophylline is associated with an increase in coronary sinus oxygen saturation [34].

Many questions that relate to the effects of aminophylline on the coronary circulation have not been addressed. These include the effects of this drug on large and small coronary vessels, native and mature coronary collaterals, and the transmural distribution of left ventricular perfusion. Also, little is know about the effects of aminophylline on the coronary circulation of human beings [41].

Aminophylline has one action that is very unusual: it specifically antagonizes the effects of exogenous adenosine [42–48]. As a consequence, aminophylline severely attenuates the prominent coronary vasodilator effects of exogenous adenosine and dipyridamole [42–48]. Surprisingly, most studies indicate that either aminophylline does not influence the actions of endogenous adenosine [44–46] or endogenous adenosine plays a minimal role in the regulation of coronary vascular resistance [44–46]. The controversy concerning this area is discussed more fully in Chapter 3.

Dobutamine

By systematically modifying the chemical structure of isoproterenol, Tuttle and Mills [49] developed a synthetic catecholamine which acts primarily as a potent inotropic agent. Dobutamine stimulates $beta_1$,$beta_2$, and $alpha_1$ receptors but does not induce neural or adrenal release of catecholamines [49–54]. Furthermore, dobutamine does not interact with dopaminergic receptors [53]. Unlike isoproterenol, dobutamine's potent inotropic effects are not accompanied by significant tachycardia or peripheral vasodilation [49–54]. The remarkably modest tachycardia associated with dobutamine's potent inotropic effects has been partly attributed to activation of the baroreceptor reflex [54,55] and may be partly related to the selective effects of dobutamine on sinus node $beta_1$ receptors versus myocardial $beta_1$ receptors [51]. The alpha-adrenergic effects of dobutamine are minor compared with those of norepinephrine [49,52–54].

The effects of dobutamine on the coronary circulation have been studied in animals [54–59] and human beings [60,61]. By stimulating $beta_1$ receptors, dobutamine increases myocardial contractility and heart rate and thereby increases myocardial oxygen consumption [55,57,61]. This indirectly produces coronary dilation (Figure 22-4) (see Chapter 3). In addition, dobutamine activates $beta_2$ and $alpha_1$ receptors in the coronary circulation (Figure 22-4) [54,55,57]. The net effect of these actions is that progressively increasing doses of dobutamine infused intravenously produces a substantial augmentation of coronary flow and a significant diminution in coronary vascular resistance [54–61]. In normal dogs, the increase in coronary flow that occurs in response to dobutamine administration is accompanied by a significant increase in coronary sinus O_2 saturation [55,57,59].

Dobutamine does not alter the transmural distribution of left ventricular perfusion [59]. Also, dobutamine tends to maintain [56] or slightly improve perfusion to ischemic myocardium [59]. Furthermore, this drug may limit infarct size [59].

The effects of dobutamine on large conduit coronary vessels have not been reported. Furthermore, sophisticated studies that relate to the effects of dobutamine on flow through native or mature coronary collateral vessels are unavailable.

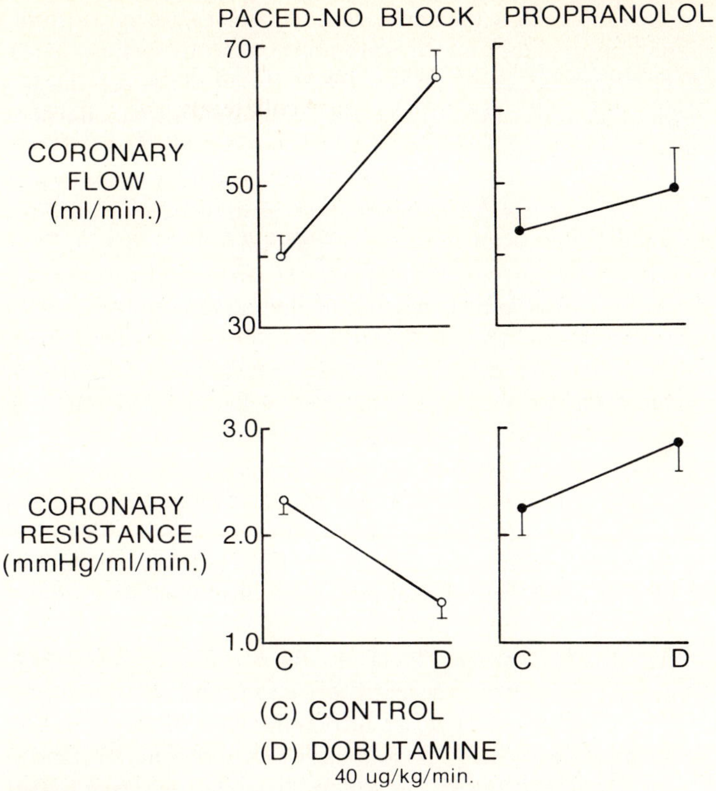

FIGURE 22-4
Effects of intravenous dobutamine on coronary hemodynamics in conscious dogs. Dobutamine produces net coronary dilation. If beta-adrenergic receptors are blocked by propranolol, dobutamine produces coronary constriction because of activation of alpha-adrenergic receptors in coronary vessels. Paced-no block = hearts were paced to keep heart rate constant during control and dobutamine and no blocking agents were administered. C = control; D = dobutamine 40 μg/kg/min. (*Redrawn from data originally presented by SF Vatner et al* [54].)

Endogenous Catecholamines

The effects of the three endogenous catecholamines (epinephrine, norepinephrine, and dopamine) on the coronary circulation have been described in Chapter 8.

NITROGLYCERIN

In 1879, Murrel suggested that nitroglycerin might possibly be of value in the treatment of angina pectoris [1]. Although there is no doubt about the effectiveness of nitroglycerin in angina, some controversy about its mechanism of action persists. Much of the argument concerning the hemodynamic effects of nitroglycerin can be resolved if one recognizes that the biphasic effects of the drug are time-dependent and modulated appreciably by the autonomic nervous system. In addition, the overall effect of nitroglycerin on the coronary circulation is largely dependent on the peripheral actions of the drug rather than on its direct effects on coronary smooth muscle.

When nitroglycerin is administered sublingually or intravenously to an awake, normal dog, coronary flow increases by 50 to 75 percent within the first minute and coronary vascular resistance declines substantially (Figure 22-5) [62]. Within 3 to 5 min following administration of nitroglycerin, coronary flow is normal or decreased and coronary vascular resistance is normal or increased (Figure 22-5). A similar biphasic pattern of response also occurs in the systemic circulation (total cardiac output, mesenteric, renal, and iliac beds [62]). Simultaneously, arterial pressure and left ventricular dimensions fall and then rise, whereas left ventricular *dp/dt* and heart rate rise and then fall. *For decades the striking, biphasic nature of the circulatory response to nitroglycerin has served as a source of confusion to investigators in this area.* The initial segment of the biphasic response primarily reflects the direct effects of nitroglycerin on vascular smooth muscle. Nitroglycerin relaxes smooth muscle by inhibiting the slow Ca^{2+} inward current [63]. The second phase of the response is modulated by reflex mechanisms and can be markedly attenuated by section of the carotid sinus, aortic, and vagal nerves [62].

Nitroglycerin exerts its effects at several levels in the coronary vascular bed. Three types of studies indicate that nitroglycerin dilates large conductive coronary vessels. Following administration of nitroglycerin intravenously or intracoronarily, large vessel coronary resistance decreases [2–4] and large vessel coronary diameter enlarges as measured by angiography [64–67] or sonomicrometers [68] (see Figure 1-3). The increase in coronary cross-sectional area can be as much as 30 to 50 percent [64–68]. Coronary arteries as small as 0.5 mm in diameter and coronary vessels that are collateral-dependent dilate in response to nitrates [66]. Studies by Brown et al. [67] indicate that stenotic coronary segments dilate almost as much as normal segments in response to nitroglycerin. This probably occurs because the atherosclerotic plaque that produces the coronary obstruction is not completely circumferential. This allows the normal segment of the wall to respond to pharmacologic dilation. It is notable that the large vessel diameter response to nitroglycerin may persist for 45 min, whereas the increase in coronary flow is transitory [62,68].

The brief increase in coronary flow that occurs in response to nitrates is due in part to the dilation of small coronary resistance vessels [2–4,62,68,69]. In addition, changes in coronary flow in response to nitroglycerin's effect on cardiac metabolism and the autonomic nervous system are also mediated by the small resistance coronary vessels [70,71].

Many studies suggest that nitroglycerin dilates coronary collateral vessels [72–93]. In dogs without preexisting coronary obstruction, resistance via native or unstimulated collaterals is only slightly decreased by nitroglycerin [72–79,81–83, 85–87]. This small change, which is not consistent [80,84], may result from alterations in the extravascular compressive forces (see Chapter 10). Studies in patients

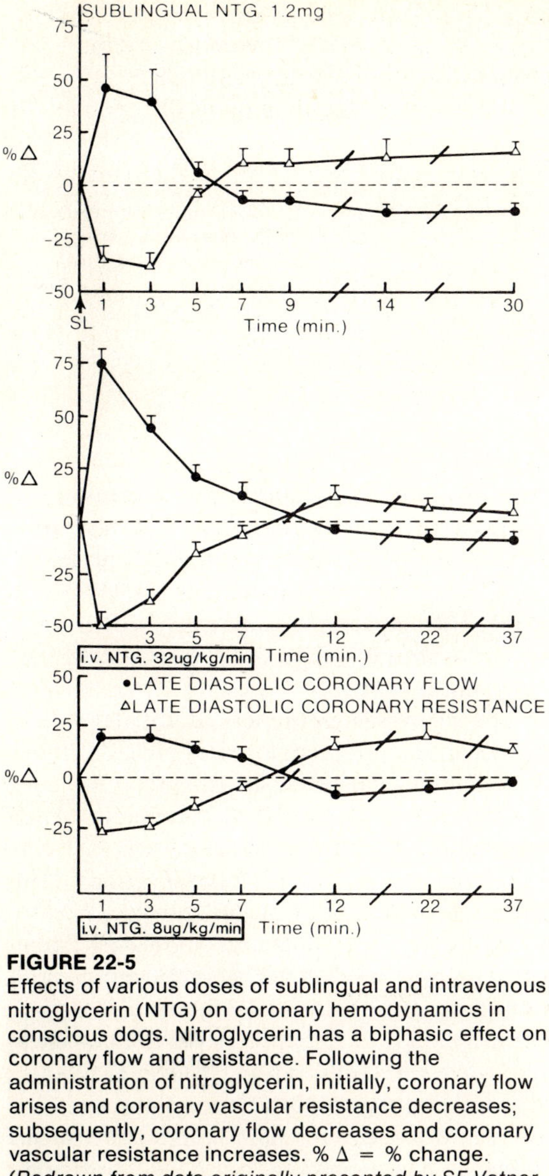

FIGURE 22-5
Effects of various doses of sublingual and intravenous nitroglycerin (NTG) on coronary hemodynamics in conscious dogs. Nitroglycerin has a biphasic effect on coronary flow and resistance. Following the administration of nitroglycerin, initially, coronary flow arises and coronary vascular resistance decreases; subsequently, coronary flow decreases and coronary vascular resistance increases. % Δ = % change. (*Redrawn from data originally presented by SF Vatner et al* [62].)

have yielded similar results [76]. In contrast, mature or stimulated collaterals dilate substantially in response to nitroglycerin [78,89,91–93]. Studies by Goldstein et al. [92] are of particular importance. These investigators demonstrated that collateral channels in patients with chronic ischemic heart disease dilate substantially following the administration of nitroglycerin [92].

In addition to altering conductance in large arteries, small resistance vessels,

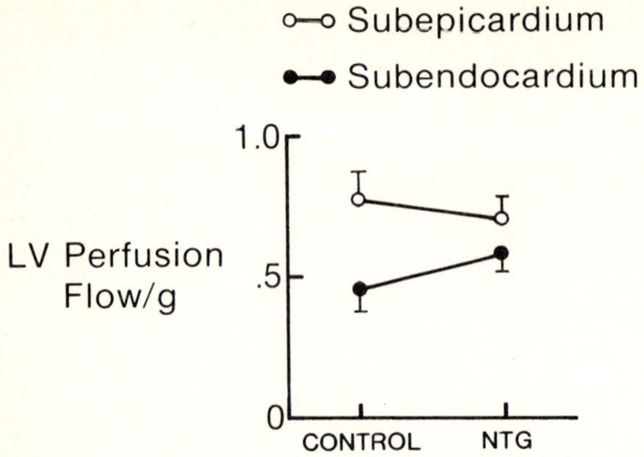

FIGURE 22-6
Effects of intravenous nitroglycerin (NTG) on the transmural distribution of left ventricular (LV) perfusion in moderately ischemic myocardium of conscous dogs. Following administration of nitroglycerin, subepicardial flow decreases slightly and subendocardial flow increases significantly. (*Based on data originally presented by JL Swain et al* [88].)

and collateral channels, nitroglycerin also alters the transmural distribution of myocardial perfusion. In normally perfused myocardium, nitroglycerin has equivocal effects on the transmural distribution of left ventricular perfusion [81–83,86,88]. In ischemic myocardium perfused via native [81,84–88] or stimulated [89,93] collaterals, however, nitroglycerin significantly redistributes flow toward the left ventricular subendocardium (Figure 22-6). Although the mechanism of this redistribution is unclear, it probably represents either a selective pharmacologic effect of nitroglycerin on vessels in the left ventricular subendocardium or alterations in the extravascular compressive forces induced by nitroglycerin which favor perfusion of the subendocardium (see Chapter 10).

The predominant mechanism by which nitroglycerin relieves angina is related to the cause of the angina. If angina is secondary to metabolic stress, such as pacing in a patient with severe fixed coronary obstructions, the peripheral actions of nitroglycerin are predominantly responsible for the relief of the chest discomfort. Under such conditions (angina induced by pacing), Ganz and Marcus [94] demonstrated that intracoronary nitroglycerin was ineffective, whereas intravenous nitroglycerin promptly relieved the angina. If angina is secondary to coronary vasospasm, intracoronary nitroglycerin is equal to or more effective than intravenous nitroglycerin in ameliorating the chest discomfort (see Chapter 12).

In addition to relieving myocardial ischemia, nitroglycerin may also decrease infarct size [86,95–100]. Data in this regard are controversial and subject to the criticisms discussed in Chapter 9 concerning pharmacologic approaches to altering infarct size.

BETA BLOCKERS

In 1948, Ahlquist [101] postulated the existence of two distinct types of adrenergic receptors, alpha and beta. Ten years later, the first beta-receptor antagonist, dichloroisoproterenol, was synthesized by Powell and Slater [102]. Propranolol, the first clinically useful beta blocker, was introduced by Black et al. [103]

in 1964. Since then, many drugs with beta-blocking activity have become available [104]. The newer beta blockers differ with respect to the following properties: specificity (selective $beta_1$ blockers vs. $beta_1$ and $beta_2$ blockers), intrinsic sympathomimetic activity, nonspecific membrane stabilizing effects, primary route of metabolism (renal vs. hepatic), and solubility (hydrophilic vs. lipophilic) [104]. Because propranolol is the beta blocker that has been most extensively studied, this section will be restricted to the effects of propranolol on the coronary circulation.

Effects on Coronary Blood Flow in Normal Myocardium

Because propranolol is a competitive antagonist, its effects markedly depend on the existing level of sympathetic tone. In young, healthy subjects [105] and in awake, well-conditioned dogs [106], sympathetic tone is minimal. Under these conditions, propranolol has minimal effects on hemodynamics, myocardial oxygen consumption, or coronary blood flow. If sympathetic tone is increased in a normal cardiovascular system, propranolol will decrease heart rate, myocardial contractility, systolic blood pressure, and cardiac output and will slightly increase ventricular filling pressure and ventricular volume (Figure 22-7) [105,107–117]. The net effect of these perturbations will be to limit increases in myocardial oxygen consumption and coronary flow in response to increases in sympathetic stimulation (Figure 22-8) [117a]. The magnitude of the decrement in myocardial oxygen consumption and coronary flow will depend on the level of sympathetic tone and the dose of the beta blocker administered.

Following acute administration of propranolol to subjects at rest, arterial pressure changes are usually modest [105,107–114]. Long-term administration of propranolol decreases arterial pressure, particularly if hypertension is present [118].

Because changes in myocardial oxygen consumption are closely coupled to changes in coronary vascular resistance (see Chapter 3), when beta blockers are administered in the presence of significant symphathetic tone, coronary flow decreases and calculated coronary vascular resistance increases [116]. Most studies indicate that propranolol does not change the transmural distribution of left ventricular perfusion in normal animals [119,120]. The effects of propranolol on the resistance of large and small coronary arteries have not been reported. Although propranolol blocks the mild coronary dilation that occurs in response to $beta_2$ stimulation (see Chapter 5), the clinical importance of this effect is probably minimal.

Effects on Coronary Blood Flow in Ischemic Myocardium

In many ways, the effects of beta blockade on myocardial function and perfusion of ischemic muscle are the opposite of those observed in normal myocardium [82,84,88,119–125]. For example, function of acutely ischemic myocardium is either unchanged or increased by beta blockade [82,84,88,119–125]. Furthermore, perfusion of the ischemic subendocardium of the left ventricle is often improved

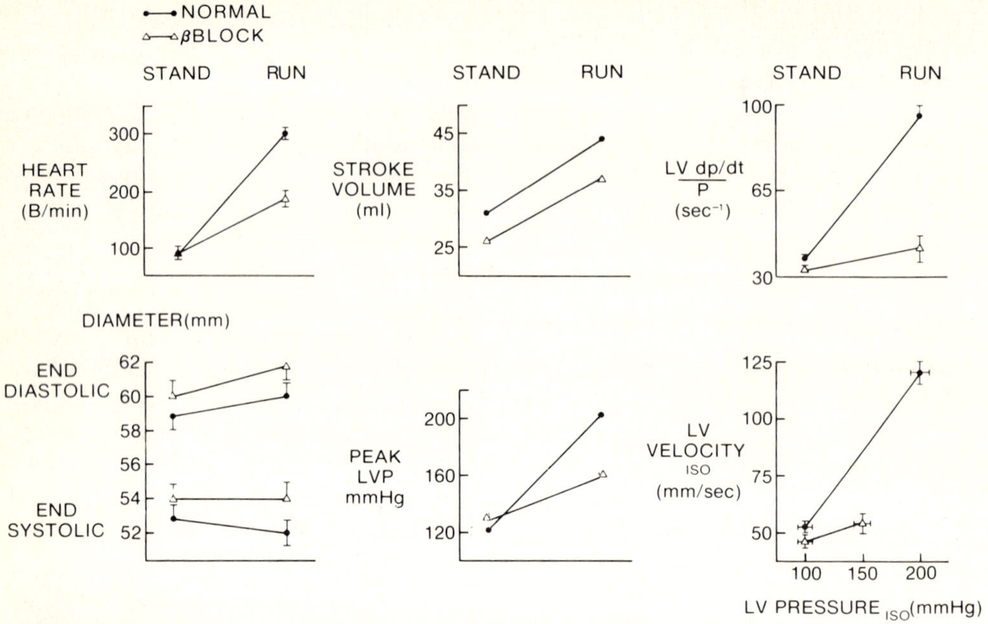

FIGURE 22-7
Effects of beta blockade (β block) on hemodynamic responses to intense exercise in dogs. Beta blockade, decreased heart rate, stroke volume, peak left ventricular pressure (LVP), and two indices of myocardial contractility (left ventricular, LV, $\frac{dp/dt}{P}$) and LV velocity (mm/s) that occur in response to exercise. However, left ventricular end-systolic and end-diastolic diameters both at rest and during exercise were increased during beta blockade. Stand = dog standing quietly; run = maximal exercise; B/min = beats per minute; diameter mm = left ventricular diameter in millimeters. (*Redrawn from data originally presented by SF Vatner et al* [*116*].)

by the administration of propranolol [82,84,88,119–125]. Finally, metabolic indices of ischemia often improve following beta blockade [126]. If perfusion to the myocardium is blunted by a coronary obstructive lesion, beta blockade almost always either prevents ischemia from developing during stress or limits the severity of ischemia that does develop [104,109,112,117].

The effects of beta blockade on mature coronary collateral vessels have not been evaluated. However, Neill et al. [127] have shown that chronic administration of propranolol to dogs does not limit the development of collateral vessels in response to an ischemic stress.

Other Effects That Could Alter Myocardial Perfusion or Oxygenation

Scattered reports suggest that propranolol has many ancillary effects which could modulate myocardial perfusion or oxygenation. For example, under some condi-

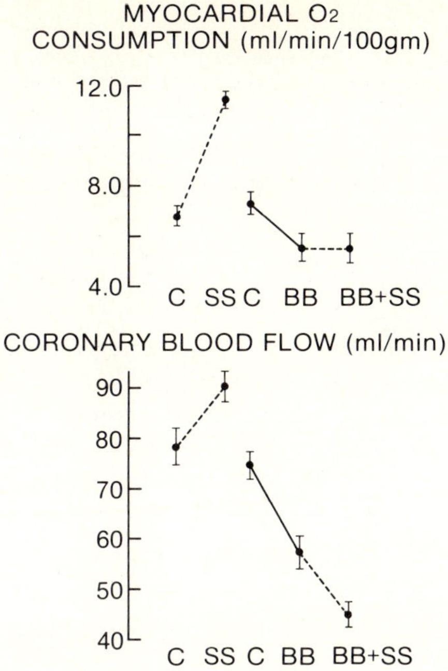

FIGURE 22-8
Effects of sympathetic stimulation (SS) on myocardial oxygen (O_2) consumption and coronary blood flow before and after beta blockade (BB) with propranolol in dogs on right heart bypass. Sympathetic stimulation was produced by electrically stimulating the right stellate ganglion (5 Hz, 15 v, 2 ms). During sympathetic stimulation, myocardial oxygen consumption increased and coronary blood flow increased substantially. During beta blockade, sympathetic stimulaton had no effect on myocardial oxygen consumption and decreased coronary blood flow probably because of alpha-adrenergic coronary constriction. C = control. (*Redrawn from data originally presented by WG Nayler and V Carson [117a].*)

tions, beta blockade can alter myocardial substrate utilization in a manner that would conserve oxygen (increase carbohydrate utilization and decrease lipid uptake) [128]. Also, propranolol decreases platelet aggregation [129], favorably shifts the oxygen-hemoglobin dissociation curve [130], decreases renin levels [118], and may decrease left ventricular mass under some conditions [131]. A recent study suggests that beta blockade decreases oxygen extraction across the myocardium and may tend to minimize microregional heterogeneity of oxygen extraction in both normal and ischemic myocardium [125]. Although all these various effects of propranolol are interesting, their relative importance remains to be defined.

Finally, many studies suggest that beta blockade may decrease infarct size or prevent recurrent infarction or sudden death in patients who have survived a myocardial infarction [132,133]. Investigations that relate to infarct size modification by propranolol have been associated with many problems (see Chapter 10). The mechanism by which long-term beta blockade prevents recurrent infarction or sudden death awaits definition.

Although there are many mechanisms by which propranolol could favorably influence the perfusion and oxygenation of ischemic myocardium, this drug's salutary actions in patients with angina probably occur because (1) myocardial oxygen consumption decreases, (2) extravascular compression of coronary vessels is attenuated, and (3) perfusion may redistribute toward the ischemic subendocardium of the left ventricle.

POTENT CORONARY VASODILATORS

Many endogenous (see Chapter 8) and exogenous coronary dilators (papavarine, dipyridamole, and carbochromen) can produce intense coronary dilation; however, only three potent coronary dilators—adenosine, dypridamole, and carbochromen—are frequently employed. When administered in sufficient dosage, each of these drugs can produce maximal coronary dilation. Specific characteristics of these three agents are listed in Table 22-1 (Figure 22-9).

Adenosine causes intense dilation in many vascular beds [42,43] (see Chapter 8). Therefore, intravenous administration of this drug to conscious animals produces marked systemic hypotension and reflex tachycardia [135,138,139] (See Table 22-1 and Figure 22-9). If reflex mechanisms are impaired, adenosine can produce striking bradycardia by its direct action on the SA and AV nodes [42,43]. Also, at intermediate doses, adenosine strikingly increases the subendocardial/subepicardial ratio of left ventricular perfusion [135]. Because of the hypotensive effects of adenosine, it is not utilized clinically to produce maximal coronary dilation. Although adenosine primarily dilates small resistance coronary vessels [63], it also dilates larger conduit coronary arteries [151a].

FIGURE 22-9
Diagrammatic presentation of the effects of three potent coronary dilators (dypridamole, carbochromen, and adenosine) on coronary flow and mean arterial pressure. Each drug has been hypothetically infused intravenously for a similar time period (drug administration) in a dose that would produce maximal coronary dilation (maximal). The diagram emphasizes that the time course of changes in coronary blood flow and mean arterial pressure and the magnitude of the changes in mean arterial pressure produced by these three potent coronary dilators vary considerably. Time Min = time in minutes. (For additional details and references see Table 22-1.)

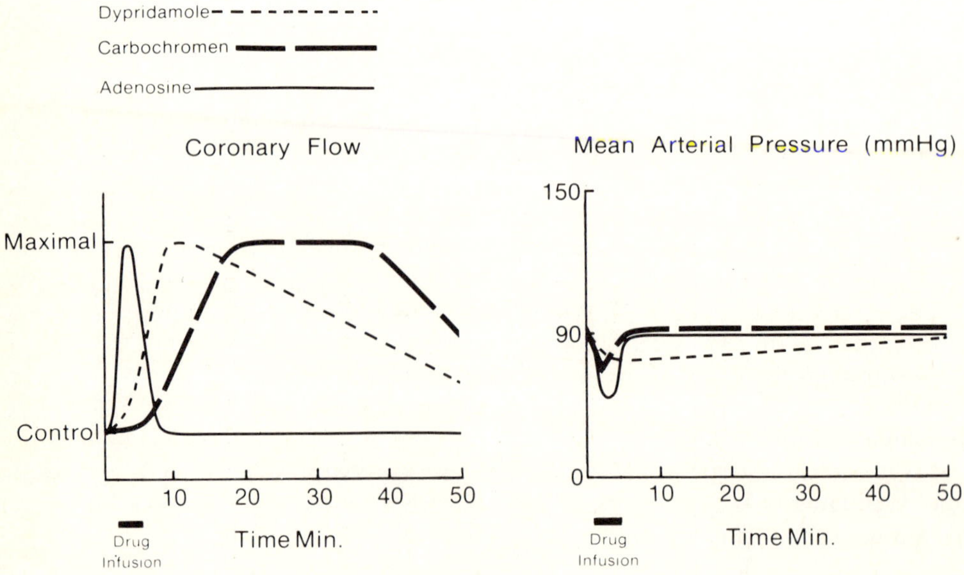

TABLE 22-1
CHARACTERISTICS OF POTENT CORONARY DILATORS

Dilator	Time to peak response following onset of IV administration, min	Duration of action (half-life) following cessation of infusion, min	Dose required for maximal coronary dilation, IV administration	Hemodynamic effects at maximal coronary dilation		Alterations in myocardial oxygen consumption at peak dilation	Transmural left ventricular perfusion at maximal coronary dilation, endocardial/epicardial flow ratio, %
				Heart rate, beats/min	Arterial pressure, mmHg		
Adenosine	1–4	1.5–2.5	4.5–9.0 μM/kg/min IV	↑20–60	↓20–50	+/–	↓10–20
Dipyridamole	2–6	30–40	0.12–0.25 mg/kg/min IV	↑10–15	↓10	↓20% (?)	↓10–20
Carbochromen	5–20	40	Bolus 7–10 mg/kg IV	↑5	↓5	+/–	↓10–20

Source: The data summarized in this table are based upon published reports for adenosine [42,43,134–142], dipyridamole [44,45,47,48,142–151a], and carbochromen [152–161], the author's experience, and the unpublished experience of F Klocke, Professor of Medicine, University of Buffalo, and G Gross, Professor of Pharmacology, Medical College of Wisconsin.

Dipyridamole is a relatively selective coronary dilator. In awake dogs or patients, infusion of the drug has only modest effects on systemic pressure [47,48,146–151] (see Table 22-1 and Figure 22-9). In anesthetized dogs, administration of dipyridamole in doses sufficient to produce maximal coronary dilation is usually associated with significant hypotension [148]. Dipyridamole has two specific advantages when used to produce maximal coronary dilation in human beings. First, the coronary dilation produced is reasonably well sustained (half-life = 33 min) [48] (see Table 22-1, Figure 22-9). Therefore, maximal coronary flow in response to drug administration is sufficiently sustained to be measured with a washout technique (see Chapter 2). Second, the safety of intravenous dipyridamole in doses that produce intense coronary dilation is based on experience with hundreds of patients with heart disease. In 99 percent of patients, side effects are mild, transient in nature, or nonexistent [47,48,146–151]. In the occasional patient who develops severe nausea, chest pain, or hypotension, the action of dipyridamole can be abruptly terminated by administration of an antidote intravenous aminophylline (125 to 250 mg IV) [44,45,48,149,150] (see the section in this chapter on methyxanthines).

Recent studies suggest that dipyridamole dilates both large and small vessels [151a].

Carbochromen has the smallest effect on systemic hemodynamics and is the most selective coronary dilator in this group [152–160] (Table 22-1, Figure 22-9). Unfortunately, the time to peak effect of this drug is variable. As a consequence, when carbochromen is used, coronary flow must be monitored continuously and repeated reactive hyperemic responses (see Chapter 3) must be performed to demonstrate that coronary dilation is maximal. Also, experience with intravenous administration of this drug in humans to produce intense coronary dilation is limited [160]. Although the drug in oral form has been used in the treatment of angina [161], the efficacy of this antianginal agent is open to serious question.

The effects of carbochromen on large coronary vessels have not been reported.

Although none of the potent coronary dilators is ideal for application in experimental or clinical research, these agents provide investigators with several alternative pharmacologic approaches to producing maximal coronary dilation. None of the potent coronary dilators in their intravenous form has been approved for clinical use in the United States. These drugs are available only for investigational applications.

POTENT CORONARY VASOCONSTRICTORS

The actions of the potent coronary vasoconstrictors (vasopressin, thromboxane A_2, angiotensin II) have been described in Chapter 8.

CALCIUM CHANNEL BLOCKERS

The calcium antagonists or calcium channel blockers have recently become available in the United States for clinical use. The prototype drug in this class, verapamil, was introduced in 1962 [162]. However, the ability of verapamil to block slow calcium channels was not known until 1969 [163]. The clinical applications of calcium blockers have been extensively reviewed [164–175].

The effects of the calcium channel blockers on the coronary circulation are exceedingly complex because these agents influence numerous factors that indirectly modulate coronary vascular resistance (heart rate myocardial contractility, arterial pressure, and autonomic tone) [164–175]. In addition, the calcium blockers have direct effect at various levels in the coronary vascular tree (large vessels, small resistance channels, and collaterals) [164–175]. The interactions of the calcium channel blockers on the coronary circulation are further complicated by: (1) the vasodilator, chronotropic, dromotropic, and inotropic effects of the calcium blockers become manifest at different drug concentrations [164–175], and these relationships vary among the various calcium blockers [164–175]; (2) the rate of onset and duration of action on different segments of the coronary vasculature vary considerably when calcium blockers are administered [176]; (3) the net effect of the calcium channel blockers on the coronary circulation are remarkably altered in the presence of pathophysiologic states (see below).

To understand the actions of the calcium antagonists on the coronary circulation in a comprehensive manner, it is instructive to begin with the effects of these agents in simple, relatively isolated systems and then progress to pathological states.

Effects in Isolated Systems

The slow inward calcium current influences the function of cardiac myocytes and excitable tissues in the heart (SA node, AV node, Purkinje fibers) [163,177,177a]. The role of the slow calcium current in vascular smooth muscle is less well defined [163,174,177–179]

When isolated tissue preparations are exposed to calcium channel blockers, the following actions are noted: myocardial contractility declines [166], vascular smooth muscle relaxes [165,166,180], SA node discharge rate is diminished [181], and AV node conduction time is prolonged [181] (Figure 22-10). In isolated systems, the effects of nifedipine and verapamil on coronary smooth muscle and AV nodal conduction are 10 to 100 times more potent than their depressant effects on myocardial contractility and heart rate (see Figure 22-10).

Effects of Intracoronary Injection

By examining the effects of intracoronary administration of calcium channel blockers, one can partially dissociate the cardiac actions of these agents from their peripheral actions [182–185]. In normal hearts, intracoronary administration of verapamil or nifedipine causes a substantial decrease in myocardial contractility and little or no change in heart rate [185]. In addition, intracoronary administration of verapamil does not alter systemic arterial pressure [185]. When intracoronary nifedipine is administered, coronary sinus oxygen saturation rises strikingly

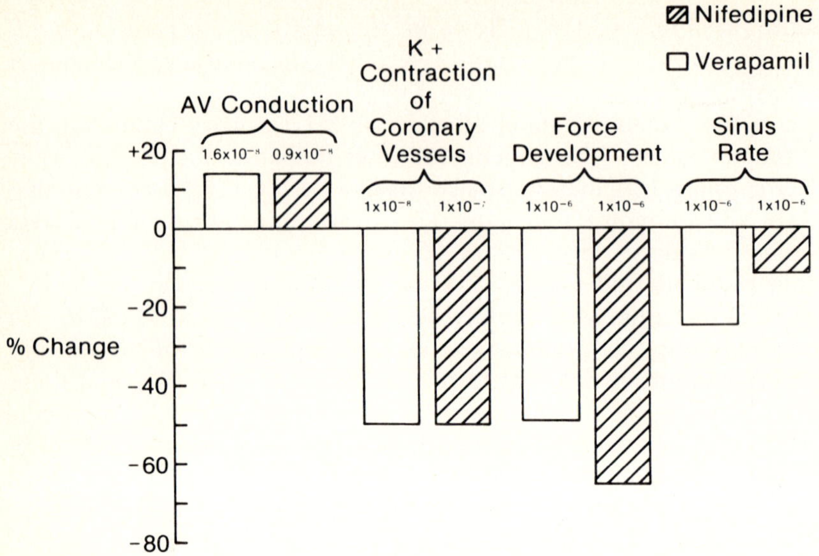

FIGURE 22-10
Effects of two calcium channel blockers (nifedipine and verapamil) on four aspects of cardiovascular function: AV conduction, coronary dilation, forced development in the myocardium, and sinus rate. All data were obtained in relatively isolated systems. Note that the drug concentrations necessary to produce significant effects on forced development and sinus rate are 10 to 100 times greater than those necessary to produce significant effects on AV conduction and relaxation of coronary smooth muscle. AV = atrioventricular node. (*Based on data obtained from several studies* [*166,180,181*].)

and then returns to control within minutes [182]. In addition, intracoronary administration of calcium antagonists induces the large coronary arteries to dilate slightly [164,165].

Effects of Systemic Administration

When calcium antagonists are given systemically, the direct cardiac effects (negative inotropic, chronotropic, and dromotropic responses) are blunted by peripheral actions of the drugs and reflex phenomena (Figure 22-11). [185–192]. Both verapamil and nifedipine produce peripheral vasodilation, which is associated with modest decreases in arterial pressure [176,182,185–192] (Figure 22-11). It should be noted, however, that the coronary dilator effects of the calcium channel blockers are considerably more potent than their vasodilator effects in other vascular beds [165]. The decrease in systemic pressure that occurs in response to the calcium blockers decreases ventricular afterload and thereby improves ventricular performance. This effect then counterbalances the direct negative inotropic effect of the calcium blockers. By decreasing arterial pressure, the calcium antagonists also activate the baroreceptor reflex. As a consequence, sympathetic activity increases and vagal tone is withdrawn [185,187,190,192]. These effects improve

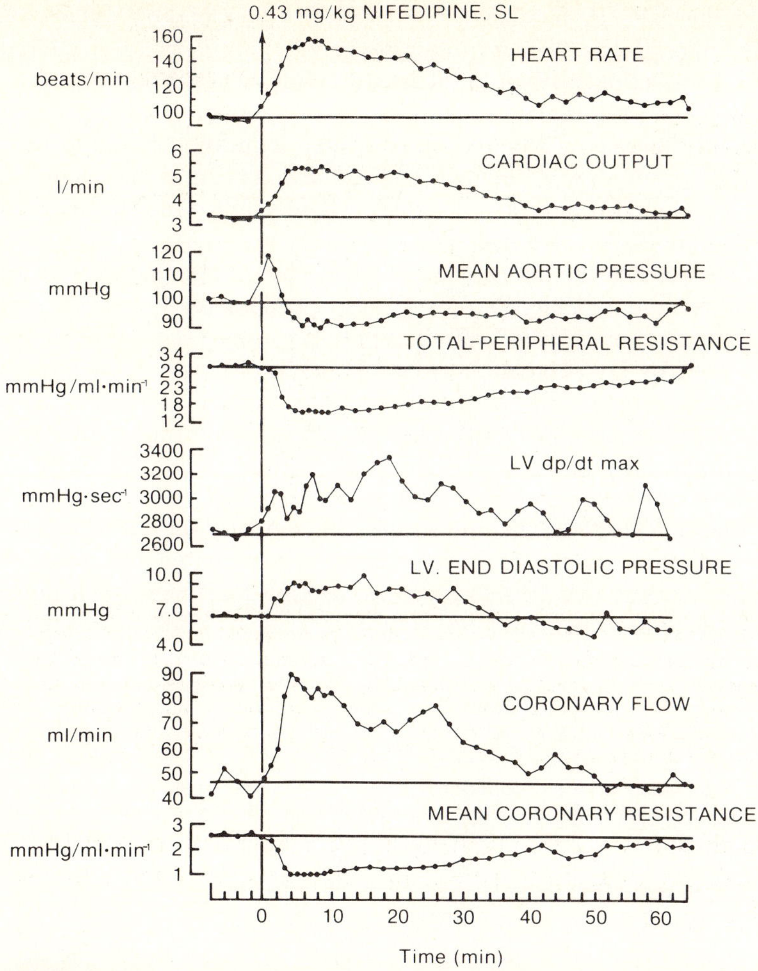

FIGURE 22-11
Effects of sublingual (SL) nifedipine on systemic and coronary hemodynamics in conscious dogs. Nifedipine increased heart rate, cardiac output, left ventricular (LV) *dp/dt* max, left ventricular end-diastolic pressure, and coronary flow. Simultaneously, nifedipine decreased aortic pressure, total peripheral resistance, and mean coronary resistance. *dp/dt* = maximal first derivative of LV pressure. (*Redrawn from data originally presented by R Gross et al* [*187*].)

ventricular performance and also tend to counteract the direct negative chronotropic and dromotropic actions of the calcium blockers [185,187,190].

The calcium blockers have one other important neural effect: they modify the gain of the baroreceptor reflex [193–195]. Nifedipine augments and verapamil diminishes the gain of the baroreceptor reflex [195].

The actions of the calcium blockers on the coronary circulation reflect the aggregate of these phenomena. When nifedipine or verapamil are administered systemically, in the absence of superimposed disease states, typically coronary flow rises transiently [176,186,187]. Intravenous infusions of verapamil, nifedipine, or diltiazem significantly increase coronary sinus oxygen saturation [182,186,188]. Following intravenous nifedipine, myocardial oxygen consumption decreases [191,195a]. Large conduit coronary arteries dilate slightly following intravenous injection of the calcium blockers [195b,195c].

It is important to note that the time course of the effects of the calcium channel blockers on coronary flow and large coronary vessel caliber are quite different [176]. Following intravenous injection of nifedipine (20 μg/kg IV) for example, coronary flow increases by 170 percent almost immediately (10 to 30 s) and returns to control levels in 15 min [176]. In contrast, large coronary artery diameter changes are maximal (increase 6 percent) 2 to 5 min following intravenous injection of nifedipine and persist for 45 min [176].

In normal animals intravenous administration of diltiazem has another action which warrants attention [196]. Bache and Dymek have demonstrated that, after transient coronary dilator responses to intravenous diltiazem abated, the coronary reactive hyperemic response to a 10-s coronary occlusion (debt/repayment ratio) was decreased as much as 50 percent [196] (Figure 22-12). It is not known if the decrease in vasodilator responsiveness is selective to ischemia or represents a

FIGURE 22-12
Effects of intravenous diltiazem on the coronary reactive hyperemic response in a conscious dog. The coronary reactive hyperemic response was substantially attenuated 30 min following administration of diltiazem. For definition of debt/repayment see Figure 3-10. (*Modified from a figure originally presented by RJ Bache and DJ Dymek* [*196*].)

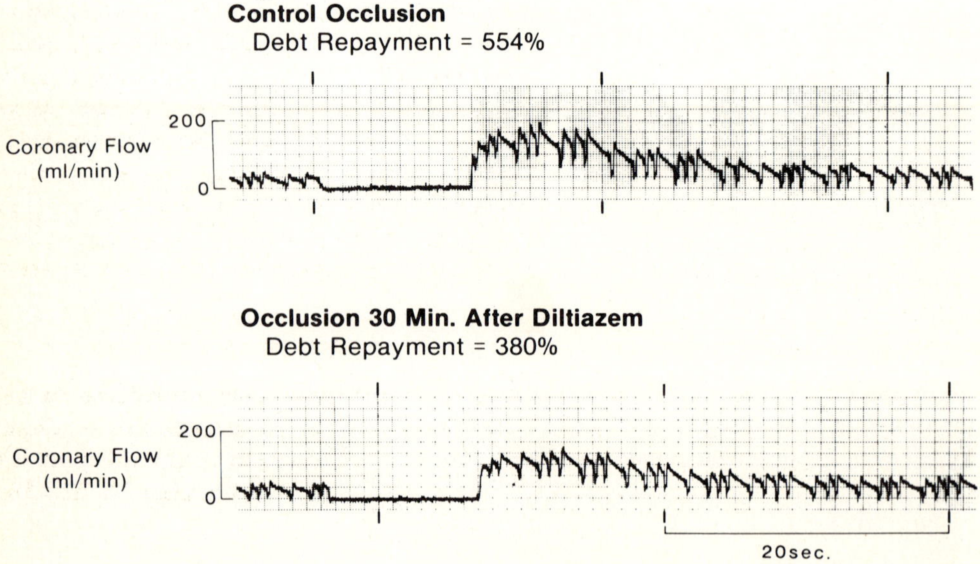

generalized decrease in responsiveness to all dilator stimuli (increases myocardial oxygen consumption, pharmacologic dilation). Furthermore, it is not known if other calcium channel blockers have a similar effect. The action of diltiazem on coronary reactive hyperemia is no longer present 2 h following intravenous administration of the drug [196].

When nifedipine is administered to normal animals, the transmural distribution of left ventricular perfusion is not altered [197,198].

Effects in the Presence of Pathological States

Because the net effect of calcium channel blockers on the coronary circulation depends on the interaction of several physiological systems, when these systems are altered by a disease process the net action of the calcium blockers is changed. This is particularly so with respect to seven pathological states: coronary spasm, myocardial ischemia, heart failure, atrial fibrillation, idiopathic hypertrophic subaortic stenosis, sick sinus node syndrome, and Wolf-Parkinson-White syndrome. Each will be described briefly.

Coronary Spasm Many clinical trials have demonstrated that the calcium channel blockers are extremely effective in the treatment of patients with coronary spasm [199–205]. Although calcium channel blockers cause slight dilation of large coronary vessels under normal conditions [195b,195c], they have much greater dilator effects when the large coronary arteries are constricted (Figure 22-13) [195c]. When coronary constriction occurs spontaneously or in response to pharmacologic or adrenergic stimulation, it is readily reversed by the calcium channel blockers [195c]. Also, calcium channel blockers effectively prevent recurrences of spontaneous coronary spasm or spasm induced by pharmacologic means [164–173,199–205].

Myocardial Ischemia In the presence of myocardial ischemia, the net actions of the calcium blockers are modified substantially. Although these drugs decrease ventricular function under normal conditions, the function of ischemic cardiac muscle improves following administration of the calcium blockers [172,197, 206,207]. The precise mechanisms responsible for this paradox are not clear. Calcium blockers may limit the intensity of ischemia that occurs when exercise stress is superimposed on ventricular muscle perfused by a coronary vessel with a fixed obstructive lesion. This would prevent the expected decline in ventricular performance. This effect is probably mediated by a decrease in myocardial oxygen consumption that often accompanies administration of calcium blockers [195a]. Thus, this action would favorably alter the supply/demand ratio in the ischemic zone. In addition, although calcium blockers do not alter the transmural distribution of left ventricular perfusion under normal conditions [197,198], in ischemic zones some studies suggest left ventricular perfusion redistributes toward the left ventricular subendocardium [196,198]. This effect, however, has not been consistently observed [197,208,209].

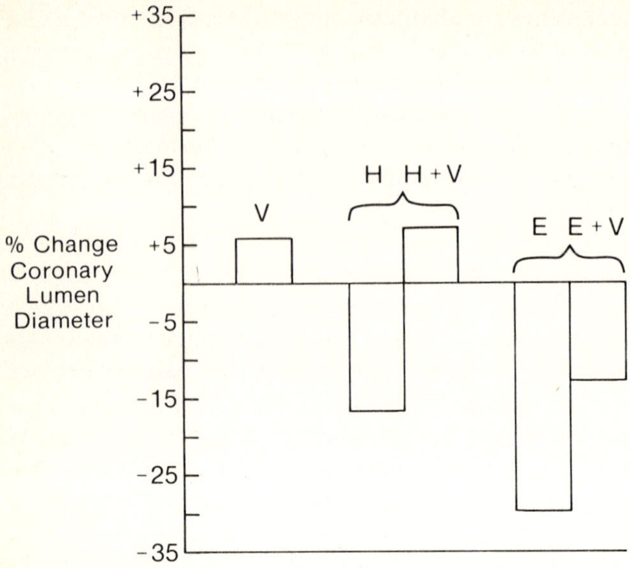

FIGURE 22-13
Effects of verapamil on coronary lumen diameter determined angiographically in patients. Coronary arteries examined were greater than 1.5 mm in diameter. Under control conditions intravenous verapamil increased coronary diameter slightly. However, when coronary constriction occurred in response to hand grip (H) or intravenous ergonovine (E), the coronary dilation produced by verapamil was augmented. *(Based on data presented by BG Brown et al* [195c].)

The coronary dilator properties of the calcium blockers also favorably influence the myocardium when it is subjected to a potentially ischemic stress. Although the calcium blockers may not significantly dilate native coronary collaterals [197,208, 209], these drugs presumably dilate mature coronary collaterals [210] and minimize superimposed spasm [164–175] if it coexists in the presence of a fixed coronary obstruction.

Many studies suggest that the calcium blockers may limit infarct size [198, 208,210–215]. Although the interpretation of this data is often controversial (see Chapter 10), one recent study indicates that the administration of calcium blockers several hours after coronary occlusion shifts the infarct-risk relationship in a favorable fashion [216]. Additional studies in this regard should be encouraged. Also, calcium channel blockers improve left ventricular diastolic function in patients with coronary disease [217]. This effect could decrease left ventricular diastolic pressure and thereby improve coronary driving pressure. This would improve perfusion to ischemic myocardium.

Thus, the calcium antagonists have a host of actions that in the main tend to favorably affect myocardial ischemia. Clinical studies suggest that multiple actions of these drugs probably contribute to the amelioration of myocardial ischemia in patients with coronary artery disease [164–173].

Heart Failure In the presence of heart failure, the effects of the calcium channel blockers are modified in several ways. First, if heart failure is severe (left ventricular ejection fraction less than 30 percent), the negative inotropic properties of the calcium blockers can precipitate profound left ventricular dysfunction and pulmonary edema [218,219]. If systemic pressure falls and left ventricular end diastolic pressure rises precipitously, coronary driving pressure can be critically compromised. This would adversely affect myocardial perfusion, particularly if severe coronary obstructions were present. Second, because reflex mechanisms are attenuated in patients with heart failure [220], this effect would tend to augment the direct negative inotropic, chronotropic, and dromotropic effects of the calcium blockers. This occurs because intact reflex mechanisms counterbalance these direct actions of the calcium antagonists. Third, in selected patient groups in whom heart failure. Direct measurements of coronary hemodynamics obtained when calcium favorably influence diastolic left ventricular function and thereby decrease left ventricular end diastolic pressure [221]. Theoretically, this effect would improve coronary driving pressure and may under some conditions improve myocardial perfusion. In view of the above, it is likely that the interaction between calcium antagonists and coronary hemodynamics is altered in the presence of cardiac failure. Direct measurements of coronary hemodynamics obtained when calcium blockers are administered to patients with heart failure are unavailable.

Atrial Fibrillation Because clinically relevant doses of some calcium blockers (verapamil) produce significant AV block, they slow the ventricular response in patients with atrial fibrillation [222]. Furthermore, unlike the digitalis glycosides, the calcium blockers limit the ventricular response in patients with atrial fibrillation both at rest and during exercise [222]. No doubt this dromotropic effect modifies coronary hemodynamics in patients with atrial fibrillation. In turn, this effect could contribute to the alleviation of angina in patients with coronary artery disease and atrial fibrillation. Studies that relate to the effects of calcium blockers on coronary hemodynamics in patients with atrial fibrillation have not been reported.

Idiopathic Hypertrophic Subaortic Stenosis The calcium blockers have several favorable effects in patients with idiopathic hypertrophic subaortic stenosis [175,221,223–225]. These include: (1) decreasing the severity of left ventricular outflow obstruction at rest and during provocative maneuvers [224], (2) diminishing myocardial contractility [175,224], and (3) improving left ventricular diastolic function [221]. These actions would all tend to modify coronary hemodynamics. Again, the effects of calcium blockers on coronary hemodynamics in patients with idiopathic hypertrophic subaortic stenosis have not been reported.

Sick Sinus Node Syndrome and Wolf-Parkinson-White Syndrome The arrhythmias associated with these syndromes can be exaggerated by calcium blockers [226,227]. One could therefore anticipate that these arrhythmias would modify coronary hemodynamics.

Other Interactions

Several drugs that are often prescribed for patients with heart disease or hypertension have important interactions with the calcium channel blockers. For example, the calcium channel blockers alter the renal excretion of digoxin and thereby increase serum levels of digoxin [228,229]. Since the digitalis glycosides have many effects on the coronary circulation, increasing the concentration of digoxin in the blood will augment these effects (see section on cardial glycosides). The beta blockers and calcium blockers share certain actions, that is, negative inotropic, chronotropic, and dromotropic effects. The additive effects of these agents can sometimes produce profound adverse responses such as heart failure or advanced AV block. It should be noted, however, that in patients with angina and normal left ventricular function, beta blockers and calcium antagonists can interact favorably and markedly ameliorate episodes of myocardial ischemia [230]. Finally, sympatholytic agents and anesthetics blunt the normal reflex responses to the administration of calcium blockers and thereby modify the net action of the calcium antagonists on the coronary circulation.

SUMMARY

Although much has been learned about the effects of the calcium channel blockers on the coronary circulation in the presence and absence of disease states, many important questions remain unanswered. No doubt, during the next 5 to 10 years, knowledge in this area will expand considerably.

REFERENCES

1 Murrel W: Nitro-glycerin as a remedy for angina pectoris. *Lancet* 1: 80, 1879.

2 Fam WM, McGregor M: Effect of nitroglycerin and dipyridamole on regional coronary resistance. *Circ Res* 22: 649, 1968.

3 Winbury MM, Howe BB, Hefner MA: Effect of nitrates and other coronary dilators on large and small coronary vessels: An hypothesis for the mechanism of action nitrates. *J Pharmacol Exp Ther* 168: 70, 1965.

4 Cohen MV Kirk ES: Differential response of large and small coronary arteries to nitroglycerin and angiotensin. *Circ Res* 33: 445, 1973.

4a Rahimtoola SH: Digitalis and William Withering, the clinical investigator. *Circulation* 52: 969, 1975.

5 Gilbert NC Fenn GK: Effect of digitalis on the coronary flow. *Arch Intern Med* 50: 668, 1932.

6 Coleman HN: Role of acetylstrophanthidin in augmenting myocardial oxygen consumption. *Circ Res* 21: 487, 1967.

7 Bellett S: Atrial fibrillation (clinical manifestations), in *Clinical Disorders of the Heart Beat* (3rd ed). Philadelphia, Lea & Febiger, 1971.

8 Gillis RA, Pearle DL, Levitt B: Digitalis: A neuroexcitatory drug. *Circulation* 52: 739, 1975.

9 Ross J Jr, Waldhsusen JA, Braunwald E: Studies on digitalis. I. Direct effects on peripheral vascular resistance. *J Clin Invest* 39: 930, 1960.

10 Stark JJ, Sanders CA, Powell W Jr: Neurally mediated and direct effects of acetylstrophanthidin on canine skeletal muscle vascular resistance. *Circ Res* 30: 274, 1972.

11 Levinsky RA, Lewis RM, Bynum TE, Hanley HG: Digoxin induced intestinal vasoconstriction. The effects of proximal arterial stenosis and glucagon administration. *Circulation* 52: 130, 1975.

12 Ferrer MI, Bradley SE, Wheeler HO, Enson Y, Preisig R, Harvey RM: The effect of digoxin in the splanchnic circulation in ventricular failure. *Circulation* 32: 524, 1965.

13 Vatner SF, Higgins CB, Franklin D, Braunwald E: Effects of a digitalis glycoside on coronary and systemic dynamics in conscious dogs. *Arch Pharmacol* 299: 61, 1977.

14 Bloor CM, Walker DE, Pensinger RR: Ouabain induced primary coronary vasoconstriction. *Proc Soc Exp Biol Med* 140: 1409, 1972.

15 Sagar KB, Hanson EC, Powell WJ Jr: Neurogenic coronary vasoconstrictor effects of digitalis during acute global ischemia in dogs. *J Clin Invest* 60: 1248, 1977.

16 Hamlin NP, Willerson JT, Garan H, Powell WJ Jr: The neurogenic vasoconstrictor effect of digitalis on coronary vascular resistance. *J Clin Invest* 53: 288, 1974.

17 Garan H, Smith TW, Powell WJ Jr: The central nervous system as a site of action for the coronary vasoconstrictor effect of digoxin. *J Clin Invest* 54: 1365, 1974.

18 Grun G, Weder U: Augmentation of coronary smooth muscle tone and sensitization to Ca^{++} by cardiac glycosides. *Arch Pharmacol* 282: 28, 1974.

19 Fleckenstein A, Fleckenstein-Grun G: Further studies on the neutralization of glycoside-induced contractures of coronary smooth muscle by Ca^{++}-antagonistic compounds. *Arch Pharmacol* 287: 38, 1975.

20 Vatner SF, Baig H: Comparison of the effects of ouabain and isoproterenol on ischemic myocardium of conscious dogs. *Circulation* 58: 654, 1978.

21 Vatner SF, Baig H, Manders WT, Murray PA: Effects of a cardiac glycoside in combination with propranolol on the ischemic heart of conscious dogs. *Circulation* 57: 568, 1978.

22 Zimpfer M, Schutz W, Raberger G: Haemodynamic and coronary actions of ouabain during coronary infusion. *Arch Pharmacol* 299: 61, 1977.

23 DeMots H, Rahimtoola SH, Kremkau EL, Bennett W, Mahler D: Effects of ouabain on myocardial oxygen supply and demand in patients with chronic coronary artery disease. *J Clin Invest* 58: 312, 1976.

24 Moran NC: Contraction dependency of the positive inotropic action of cardiac glycosides. *Circ Res* 21: 727, 1967.

25 Balcon R, Hoy H, Sowton E: Haemodynamic effects of rapid digitalization following acute myocardial infarction. *Br Heart J* 30: 373, 1968.

26 Cohn JN, Fristani FE, Khatri IM: Cardiac and peripheral vascular effects of digitalis in clinical cardiogenic shock. *Am Heart J* 78: 318, 1969.

27 Lipp H, Denes P, Gambetta M, Resnekov L: Hemodynamic response to acute intravenous digoxin in patients with recent myocardial infarction and coronary insufficiency with and without heart failure. *Chest* 63: 862, 1973.

28 Forrester J, Bezdek W, Chatterjee J, Levin P, Parmley WW, Swan HJC: Hemodynamic effects of digitalis in acute myoardial infarction. *Ann Intern Med* 76: 863, 1972.

29 Crawford MH, LeWinter MM, O'Rourke RA, Karliner JS, Ross J Jr: Combined propranolol and digoxin therapy in angina pectoris. *Ann Int Med* 83: 449, 1975.

30 Rall TW: Central nervous system stimulants, in *The Pharmacological Basis of Therapeutics*, AG Gilman, LS Goodman, A Gilman (eds). New York, Macmillan, 1980, chap 25.

31 Atuk NO, Blaydes MC, Westervelt FE, Wood JE: Effect of aminophylline on urinary excretion of epinephrine and norepinephrine in man. *Circulation* 35: 745, 1967.

32 Marcus ML, Skelton CL, Grauer LE, Epstein SE: Effects of theophylline on myocardial mechanics. *Am J Physiol* 222: 1361, 1972.

33 Rutherford JD, Stephen MB, Vatner F, Braunwald E: Effects and mechanism of action of aminophylline on cardiac function and regional blood flow distribution in conscious dogs. *Circulation* 63: 378, 1981.

34 Oei HH, Hale TH, Gandhi SS, Pilla TJ, Wegria R: Effect of aminophylline on coronary circulation and cardiac metabolism. *Arch Int Pharmacodyn Ther* 229: 95, 1977.

35 Gilbert NC, Fenn GK: The effect of the purine base diuretics on the coronary flow. *Arch Intern Med* 44: 118, 1929.

36 Stoland OO, Ginsberg AM, Loy DL, Hiebert PE: Studies on the coronary circulation. IV. A. The duration of the coronary dilator action of theophylline ethylenediamine. B. The effect of insulin-free pancreatic extract on the coronary circulation. *J Pharmacol Exp Ther* 51: 387, 1934.

37 Wegria R, Essex HE, Herrick JF, Mann FC: The simultaneous action of certain drugs on the blood pressure and on the flow in the right and left coronary arteries. *Am Heart J* 20: 557, 1940.

38 Boyer NH, Green HD: The effects of nitrites and xanthines on coronary inflow and blood pressure in anesthetized dogs. *Am Heart J* 21: 199, 1941.

39 Melville KI, Lu FC: Effects of epinephrine, aminophylline, nitroglycerine, and papaverine on coronary inflow and on heart contraction, as recorded concurrently. *J Pharmacol Exp Ther* 99: 286, 1950.

40 Takeda K, Katono Y, Nakagawa Y, Tsukada T, Nakazawa M, Otorii T, Imai S: Effects of aminophylline, proxphylline and proxphylline-mililotus extract-rutin mixture (theoesberiven) on the heart and the coronary circulation. *Jap J Pharmacol* 27: 709, 1977.

41 Maxwell GM, Crumpton CW, Rowe GG, White DH, Castillo CA: The effects of theophylline ethylenediamine (aminophylline) on the coronary hemodynamics of normal and diseased hearts. *J Lab Clin Med* 54: 88, 1959.

42 Berne RM, Rubio R: Coronary circulation, in *Handbook of Physiology*, Bethesda, Maryland, American Physiological Society, 1979, vol 1, sect 2, The cardiovascular system, chap 25, p 873.

43 Berne RM: The role of adenosine in the regulation of coronary blood flow. *Circ Res* 47: 807, 1980.

44 Afonso S: Inhibition of coronary vasodilating action of dipyridamole and adenosine by aminophylline in the dog. *Circ Res* 26: 743, 1970.

45 Eikens E, Wilcken DEL: Myocardial reactive hyperemia in conscious dogs: Effect of dipyridamole and aminophylline on responses to four and eight second coronary artery occlusions. *Aust J Exp Biol Med Sci* 51: 617, 1973.

46 Jones C, Hurst TW, Randall JR: Effect of aminophylline on coronary functional hyperemia and myocardial adenosine. *Am J Physiol* 243: H480, 1982.

47 Gould KL: Noninvasive assessment of coronary stenosis by myocardial perfusion imaging during pharmacologic coronary vasodilation. I. Physiological basis and experimental vasodilation. *Am J Cardiol* 41: 267, 1978.

48 Brown BG, Josephson MA, Petersen RB, et al: Intravenous dipyridamole combined with isometric handgrip for near maximal acute increase in coronary flow in patients with coronary artery disease. *Am J Cardiol* 48: 1077, 1981.

49 Tuttle RR, Mills J: Dobutamine: Development of a new catecholamine to selectively increase cardiac contractility. *Circ Res* 36: 185, 1975.

50 Robie NW, Nutter DO, Moody C, McNay JL: In vivo analysis of adrenergic receptor activity of dobutamine. *Circ Res* 24: 663, 1974.

51 Tuttle RR, Hillman CC, Toomey RE: Differential beta adrenergic sensitivity of atrial and ventricular tissue assessed by chronotopic, inotropic, and cyclic AMP responses to isoprenaline and dobutamine. *Cardiovasc Res* 10: 452, 1976.

52 Sonnenblick EH, Frishman WH, LeJemtel TH: Dobutamine: A new synthetic cardioactive sympathetic amine. *N Engl J Med* 300: 17, 1979.

53 Goldberg LI, Hsieh YY, Resnekov L: Newer catecholamines for treatment of heart failure and shock; an update on dopamine and a first look at dobutamine. *Prog Cardiovasc Dis* 19: 327, 1977.

54 Vatner SF, McRitchie RJ, Braunwald E: Effects of dobutamine on left ventricular performance, coronary dynamics, and distribution of cardiac output in conscious dogs. *J Clin Invest* 53: 1265, 1974.

55 Liang C-S, Hood WB Jr: Dobutamine infusion in conscious dogs with and without autonomic nervous sytem inhibition: Effects on systemic hemodynamis, regional blood flows and cardiac metabolism. *J Pharmacol Exp Ther* 211: 698, 1979.

56 Vatner SF, McRitchie RJ, Maroko PR, Patrick TA, Braunwald E: Effects of catecholamines, exercise, and nitroglycerin on the normal and ischemic myocardium in conscious dogs. *J Clin Invest* 54: 563, 1974.

57 Willerson JT, Hutton I, Watson JT, Platt MR, Templeton GH: Influence of dobutamine on regional myocardial blood flow and ventricular performance during acute and chronic myocardial ischemia in dogs. *Circulation* 53: 828, 1976.

58 von Restorff W, Bassenge E: Effect of dobutamine, a new cardioselective sympathomimetic drug, on myocardial oxygen balance in conscious dogs. *Arzneim-Forsch* 28: 6, 1978.

59 Tuttle RR, Pollock GD, Todd G, McDonald B, Tust R, Dusenberry W: The effect of dobutamine on cardiac oxygen balance, regional blood flow, and infarction severity after coronary artery narrowing in dogs. *Circ Res* 41: 357, 1977.

60 Meyer SL, Curry GC, Donsky MS, Twieg, DB, Parkey RW, Willerson JT: Influence of dobutamine on hemodynamics and coronary blood flow in patients with and without coronary artery disease *Am J Cardiol* 38: 103, 1976.

61 Bendersky R, Chatterjee K, Parmley WW, Brundage BH, Ports TA: Dobutamine in chronic ischemic heart failure: Alterations in left ventricular function and coronary hemodynamics. *Am J Cardiol* 48: 554, 1981.

62 Vatner SF, Massimo P, Rutherford RW, Millard RW, Manders WT: Effects of nitroglycerin on cardiac function and regional blood flow distribution in conscious dogs. *Am J Physiol* 234: H244, 1978.

63 Harder DR, Belardinelli L, Sperelakis N, Rubio R, Berne RM: Differential effects of adenosine and nitroglycerin on the action potentials of large and small arteries. *Circ Res* 44: 176, 1979.

64 Likoff W, Kasparian H, Lehman JS, Segal BL: Evaluation of "coronary vasodilators" by coronary arteriography. *Am J Cardiol* 13: 7, 1964.

65 Feldman RL, Pepine CJ, Curry RC Jr, Contri CR: Coronary arterial responses to graded doses of nitroglycerin. *Am J Cardiol* 43: 91, 1979.

66 Feldman RL, Pepine CJ, Conti CR: Magnitude of dilation of large and small coronary arteries by nitroglycerin. *Circulation* 64: 324, 1981.

67 Brown BG, Petersen RB, Pierce CD, Bolson EL, Dodge HT: Dynamics of human

coronary stenosis: Interaction among stenosis flow, distending pressure and vasomotor tone, in *Coronary Artery Disease*, WP Santamore, AA Bove (eds). Baltimore-Munich, Urban & Schwarzenberg, 1982, p 199.

68 Macho P, Vatner SF: Effects of nitroglycerin and nitroprusside on large and small coronary vessels in conscious dogs. *Circulation* 64: 1101, 1981.

69 Mehta J, Pepine CJ: Effect of sublingual nitroglycerin on regional flow in patients with and without coronary disease. *Circulation* 58: 803, 1978.

70 Greenberg H, Dwyer EM Jr, Jameson AG, Pinkernell BH: Effects of nitroglycerin on the major determinants of myocardial oxygen consumption: An angiographic and hemodynamic assessment. *Am J Cardiol* 36: 426, 1975.

71 Strauer BE, Scherpe A: Ventricular function and coronary hemodynamics after intravenous nitroglycerin in coronary artery disease. *Am Heart J* 95: 210, 1978.

72 Kattus AR, Gregg DE: Some determinants of coronary collateral blood flow in the open-chest dog. *Circ Res* 7: 628, 1959.

73 Wiggers CJ, Green HD: The ineffectiveness of drugs upon collateral flow after experimental coronary artery occlusion in the dog. *Am Heart J* 11: 527, 1936.

74 Fam WM, McGregor M: Effect of coronary vasodilator drugs on retrograde flow in areas of chronic myocardial ischemia. *Circ Res* 15: 355, 1964.

75 Pasyk S, Bloor CM, Khouri EM, Gregg DE, et al: Systemic and coronary effects of coronary artery occlusion in the unanesthetized dog. *Am J Physiol* 220: 646, 1971.

76 Goldstein RE, Michaelis LL, Morrow AG, et al: Coronary collateral function in patients without occlusive coronary artery disease. *Circulation* 51: 118, 1975.

77 Becker LC: Effect of nitroglycerin and dipyridamole on regional left ventricular blood flow during coronary artery occlusion. *J Clin Invest* 58: 1287, 1976.

78 Goldstein RE: Coronary vascular responses to vasodilator drugs. *Prog Cardiovasc Dis* 24: 419, 1982.

79 Diemer HP, Wichmann J, Lochner W: Coronary collateral flow: Effect of drugs and perfusion pressure. *Basic Res Cardiol* 72: 332, 1977.

80 Becker C: Conditions for vasodilator-induced coronary steal in experimental myocardial ischemia. *Circulation* 57: 1103, 1978.

81 Capurro NL, Kent KM, Smith HJ, Aamodt R, Epstein SE: Acute coronary occlusion: Prolonged increase in collateral flow following brief administration of nitroglycerin and methoxamine. *Am J Cardiol* 39: 679, 1977.

82 Gross GJ, Warltier DC: Endocardial viability ratio: An effect of nitroglycerin and propranolol on regional myocardial blood flow in intact canine hearts. *J Pharm Exper Ther* 203: 664, 1977.

83 Gross GJ, Warltier DC: Intracoronary versus intravenous nitroglycerin on the transmural distribution of coronary blood flow. *Cardiovasc Res* 11: 499, 1977.

84 Becker LC, Fortuin NJ, Pitt B: Effect of ischemia and antianginal drugs on the distribution of radioactive microspheres in the canine left ventricle. *Circ Res* 28: 263, 1971.

85 Mathes P, Rival J: Effect of nitroglycerin on total and regional coronary blood flow in the normal and ischaemic canine myocardium. *Cardiovasc Res* 5: 54, 1971.

86 Fukuyama T, Roberts R: The effect of intravenous nitroglycerin on coronary blood flow and infarct size during myocardial infarction in conscious dogs. *Clin Cardiol* 3: 317, 1980.

87 Bache RJ: Effect of nitroglycerin and arterial hypertension on myocardial blood flow following acute coronary artery occlusion in the dog. *Circulation* 57: 557, 1978.

88 Swain JL, Parker JP, McHale PA, Greenfield JC Jr: Effects of nitroglycerin and propranolol on the distribution of transmural myocardial blood flow during ischemia in the absence of hemodynamic changes in the unanesthetized dog. *J Clin Invest* 63: 947, 1979.

89 Capurro NL, Kent KM, Epstein SE: Comparison of nitroglycerin-, nitroprusside-, and phentolamine-induced changes in coronary collateral function in dogs. *J Clin Invest* 60: 295, 1977.

90 Moir TW: Subendocardial distribution of coronary blood flow and the effect of antianginal drugs. *Circ Res* 30: 621, 1972.

91 Horowitz LD, Gorlin R, Taylor WJ, Kemp HG, et al: Effects of nitroglycerin on regional myocardial blood flow in coronary artery disease. *J Clin Invest* 50: 1578, 1971.

92 Goldstein RE, Stinson EB, Scherer JL, Sehingen RP, Grehl TM, Epstein SE, et al: Intraoperative coronary collateral function in patients with coronary occlusive disease: Nitroglycerin responsiveness and angiographic correlations. *Circulation* 49: 298, 1974.

93 Myers RW, Scherer JL, Goldstein RA, Goldstein RE, Kent KM, Epstein SE, et al: Effects of nitroglycerin and nitroglycerin-methoxamine during acute myocardial ischemia in dogs with pre-existing multivessel coronary occlusive disease *Circulation* 51: 632, 1975.

94 Ganz W, Marcus HS: Failure of intracoronary nitroglycerin to alleviate pacing-induced angina. *Circulation* 46: 880, 1972.

95 Hirshfeld JW Jr, Borer JS, Goldstein RE, Barrett MJ, Epstein SF, et al: Reduction in severity and extent of myocardial infarction when nitroglycerin and methoxamine are administered during coronary occlusion. *Circulation* 49: 291, 1974.

96 Jugdutt B, Hutchins G, Bulkley BH, Becker L: Reduction of infarct size by intravenous nitroglycerin infusion in conscious dogs. *Circulation* 58(suppl II): 98, 1978.

97 Epstein SE, Kent KM, Goldstein RE, Borer JS, Redwood DR, et al: Reduction of ischemic injury by nitroglycerin during acute myocardial infarction. *N Engl J Med* 292: 29, 1975.

98 Borer JS, Redwood DR, Levitt B, Cagin N, Bianchi C, Vallin H, Epstein SE, et al: Reduction in myocardial ischemia with nitroglycerin or nitroglycerin plus phenylephrine administered during acute myocardial infarction in man. *N Engl J Med* 293: 1008, 1975.

99 Bussman WD, Passek D, Seidel W, Kaltenbach M: Prospective randomized trial of intravenous nitroglycerin in acute myocardial infarction. *Circulation* 60(suppl II): 164, 1979.

100 Chiche P, Baligadoo SJ, Derrida JP: A randomized trial of prolonged nitroglycerin infusion in acute myocardial infarction. *Circulation* 60(suppl II): 164, 1979.

101 Ahlquist RP: Study of the adrenotropic receptors. *Am J Physiol* 153: 586, 1948.

102 Powell CE, Slater IH: Blocking of inhibitory adrenergic receptors by a dichloro analog of isoproterenol. *J Pharmacol Exp Ther* 122: 480, 1958.

103 Black JW, Crowther AF, Shanks RG, Smith LH, Dornhorst AC: New adrenergic beta-receptor antagonist. *Lancet* 1: 1080, 1964.

104 Koch-Weser J, Frishman WH: β-adrenoceptor antagonists: New drugs and new indications. *N Engl J Med* 305: 500, 1981.

105 Marcus ML, Ehrhardt JC, Verani MS: Reproducibility and sensitivity of the exercise isotope ventriculogram. *Clin Res* 25: 556A, 1977.

106 Chilian WM, Boatwright RB, Shoji T, Griggs DM, Jr: Evidence against significant resting sympathetic coronary vasoconstrictor tone in the conscious dog. *Circ Res* 49: 866, 1981.

107 Schang SJ Jr, Pepine CJ: Coronary and myocardial metabolic effects of combined glyceryl trinitrate and propranolol administration. Observations in patients with and without coronary disease. *Br Heart J* 40: 1221, 1978.

108 Lewis CM, Brink AJ: Beta adrenergic blockade: Hemodynamics and myocardial energy metabolism in patients with ischemic heart disease. *Am J Cardiol* 21: 846, 1968.

109 Frishman W, Smithen C, Befler B, Kligfield P, Killip T: Noninvasive assessment of clinical response to oral propranolol therapy. *Am J Cardiol* 35: 635, 1975.

110 Shubrooks SJ Jr, Zir LM, Dinsmore RE, Harthorne JW: Left ventricular wall motion response to intravenous propranolol. *Circulation* 52: 124, 1975.

111 Weiner N: Drugs that inhibit adrenergic nerves and block adrenergic receptors, in *The Pharmacological Basis of Therapeutics*, AG Gilman, LS Goodman, A Gilman (eds). New York, Macmillan, 1980, chap 9.

112 Epstein SE, Braunwald E: Beta-adrenergic receptor blocking drugs: Mechanisms of action and clinical applications. *N Engl J Med* 275: 1106, 1966.

113 Sonnenblick E, Braunwald E, Williams JF Jr, Glick G: Effects of exercise on myocardial force-velocity relations in intact unanesthetized man: Relative roles of changes in heart rate, sympathetic activity and ventricular dimensions. *J Clin Invest* 44: 2051, 1965.

114 Epstein S, Robinson BF, Kahler RL, Braunwald E: Effects of beta-adrenergic blockade on cardiac response to maximal and submaximal exercise in man. *J Clin Invest* 44: 1745, 1965.

115 Chamberlain DA: Effects of beta-adrenergic blockade on heart size. *Am J Cardiol* 18: 321, 1966.

116 Vatner SF, Franklin D, Higgins CB, Patrick T, Braunwald E: Left ventricular response to severe exertion in untethered dogs. *J Clin Invest* 51: 3052, 1972.

117 Thadani W, Davidson C, Singleton W, Taylor SH: Comparison of the immediate effects of β-adrenoreceptor-blocking drugs with different ancillary properties in angina pectoris. *N Engl J Med* 300: 750, 1979.

117a Nayler WG, Carson V: Effect of stellate ganglion stimulation on myocardial blood flow, oxygen consumption, and cardiac efficiency during beta-adrenoreceptor blockade. *Cardiovasc Res* 7: 22, 1973.

118 Tarazi RC, Dustan HP, Bravo EL: Haemodynamic effects of propranolol in hypertension: A review. *Postgrad Med J* 52(suppl 4): 92, 1976.

119 Pitt B, Craven P: Effect of propranolol on regional myocardial blood flow in acute ischaemia. *Cardiovasc Res* 4: 176, 1970.

120 Becker LC, Ferreira R, Thomas M: Effect of propranolol and isoprenaline on regional left ventricular blood flow in experimental myocardial ischaemia. *Cardiovasc Res* 9: 178, 1975.

121 Kloner RA, Reimer KA, Jennings RB: Distribution of coronary collateral flow in acute myocardial ischaemic injury: Effect of propranolol. *Cardiovasc Res* 10: 31, 1976.

122 Fox K, Welman E, Selwyn A: Myocardial infarction in the dog: Effects of intravenous propranolol. *Am J Cardiol* 45: 769, 1980.

123 Melby K, Bache RJ: Effect of selective beta-adrenergic blockade and stimulation on regional myocardial blood flow following acute coronary artery occlusion in the awake dog. *Cardiovasc Res* 14: 192, 1980.

124 Vatner SF, Baig H, Manders WT, Ochs H, Pagani M: Effects of propranolol on regional myocardial function, electrograms, and blood flow in conscious dogs with myocardial ischemia. *J Clin Invest* 60: 353, 1977.

125 Conway RS, Weiss HR: Role of propranolol in improvement of the relationship between O_2 supply and consumption in an ischemic region of the dog heart. *J Clin Invest* 70: 320, 1982.

126 Goodlett M, Dowling K, Eddy LJ, Downey JM: Direct metabolic effects of isoproterenol and propranolol in ischemic myocardium of the dog. *Am J Physiol* 239: H469, 1980.

127 Neill WA, Nakornchai V, Oxendine J, Paul MS: Effect of beta-adrenergic suppression by propranolol on coronary collateral development in response to chronic coronary ischemia in dogs. *Circulation* 59: 280, 1979.

128 Lydtin H, Lohmöller G: Pharmacological effects of beta blockers, in *Beta Blockers*. Bern, Hans Huber, 1980.

129 Frishman WH, Weksler B, Christodoulou JP, Smithen C, Killip T: Reversal of abnormal platelet aggregability and change in exercise tolerance in patients with angina pectoris following oral propranolol. *Circulation* 50: 887, 1974.

130 Schrumpf JD, Sheps DS, Wolfson S, Aronson AL, Cohen LS: Altered hemoglobin-oxygen affinity with long-term propranolol therapy in patients with coronary artery disease. *Am J Cardiol* 40: 76, 1977.

131 Sen S, Tarazi RC, Bumpus FM: Cardiac hypertrophy and antihypertensive therapy. *Cardiovasc Res* 11: 427, 1977.

132 Sobel BE: Propranolol and threatened myocardial infarction. *N Engl J Med* 300: 191, 1979.

133 Shand DG: Beta-adrenergic blocking drugs after acute myocardial infarction. *Mod Concepts Cardiovasc Dis* 51: 103, 1982.

134 Drury AN, Szent-Gyorgyi A: The physiological activity of adenine compounds with special reference to their action upon the mammalian heart. *J Physiol* (London) 68: 213, 1929.

135 Rembert JC, Boyd LM, Watkinson WP, Greenfield JC Jr: Effect of adenosine on transmural myocardial blood flow distribution in the awake dog. *Am J Physiol* 239: H7, 1980.

136 Hoffman JIE: Transmural pressure-flow relations during diastole in the canine left ventricle. *Circulation* 62(suppl III): 62, 1980.

137 Wusten B, Buss DD, Deist H, Schaper W: Dilatory capacity of the coronary circulation and its correlation to the arterial vasculature in the canine left ventricle. *Basic Res Cardiol* 72: 636, 1977.

138 Mueller TM, Marcus ML, Kerber RE, Young YA, Barnes RW, Abboud FM: Effect of renal hypertension and left ventricular hypertrophy on the coronary circulation in dogs. *Circ Res* 42: 543, 1978.

139 Bache RJ, Vrobel TR, Arentzen CE, Ring WS: Effect on maximal coronary vasodilation on transmural myocardial perfusion during tachycardia in dogs with left ventricular hypertrophy. *Circ Res* 49: 742, 1981.

140 Marcus JL, Mueller TM, Eastham C: The effect of short- and long-term left ventricular hypertrophy on the coronary circulation. *Am J Physiol* 10: H358, 1981.

141 Patterson RE, Kirk ES: Apparent improvement in canine collateral myocardial blood flow during vasodilation depends on criteria used to identify ischemic myocardium. *Circ Res* 47: 108, 1980.

142 Schaper W: *The Collateral Circulation of the Heart.* Amsterdam, North Holland, 1971.

143 West JW, Bellet S, Manzoli VC, Muller OF: Effects of persantin (RA8), a new coronary vasodilator, on coronary blood flow and cardiac dynamics in the dog. *Circ Res* 10: 35, 1962.

144 Kinsella D, Troup W, McGregor M: Studies with a new coronary vasodilator drug: persantin. *Am Heart J* 63: 146, 1963.

145 Strauss HW, Harrison K, Langan JK, et al: Thallium-201 for myocardial imaging. *Circulation* 51: 641, 1975.

146 Tauchert M, Kochsiek K, Heiss HW, et al: Measurement of coronary blood flow in man by the argon method, in *Myocardial Blood Flow in Man,* A Maseri (ed). Torino, Italy, Minerva Medica, 139, 1972.

147 Strauer BE: Coronary blood flow, coronary reserve and myocardial oxygen consumption, in *Hypertensive Heart Disease,* Berlin, Springer-Verlag, 1980.

148 Gould KL, Wescott RJ, Albro PC, Hamilton GW: Noninvasive assessment of coronary stenoses by myocardial imaging during phamacological coronary vasodilation. II. Clinical methodology and feasibility. *Am J Cardiol* 41: 279, 1978.

149 Francisco DA, Collins SM, Go RT, Ehrhardt JC, VanKirk OC, Marcus ML: Tomographic thallium-201 myocardial perfusion scintigrams after maximal coronary artery vasodilation with intravenous dipyridamole. *Circulation* 66: 370, 1982.

150 Leppo J, Boucher CA, Okada RD, Newell JB, Strauss W, Pohost GM: Serial thallium-201 myocardial imaging after dipyridamole infusion: Diagnostic utility in detecting coronary stenoses and relationship to regional wall motion. *Circulation* 66: 649, 1982.

151 Feldman RL, Nichols WW, Pepine CJ, Conti CR: Acute effect of intravenous dipyridamole on regional hemodynamics and metabolism. *Circulation* 64(2): 333, 1981.

151a Hintz TH, Vatner SF: Adenosine and dipyridamole dilate large coronary arteries in the conscious dog. *Circulation* 66(suppl II): 154, 1982.

152 Rowe GG, Terry W, Stenlund RR, Thomsen JH, Querimit AS: Systemic and coronary hemodynamic effects of 3-(β-diethylaminoethyl (4-methyl-7-carbethoxymetoxy-2-oxo(1,2-chromen)-hydrochloride(Intensain, A-27053)). *Arch Int PharmacodynTher* 178: 99, 1969.

153 Scholtholt V, Fiedler V, Göbel R, Neitz E, Pötzch E: Wirkungen von Carbocromen auf toxische Digitaliseffekte. *Arzneim Forsch* 26: 876, 1976.

154 Freise G, Eisenbarth D: Die Behandlung der schweren Koronarisuffizienz mit Intensain. *Med Welt* 36: 1896, 1968.

155 Grayson J, Irvine M, Parratt R: Effects of carbochromen and dipyridamole on blood flow and heat production in the normal and ischemic canine myocardium. *Cardiovasc Res* 5: 41, 1971.

156 Nitz RE, Poetzch E: 3(β-diethylaminoethyl)4-methyl-7-carboehoxy-methoxy-2-oxo-(1,2 chromen)–a specific, long acting coronary dilator. *Arzneim Forsch* 13: 243, 1963.

157 Gross GJ, Warltier DC: Coronary steal in four models of single or multiple vessel obstruction in dogs. *Am J Cardiol* 48: 84, 1981.

158 O'Keefe DD, Hoffman JIE, Cheitlin RJ, O'Neill MJ, Allard JR, Shapkin E: Coronary blood flow in experimental canine left ventricular hypertrophy. *Circ Res* 43: 43, 1978.

159 Klocke FJ, Weinstein IR, Klocke JF, Ellis AK, Kraus DR, Mates RE, Canty JM, Anbar RD, Romanowski RR, Wallmeyer KW, Echt MP: Zero-flow pressures and pressure-flow relationship during single long diastoles in the canine coronary bed before and during maximal vasodilation; limited influences of capacitive effects. *J Clin Invest* 68: 970, 1981.

160 Kjekshus JK, Simonsen S, Bohmer T: Effect of carbocromen induced coronary vasodilatation on myocardial metabolism in coronary artery disease. *Clin Cardiol* 1: 74, 1978.

161 Bing RJ, Bender SR, Dunn ME, Fry GA, Fuller WM, Liu SCK, Miller HS, Moses JW, Ritzmann LW, Segal JP, Shugoll GE, Tillmanns H, Wallace A: Antianginal effects of chromonar. *Clin Pharmacol Ther* 16: 4, 1974.

162 Haas H, Hartfelder G: α-isopropyl-α-(N-methyl-N-homoveratryl-α-amino propyl) 3-4 dimethoxyphenylacetonitril, eine Aulstanz mit coronasgefassen Eigenschaften. *Arzneim Forsch* 12: 549, 1962.

163 Fleckenstein A, Tritthart H, Fleckenstein B, et al: Eine neue Gruppe Kompetitieur Ca^{++} antagonisten (iproveratril, D600, Prenylamin)mit starken Hemmoffekten auf die elektromechanische Koppelung im Warmblutermyokard. *Pfluegers Arch* 307: 25, 1969.

164 Antman EM, Stone PH, Muller JE, Braunwald E: Calcium channel blocking agents in the treatment of cardiovascular disorders. Part I: Basic and clinical electrophysiologic effects. *Ann Intern Med* 93: 875, 1980.

165 Stone PH, Antman EM, Muller JE, Braunwald E: Calcium channel blocking agents in the treatment of cardiovascular disorders. Part II: Hemodynamic effects and clinical applications. *Ann Intern Med* 93: 886, 1980.

166 Henry PD: Comparative pharmacology of calcium antagonists: Nifedipine, verapamil and diltiazem. *Am J Cardiol* 46: 1047, 1980.

167 Mitchell LB, Schroeder JS, Mason JW: Comparative clinical electrophysiologic effects of diltiazem, verapamil and nifedipine: A review. *Am J Cardiol* 49: 629, 1982.

168 Pepine CJ, Conti CR: Calcium blockers in coronary heart disease. *Mod Concepts Cardiovasc Dis* 50: 61, 1981.

169 Low RE, Takeda P, Mason DT, DeMaria AN: The effects of calcium channel blocking agents on cardiovascular function. *Am J Cardiol* 49: 547, 1982.

170 McAllister RG, Jr: Clinical pharmacology of slow channel blocking agents. *Prog Cardiovasc Dis* 25: 83, 1982.

171 Packer M, Frishman WH: Verapamil therapy for stable and unstable angina pectoris: Calcium channel antagonists in perspective. *Am J Cardiol* 50: 881, 1982.

172 Singh BN, Chew CYC, Josephson MA, Packer M: Pharmacologic and hemodynamic mechanisms underlying the antianginal actions of verapamil. *Am J Cardiol* 50: 886, 1982.

173 McGoon MD, Vlietstra RE, Holmes DR Jr, Osborn JE: The clinical use of verapamil. *Mayo Clin Proc* 57: 495, 1982.

174 Weiss GB: *New Perspectives on Calcium Antagonists.* Bethesda, Maryland, American Physiological Society, 1981.

175 Kaltenbruh M, Epstein SE: Hypertrophic cardiomyopathy: The therapeutic role of calcium antagonists. Berlin, Springer-Verlag, 1982.

176 Vatner SF, Hintze TH: Effects of a calcium-channel antagonist on large and small coronary arteries in conscious dogs. *Circulation* 66: 579, 1982.

177 Allen JC: The current status of the mechanism of the calcium channel antagonists. *Prog Cardiovasc Dis* 25: 133, 1982.

177a Mangiardi LM, Hariman RJ, McAllister RG Jr, Bhargava V, Surawicz B, Shabetai R: Electrophysiologic and hemodynamic effects of verapamil. *Circulation* 57: 366, 1978.

178 Singh BN, Hecht HS, Nademanne K, Chew CYC: Electrophysiologic and hemodynamic effects of slow-channel blocking drugs. *Prog Cardiovasc Dis* 25: 103, 1982.

179 Flaim SF, Irwin JM, Ratz PH, Swigart SC: Differential effects of calcium channel

blocking agents on oxygen consumption rate in vascular smooth muscle. *Am J Cardiol* 49: 511, 1982.

180 Fleckenstein A: Specific pharmacology of calcium in myocardium, cardiac pacemakers, and vascular smooth muscle. *Ann Rev Pharmacol Toxicol* 17: 149, 1977.

181 Narimatsu A, Taira N: Effects on atrio-ventricular conduction of calcium-antagonistic coronary vasodilators, local anaesthetics and quinidine injected into the posterior and the anterior septal artery of the atrio-ventricular node preparation of the dog. *Arch Pharmacol* 294: 169, 1976.

182 Kaltenbach M, Schulz W, Kober G: Effects of nifedipine after intravenous and intracoronary administration. *Am J Cardiol* 44: 832, 1979.

183 Serruys PW, Brower RW, TenKaten HJ, Bom AH, Hugenholtz PG: Regional wall motion from radiopaque markers after intravenous and intracoronary injections of nifedipine. *Circulation* 63: 584, 1981.

184 Rousseau MF, Pouleur H, Detry J-M, Brasseur LA: Relationship between changes in left ventricular inotropic state and relaxation in normal subjects and in patients with coronary artery disease. *Circulation* 64: 736, 1981.

185 Walsh RA, Badke FR, O'Rourke RA: Differential effects of systemic and intracoronary calcium channel blocking agents on global and regional left ventricular function in conscious dogs. *Am Heart J* 102: 341, 1981.

186 Simonsen S: Effect of verapamil on coronary hemodynamics in patients with coronary heart disease. *Eur J Cardiol* 9, 1978.

187 Gross R, Kirchheim H, Von Olshausen J: Effects of nifedipine on coronary and systemic hemodynamics in the conscious dog. *Arzneim-Forsch* 29: 1861, 1979.

188 Yabe Y, Abe H, Yoshimura S, Tsuzuku A, Hasegawa M, Kashiwakura Y, Arai C, Kawasaki T, Abe M: Effect of diltiazem on coronary hemodynamics and its clinical significance. *Jpn Heart J* 20: 83, 1979.

189 Vincenzi M, Allegri P, Gabaldo S, Maiolino P, Ometto R: Hemodynamic effects caused by i.v. administration of verapamil in healthy subjects. *Arzneim Forsch* 26: 1223, 1976.

190 Newman RK, Bishop VS, Peterson DF, Leroux EJ, Horwitz LD: Effect of verapamil on left ventricular performance in conscious dogs. *J Pharmacol Exp Ther* 201: 723, 1977.

191 Bourassa MG, Cote P, Theroux P, Tubau JF, Genain C, Waters DD: Hemodynamics and coronary flow following diltiazem administration in anesthetized dogs and in humans. *Chest* 78: 224, 1980.

192 White SW, Porges WL, McRitchie RJ: Coronary haemodynamic effects of nifedipine (Bayer 1040) and glyceryl trinitrate in unanaesthetized dogs. *Clin Exp Pharmacol Physiol* 1: 77, 1974.

193 Millard RW, Gabel M, Fowler NO, Schwartz A: Baroreceptor reflex sensitivity reduced by diltiazem and verapamil. *Fed Proc* 41: 1632, 1982.

194 Taylor DG, Kowalski TE: Effects of Ca^{2+}-entry blockers on vagal mediated heart rate responses elicited by baroreceptor reflex activation. *Fed Proc* 41: 1588, 1982.

195 Heesch CM, Thames MD, Abboud FM: Effects of calcium antagonists on carotid sinus baroreceptors. *Fed Proc* 41: 1116, 1982.

195a Nayler WG, McInnes I, Swann JB et al: Some effects of iproveratil (Isoptin) on the cardiovascular system. *J Pharmacol Exp Ther* 161: 247, 1986.

195b Chew CYC, Brown BG, Wong W, Shah PM, Singh BN, Bolson EL, Dodge HT: The effect of verapamil on coronary hemodynamics and vasomobility in patients with coronary artery disease. *Am J Cardiol* 45: 389, 1980.

195c Brown BG, Pierce CD, Peterson RB, Singh BN, Bolson EL, Dodge HT: Verapamil: A mild epicardial coronary dilator inhibits sympathetic and ergonovine-induced coronary constriction in humans. *Circulation* 64(suppl IV): 150, 1981.

196 Bache RJ, Dymek DJ: Effect of diltiazem on myocardial blood flow. *Circulation* 65 (suppl 1): 19, 1982.

197 Weintraub WS, Hattori S, Agarwal JB, Bodenheimer MM, Banka VS, Helfant RH: The effects of nifedipine on myocardial blood flow and contraction during ischemia in the dog. *Circulation* 65: 49, 1982.

198 Henry PD, Shuchleib R, Borda LJ, Roberts R, Williamson JR, Sobel BE: Effects of nifedipine on myocardial perfusion and ischemic injury in dogs. *Circ Res* 43: 372, 1978.

199 Antman E, et al: Nifedipine therapy for coronary-artery spasm. *N Engl J Med* 302: 1269, 1980.

200 Gerstenblith G et al: Nifedipine in unstable angina: A double-blind, randomized trial. *N Engl J Med* 306: 885, 1982.

201 Parodi O, Maseri A, Simonetti I: Management of unstable angina at rest by verapamil: A double-blind cross-over study in coronary care unit. *Br Heart J* 41: 167, 1979.

202 Johnson SM, Mauritson DR, Willerson JT, Hillis LD: Comparison of verapamil and nifedipine in the treatment of variant angina pectoris: Preliminary observations in 10 patients. *Am J Cardiol* 47: 1295, 1981.

203 Hill JA, Feldman RL, Pipine CJ, Conti CR: Randomized double-blind comparison of nifedipine and isosorbide dinitrate in patients with coronary arterial spasm. *Am J Cardiol* 49: 431, 1982.

204 Feldman RL, Pepine CJ, Whittle J, Conti CR: Short- and long-term responses to diltiazem in patients with variant angina. *Am J Cardiol* 49: 554, 1982.

205 Mueller HS, Chahine RA: Interim report of multicenter double-blind, placebo-controlled studies of nifedipine in chronic stable angina. *Am J Med* 71: 645, 1981.

206 Tan ATH, Sadick N, Kelly DT, Harris PJ, Freedman SB, Bautovich G: Verapamil in stable effort angina: Effects on left ventricular function evaluated with exercise radionuclide ventriculography. *Am J Cardiol* 49: 425, 1982.

207 Osakada G, Kumada T, Gallagher KP, Kemper WS, Ross R Jr: Reduction of exercise-induced ischemic regional myocardial dysfunction by verapamil in conscious dogs. *Am Heart J* 101: 707, 1981.

208 Nakamura M, Kikuchi Y, Senda Y, Yamada A, Koiwaya Y: Myocardial blood flow following experimental coronary occlusion. *Chest* 78: 205(suppl I), 1980.

209 Millard RW: Changes in cardiac mechanics and coronary blood flow of regionally ischemic porcine myocardium induced by diltiazem. *Chest* 78: 193(suppl I), 1980.

210 Franklin D, Millard RW, Nagao T: Responses of coronary collateral flow and dependent myocardial mechanical function to the calcium antagonist, diltiazem. *Chest* 78: 200(suppl I), 1980.

211 Wende W, Bleifeld W, Meyer J, Stuhlen HW: Reduction of the size of acute, experimental myocardial infarction by verapamil. *Basic Res Cardiol* 70: 198, 1975.

212 Smith HJ, Singh BN, Nisbet HD, Norris RM: Effects of verapamil on infarct size following experimental coronary occlusion. *Cardiovasc Res* 9: 569, 1975.

213 Selwyn AP, Welman E, Fox K, Horlock P, Pratt T, Klein M: The effects of nifedipine on acute experimental myocardial ischemia and infarction in dogs. *Circ Res* 44: 16, 1979.

214 Reimer KA, Lowe JE, Jennings RB: Effect of the calcium antagonist verapamil on necrosis following temporary coronary artery occlusion in dogs. *Circulation* 55: 581, 1977.

215 Nayler WG, Grau A, Slade A: A protective effect of verapamil on hypoxic heart muscle. *Cardiovasc Res* 10: 650, 1976.

216 Melin J, Bulkley BH, Hutchins GM, Becker LC: Effectiveness of delayed treatment by nifedipine in reducing the size of experimental myocardial infarction in the conscious dog. *Circulation* 66(suppl II): 85, 1982.

217 Urquhart J, Patterson RE, Bacharach S, Green MV, Epstein SE: Comparative effects of verapamil, diltiazem and nifedipine on hemodynamics and left ventricular function. *Circulation* (suppl IV) 64: 230, 1981.

218 Sacks H, Kennelly BM: Verapamil in cardiac arrhythmias, *Br Med J* 2: 716, 1972.

219 Witchitz S, Haiat R, Tarrade T, Chiche P: Accidents cardiovasculaires au cours des traitements par le verapamil. A propos de 6 observations. *Nouv Presse Med* 4: 337, 1975.

220 Eckberg WW, Drabinsky M, Braunwald E: Defective cardiac sympathetic control in patients with heart disease. *N Engl J Med* 285: 877, 1971.

221 Bonow RO, Rosing DR, Bacharach SL, Green MV, Kent KM, Lipson LC, Maron BJ, Leon MB, Epstein SE: Effects of verapamil on left ventricular systolic function and diastolic filling in patients with hypertrophic cardiomyopathy. *Circulation* 64: 787, 1981.

222 Klein HO, Kaplinsky E: Verapamil and digoxin: Their respective effects on atrial fibrillation and their interaction. *Am J Cardiol* 50: 894, 1982.

223 Kaltenbach M, Hopf R, Keller M: Calciumantagonistische Therapie bei hypertrophobstruktiver Kardiomyopathie. *Dtsch Med Wschr* 101: 1284, 1976.

224 Rosing DR, Kent KM, Borer JS, Seides SF, Maron BJ, Epstein SE: Verapamil therapy: A new approach to the pharmacologic treatment of hypertrophic cardiomyopathy. I. Hemodynamic effects. *Circulation* 60: 1201, 1979.

225 Rosing DR, Kent KM, Maron BJ, Epstein S: Verapamil therapy: A new approach to the pharmacologic treatment of hypertrophic cardiomyopathy. II. Effects on exercise capacity and symptomatic status. *Circulation* 60: 1208, 1979.

226 Breithardt G, Seipel L, Wiebringhaus E: Dual effect of verapamil on sinus node function in man, in *The Sinus Node Structure, Function and Clinical Relevance*, FIM Bonke (ed). The Hague, Martinus Nijhoff, 1978.

227 Spurreli R, Krikler DM, Sowton E: Effects of verapamil on electrophysiological properties of anomalous atrioventricular connection in Wolff-Parkinson-White syndrome. *Br Heart J* 36: 256, 1974.

228 Klein HO, Lang R, Weiss E, et al: The influence of verapamil on serum digoxin concentration. *Circulation* 65: 998, 1982.

229 Belz GG, Aust PE, Munkes R: Digoxin plasma concentrations and nifedipine. *Lancet* 1: 844, 1981.

230 Dargie HJ, Lynch PG, Krikler DM, Harris L, Krikler S: Nifedipine and propranolol: A beneficial drug interaction. *Am J Med* 71: 676, 1981.

INDEX

INDEX

Page numbers in *italic* indicate illustrations or tables.